Handbook
of Pharmaceutical
Public Policy

Handbook
of Pharmaceutical
Public Policy

Thomas R. Fulda, BA, MA
Albert I. Wertheimer, PhD
Editors

informa
healthcare

New York   London

Informa Healthcare USA, Inc.
52 Vanderbilt Avenue
New York, NY 10017

No claim to original U.S. Government works
Printed in the United States of America on acid-free paper
10 9 8 7 6 5 4 3 2

International Standard Book Number-10: 0-7890-3058-6 (Hardcover)
International Standard Book Number-13: 978-0-7890-3058-0 (Hardcover)

Library of Congress Cataloging-in-Publication Data

Handbook of pharmaceutical public policy / Thomas R. Fulda, Albert I. Wertheimer, eds.
 p. ; cm.
 Includes bibliographical references and index.
 ISBN-13: 978-0-7890-3058-0 (hard : alk. paper)
 ISBN-13: 978-0-7890-3059-7 (soft : alk. paper)
 1. Pharmaceutical policy--United States. I. Fulda, Thomas R. II. Wertheimer, Albert I.
 [DNLM: 1. Drug and Narcotic Control--legislation & jurisprudence--United States. 2.
 2. Drug Industry--legislation & jurisprudence--United States. QV 33 AA1 H236 2007]

 RA401.A3H36 2007
 362.17'82--dc22   2007000495

Visit the Informa Web site at
www.informa.com

and the Informa Healthcare Web site at
www.informahealthcare.com

To our spouses, Martha Fulda and Joaquima Wertheimer,
our mentors the late Dr. Irene Till and Dr. Larry Weaver,
and to Dr. Hans Hogerzeil, T. Donald Rucker,
and the contributing authors without whom this book
could not have happened.

CONTENTS

ABOUT THE EDITORS

Thomas R. Fulda, BA, MA, a federal civil servant for 30 years, held positions at the Social Security Administration and the Health Care Financing Administration. He conducted research on prescription drug pricing, participated in the development and implementation of the Federal Maximum Allowance Program planning for the implementation of the prescription drug provisions of the Medical Catastrophic Coverage Act of 1988, and had lead responsibilities for implementation of the Medicaid Drug Utilization Review provisions of the Omnibus Budget Reconciliation Act of 1990. He has published articles in the *Journal of Managed Care Pharmacy, Journal of the American Pharmacist Association,* and other journals. In 1995 he was made an honorary pharmacist by APhA (American Pharmacy Association).

Albert I. Wertheimer, PhD, RPh, MBA, is Professor and Research Center Director at Temple University School of Pharmacy. He is a former Director of Outcomes Research and Management at Merck & Co., Inc., in West Point, Pennsylvania, and a former Vice President of Pharmacy Managed Care at First Health Service Corporation in Glen Allen, Virginia. Prior to his work with pharmaceutical companies, he held academic appointments at the University of Minnesota and the Philadelphia College of Pharmacy where he served as Dean. He has also served as a consultant to governmental and international agencies, such as the World Health Organization, United States Congress, and the World Bank, as well as to pharmaceutical manufacturers, managed care organizations, and professional societies. He is the author or co-editor of 13 books and the author or co-author of 300 journal articles as well as being a reviewer or editorial board member of 13 journals. Dr. Wertheimer has lectured and consulted in more than 40 countries. His current research interests are pharmacoeconomics and outcomes related to disease state management.

Contributors

Syed Rizwannaddin Ahmad, MD, MPH, FIPC, Medical Epidemiologist, Silver Spring, Maryland.

Dr. Katja Borchardt, Head of Health Affairs Policy, German Pharmaceutical Industry Association (BPI), Berlin, Germany.

Susan Canny, Research Assistant, Program in Human Biology, School of Humanities and Sciences, Stanford University, Palo Alto, California.

Theodore P. Chiappelli, Dr PH, MHA, MSSM, Captain–Retired, United States Public Health Service; Associate Professor, Western Carolina University, Cullowhee, North Carolina.

Dale B. Christensen, RPh, PhD, Professor Emeritus, School of Pharmacy, University of North Carolina, Chapel Hill, North Carolina.

Theodore M. Collins, RPh, Consultant Pharmacist, Center for Health Systems Research and Analysis, University of Wisconsin-Madison, Madison, Wisconsin.

Robert L. Dupont, MD, FASAM, President, Institute for Behavior and Health, Rockville, Maryland.

Linda Elam, PhD, MPH, Senior Policy Analyst, Kaiser Commission on Medicaid and the Uninsured, Washington, DC.

Bill Felkey, MS, Professor, Department of Pharmaceutical Care Systems, Harrison School of Pharmacy, Auburn University, Auburn, Alabama.

Kimberly Fox, MPH, Institute for Health Policy, Muskie School of Public Service, University of Southern Maine, Portland, Maine.

Louis P. Garrison Jr., PhD, Professor of Pharmaceutical Outcomes Research and Program Policy, Department of Pharmacy, University of Washington, Seattle, Washington.

David Gross, PhD, Manager, Health and Support Services, AARP, Washington, DC.

Jeff J. Guo, BPharm, PhD, Associate Professor of Pharmacoeconomics and Pharmacoepidemiology, College of Pharmacy, University of Cincinnati Medical Center, Cincinnati, Ohio.

W. Mike Heath, Colonel (Retired) U.S. Army, Former U.S. Army Chief Pharmacist and Former Pharmacy Consultant to the Army Surgeon General, Martinez Georgia.

John D. Jones, RPh, JD, Prescription Solutions, Costa, Mesa, California.

Judith K. Jones, MD, PhD, President & CEO, The Degge Group Ltd., Arlington, Virginia.

Christina M.L. Kelton, PhD, Professor of Economics, Economics Center for Education & Research, College of Business, University of Cincinnati, Cincinnati, Ohio.

Duane Kirking, PharmD, PhD, Professor, Director, Center for Medication Use, Policy and Economics, Department of Social and Administrative Sciences, College of Pharmacy, University of Michigan, Ann Arbor, Michigan.

Brendan Krause, BA, Senior Policy Analyst, Health Division, National Governors Association, Washington, DC.

David H. Kreling, PhD, Professor, Sonderegger Research Center, School of Pharmacy, University of Wisconsin, Madison, Wisconsin.

Paul C. Langley, PhD, Director, Maimon Research LLC, Woodbury, Minnesota.

Philip R. Lee, MD, Professor of Social Medicine (Emeritus), School of Medicine, University of California, San Francisco, San Francisco, California.

Earle "Buddy" Lingle, RPh, PhD, Associate Professor, College of Pharmacy, University of South Carolina, Columbia, South Carolina.

Earlene Lipowski, PhD, Associate Professor, Department of Pharmacy Health Care Administration, College of Pharmacy, University of Florida, Gainesville, Florida.

Helene L. Lipton, PhD, Professor of Pharmacy and Health Policy, Schools of Pharmacy and Medicine, University of California at San Francisco, San Francisco, California.

Eva Lydick, PhD, Epidemiology and Applied Health Economics, Lovelace Clinic Foundation, Albuquerque, New Mexico.

C. Allen Lyles, ScD, MPH, BS Pharm, Henry A Rosen Professor of Public and Non Profit Partnerships, Division of Government and Public Administration, University of Baltimore, Baltimore, Maryland.

Melissa Madigan, PharmD, JD, Professional Affairs Senior Manager, National Association of Boards of Pharmacy, Mt Prospect, Illinois.

Kimberly P. McDonough, PharmD, President, Advance Pharmacy Concepts, North Kingston, Rhode Island.

Patrick L. McKircher, PhD, Adjunct Professor, University of Maryland, School of Pharmacy, Center on Drugs and Public Policy, Baltimore, Maryland.

Louis A. Morris, PhD, Louis A. Morris and Associates Inc., Dix Hills, New York.

David P. Nau, PhD, RPh, CPHQ, Associate Professor, Coordinator, Pharmaceutical Policy Ph.D. Programs, College of Pharmacy & School of Public Policy, University of Kentucky, Lexington Kentucky.

Thomas R. Oliver PhD, MHA, Associate Professor and Director, MHS Program in Health Policy, Bloomberg School of Public Health, Johns Hopkins University, Baltimore, Maryland.

Jonathan B. Perlin, MD, PhD, MSHA, FACP, Former Acting Under Secretary for Health, Department of Veterans Affairs,Chief medical Officerand Senior Vice President for Quality, HCA, Inc. Nashville Tennessee

Ed Rickert, BS Pharm, JD, Partner, Smith, Rickert, and Smith, Downers Grove, Illinois.

John Santa, MD, MPH, Medical Director, Center for Evidence Based Policy, Oregon Health Sciences University, Portland, Oregon.

Thomas Santella, BS, Center for Pharmaceutical Health Services Research, School of Pharmacy, Temple University, Philadelphia, Pennsylvania.

Prof. Dr. Marion Schaefer, Institute fur Klinische Pharmakologie, Humboldt University, Berlin, Germany.

Gordon Schiff, MD, Department of Medicine, Cook County Hospital, Chicago, Illinois.

Jon C. Schommer, PhD, Professor, College of Pharmacy, University of Minnesota, Minneapolis, Minnesota.

Sarah Schulman, Research Assistant, Program in Human Biology, School of Humanities and Sciences, Stanford University, Palo Alto, California.

Reshmi L. Singh, PhD, Assistant Professor, Department of Pharmaceutical Science, Massachusetts College of Pharmacy and Health Sciences, Boston, Massachusetts.

Richard N. Spivey, PharmD, PhD, Senior Vice President, Research and Development, MedPointe Pharmaceuticals, Somerset, New Jersey.

Michael A. Valentino, RPh, MHSA, Chief Consultant, Pharmacy Benefit Management, Strategic Health Care Group, Department of Veterans Affairs, Washington, DC.

William W. Vodra, Esq, Senior Partner, Arnold and Porter, Washington, DC.

William Wardell, MD, PhD, Wardell Associates International, Princeton, New Jersey.

Bonnie B. Wilford, MS, Director, Center for Health Services and Outcomes Research, JBS International, Inc., Silver Spring, Maryland.

Susan C. Winckler, RPh, Esq, Acting Chief of Staff, Office of the Commissioner, FDA, Rockville, Maryland.

Foreword

The World Health Organization (WHO) defines essential medicines as "... those that satisfy the priority health care needs of the population. They are selected with due regard to disease prevalence, evidence on efficacy and safety, and comparative cost-effectiveness. They are intended to be available at all times, in adequate amounts, in the appropriate dosage forms, with assured quality, and at a price the individual and the community can afford."[1]

This carefully constructed definition says it all, especially if one also looks at the next statement from WHO: "The implementation of the concept of essential medicines is intended to be flexible and adaptable to many different situations; exactly which medicines are regarded as essential remains a national responsibility." Note: Source on this quote is same as first one.

My predecessor as director of the department of Essential Drugs and Medicine Policy at WHO, Dr. Jonathan Quick, used to say that if we define a national essential medicines program as a pharmaceutical system in which most of the medicines are prescribed within restricted formularies and dispensed as generic products, the United States is the largest essential medicines program in the world. Indeed, more than half of all U.S. prescriptions (in volume terms) are filled as generic products, one of the highest percentages in the industrialized world.

However, in value terms the percentage is quite different, and this discrepancy shows one of the political tensions that make a national medicine policy a necessity. In a recent article I have argued that industrialized countries can learn from developing countries in this regard.[2] Essential medicines are not cheap, second-rate medicines for poor people in rural areas of developing countries; on the contrary, they are the most cost-effective medicines for a given condition, they represent the "best bang for your buck."

The three objectives of a national essential medicines policy are that essential medicines are available to all who need them, are of good quality, and are used in a scientifically sound and cost-effective way by prescribers and consumers. The problem is that some of these objectives may contradict one another, or may not be in line with other national objectives, such as industrial development. For example, evidence-based clinical guidelines and restricted formularies are known to lead to better health outcomes and more cost-effective services, yet some doctors do not like to be restricted in their prescribing. The pharmaceutical industry speaks of "the fourth hurdle." High medicine prices hamper access to essential medicines by the poor, or semi-poor, especially if they have to pay for the medicines out-of-pocket; however, the risky and costly research and development costs also have to be paid back. The question then rises, paid by whom? And is market-driven research really covering all medical needs of the society, or only those which will bring economic benefits? Medicine quality comes at a price, and further reduction in level of impurities may add a disproportionate cost to the product, thus inviting questions about the clinical relevance and cost-effectiveness of the final risk-reduction achieved. Or, as a final example, the national pharmaceutical industrial interests may not necessarily be in line with the public interest if better prices for good quality products can be achieved by importing the medicines from overseas. Because of these conflicting interests, which usually represent considerable economic interests as well, it is not really possible to fulfill all pharmaceutical objectives equally or at the same time.

One approach would be to let the market "sort itself out." It is my personal opinion that the pharmaceuticals are too complicated for that approach to work, mainly because of the inbalance in the information: individual consumers simply cannot judge for themselves the efficacy, safety, quality, and price of the medicines; independent professional and regulatory bodies are needed to advice and protect them.

The public health approach recommended by the World Health Organization is therefore that countries should bring all stakeholders, including the consumers, together in an open and honest forum, and prepare a national medicine policy to sort these differences out. This policy should then be endorsed by the government as a public commitment and should serve as a guide for action. Many countries have gone this way, with Australia and South Africa as shining examples.

Where do pharmacy students and pharmacists stand in all this? Well, they can no longer turn a blind eye on these issues and restrict themselves to physical sciences or clinical aspects. They must understand the environment in which their profession is practiced and must understand the rationale for policies, rules, and regulations. They must understand why so many patients vote with their feet and buy medicines in Canada or via the Internet. They must understand why so many people in the country are not covered by health insurance, and why their patients ask for specialty medicines they never thought they would know the name of. And, finally, they must understand that the pharmaceutical sector can be made more equitable and more cost effective, and how this can be done.

It is for this reason that I very much welcome this new book, which addresses these issues in an operational rather than academic way. It contains a wealth of information and should quickly establish itself as an essential resource for training and reference in pharmaceutical policy.

Hans V. Hogerzeil, MD, PhD, FRCP Edin
Director for Medicines Policy and Standards
World Health Organization
Geneva, Switzerland

NOTES

1. The Selection and Use of Essential Medicines. Report of the 14th WHO Expert Committee, including the 14th WHO Model List of Essential Drugs (revised March 2005). Geneva: WHO; 2006. Available at: www.who.int/medicines.

2. Hogerzeil HV. The concept of essential medicines: Lessons for rich countries. *British Medical Journal* 2004; 329: 1169-1172.

Preface

It is more than thirty-five years since we first became interested in how pharmaceutical issues are dealt with in the public policy arena. Over that period of time much has changed. The cost of and expenditures for prescription drugs have significantly increased. As a reaction, pharmaceuticals are covered by collective bargaining agreements and governmental programs. Consequently, pharmaceuticals account for a large share of the health care budget and receive more attention from policymakers than they used to.

Coverage of prescription drugs, which was then almost nonexistent, is now widespread. Pharmaceutical benefits managers and managed care are increasingly important in the management of these programs. Medicare has finally added a prescription drug benefit. The pharmaceutical industry has globalized and is moving rapidly to develop biotechnology and pharmacogenetics.

Pharmacoeconomics and outcomes research have become increasingly important to pharmaceutical companies in demonstrating the value of their products,and to payers in making coverage decisions. For pharmacists, although retail outlets remain important, relatively new educational requirements for PharmD degrees, drug utilization review, and pharmaceutical care are slowly changing the focus of the profession, not to mention the use of credentialed technicians and new levels of automation.

We decided to prepare this book because, to the best of our knowledge, we knew of no other book that would help pharmacy students, other health professionals, trade association leaders, academics, and policymakers understand who the players are and the complexity of the issues that are examined in most pharmaceutical policy debates. Many of the issues you will see listed in the table of contents will appear over and over again in different contexts in various chapters of this book. Two issues have become particularly important.

First, growing expenditures for drugs and rising drug costs have focused particular attention on how to control costs. Second, more recently, growing evidence that drugs are sometime used inappropriately has increased interest in trying to understand how drugs are prescribed, dispensed, and used by patients and to develop policies that will both reduce the incidence of drug morbidity and contain utilization increases.

We know that little or no definitive answers can be given to many of the policies considered in our book. Drug makers, prescribers, dispensers, and patients have different goals and different interests. We expect that in the coming years as the policy debates continue new answers will be posed to old questions, and new questions that have no answers will arise. For us this is what has made the study of pharmaceutical public policy sometimes frustrating, but always of such abiding interest. We hope that use of this book will stimulate your interest as well as make you aware of the variety of ways in which you can contribute to what may happen in the future. Your suggestions and comments to us are always welcome.

Chapter 1

Policy, Law, and Regulation

Susan Winckler

INTRODUCTION

One cannot understand the field of pharmaceutical policy without first knowing the policies, the relationship of law to policy, and how regulations relate to each of the other terms. By definition, policy is intended to influence action. Policy is defined as "a plan or course of action . . . intended to influence and determine decisions and action" (*Webster's New World College Dictionary,* Third Edition). Policies may be put in place by individuals or by organizations. An employer may, for example, adopt policies about a dress code for the workplace or establish a policy policies regarding how long employees may take lunch. Within the context of this book, prescription drug buyers may insist that drug insurance have in place policies to limit the cost of drugs that are provided.

Laws "are the rules of conduct established and enforced by the authority, legislation...of a given community, state or other group" (*Webster's New World College Dictionary,* Third Edition). Policies are given the force of law when they are adopted by the legislative branch of the state or federal government and signed by the executive (president or governor) or passed by the legislative branch over the veto of the executive. Federal laws, for example, require that prescription drugs be proven safe and effective for their intended use before they can be marketed, and they establish parameters for government-operated health care programs such as Medicare. State laws called pharmacy practice acts establish policies for licensure and how pharmacists practice their profession. Often laws at the federal and state level create overlapping responsibilities, requiring state and federal courts to further interpret the laws and resolve conflicts between them.

Regulations are written rules, usually issued by government agencies responsible for implementation of laws, providing the details necessary to implement policies set forth in laws. The Centers for Medicare and Medicaid

Services issued rules implementing the new Medicare prescription drug benefit. The law required a formulary to specify which drugs would be covered, and the regulations specified how to determine what the formulary would include. Similarly, state lawmakers establish the overarching structures that govern pharmacy practice and decide which activities pharmacists may engage in. State licensing bodies then define by regulation how these rules apply to pharmacists and pharmacies. This chapter will provide an overview of these policy sources and will consider particularly the process for developing law and regulation at the federal level.

ROLE OF FEDERAL AND STATE GOVERNMENTS

As discussed elsewhere in this book (see Chapter 11), laws affecting pharmacy practice emanate from both federal and state lawmakers. The laws implement the policy positions of the respective legislative bodies. The division of powers among these lawmakers is established in the United States Constitution. Federal lawmakers focus on activity that occurs between states by exercising authority under the "commerce clause," Section 8 of Article I of the Constitution. In pharmacy practice, this interstate commerce most commonly affects the review and approval of prescription and nonprescription drugs for marketing, including designation and regulation of controlled substances under the Controlled Substances Act. State lawmakers must address all areas beyond those designated for the federal government in the Constitution, resulting in broad so-called "police powers" to regulate health care practitioners and protect the public health and safety. These police powers authorize states to determine who may engage in what activity, and under what circumstances.

The distinction between the role of federal and state lawmakers is not always clear. One might argue, for example, that the practice of pharmacist compounding (the preparation of individualized medication at the direction of a prescriber) is appropriately directed by state-based policy, established by the state legislature and administered by state regulators as a component of pharmacy practice. Compounding is conducted by or under the direction of pharmacists or physicians, and provided to individual patients. Although the patient may reside in another state, and thus introduce some interstate component of practice, compounding is an essential companion service to the dispensing and patient care services provided by pharmacists. Others, however, may observe that pharmacist compounding is more analogous to the creation, manufacture, and marketing of drugs, as controlled by the federal government under the Federal Food, Drug, and Cosmetic Act and administered by the Food and Drug Administration (FDA). Federal authority to regulate drug approval and marketing was established upon recognition of the inherent interstate nature of compiling appropriate ingredients to formulate the product and the need for uniformity in the medications available in each state. Unfortunately, no clear answer exists: attempts to clarify the roles of state and federal lawmakers in this area were struck down by the United States Supreme Court in 2002 because of unconstitutional speech restrictions. Regardless of questions about the role of federal and state governments, both have a role in directing pharmacy practice.

THE DEVELOPMENT OF FEDERAL LAWS

The development of laws at the state and federal level is a relatively straightforward process, with the potential for many detours.[1] At the federal level, a legislative proposal (a "bill") becomes federal public law if it is passed by both the House of Representatives and the Senate and signed into law by the president (or the Senate and House override the president's veto with approval from two-thirds of each house). That process, however, is rarely quick, and often involves many stops along the way. Throughout the process described in the following section, lobbyists representing various interest groups work with lawmakers and their staff to craft the legislation—providing relevant technical expertise, identifying unintended consequences, and attempting to gain advantage for (or at least minimize negative effects against) their constituent group. In addition to the process discussed in the next section, many other routes and parliamentary maneuvers exist that may affect a particular proposal.

The concept for a bill may come from anyone, including individuals, businesses, or trade groups, a representative or senator, government agencies, and even the president. A representative or senator, however, must convert the concept into a bill and then introduce it in the House of Representatives or the Senate. Creation of the bill includes identifying the existing law to be amended, such as the federal Food, Drug, and Cosmetic Act, and the exact revisions to the law needed. Bills often include directives regarding when the revision should become effective, as well as a deadline for the development of implementing regulations. The representative or senator who introduces, or sponsors, the bill then becomes the de facto champion for moving the bill through the legislative process and will seek to gain support for the bill from other legislators. Once introduced, the bill is active for the remainder of the current two-year congressional session. Because of the magnitude of bills introduced in a typical two-year session of Congress, many bills are introduced but do not move further in the process. For example, in the 108th session of Congress (2003 to 2004), more than 8,000 bills were introduced in either the House or the Senate.[2] Those bills yielded nearly five hundred separate laws,[3] although many bills are often combined to create one law.

Upon introduction by a senator or representative, the bill is assigned a number in the format of "S. (insert number)"or "H.R. (insert number)," respectively. In the Senate, the parliamentarian, and in the House, the speaker of the House (with assistance from their chamber's parliamentarian) refers the bill to the committee(s) of jurisdiction. For example, a bill intended to amend the Food, Drug, and Cosmetic Act (FD&C Act) to change the standards for reviewing and approving new prescription drugs would be referred to the Energy and Commerce Committee in the House of Representatives and to the Health, Education, Labor, and Pensions Committee in the Senate. Much of the analysis of a bill occurs in committee deliberations rather than requiring the entire legislative body to exhibit expertise on a particular issue, the committee system allows a subset of the Congress to focus on similar proposals. Committees have varying numbers of members, although the ratio of majority political party members to minority party members depends on the margin of majority in the House or the Senate.

The scope of committee assignments, although smaller than the scope of general congressional responsibility, is still quite large. The House Energy and Commerce Committee, for example, considers proposals on issues ranging from biomedical research and development to interstate and foreign commerce to national energy policy to public health and quarantine. Such a broad scope of authority and the aforementioned significant number of bills introduced each year affects the opportunity for concerted action on each bill.

Once referred to the committee(s) of jurisdiction, the bill faces a number of different fates, most determined at some level by the chairperson of the committee. The chairperson, a member of the majority political party, oversees the operation of the committee, including what bills the group will consider for action. The bill may sit dormant and face no committee action, a process often described as "dying" in committee. A bill may face this fate if the sponsor fails to generate enough support for the proposal to stimulate the chairperson of the committee to take action on the proposal or if the chairperson opposes the proposal. If the proposal has sufficient support, the committee may hold a hearing to consider comments on and gather additional information about the topic from interest groups and individuals impacted by the proposed legislation.

If further action is supported by the chairperson and a majority of the other members of the committee, a "markup" session will be held. During this session, committee members will discuss and vote on amendments to the bill. This process can occasionally result in a complete revision of the bill, perhaps even revising it to produce a completely different result than originally intended by the sponsor. In addition, the markup may also involve combining the bill with a number of other similar bills, often bills amending the same underlying statute. For example, a number of individual bills amending the FD&C Act were combined in the Food and Drug Administration Modernization Act of 1997, a bill spanning hundreds of pages. In the consolidation process—which can facilitate moving bills by improving efficiency, allowing the committee to vote once on a bill containing the objectives of ten or fifteen underlying bills—the original sponsor of one section of the legislation may find himself or herself opposing another section. In such situations, the sponsor must assess the relative merits of each section and determine whether the support for one section outweighs opposition for another. If not, the sponsor may need to oppose the consolidated bill. The consolidation and amendment process are designed to yield support from a majority of committee members. If such support is secured, the chairperson will take a vote on the consolidated bill and pass it out of committee to the full House or Senate for consideration. If sufficient support does not exist, and no additional successful amendments secure such support, the bill may die without further action or may be voted down by the committee.

A consolidated bill passed out of committee then moves to consideration by the full House or Senate. Once again, the bill is subject to death by inaction if neither chamber acts on the proposal. If the speaker of the House or majority leader of the Senate schedules consideration of the bill, it will face debate and a vote on the floor of the relevant chamber. In the House, significant limits exist on what action may occur during this debate and vote, including limits on acceptable amendments and on the time for debate. In the Senate, far fewer limits exist, and one senator may halt consideration of a bill.

Assuming the bill is passed out of the House or Senate, the bill then moves to the other chamber for consideration—and must navigate the process again. It is unlikely that the bill will make it through this process unchanged. If changes are made, the differences between the two bills must be addressed via a conference committee. This committee, composed of members of both chambers, resolves the differences between the bills and issues a compromise bill (technically a conference report) that returns to both the House and the Senate for passage. Although conference committee discussions should technically work from the two bills at issue, the final conference report may have little resemblance to the original bills. When passed by both the House and the Senate in the same version, the bill proceeds to the president for his signature.

IMPLEMENTING FEDERAL LAW: REGULATION

Successful implementation of a federal statute depends on regulations developed by the appropriate federal agency. Regulations provide important details that clarify language contained in the statute. Regulations implementing changes to the Social Security Act and the Medicare program, for example, are prepared by the Centers for Medicare and Medicaid Services (CMS). The regulations develop the detail necessary to interpret and apply a new law. Although the regulations must be consistent with the authorizing law, the detail provided in regulations may yield a substantially different interpretation of that law than originally intended. The law establishing drug coverage under the Medicare program, for example, required many pages of regulation to interpret and make the program operational. A provision of the Medicare drug benefit law required prescription drug program sponsors to offer medication therapy management programs to targeted beneficiaries. This required regulation to identify those beneficiaries. Regulation could set explicit parameters for the programs, or set a basic structure.

Developing those regulations follows an explicit process, documented in the Federal Register published daily by the federal government. Generally, the relevant agency will publish their initial approach as a proposed rule. Interested groups, such as associations and affected companies and individuals, submit comments on the proposal, suggesting changes and supporting relevant elements. The agency considers these comments and publishes the revised version as the final regulation. The final regulation binds the agency and the regulated community.

Although regulation provides much more detail than the typical federal law, neither legislation nor regulation will anticipate every possible situation nor answer every potential question. Occasionally agencies will issue interpretive guidance to provide further detail, but interpretation of regulation is often required.

INTERPRETING LEGISLATION
AND REGULATION IN THE COURTS

Disputes about interpreting legislation and regulation often involve the judicial system. An affected party sues the relevant agency and the federal courts are asked to resolve the difference. Although federal agencies and their regulations and other interpretations are granted significant deference by the courts, their positions may be overturned. In 2005, the U.S. Supreme Court reversed the attorney general's interpretation of the Controlled Substances Act (CSA). The attorney general had interpreted the CSA to prohibit the use of controlled substances, such as barbiturates, to carry out physician-assisted suicide as authorized by state law in Oregon. The Court, however, determined that the act did not support the interpretation of the attorney general. Similarly, federal statutes are granted significant deference, but are subject to the limits of the Constitution. As noted previously in this chapter, congressional attempts to distinguish between drug compounding and drug manufacturing contained a prohibition on advertising specific compounded products. This prohibition was found to violate the free speech requirements of the Constitution, as advertising is a form of speech. The potential for judicial review of laws and regulations requires careful consideration. Even with such care, however, the courts serve as a check on the power of Congress and the administration.

Judicial action is sometimes interpreted as creating new law, although its domain is limited to interpreting the law and regulations and, when questions of constitutionality arise, comparing those laws, regulations, and administrative actions with the scope of the Constitution.

POLICY FROM THE PRIVATE SECTOR

Employers have rights that are often stated as policies. They can require drug testing or monitor or limit employees use of the telephone or Internet. Employers or professional societies can require a specified amount of continuing education to maintain one's certification or to keep one's job. Schools may require their teachers to earn a master's degree within five years of being hired. Group practices of physicians or dentists may require each member of the practice to provide weekend coverage on a specific schedule.

Business policy also affects pharmacy practice, establishing the parameters for employee activities. Whether establishing staffing structures or duty-to-dispense requirements, failure to follow business policies can result in sanctions or termination. Businesses sometimes establish policy that is more rigorous than what is required in order to comply with existing laws and regulations.

Some business policies may limit the availability of products or services to avoid having to comply with certain laws and regulations. A pharmacy, for example, may choose not to carry Schedule II controlled substances because of the procedures required to comply with regulations applicable to those products. In other situations, compliance is required for general pharmacy operations, but business policies implementing the same laws or regulations may vary. One pharmacy, for example, may comply with state requirements to assure dispensing of contraception prescriptions "without delay" by providing additional staffing, but with backup pharmacists who choose not to dispense such prescriptions. Another pharmacy may compel its pharmacists to dispense such prescriptions to assure compliance with such requirements. Different approaches are typically established by business management, but knowing how such approaches are developed allows employees or future employees the opportunity to influence the outcome.

If we step back and think about it, most policies, laws, and regulations have a purpose and are nearly always well intentioned, aiming to prevent harm and exploitation, to avoid confusion, and to address the needs of the community or the nation. Following such policies, although not always agreeable, benefits the common good, and are examples of constraints placed on the individual for the betterment of the entire community or society.

NOTES

1. Adapted from How Our Laws Are Made, revised and updated by Charles W. Johnson, Parliamentarian, United States House of Representatives June 30, 2003. Available at: http://thomas.loc.gov/home/lawsmade.toc.html.

2. Listing of Bills Introduced in the 108th Congress. Available at: http://thomas .loc.gov/ home/c108bills.html.

3. Public Laws of 108th Congress (2003-2004). Available at: http://thomas .loc.gov/bss/d108/ d108laws.html.

Chapter 2

The Political Evolution of Medicare and Prescription Drug Coverage

Thomas R. Oliver
Philip R. Lee
Sarah B. Schulman
Susan P. Canny
Helene L. Lipton

A POLITICAL HISTORY OF MEDICARE AND PRESCRIPTION DRUG COVERAGE

This chapter will deal with the major policy and programmatic changes in Medicare related to prescription drugs since its enactment in 1965, as well as the factors influencing the health policy process that created Medicare in 1965 and that failed to add an outpatient prescription drug benefit until November 2003. We have dealt with these issues in detail in other publications.[1] The politics of Medicare have been more broadly considered.in other publications as well.[2,3] Health policies that seemed far removed from Medicare, such as the Food and Drug Administration (FDA)'s process for the approval of new drugs, the National Institutes of Health (NIH) investments in biomedical research, and legislation to strengthen ties between NIH and the pharmaceutical industry all played a part in the exclusion of outpatient prescription drugs from Medicare prior to November 2003 We will not address these issues here because they are dealt with in Chapters 3 and 18.

Politics played the critical role in shaping the Social Security Amendments of 1965 that created Medicare (Title XVIII) and, at the same time, Medicaid (Title XIX). Repeated efforts to enact programs of universal health insurance occurred in the period before World War I (the progressive era), and from the mid-1930s, when the Social Security Act was passed, until the late 1940s, when President Truman attempted to enact a single payer national health insurance plan. After 1949, the focus shifted away from universal health insurance to a limited plan for hospital insurance for the elderly and retired beneficiaries of Social Security.[4]

The strategy that evolved in the 1950s that resulted in Medicare was to develop a politically viable plan that met a critical need for the elderly, a social group that was viewed as especially deserving (having worked and paid into Social Security prior to retirement) and especially needy (having been insured during their working years but now facing a combination of lower incomes and very limited access to health insurance coverage after retirement).

Although proposals to provide health insurance for the elderly were submitted to Congress during the 1950s, they had little chance of enactment. After the election of President Kennedy in 1960, the proposal for hospital insurance for retired, elderly Social Security beneficiaries (King-Anderson bill) generated widespread support, particularly from organized labor and organized groups of the elderly, but even with the president's support it never emerged from the Ways and Means Committee of the U.S. House of Representatives, the key committee in Congress that, along with the Senate Finance Committee, dealt with taxes and Social Security.

What happened that changed the politics so dramatically? President Kennedy was assassinated on November 22, 1963, and Lyndon Johnson, the vice president, was sworn in as president that day aboard Air Force One in Dallas, Texas. President Johnson soon began to advocate a very progressive domestic policy agenda in the memory of the late president, led by the Civil Rights Act, the poverty programs, federal aid for elementary and secondary education, and hospital insurance for the elderly. In November 1964, President Johnson was elected by a landslide and the Democrats had their largest majority in Congress in twenty-eight years. The passage of hospital insurance for the elderly became President Johnson's first priority after his inauguration in January 1965.

The result was prompt consideration of the King-Anderson bill by the Ways and Means Committee. Soon known as Part A of Medicare, it paid for inpatient hospital care after an initial deductible. Part A was financed by a payroll tax on employees and employers, the same as Social Security, but was earmarked for Part A. Also included in Title XVIII of the Social Security Act was a dramatic expansion of Medicare to include physician services to be paid for by general revenues (50 percent) and premiums paid by the beneficiaries (50 percent). This expansion was proposed by the Republicans as an alternative to the hospital insurance program, but in the new package of legislation it was combined and became Part B of Medicare. Finally, because the American Medical Association (AMA) favored a means-tested program to cover the poor, Medicaid was added as Title XIX of the Social Security Act.[5]

Why did Medicare take the dramatically expanded form that it did in 1965, when the Democrats had proposed only limited hospital insurance for the elderly, financed through a universal social insurance mechanism? Two counter proposals were made before the Ways and Means Committee in early 1965 that went beyond the King-Anderson bill. The counter proposal put forward by Republicans, the Byrnes bill, called for voluntary enrollment in a health insurance program financed by premiums paid by beneficiaries and subsidized by general revenues. It included an expanded set of benefits, including physician services and prescription drugs. In addition, the AMA proposed a state-based, means-tested program of comprehensive benefits to expand the Kerr-Mills program first enacted in 1960. This also included hospital inpatient care, physician services, and prescription drugs.

Representative Wilbur Mills, then chairman of the House Ways and Means Committee, made the surprise suggestion that Democratic and Republican proposals (King-Anderson and Byrnes) essentially be combined into Title XVIII of the Social Security Act, a new Medicare program with both Part A (Hospital Insurance) and Part B (Supplementary Medical Insurance). Chairman Mills favored adding Part B, financed by general revenues and premium payments, because he felt it would prevent the further expansion of Social Security. President Johnson supported this proposal. As the Ways and Means Committee marked up the combined bill in March 1965 (and also added what would become Medicaid), the outpatient prescription drug benefit for Part B was dropped, according to Marmor, "on the grounds of unpredictable and potentially high costs."[6] An additional barrier to adding an outpatient prescription drug benefit was the relatively high administrative cost of paying for each prescription drug dispensed compared with the relatively low administrative costs of paying for a hospital stay of seven to ten days or physician payments for many expensive procedures.

The principal architects of the program were focused primarily on providing financial protection for the elderly against the high cost of inpatient hospital care after retirement, not on meeting the chronic care needs of the elderly. Long term, their goal was for Medicare to be the foundation on which universal health insurance for all Americans would be based.

Included in the original Medicare law was a provision that covered pharmaceuticals administered by a physician and incidental to a visit to the physician in his or her office. When Part B, Section 1832 of Title 18 of the Social Security Act came into effect on July 1, 1966, retired, elderly (age sixty-five years and older) Social Security beneficiaries became entitled to "medical and other health services" that included "services and supplies [including drugs and biologics not usually self-administered by the patient] furnished as an incident to a physician's professional service, of kinds which are commonly furnished in physicians' offices and are commonly either rendered without charge or included in the physicians' bills."[7] This seemingly innocuous provision had little initial impact, but as an increasing number of prescription drugs administered intravenously or intramuscularly were approved by the FDA, the costs of this benefit began to rise. The most significant addition was Epoetin alfa, which was approved on January 1, 1989, to treat anemia, particularly in patients with end stage renal disease. Recognizing the cost impact of adding epoetin to the Part B benefit package, the Reagan administration negotiated a price (80 percent of the market price) for epoetin in advance of FDA approval of the drug for marketing.[8] The addition of the disabled and persons with end stage renal disease to the Medicare program in 1972 set the stage for a rapid increase in the expenditures for prescription drugs administered in the physicians' office because anemia was one of the features of end stage renal disease. We will return to this issue.

Other important developments in Medicare occurred after its implementation on July 1, 1966. Eight developments have related particularly to Medicare and prescription drug policies.[9] They are described in the following sections.

HEW Task Force on Prescription Drugs

The Task Force on Prescription Drugs was appointed in May 1967 by John Gardner, the Secretary of Health, Education, and Welfare, following a directive by President Johnson. The Task Force was chaired by the Assistant Secretary for Health and Scientific Affairs, and included the Surgeon General of the U.S. Public Health Service, the Commissioner of Social Security, and the Commissioner of the Food and Drug Administration. The primary objective of the task force was to determine whether it was feasible or advisable for Medicare to cover prescription drugs as a new benefit, beyond the limited coverage of drugs administered by the physician in his or her office.

The mission of the task force was not a simple one. It was to undertake a comprehensive study of the problems of including the cost of prescription drugs, both in hospital and out of hospital, under the Medicare program. The goal was clear: the provision of the highest quality of medical care to the elderly at a reasonable cost. The task force examined a range of issues—generic equivalency, antisubstitution laws, physician prescribing, adverse drug reactions, dispensing by pharmacists, insurance coverage, foreign drug insurance programs, state programs, drug regulation, drug reimbursement, and costs. The Task Force's most significant conclusion was: "a drug insurance program under Medicare is needed by the elderly and would be medically feasible."[10] To expand out of hospital prescription drug coverage would require decisions about the scope of the coverage, price controls, beneficiary cost sharing and the possible role of Medicare as purchaser, similar to the role by the Department of Defense, the Department of Veterans Affairs, and the U.S. Public Health Service.[11]

While President Nixon's Secretary of HEW, Robert Finch, accepted the Task Force Report and its recommendations, the president did not, in part because he was developing a proposal for universal health insurance, based on an employer mandate. President Nixon did not favor the Medicare expansion because it would be a direct federal expenditure increase.

Many of the recommendations of the Task Force related to prescription drug coverage in Medicare were introduced in the Congress in subsequent years, but remained matters of heated debate rather than legislation until 1988 when the Medicare Catastrophic Coverage Act (MCCA) was enacted.

Social Security Amendments of 1972

The Social Security Amendments of 1972 extended Medicare benefits to individuals under age 65 years, who were Social Security Disability Insurance (SSDI) beneficiaries, and it also added individuals with end stage renal disease (ESRD) to the program. The unintended consequence of adding the ESRD program was that anemia was a serious problem among these patients and when Epoetin Alfa became available in 1989, it resulted in a dramatic increase in expenditures for prescription drugs administered in the doctor's office.

Enactment (1988) and Subsequent Repeal (1989)
of the Medicare Catastrophic Coverage Act,
Including a Prescription Drug Benefit

In 1988, Congress enacted the Medicare Catastrophic Coverage Act to provide protection for catastrophic medical costs, to add a limited long-term care benefit, and to add a limited prescription drug benefit. Because President Reagan refused to consider a tax increase to pay for this benefit, and the laws then in effect required any new program to not increase the deficit (called PAYGO), Congress required the beneficiaries, particularly those with high incomes, to pay for the benefit. The beneficiaries, including the low-income beneficiaries who would receive the drug benefit without added premiums, rebelled, and Congress repealed the benefit in 1989. As previously observed, "In the eyes of many beneficiaries and advocacy groups . . . the income-related premium violated the original social contract, under which individuals earned benefits during their working years and so would not have to pay for added benefits during their retirement; and all seniors would have the same set of benefits from and financial obligations to the Medicare program."[12]

The repeal of the MCCA in 1989 had an enduring effect on the minds of the members of Congress and almost all experts on Medicare policy. The outcome was the result of politics, not substance. The point was made very clearly by Rovner:

> The real story of the rise and fall of the Medicare Catastrophic Coverage Act sends several ominous messages about the state of Congress and our political system, but the power of the senior citizens' lobby is not one of them. Those who lived through this nightmare instead learned a lot more about the power of direct mail, the ease of manipulating the public with information that is simply wrong, the resistance recipients of federal entitlement programs feel toward change, and the lack of knowledge Americans have about programs that so directly affect their lives.[13]

Adoption of Policies Regulating Private Insurance for Benefits Not Covered by Medicare (Medigap Policies) in 1990

Because of the rapid growth of a wide range of private health insurance policies to cover Medicare deductibles, copayments, and in some cases, prescription drugs, Congress began to regulate these policies, enacting legislation to limit the number of benefit packages and to include coverage of prescription drugs in a limited number of those policies. The Medigap policies had to conform to ten standardized benefit packages approved by the National Association of Insurance Commissioners. The law was implemented in 1992.

Prescription Drug Coverage in the Health Security Act—1993

The first opportunity to add a prescription drug benefit to the Medicare program after 1988 came in 1993, as part of the Health Security Act proposed by President Clinton. The addition of a drug benefit to Medicare made political and policy sense because it was to be included for those under age sixty-five years of age, as part of the Health Security Act. To help control the added costs of the prescription drug benefit, the president proposed that Medicare use its purchasing power to get discounts from the pharmaceutical companies. The pharmaceutical manufacturers would have to sign rebate agreements with the Department of Health and Human Services as a condition of their participation in the Medicare and Medicaid Programs. The Health Security Act also included provisions to encourage the use of generic drugs to lower costs. These provisions reflected the necessity of using a regulatory approach to control the costs of prescription drugs, even as "managed competition" was a key element proposed to control the costs of hospital and physician services.

The Health Security Act died in Congress in 1994 without ever reaching the floor of the House of Representatives or the Senate for a vote on its merits. The politics of this process have been described in detail.[14,15,16] Although the defeat of the Health Security Act was not related to the proposals for prescription drug coverage, the provisions raised concerns among the pharmaceutical manufacturers that the new drug benefit would be accompanied by price controls or other regulatory measures.[17]

Balanced Budget Act of 1997

The Balanced Budget Act (BBA) of 1997 represented compromise by both the president and Congress. Projected spending on Medicare was to be reduced by $115 billion over five years. Among its many provisions, the BBA created a Medicare Part C program (Medicare+Choice*) to expand options for enrollment in managed care. The growth of managed-care enrollment throughout the 1990s was fueled in part because health plans offered prescription drug coverage and other benefits, including lower cost sharing, to Medicare beneficiaries. Building on the establishment of Part C, the legislation also created a National Bipartisan Commission on the Future of Medicare to consider broad restructuring of the entire Medicare program.

National Bipartisan Commission on the Future of Medicare 1998 to 1999

The National Bipartisan Commission on the Future of Medicare developed proposals to change the nature of the Medicare entitlement and add prescription drug coverage. The prescription drug benefit was added as a "sweetener" to persuade some members of the commission to support the massive conversion of Medicare from a defined benefit to a defined contri-

---

*Medicare+Choice was renamed Medicare Advantage as part of the Medicare Prescripton Drug Improvement and Modernization Act of 2003.

bution plan. The commission failed to achieve enough support to send formal recommendations to Congress. After the failure of the Commission to reach an agreement, President Clinton and various members of Congress proposed outpatient prescription drug coverage for Medicare.[18]

Medicare Prescription Drug Improvement and Modernization Act of 2003

The Medicare Prescription Drug Improvement and Modernization Act (MMA) of 2003 was enacted in a very divisive political environment and included many provisions unrelated to prescription drugs or Medicare modernization because they seemed necessary to assure passage of the legislation.

The importance of having private health plans contract with Medicare to provide prescription drug coverage as part of the Part C program is underscored by a name change and enhanced payments to Part C plans. The Medicare+Choice managed care program has been renamed the Medicare Advantage program. The law guarantees beneficiaries a choice of at least two managed care plans in their area of residence. Participating plans will begin to receive payment increases averaging 10.6 percent in fiscal year 2005. For the first time, Medicare will pay more to private managed care plans than it does for fee-for-service Medicare.[19] The Congressional Budget Office estimates that this will cost $500 million this year. A "stabilization" fund for Medicare Advantage plans has also been created that will provide subsidies of $12.5 billion over a decade.

The prescription drug benefit was the most controversial provision in MMA. The cost estimates rose from $400 billion to $520 billion a few months after enactment. The costs are now projected to be $720 billion in the period from 2006 to 2015. General revenues and beneficiary premiums will be the source of financing for the prescription drug benefit. The benefit was not scheduled to begin until 2006, but in the interim, the Department of Health and Human Services established a temporary drug discount program. The law provides that the drug benefit be administered by private health plans, including pharmacy benefit management companies. It prohibits the government from directly negotiating drug prices with the drug industry, as is done by the Department of Defense and the Department of Veterans Affairs.

In the debate on the MMA of 2003, few paid much attention to the rising costs of prescription drugs administered in the physician's office. In 1992, Medicare spent $700 million for prescription drugs administered in the physician's office (which totaled 2 percent of physicians and clinical services expenditure under Part B). By 1993, the prescription drug expenditure reached one billion dollars and represented 2.9 percent of physician-related expenditures. By 1997, the year the Balanced Budget Act of 1997 was passed, prescription drug expenditures had reached $2.6 billion and were 6.3 percent of physician and clinical service expenditures. In 2000, the expenditures for physician-administered prescription drugs rose to $4.9 billion, or 8 percent of physician and clinical service expenditures. By 2001, the expenditure was $6.5 billion, an increase of 32 percent since 2000 and 10 percent of physician and clinical services expenditures.[20] The rapid increase in costs reflected the increased number of drugs included in Part B and the rising costs of prescription drugs. Part of these increases was the result of the inclusion of injectable anticancer drugs and oral antinausea drugs as Medicare benefits. The addition of these drugs reflected the efforts of the cancer lobby.

Compared to Medicare, the VA Hospital System paid between 15 and 91 percent less for outpatient prescription drugs. After comparing the Medicare reimbursement with the VA Health System acquisition costs for twenty-four drugs, the DHHS Inspector General's Office estimated that Medicare would save $1.6 billion if the same payment structure were adopted.[21] Congress took quite a different approach in the Medicare Prescription Drug Improvement and Modernization Act of 2003. The decision by Congress to prohibit Medicare's direct purchase of prescription drugs, with billions of dollars of savings, was in direct response to the interests of the pharmaceutical manufacturers by members of Congress. At the same time, Congress introduced new price controls for prescription drugs administered in the physician's office under Part B of Medicare.

The new drug benefit (Part D of Medicare) will begin to pay for outpatient prescription drugs through private plans, giving beneficiaries access to a standard drug benefit or its actuarial equivalent. After the patient pays a $250 deductible, Medicare will pay 75 percent of the annual costs of covered drugs, from $250 to $2,250. Between $2,250 and $5,100, Medicare will pay nothing. This is referred to as the "donut hole" in the benefit. After prescription drug costs exceed $5,100 (with $3,600 out of pocket), Medicare will pay 95 percent of the costs. It is anticipated that about 27 percent of Medicare beneficiaries will fall into the "donut hole," and an additional 15 percent, whose expenditures on prescription drugs exceed $5,100, will be affected by the donut hole because of the lack of coverage between $2,250 and $5,100.[22] Low-income Medicare beneficiaries who are currently also eligible for Medicaid will now receive prescription drug coverage under Medicare Part D, not under their state Medicaid programs. Participants who are not eligible for Medicaid, but have incomes below 135 percent of poverty, will have their costs subsidized and will only pay $2 and

$5 copayments for generic and brand-name prescriptions. They will need to apply for the low-income subsidies, with eligibility determined by both income and asset tests similar to the Medicaid program. Currently, 42 million Medicare beneficiaries exist, and 29 million are expected to participate, including 8.7 million who will receive the low-income subsidy.[23] It is anticipated that about 27 percent of Medicare beneficiaries will fall into the category receiving subsidies.

THE POLITICS OF MEDICARE
AND THE HEALTH POLICY PROCESS

Theories of the policy process can help us understand how and why opportunities for policy change arose and explain why an extraordinary political window of opportunity was available in 2003. Political and economic forces outside of Medicare have as much or more influence on policies as the conditions inside Medicare itself. Shifts in control of the presidency and Congress create or close down opportunities for reform and, in addition, dictate what kinds of reforms are possible. Another important contextual factor is the nearly perennial budget deficit, which grew dramatically after President Reagan's tax cuts in the early 1980s and had a dominant influence on Medicare policies until the short-lived budget surplus of the late 1990s.

The enactment of the Medicare Prescription Drug Improvement and Modernization Act of 2003 represents an example of the model of the public policymaking process as described by John Kingdon in his classic book *Agendas, Alternatives, and Public Policies.*[24] In his book, Kingdon focuses on how an idea gets on the policy agenda. He argues that issues rise to the top of the policy agenda when two conditions are met: The first condition is an abrupt shift in how a problem is perceived or in who controls the levers of governmental power, which opens a "window of opportunity" for policy innovation. Second is a convergence of three relatively independent "streams" in the policy process: problems, policies, and politics.

A problem may be recognized for many years, but no agreed-upon policy choice is available. Even when the problem is recognized and the policy choices are clear, the politics stream may not be favorable. This was certainly true for the Medicare prescription drug benefit after repeal of the Medicare Catastrophic Coverage Act in 1989.

The most notable examples of the opening of "windows of opportunity" are during periods with large-scale problems and a major shift in political values. Reforms instigated at the turn of the century that led to the Pure Food and Drug Act, the Depression era policies of the New Deal that led to the enactment of the Social Security Act in 1935, and the many programs, including Medicare and Medicaid, the Civil Rights Act, health professions education, cigarette labeling, neighborhood health centers, and highway and auto safety during the Great Society initiatives from 1964 to 1969, come to mind.

The prescription drug benefit and the other Medicare reforms enacted in November 2003 resulted from a much narrower window of opportunity and are notable since the political stream has been largely controlled by Republicans, who generally have opposed significant expansions in the role of government and entitlement programs such as Medicare in particular. In addition to the Republicans' control of the White House, the Senate, and the House of Representatives after the 2002 election (when Republicans regained control of the Senate) and the inadequacy of prescription drug coverage for Medicare beneficiaries, several other issues arose, such as automatic patent extensions, reduced drug coverage for retirees by employers, and reimportation of drugs from other countries (e.g., Canada), that contributed to the debate in 2002-2003. In clear violation of federal law, elderly were crossing the Canadian and Mexican to buy lower-cost drugs. In addition, drug prices and expenditures had been rising at record rates. These controversies were mutually reinforcing and put the pharmaceutical industry and the Bush Administration on the defensive. Finally, the election of 2004 loomed, and a perception grew that the Republicans, particularly with the tax cuts, were passing laws benefiting the upper income groups and not the elderly or the middle class. We have described these developments in detail in an earlier publication.[25]

Mark Peterson's model of social learning builds on the work of Paul Pierson, who found that a change in public policy creates "feedback" or "legacies" in two ways:[26,27] first, by altering existing institutions or creating new ones, it can have "structural effects" on the resources and incentives of participants in the policy process: social groups, government elites, or the mass public; and second, policy changes can produce "learning effects" that alter the distribution of information and interpretations of social conditions and government actions.

Perhaps the most powerful structural effect of Medicare's evolution has been the incentive for Medicare beneficiaries to mobilize politically to defend their existing benefits in a program that, despite its defects, gives them greater access to care and greater overall satisfaction than nonelderly adults have with private insurance.

Medicare's limited benefits resulted in the creation of other sources of supplementary coverage, including a variety of forms of prescription drug coverage either bought by former employers, paid by Medicaid, or purchased out of pocket. The development of this supplementary coverage then stalled the development of broader benefits within the Medicare program.

This is a structural effect in Peterson's model and helps explain why policymakers could ignore inadequate prescription drug coverage for so long: large numbers of beneficiaries, especially the most well-off and politically active, had decent benefits from their retiree programs or Medigap or Medicare+Choice/Medicare Advantage plans.

The history of Medicare also illustrates a number of learning effects on the current handling of the issues of prescription drug coverage. Peterson makes the important distinction between *substantive learning* about the need for new policies and the relative effectiveness of policy options and *situational learning* about the political and social consequences of policies. Substantive learning tends to be dominated by experts, whereas situational learning is dominated by politicians and organized interests.[28] The evolution of Medicare has numerous examples of each form of policy learning.

The repeal of the Medicare Catastrophic Coverage Act (MCCA) in 1989 is an enduring event in the minds of almost all experts in Medicare policy and a prominent example of situational learning. A number of the provisions of the Medicare Prescription Drug Improvement and Modernization Act of 2003 reflect situational learning from the demise of the MCCA of 1988. None of the proposals, including the final bill, imposed the full cost of the drug benefit on the elderly, as happened in 1988. Instead, the costs of the program were to be paid out of general revenues, with a huge increase in the deficit during the next ten years, and out of enrollee premiums and out-of-pocket expenses. Another lesson was that the participation in the new prescription drug coverage had to be voluntary.[29]

On the other hand, many of the provisions of the MMA of 2003 were not consistent with lessons learned from the MCCA of 1988, and these may haunt Congress in the future. The Part D benefit is incomplete, complex, and confusing. Many of the elderly, particularly those with supplementary coverage from their former employers, will not see any improvement in their coverage, and indeed, some may be worse off. That neither the elderly nor their former employers may buy supplementary coverage for costs not covered by Medicare is likely to cause a problem. Finally, the MMA of 2003 reintroduces income-related premiums and direct means testing for low-income subsidies. Both policies are contrary to long-agreed upon policies in Medicare.

Situational learning by the pharmaceutical manufacturers is also evident in the 2003 law. The pharmaceutical manufacturers noted their public opposition to a prescription drug benefit and were able to support a stand-alone drug benefit, first proposed by President Clinton in 1999, and were able to preclude direct control of drug prices by the federal government. Similar to Part A and Part B when they were first implemented in 1966, the drug benefit (Part D) will be administered by a private sector intermediary, either a pharmaceutical benefit management company or a health plan. The short experience with pharmacy benefit management companies and a freestanding drug benefit suggests that the policies in the MMA of 2003 are based more on situational learning than on substantive learning from experience.

Finally, although Republicans favor Medicare Advantage plans, the backlash against managed care that began with the rejection of Clinton's health care reform proposals in 1994 convinced them to include equal drug benefits for Medicare enrollees who remained in fee-for-service plans and Medicare Advantage plans. The politics of the Clinton health plan drastically changed the politics of Medicare in 1993-1994. Although President Clinton had seized upon "managed competition" as a synthesis of liberal goals and conservative methods, the health insurance industry, small business groups, pharmaceutical companies, and other opponents successfully attacked the reforms on the grounds that they represented heavy-handed intrusion on individual choice and created sizable new bureaucracies to manage the system and constrain costs if competition failed to do so.

Republicans helped kill the "big government" Clinton plan, then moved to dismantle many existing governmental programs once they captured control of the Congress in 1994. As Haynes Johnson and David Broder observed:

> It was not consensus politics being practiced in Washington, or even conservative politics as previously defined. This was ideological warfare, a battle to destroy the remnants of the liberal, progressive brand of politics that had governed American throughout most of the twentieth century.[30]

In 2004, we summarized our views on this subject:

> In 2003 policymakers seized a historic opportunity to integrate prescription drug benefits into a program that 41 million older and disabled Americans admire and rely on. Despite this opportunity, the effort to establish a Medicare drug benefit was boxed in by current sources of coverage, by ideological insistence on market "solutions" for a massive social problem, by arbitrary budgetary constraints, and by the failure of managed care in rural America. The resulting program design may make it more difficult for Medicare administrators and private organizations to implement the policy successfully, satisfy the expectations of millions of Medicare beneficiaries, and protect the public purse. In our view, several challenges remain for those trying to implement the new law.[31]

We still hold these views today.

During the past forty years Medicare has been a great benefit to the elderly and disabled beneficiaries and those with end stage renal disease. At the same time, the costs of these programs have been a major driver of health policies during this period. In recent years, partisan politics have replaced the years of bipartisanship that guided Medicare policy. Medicare will undoubtedly remain a major political issue, particularly when the baby boomers retire.

NOTES

1. Oliver, TR, Lee, PR, and Lipton, HL. (2004). A Political History of Medicare and Prescription Drugs Coverage. *The Milbank Quarterly* 82(2): 283-354.
2. Marmor, T. (2000). *The Politics of Medicare,* 2nd Edition. Hawthorne, New York: Aldine De Gruyter.
3. Oberlander, J. (2003). *The Political Life of Medicare.* Chicago. University of Chicago Press.
4. Marmor, T. (2000), pp.1-27.
5. Marmor, T. (2000), pp. 45-61.
6. Marmor, T. (2000), p. 49.
7. Social Security Administration, Office of Disability and Income Security Programs, Office of Income Security Programs, Office of Technology and Services Policy, Center for Policynet Management. Compilation of the Social Security Laws, Including the Social Security Act as Amended, and Related Enactments. Baltimore, MD. Available at http://www.ssa.gov/OP_Home/ssact/title 18/1861.htm.
8. Schulman, S. (2003). *No More Refills: The Past, Present, and Future of Physician-Administered Prescription Drug Coverage.* Unpublished.
9. Oliver, TR, Lee, PR, and Lipton, HL. (2004).
10. U.S. Department of Health, Education, and Welfare (U.S. DHEW). (1969). Task Force on Prescription Drugs, Final Report. Washington, DC: Office of the Secretary, U.S Department of Health, Education and Welfare, p. xxi.
11. U.S. Department of Health, Education, and Welfare (U.S. DHEW). (1969).
12. Oliver, TR, Lee, PR, and Lipton, HL. (2004), pp. 299-300.
13. Rovner, J. (1995). Congress' "Catastrophic" Attempt to Fix Medicare. In *Intensive Care: How Congress Shapes Health Policy,* edited by TE Mann and N Ornstein, pp. 145-178. Washington, DC: American Enterprise Institute and Brookings Institution, pp. 145-146.
14. Hacker, JS. (1997). *The Road to Nowhere: The Genesis of President Clinton's Plan for Health Security.* Princeton, NJ: Princeton University Press.
15. Johnson, H and Broder, DS (1996). *The System: The American Way of Politics at The Breaking Point.* Boston, MA: Little Brown.

16. Skocpol, T. (1996). *Boomerang: Clinton's Health Security Effort and the Turn Against Government in U.S. Politics.* New York: Norton.

17. Newhouse, JP. (2002). Medicare. In *American Economic Policy in the 1990s,* edited by J Frankel and P Oszag, pp. 899-955. Cambridge, MA: MIT Press.

18. Oliver, TR, Lee, PR, and Lipton, HL. (2004), pp. 302-306

19. Biles, B, Nicholas, LH, and Cooper, BS. (May 2004). The Cost of Privatization: Extra Payments to Medicare Advantage Plans. Commonwealth Fund Issue Brief (#750). Available at http://www.cmwf.org.

20. Schulman, S. (2003).

21. Schulman, S. (2003).

22. Moon, M. (June 2004). How Beneficiaries Fare Under the New Medicare Drug Bill. Commonwealth Fund Issue Brief (#730). Available at http://www.cmwf.org.

23. Oliver, TR, Lee, PR, and Lipton, HL. (2004), pp. 316-323.

24. Kingdon, JW. (1995). *Agendas, Alternatives, and Public Policies,* 2nd Edition. New York: HarperCollins.

25. Oliver, TR, Lee, PR, and Lipton, HL. (2004), pp. 327-329.

26. Peterson, MA. (1997). The Limits of Social Learning: Translating Analysis into Action. *Journal of Health Politics, Policy and Law* 22 (Aug.): 1077-1114.

27. Pierson, P. (1993). When Effect Becomes Cause: Policy Feedback and Political Change. *World Politics* 45: 595-628.

28. Peterson, M.A. (1997). The Limits of Social Learning: Translating Analysis into Action. *Journal of Health Politics, Policy and Law* 22 (Aug.): 1077-1114.

29. Dalleck, G. (December 7, 2003). Thanks for the Medicare Muddle. *Washington Post,* B1.

30. Johnson, H. and Broder, DS. (1996). *The System: The American Way of Politics at The Breaking Point.* Boston, MA: Little Brown, p. 569.

31. Oliver, TR, Lee, PR, and Lipton, HL. (2004), p. 341.

Chapter 3

Evolution of the FDA Drug Approval Process

Syed Rizwanuddin Ahmad

The United States Food and Drug Administration (FDA) is the U.S. consumer protection agency that has the regulatory responsibility for ensuring safety of all marketed medical products.[1] The FDA is comprised of five product-specific centers, Center for Drug Evaluation and Research (CDER), which regulates drugs and therapeutic biologic products; Center for Biologics Evaluation and Research (CBER), which regulates vaccines, blood and blood components, gene therapy products, and cells and tissues for transplants; Center for Food Safety and Applied Nutrition (CFSAN), which regulates cosmetics, dietary supplements, and genetically engineered foods; Center for Veterinary Medicine (CVM), which regulates drugs and food additives used for animals; and Center for Devices and Radiological Health (CDRH), which regulates medical devices and radiological products. The purview of the FDA is broad, and the agency has oversight over products that make up a quarter of every dollar spent by consumers in the United States.[2] The FDA monitors the products of about 95,000 businesses, amounting to goods worth about $1 trillion each year.[3] By federal government standards, the FDA is a small agency, even with more than 10,000 employees. The FDA's budget is about $1.3 billion, which is less than one–two hundred and fiftieth that of the U.S. Department of Defense and one-fiftieth of the U.S. Department of Agriculture's (USDA) budget,[4] and the same amount that Fairfax county, Virginia, provides for its schools.[5] A chronology of the milestones in the history of drug regulation is found in the appendix at the end of this chapter.

Syed Rizwanuddin Ahmad is an employee of the U.S. Food and Drug Administration. This chapter had been approved by the FDA as an outside activity and was written in the author's private capacity.

HISTORY OF THE ESTABLISHMENT OF THE FDA, DRUG APPROVAL, AND SAFETY REGULATIONS

Regrettably, medical and therapeutic disasters and misadventures have to a large extent shaped the history and development of most drug approval and safety regulations in the United States. The Import Drugs Act of 1848 was the U.S. Congress's first attempt at drug regulation. Even though this Act did not address adulteration and contamination of domestic drugs, it was a comprehensive and ambitious attempt by Congress to solve the adulteration problem in imported drugs.[6] This law prohibited the importation of such drugs.[7] The year 1902 saw an important first step toward organizing federal research related to drugs, and eventually their regulation when Harvey W. Wiley, MD, a chemist with the Bureau of Chemistry of the U.S. Department of Agriculture announced the formation of a drug laboratory.[8] The original Pure Food and Drug Act was passed by U.S. Congress and signed into law by President Theodore Roosevelt on June 30, 1906. This act administered by the Bureau of Chemistry prohibited the interstate transport of unlawful food and drugs under penalty of seizure of the questionable products and/or prosecution of the responsible parties. The basis of the act rested on regulation of product labeling rather than a premarket approval system for food ingredients or drugs. The government could act only after products were on the market. In the first decade after its passage, accurate drug labels protected Americans from dangerous ingredients. Complete freedom to market was allowed and no requirement for testing or approval existed. In 1930, the Bureau of Chemistry became what is now the FDA.

Age of Safety

In the early 1930s a bill was introduced in the U.S. Senate to revamp the 1906 drug act but it did not receive enough congressional support. However, two drug disasters eventually facilitated major congressional action:

- Dinitrophenol (DNP): DNP was used in diet pills in the 1930s but this use was banned in 1938.[9] DNP was associated with some two hundred cases of blindness, cataracts, and at least nine deaths were reported. However, the drug-induced sufferings associated with DNP did not stimulate any public outcry or any new law.[10]
- Elixir Sulfanilamide: Elixir Sulfanilamide was an antibiotic used to treat certain infections. This product was not available in liquid formulation, which even at that time was considered the ideal form for use, especially in children. The manufacturer tried different solvents

to produce a palatable liquid form of the drug and eventually settled with diethylene glycol, a poisonous ingredient chemically related to antifreeze now used in the automobile industry. The manufacturer started shipping the liquid form of Elixir Sulfanilamide in September 1937, and within three months at least 107 people, mostly children, died after ingesting the new drug formulation. Investigation showed that diethylene glycol in Elixir Sulfanilamide was the culprit. The company regretted the deaths and claimed that the drug was extensively tested and that there was no manufacturing error. Nevertheless the company was prosecuted for mislabeling and fined $26,000, or about $240 per death.[11] This tragedy led to the passage of the 1938 Federal Food, Drug, and Cosmetic (FD&C) Act by the Congress.

President Franklin Roosevelt signed the FD&C Act into law on June 25, 1938. This law for the first time required a manufacturer to prove the safety of a drug before it could be marketed.[12] In addition, this law required manufacturers to submit a New Drug Application (NDA) to the FDA before marketing a drug and the NDA was considered approved, if the FDA did not object. The application could be refused if:

1. Investigations did not include all tests reasonably applicable to show whether the drug was safe when used under proposed labeling.
2. Results of tests showed that the drug was unsafe or did not show that it was safe.
3. Information submitted was not sufficient to determine the safety.
4. Proposed labeling appeared to be false or misleading.

Age of Effectiveness

In 1957, thalidomide, a sleep medicine which was also used by women to prevent nausea associated with pregnancy was first marketed in Germany and elsewhere, largely in European countries by the German company Chemie Grunenthal. In early 1960, Richardson-Merrell, licensee of Grunenthal in the United States started the largest human drug trial ever conducted in the United States and thalidomide was given to some 20,000 patients. Under the 1938 FD&C Act, it was perfectly legal for pharmaceutical companies to recruit doctors to conduct experiments with new drugs without getting any FDA approval or obtaining consent from patients. In September 1960, seven months after thalidomide experiments began in the United States, the company officially submitted its application to the FDA. The thalidomide application was reviewed by Dr. Frances Kelsey, an FDA medical officer who was unhappy with the lack of scientific data in support of the drug. Dr. Kelsey consulted her colleagues at FDA and asked for additional information from the company. Meanwhile, as the company was putting more pressure on the FDA to approve thalidomide, reports of thalidomide-associated malformed babies began emerging in Europe.[13] Eventually, the thalidomide tragedy of the 1960s saw the birth of thousands of babies with deformities and prompted the need for tougher national drug regulation worldwide.[14,15]

In October 1962, following an intensive media and public debate on drug safety, the U.S. Congress passed the Kefauver-Harris Amendments to the FD&C Act to address the need for a more comprehensive drug regulation. These amendments required that the pharmaceutical company demonstrate proof of efficacy, using adequate and well-controlled studies, before drug approval and marketing; required rules for investigation of new drugs, including informed consent requirement of study subjects; and for the first time, drug manufacturers were required to report adverse drug events to the FDA.[16] On October 10, 1962, President John F. Kennedy signed the bill into law.

Age of Speedy Drug Approval

In the late 1980s, more than one thousand AIDS activists staged a large demonstration in front of the FDA's headquarters building in Rockville, MD, calling the FDA to approve drugs for AIDS. The protestors carried signs that said "Federal Death Agency" and "Red Tape Kills." As a result FDA embarked on a series of reforms that enabled patient access to drugs still in the clinical trials phase.[17] In the 1990s, a series of calls were made to overhaul the FDA drug regulations from all quarters, especially the Republican-controlled Congress. House speaker Newt Gingrich called the FDA "the leading job killer in America," and called for replacing the FDA with a "council of entrepreneurs," and literally rolling back the food and drug regulation to pre-1848 years. Rep. Joe Barton, Chairman, House Committee on Energy and Commerce stated that FDA should stop ruling on the efficacy of drugs at all and stick to measuring whether they are "safe, pure, and packaged safely."[18] The principal complaint was that the FDA was too slow in approving drugs compared to other industrialized nations, and was too tough on drug companies. This was referred to as "drug lag," and the agency was labeled a "Foot Dragging Agency." Newt Gingrich called Dr. David Kessler, the Commissioner of FDA, "a bully and a thug." Dr. Kessler said that the "U.S. approves many drugs months and even years before other nations do,"[19] and a Government Accountability Office (GAO) report[20] concluded that the FDA "stacks up well against its British counterpart, process-ing applications as fast or faster."[21] The conservative Washington Legal Foundation, placed ads with messages saying, "If a murderer kills you, it's homicide. If a drunk driver kills you, it's manslaughter. If the FDA kills you, it's just being cautious," creating an impression that American consumers were deprived of life-saving drugs because of the FDA's overcautious ap-proach. A call to "streamline America's costly and archaic drug regulation system" was made in an editorial in the *Wall Street Journal* (WSJ) "because last century regulations stifle the 21st century's scientific innovators."[22] The previous sentiments created an environment leading to change, and in 1992 Congress passed landmark legislation known as the Prescription Drug User Fee Act or PDUFA, which authorized the FDA to collect user fees from pharmaceutical companies to review drug and biological applications. The funds allowed the FDA to hire more review and support staff, upgrade its computer system, and provide guidance to the industry with the overall objective to speed review.[23] In 1996, legislation was introduced in Congress to overhaul the FDA. Dr. David Kessler, said that the proposed legislation would lower the safety standards for foods, drugs, and medical devices.[24] One of the most controversial parts of the legislation was to outsource the review of new drug and device applications to outside parties. One of the fiercest opponents of the call for FDA deregulation was Dr. Sidney Wolfe, director of Public Citizen Health Research Group, who said that this reform bill would "cripple" the FDA's "ability to adequately protect Americans from dangerous drugs, medical devices" and other regulated products.[25]

In 1997, PDUFA was renewed under the FDA Modernization Act or FDAMA. FDAMA liberalized the FDA's approval criteria, reduced the number of clinical trials required to demonstrate the effectiveness of a new drug, and accelerated the drug-approval process.[26] The changes to the drug act introduced in 1992 and 1997 may have brought benefits to patients with life-threatening diseases such as AIDS or cancer. However, these "drug in-dustry-inspired and approved amendments" will mostly benefit the industry and their stockholders.[27] PDUFA was renewed again in 2002 for five more years until 2007. More than 50 percent of CDER's budget now comes from user fees. Because of PDUFA, 50 percent of new drugs are first launched in the United States compared to 8 percent in the pre–PDUFA years.[28]

Age of Heightened Safety Scrutiny

All stakeholders in drug development, drug regulation, drug marketing, drug prescribing, drug dispensing, and drug use were influenced by two landmark events in 2004: (1) the determination that the use of selective serotonin reuptake inhibitors (SSRI) antidepressants in children was associated with suicidal behavior, and (2) the withdrawal of the cyclooxygenase (COX)-2 inhibitor drug rofecoxib from the market due to its association with life threatening cardiovascular events. Both of these issues brought extensive media coverage and publicity, and as a consequence the debate on drug safety and drug regulation is again a hot topic.[29-35] Many committees in both houses of the U.S. Congress have taken immense interest in this subject and a few have also held hearings—the first of its kind in perhaps the past fifteen years.

Senator Charles Grassley, Chairman of the Senate Finance Committee organized a hearing on November 18, 2004, which had a chilling effect on the FDA and the pharmaceutical industry. At the Senate hearing, twenty-year FDA veteran, Dr. David Graham, Associate Director for Science and Medicine at the FDA's Office of Drug Safety (now Office of Surveillance and Epidemiology [OSE]), testified that the agency as currently configured was "broken" and "is incapable of protecting against another Vioxx. We are virtually defenseless." Dr. Graham said, "the FDA has let the American people down." He estimated that rofecoxib was associated with 88,000 to 139,000 heart attacks and cardiac deaths, "the rough equivalent of 500 to 900 aircraft dropping from the sky." In the summer of 2004, Dr. Graham completed a large epidemiological study that examined the cardiovascular risk of COX-2 selective and nonselective nonsteroidal anti-inflammatory drugs or NSAIDs, and found that patients on low dose rofecoxib have 50 percent greater risk of heart attack and sudden cardiac death compared to celecoxib. And the risk of heart attack and sudden cardiac death increased by three times in patients who took the highest recommended dose of rofecoxib. Dr. Graham told his supervisors that high-dose rofecoxib should be banned. They told him to be quiet. Senior managers at the FDA tried to suppress his findings and made it difficult for him to publish his study because he did not follow the agency's clearance procedure.[36] Eventually the study was published in a prestigious journal.[37]

The heightened awareness on drug safety issues brought about by the antidepressants and the COX-2s debacle is very much alive. In the U.S. Senate, one bill, the Food and Drug Administration Safety Act of 2005 (FDASA) to set up a new, independent center within the FDA to review drugs and biological products once they are on the market was introduced by Senators Charles Grassley and Christopher Dodd to give more teeth to the FDA's OSE.[38] Senator Mike Enzi, Chairman of the Health, Education, Labor, and Pensions (HELP) Committee held two hearings, the first on March 1, 2005, to examine how the agency makes decision about new drugs and to review controversies regarding the drug approval process. The second hearing on March 3, 2005, examined steps the FDA had taken to address public concerns about the safety of prescription medications and to evaluate its ability to handle the challenges it faces in order to meets its mission. Senator Enzi said that "Congress needs to encourage new methods and resources to improve and streamline the nation's drug approval and post marketing process."[39] In the House, Representative Maurice Hinchey introduced the FDA Improvement Act of 2005 (FDAIA), a sweeping reform bill that would have ended the financial link and cozy relationship between the drug industry and the FDA, eliminate conflicts of interest on FDA advisory committees, and vastly improve the agency's postmarket drug safety program. The bill was cosponsored by Congresswoman Rosa DeLauro and Congressman Bart Stupak.[40] And Representative Tom Davis, Chairman of the Government Reform Committee organized a very powerful hearing on May 05, 2005, on the subject of "Risk and responsibility: The roles of FDA and pharmaceutical companies in ensuring the safety of approved drugs, like Vioxx." During the hearing, the public got an extraordinary glimpse of the aggressive marketing tactics of a major pharmaceutical company that was trying to push its product in campaigns such as "Project Offense" even as regulators were about to strengthen the drug's labeling.[41]

An ex–FDA official described "the curse of too much caution" in the agency and wrote that "a regulator can commit an error by permitting something bad to happen (approving a harmful product), or by preventing something good from becoming available (not approving a beneficial product). Both outcomes are bad for the public, but the consequences for the regulator are very different."[42]

> A renewed debate over who is supposed to be watching and how much surveillance is necessary is another legacy of the Vioxx controversy. Some critics are finding fault with the FDA.[43]

> Analysts say that Vioxx has had a significant effect on drug approvals. . . . If 2004 was a year to celebrate for drug approvals, then 2005 was a year in which to drown one's sorrows. . . . The fallout of Vioxx has created a culture of regulatory uncertainty.[44]

The fallout from rofecoxib's withdrawal has been seen "well beyond Merck and its ledgers." Some say that FDA has taken a "defensive posture designed to avoid another safety debacle." Although the FDA has denied that any change in the decision-making process has occurred as a consequence of rofecoxib withdrawal, an agency official rightly admitted that some reviewers may be looking more closely at safety data, and this is obviously hard to avoid.[45]

Ximelagatran (Exanta), muraglitizar (Pargluva), and modafinil (Sparlon) are recent examples of drugs that were not approved by the FDA because of heightened safety scrutiny. Ximelagatran, a novel oral thrombin inhibitor was rejected by an FDA advisory panel because of concern for hepatotoxicity, including three deaths in association with liver failure, and doubts about the company's plans to monitor and manage liver complications.[46] Dr. James Lewis, a hepatologist at Georgetown University questioned the recommendations of the FDA advisory panel not to approve the drug.[47] In February 2006 the company decided to stop all trials and sale of ximelagatran in countries where it was approved because of its hepatotoxicity potential.[48]

On September 9, 2005, an FDA advisory panel recommended approval of muraglitazar for treatment of diabetes mellitus and the FDA issued an "approvable letter" to the company. Researchers from Cleveland Clinic analyzed the data obtained from the FDA Web site and concluded that the drug "should not be approved" to treat diabetes "until safety is documented in a dedicated cardiovascular events trial."[49] Dr. Sidney Wolfe also sent a letter to the FDA saying that the agency should not approve it because of increased "risk of death, congestive heart failure, and other adverse events."[50] "And on May 18, 2006, the company announced that it would stop work on the experimental diabetes drug because it would take too long to conduct additional safety tests."[51]

On March 23, 2006, an FDA advisory panel voted not to recommend approval of modafinil (Sparlon) for the treatment of attention deficit/hyperactivity disorder. In a clinical trial the drug was associated with a single case of Stevens-Johnson syndrome (SJS), a rare but potentially fatal skin disorder in a seven-year-old boy. A lower dose of the drug is already on the market to improve wakefulness under the name of Provigil. The panel recommended that additional study of at least 3,000 patients would be needed to determine the safety of the drug with respect to SJS.[52]

IS THIS PRIME TIME FOR PASSAGE OF LANDMARK LEGISLATION TO STRENGTHEN FDA?

Events of the past few years have created very fertile ground for the passage of landmark legislation to protect the health and safety of American consumers. Historically, in the past century news about drug safety scares and debacles have always played a major role in the evolution of regulations that govern the U.S. FDA. At the April 24, 2006, launch of the much awaited Government Accountability Office (GAO) report card[53] on state of affairs at the FDA with respect to drug safety, Senator Charles Grassley stated that the GAO report

> provides solid evidence that everything is not alright at the FDA and calls for long-overdue reform. The FDA's problems are systemic and cultural, not isolated or easily fixed. The public deserves to know the risks when taking a prescription drug, and the FDA's review of drugs already on the market needs to be rigorous, independent, transparent and forthcoming. The bill I introduced with Sen. Dodd would help make that happen by giving the FDA post-market review process real teeth. Consumers shouldn't have to second-guess the safety of what's in their medicine cabinets. The FDA bears tremendous responsibility as consumers grow increasingly dependent on prescription medicines to cure diseases and maintain a better quality of life.[54]

With the PDUFA reauthorization up for renewal before it expires on September 30, 2007, it is likely that additional ideas for FDA reform will be considered by the Congress including Rep. Maurice Hinchey's proposal to restructure PDUFA so that funds are deposited into the general fund of the Treasury.[55] Currently, the drug companies pay user fees directly to the FDA to review their products, and the agency has to negotiate with them constantly, and this creates "financial dependency" and "cozy relationship." PDUFA money creates an apparent conflict of interest and fosters "the perception that the drug industry is the FDA's customer" and "client" rather than the American public.[56,57]

Whatever is the outcome of legislation to reform the FDA to meet the challenges of the twenty-first century, one thing is for certain that the agency has been "chronically underfunded," wrote Donald Kennedy, ex–FDA Commissioner in a recent editorial in *Science*.[58] William Hubbard, a senior ex–FDA official recently described the funding problem in these words:

> For some years . . . the agency's budget has remained essentially flat while major new responsibilities have been piled on. The results . . . are easy to document: Food inspections have dropped from . . . 50,000 in 1972 to about 5,000 today, meaning that U.S. food processors are inspected on average about every 10 years. The chance of a food product from overseas being inspected is infinitesimal. Most raw materials for our drugs come from foreign producers that are rarely inspected. The rate of quality-control failures found in manufacturing facilities by FDA inspectors has soared.[59]

In a powerful commentary advocating the need for a strong FDA, a commentator in *JAMA* recently wrote,

> Among the many reasons for founding the FDA a century ago was that industries and businesses that had profound effects on the nation's health were placing profits over consumer safety. Sadly, that blind, and often careless, dash toward financial or political gains is again dominating the business-government nexus today. And all recent events suggest that the FDA—as it was originally conceived and allowed to develop—is needed more than ever.[60]

Over the past century drug disasters have been a catalyst for change in drug regulation. The recent rofecoxib and antidepressants debacles have emphasized the need for drastic action again. Pending legislation in Congress to create a new center for postmarketing drug evaluation and research provides a reasonable solution and is the way to go. It is up to Congress and the White House to seize the opportunity and overhaul drug regulation. No doubt it will be a difficult task for everyone because of the corporate influence everywhere. There is no time to waste and further erode the consumer confidence in the important work done by FDA scientists. It is time to act!

APPENDIX: FDA MILESTONES

Regulation of drugs in the United States dates from pre–Civil War times. Federal controls over the drug supply began with inspection of imported drugs in 1848. The following chronology describes some of the milestones in the history of drug regulation in the United States.

1862

President Abraham Lincoln appoints a chemist, Charles M. Wetherill, to serve in the new Department of Agriculture. This appointment marked the beginning of the Bureau of Chemistry, the predecessor of the Food and Drug Administration.

1883

Harvey W. Wiley, MD, becomes chief chemist, expanding the Bureau of Chemistry's food adulteration studies. Campaigning for a federal law, Dr. Wiley is called the "Crusading Chemist" and "Father of the Pure Food and Drugs Act." He retired from government service in 1912 and died in 1930.

1902

The Biologics Control Act is passed to ensure purity and safety of serums, vaccines, and similar products used to prevent or treat diseases in humans.

Congress appropriates $5,000 to the Bureau of Chemistry to study chemical preservatives and colors and their effects on digestion and health. Dr. Wiley's studies draw widespread attention to the problem of food adulteration. Public support for passage of a federal food and drug law grows.

1906

The original Pure Food and Drugs Act is passed by Congress on June 30 and signed by President Theodore Roosevelt. It prohibits interstate commerce in misbranded and adulterated foods, drinks, and drugs.

1912

Congress enacts the Sherley Amendment to prohibit the labeling of medicines with false therapeutic claims intended to defraud the purchaser, a standard difficult to prove.

1927

The Bureau of Chemistry is reorganized into two separate entities. Regulatory functions are located in the Food, Drug, and Insecticide Administration, and nonregulatory research is located in the Bureau of Chemistry and Soils.

1930

The name of the Food, Drug, and Insecticide Administration is shortened to the Food and Drug Administration (FDA) under an agricultural appropriations act.

1937

Elixir Sulfanilamide, containing the poisonous solvent diethylene glycol, kills 107 people, many of whom are children, dramatizing the need to establish drug safety before marketing and to enact the pending food and drug law.

1938

The Federal Food, Drug, and Cosmetic Act (FD&C Act) of 1938, containing the new provisions that required new drugs to be shown to be safe before marketing, is passed by Congress.

1940

The FDA transferred from the Department of Agriculture to the Federal Security Agency, with Walter G. Campbell appointed as the first Commissioner of Food and Drugs.

1951

The Durham-Humphrey Amendment defines the kinds of drugs that cannot be safely used without medical supervision and restricts their sale to prescription by a licensed practitioner.

1962

Thalidomide, a new sleeping pill, is found to have caused birth defects in thousands of babies born in Western Europe. News reports on the role of Dr. Frances Kelsey, FDA medical officer, in keeping the drug off the U.S. market, arouse public support for stronger drug regulation.

Kefauver-Harris Drug Amendments are passed to ensure drug efficacy and greater drug safety. For the first time, drug manufacturers are required to prove to the FDA the effectiveness of their products before marketing them.

1983

The Orphan Drug Act, enabling the FDA to promote research and marketing of drugs needed for treating rare diseases, is passed.

1988

The Food and Drug Administration Act of 1988 establishes the FDA as an agency of the Department of Health and Human Services with a Commissioner of Food and Drugs appointed by the president with the advice and consent of the Senate.

1992

The Prescription Drug User Fee Act requires drug and biologics manufacturers to pay fees for product applications and supplements, and other services. The act also requires the FDA to use these funds to hire more reviewers to assess applications.

1993

Revising a policy from 1977 that excluded women of childbearing potential from early drug studies, the FDA issues guidelines calling for improved assessments of medication responses as a function of gender. Companies are encouraged to include patients of both sexes in their investigations of drugs.

1994

The Dietary Supplement Health and Education Act establishes specific labeling requirements, provides a regulatory framework, and authorizes the FDA to promulgate good manufacturing practice regulations for dietary supplements. This act classifies them as food.

1997

The Food and Drug Administration Modernization Act reauthorizes the Prescription Drug User Fee Act of 1992 and mandates the most wide-ranging reforms in agency practices since 1938. Provisions include measures to accelerate review of devices, regulate advertising of unapproved uses of approved drugs and devices, and regulate health claims for foods.

1998

The FDA promulgates the Pediatric Rule, a regulation that requires manufacturers of selected new and extant drug and biological products to conduct studies to assess their safety and efficacy in children.

2004

Senator Charles Grassley, Chairman of the Senate Finance Committee, and Representative Joe Barton, Chairman, Energy and Commerce Committee, asks the Government Accountability Office, the investigative arm of Congress, to conduct a review of FDA's current organizational structure and decision-making process.

Senator Charles Grassley organizes a hearing on November 18, 2004, to discuss the issues surrounding the withdrawal of rofecoxib (Vioxx) in which Dr. David Graham, Associate Director for Science and Medicine, at the FDA's Office of Drug Safety (now Office of Surveillance and Epidemiology [OSE]) testified that the agency as currently configured was "broken" and "is incapable of protecting against another Vioxx. We are virtually defenseless."

In the wake of safety controversy, the FDA requests the Institute of Medicine to study the drug safety system in the U.S.

2005

Senators Charles Grassley and Christopher Dodd introduces a bill in the Senate, the Food and Drug Administration Safety Act of 2005 (FDASA) to set up a new, independent center within the FDA to review drugs and biological products once they are on the market.

Senator Mike Enzi, Chairman of the Health, Education, Labor and Pensions (HELP) Committee holds two hearings, the first on March 1, 2005, to examine how the agency makes decision about new drugs and on reviewing controversies regarding the drug approval process. The second hearing, on March 3, 2005, examines steps the FDA is taking to address public concerns about the safety of prescription medications and to evaluate its ability to handle the challenges it faces in order to meets its mission.

Representative Tom Davis, Chairman of the Government Reform Committee organizes a hearing on May 5, 2005, on the subject of "Risk and responsibility: The roles of FDA and pharmaceutical companies in ensuring the safety of approved drugs, like Vioxx."

2006

GAO releases its much awaited report card on the state of drug safety at the FDA and concluded that the agency "lacks a clear and effective process for making decisions about, and providing management oversight of, postmarket drug safety issues."

In May, Representative Rosa DeLauro attaches an amendment in the House appropriations bill that was passed by a House committee. To speed drug approvals, the FDA frequently defers some clinical trials after product approval, but companies frequently do not honor the postmarketing commitments made at the time of drug approval. This amendment would allow the FDA to compel drug companies to follow through these commitments and begin proceedings to stop the sale of specific drugs if promised studies are not done.

Representative Maurice Hinchey tacks an amendment onto the same House appropriations bill to sharply limit the number of outside experts with ties to the drug industry who vote in FDA advisory panels. (Modified from *FDA Consumer*, January-February 2006, Vol. 40 No. 1 pp. 36-38.)

NOTES

1. Ahmad SR, Goetsch RA, Marks NS (2005). Spontaneous reporting in the United States. In Strom BL (ed.) *Pharmacoepidemiology* (pp. 135-159). Chichester, England. John Wiley & Sons.

2. Swann JP (1988). History of the FDA. In Kurian G (ed.) *The Historical Guide to American Government* (pp. 248-254). New York: Oxford University Press.

3. Hilts PJ (2003). Protecting America's Health: The FDA, Business, and One Hundred Years of Regulation. New York: Alfred A. Knopf.

4. Hilts PJ (2003).

5. Hubbard W (2006). Wrongly blaming the FDA. *Washington Post.* May 8, p. A19.

6. Heath WJ (2004). America's first drug regulation regime: The rise and fall of the Import Drug Act of 1848. *Food Drug Law J.* 59: 169-199.

7. Ahmad SR, Ouellet-Hellstrom R, McCloskey CA (2006). Pharmacovigilance. In AG Hartzema, HH Tilson, A Chan (eds.) *Pharmacoepidemiology and Therapeutic Risk Management,* Fourth edition (in press). Cincinnati: Harvey Whitney Press, Inc.

8. Meadows M (2006). Promoting safe and effective drugs for 100 years. *FDA Consumer* 40: 14-20.

9. ASTDR (1996). ToxFAQs for Dinitrophenols. September. Available at: http://www.atsdr.cdc.gov/tfacts64.html.

10. Hilts PJ (2003).

11. Hilts PJ (2003).

12. Wax PM (1995). Elixirs, diluents, and the passage of the 1938 Federal Food, Drug and Cosmetic Act. *Ann Int Med* 122: 456-461.

13. Meadows M (2006).

14. Hilts PJ (2003).

15. Dukes MNG (1990). The importance of adverse reactions in drug regulation. *Drug Saf* 5: 3-6.

16. Currie WJ (1990). The evolving horizon of drug registration—Europe and beyond. *Eur J Clin Pharmacol.* 39: 453-456.

17. Washburn J (2001). Undue influence: How the drug industry's power goes unchecked and why the problem is likely to get worse. *American Prospect.* Available at: http://www.prospect.org/print/V12/14/washburn-j.html. Accessed May 25, 2006.

18. Applebaum A (2005). The drug approval pendulum. *Washington Post.* April 13, p. A17.

19. Schwartz J (1995). Americans receive new medicines as quickly as others, FDA asserts: Red tape does not keep lifesaving drugs off market, Kessler says. *Washington Post.* December 13, p. A03.

20. Government Accountability Office (1995). FDA Drug approval: Review time has decreased in recent years. PEMD-96-1. October 20. Available at: http://www.gao.gov/docdblite/summary.php?rptno=PEMD-96-1&accno=155572. Accessed May 27, 2006.

21. Schwartz J (1995). FDA graded highly on relative speed of review process. *Washington Post.* November 8, p. A15.

22. A 21st century FDA: streamline America's costly and archaic drug-regulation system (2001). *Wall Street Journal.* February 2, p. 10A.

23. Berndt ER, Gottschalk AH, Philipson TJ, Strobeck MW (2005). Industry funding of the FDA: Effects of PDUFA on approval times and withdrawal rates. *Nat Rev Drug Discov* 4: 545-554.

24. Burros M (1996). FDA Chief questions safety of proposals. *New York Times.* May 2, p. A21.

25. Testimony of Dr. Sidney M. Wolfe, House Subcommittee on Health and the Environment Hearings on H.R.s 3199-3201. FDA Approval Process. May 2, 1996.

26. Washburn J (2001).

27. Lurie P, Wolfe SM (1998). Troubling climate at FDA. *Washington Post.* December 30, p. A19.

28. U.S. Food and Drug Administration (2005). White Paper: PDUFA: Adding resources and improving performance in FDA review of NDAs. Rockville, MD: FDA.

29. Horton R (1995). Vioxx, the implosion of Merck, and aftershocks at the FDA. *Lancet* 364: 1995-1996.

30. Lenzer J (2004). FDA is incapable of protecting US "against another Vioxx." *BMJ* 329: 1253.

31. Edwards I (2005). What are the real lessons from Vioxx? *Drug Safety* 28: 651-658.

32. Solomon DH, Avorn J (2005). Coxibs, science and the public trust. *Arch Intern Med* 165: 158-160.

33. Waller PC, Evans SJ, Beard K (2005). Drug safety and regulation: new powers and resources are needed. *BMJ* 331: 4-5.

34. Drazen JM (2005). Cox-2 inhibitors: A lesson in unexpected problems. *N Engl J Med* 352: 1131-1132.

35. Urquhart J (2005). Some key points emerging from the COX-2 controversy. *Pharmacoepi Drug Safety* 14: 145-147.

36. Scherer M (2005). The side effects of truth. *Mother Jones* May/June. Available at: http://www.motherjones.com/news/feature/2005/05/david_graham.html. Accessed May 27, 2006.

37. Graham DJ, Campen D, Hui R, Spence M, Cheetham C, Levy G, Shoor S, Ray WA (2005). Risk of myocardial infarction and sudden cardiac death in patients treated with cyclo-oxygenase 2 selective and non-selective nonsteroidal anti-inflammatory drugs: Nested case-control study. *Lancet* 365: 475-481.

38. The Food and Drug Administration Safety Act of 2005 (FDASA). Available at: http://finance.senate.gov/press/Gpress/2005/prg042705a.pdf. Accessed May 26, 2006.

39. U.S. Senate (2005). Rapid advances in science, drug development, demand change to FDA's review process, Enzi says. Available at: http://help.senate.gov/Maj_press/2005_03_03.pdf. Accessed May 27, 2006.

40. U.S. House of Representatives (2005). Hinchey introduces sweeping FDA reform measure. Available at: http://www.house.gov/hinchey/newsroom/press_2005/050405fdareformbill.html. Accessed May 27, 2006.

41. U.S. House of Representatives (2005). Merck documents show aggressive marketing of Vioxx after studies indicated risk. Available at: http://www.democrats.reform.house.gov/story.asp?ID=848. Accessed May 27, 2006.

42. Miller HI (2000). The curse of too much caution. *Wall Street Journal.* November 26, p. A8.

43. Palmer K (2005). The Vioxx fallout. *Minn Med* 88: 26-30.

44. Frantz S (2005). 2005 approvals: Safety first. *Nature Reviews Drug Discovery.* Available at: http://www.nature.com/drugdisc/news/articles/nrd1973.html. Accessed May 20, 2006.

45. Zwillich T (2005). How Vioxx is changing U..S drug regulation. *Lancet* 366: 1763-1764.

46. Is that it, then, for blockbuster drugs? (2004). *Lancet* 364: 1100.

47. Lewis, JH (2006). "Hy's law," the "Rezulin rule," and other predictors of severe drug-induced hepatotoxicity: Putting risk-benefit into perspective. *Pharmacoepidemiol Drug Safe* 15: 221-229.

48. Ginsberg T (2005). AstraZeneca abandons blood thinner, citing risk. *Philadelphia Inquirer.* February 15, p. C1.

49. Nissen SE, Wolski K, Topol EJ (2005). Effect of muraglitazar on death and major adverse cardiovascular events in patients with type 2 diabetes mellitus. *JAMA* 294: 2581-2586.

50. Wolfe SM (2005). Letter to Dr. Andrew Von Eschenbach, acting commissioner, FDA. November 21. Available at: http://www.citizen.org/publications/release.cfm?ID=7407&secID=1660&catID=126. Accessed May 27, 2006.

51. Steyer B (2006). Bristol pulls diabetes drug. Available at: http://www.theStreet.com/stocks/pharmaceuticals/10286692.html. Accessed May 18, 2006.

52. Bridges A (2006). Panel: Drug shouldn't be used for ADHD yet. Associated Press. March 24.

53. Government Accountability Office (2006). Drug safety: Improvement needed in FDA's postmarket decision-making and oversight process. GAO-06-402. March. Available at: http://www.gao.gov/cgi-bin/getrpt?GAO-06-402. Accessed May 27, 2006.

54. U.S. Senate (2005). Grassley press conference on GAO report. Available at: http://finance.senate.gov/press/Gpress/2005/prg042406.pdf. Accessed May 27, 2006.

55. U.S. House of Representatives (2005). Hinchey calls for complete restructuring of Prescription Drug User Fee Act: says FDA must end its financial dependency and overall cozy relationship with drug companies. November 14. Available at: http://www.house.gov/hinchey/newsroom/press_2005/press_2005/111405pdufa.html. Accessed May 27, 2006.

56. U.S. House of Representatives (2005). Hinchey calls for complete restructuring of Prescription Drug User Fee Act.

57. Ray WA, Stein CM (2006). Reform of drug regulation: Beyond an independent drug safety board. *N Engl J Med* 354: 194-201.

58. Kennedy D (2006). FDA Centennial. *Science* 312: 19.

59. Hubbard W (2006). Wrongly blaming the FDA. *Washington Post.* May 8, p. A19.

60. Markel H (2005). Why America needs a strong FDA. *JAMA* 294: 2489-2491.

Chapter 4

The Market for Pharmaceuticals: The Big Picture

David H. Kreling

When considering policies related to pharmaceuticals, it is important to understand the pharmaceutical market and thus have a context for policy and policymaking and how they may affect or relate to the market. The goal of this chapter is to provide a brief introduction to some relevant characteristics of the market for pharmaceuticals; to answer some of the "who," "what," "where," and "how" questions about pharmaceuticals; and to perhaps provide a sense of the "whys" related to pharmaceuticals and pharmaceutical policy.

The market for pharmaceuticals is complex and unique. Aspects that contribute to the complexity of the market include the number and kinds of firms that operate and interact in the market and how those firms or entities interact. The uniqueness of the market is related to peculiarities in the demand for and product selection of pharmaceuticals.

THE MARKET FOR PHARMACEUTICALS: STRUCTURAL OVERVIEW

In general, the market for pharmaceuticals has structural components and a channel of distribution similar to other consumer goods. Channel members include manufacturers, distributors, retailers, and consumers. These entities engage in functions that generate the flow of consumer goods from production through consumption. Pharmaceuticals are highly regulated products, undergoing specific and special regulations and regulatory processes and procedures throughout the channel. In addition, more than just the buyer and seller can be involved in transactions for pharmaceuticals at the consumer level, adding an aspect of complexity not present in other markets. Public and private insurance-type programs and the sponsors or funders of these programs often also have a financial stake, in addition to the consumer, when individuals purchase pharmaceutical products.

Manufacturers

Two groups of companies manufacture pharmaceuticals: brand name manufacturers and generic manufacturers. Brand name manufacturers are firms that emphasize innovation and generating new drug products. They concentrate on research and development of new products for the market and promoting those products to engender market success for their innovations. Brand name manufacturers obtain patents for new drugs that result from their research and development. When a drug is covered by a patent, only the firm with the patent can produce and market the drug. This effectively establishes a monopoly for this company for the period of time (up to twenty years, maximum) that the patent is in effect. Since only the company holding the patent can produce and sell a "patent-protected" drug, these drugs often are referred to as single-source products. When the patent for a drug expires, additional firms can begin manufacturing the drug. Such drugs are referred to as off-patent or multisource drugs. After the patent for a drug expires, the brand name manufacturer that discovered the drug typically continues to market the drug, and their version of the drug is referred to as the multisource innovator product. Versions of the drug manufactured and marketed by other firms after the patent expires are referred to as multisource generic versions of the drug, and the manufacturers are referred to as generic manufacturers.

Brand name manufacturers are noted for their marketing and promotional efforts, and it can be useful to think of their "products" as being not only pharmaceutical agents and the physical drug products, but also as information about those agents and their use. Generic manufacturers focus on making off-patent drug products and seek market success by efficiently producing and competitively pricing their versions of brand name manufacturers' products. These two groups of manufacturers are counterparts to manufacturers in many other consumer good product categories, those being major label or original equipment manufacturers and secondary or "off label" manufacturers.

Brand name and generic manufacturers generally are considered distinct and separate from each other, but they are closely interrelated. In theory, the corresponding manufacturers compete for market share since they sell the same, "identical" products. However, often efforts are made to maintain a distinction between brand and generic versions of drug products. Typically, a large difference in price between brand and generic versions of a drug product develops, and consequently brand manufacturers lose considerable market share to generic competitors' products. The often dramatic reduction in the brand name manufacturer's revenue due to generic competitors' products drives brand manufacturers to divert their attention and marketing efforts to other products they sell, sometimes even to the extent of de-marketing their older, off-patent products. Another interrelationship between brand name and generic manufacturers is that brand name companies may have subsidiaries producing generic versions of their own products, or they may apply excess manufacturing capacity and contract out for production of generic versions of their product for generic firms. An important issue for manufacturers relates to how innovation and research and development can be encouraged while at the same time advantage can be taken of lower prices for generic drugs in the marketplace.

The genesis of contemporary firms in the pharmaceutical manufacturing market was with entrepreneurial efforts of individual pharmacists, physicians, or drug distributors as they moved into standardized manufacturing of drug products and discovery of novel therapies. Companies such as Merck, Lilly, and Pfizer all have this common theme in their history. The Pharmaceutical Research and Manufacturers of America (PhRMA) lists thirty-four companies (with affiliates) as members. These firms comprise the brand name manufacturer segment of the U.S. pharmaceutical market. The Generic Pharmaceutical Association (GPhA) is a counterpart trade organization for manufacturers of generic drugs. According to the GPhA, roughly fifty generic manufacturers exist, including companies that make only generics and those that produce generics and some proprietary products or branded versions of multiple-source drugs. In both segments of the pharmaceutical market, the number of firms has decreased over the past few decades as mergers and acquisitions have occurred. Competitive factors that have contributed to these mergers and acquisitions include fewer new products and shorter product life cycles, changing customers, and globalization.

According to IMS Health, a market research firm concentrating on the pharmaceutical market and health care, the total U.S. market for prescription drugs in 2004 was $235.4 billion, valued at the ex-factory (the price at which the factory sells to the wholesaler) wholesale price level. The vast majority of these sales accrue to brand name products and their companies; in 2004 less than 8 percent ($18.1 billion) of sales were for generic drug products. A ranking of the top twenty companies, by sales, is shown in Table 4.1. Brand name companies dominate the top-twenty list; only two generic-drug firms, Teva and Watson, are included in the top-twenty list.

Slightly different results occur when the market is restricted to only prescription activity in the retail pharmacy sector in the channel of distribution.

TABLE 4.1. Top 20 Pharmaceutical Manufacturers, Ranked by U.S. Sales, 2004

Rank	Corporation	Total dollars (U.S. $billions)*	Percent market share
1	Pfizer	$30.7	13.1
2	GlaxoSmithKline	$18.8	8.0
3	Johnson & Johnson	$16.2	6.9
4	Merck & Co	$15.0	6.4
5	AstraZeneca	$11.3	4.8
6	Novartis	$10.2	4.3
7	Sanofi-Aventis	$10.0	4.3
8	Amgen	$9.5	4.1
9	Bristol-Myers Squibb	$9.2	3.9
10	Wyeth	$8.2	3.5
11	Lilly	$8.0	3.4
12	Abbott	$6.5	2.8
13	Hoffman-Laroche	$6.1	2.6
14	TAP Pharmaceutical	$4.7	2.0
15	Boehringer Ingelhein	$3.7	1.6
16	Forest Lab	$3.4	1.4
17	Teva	$3.4	1.4
18	Schering Plough	$2.9	1.2
19	Eisai	$2.5	1.1
20	Watson	$2.4	1.0

* Represents prescription pharmaceutical purchases, including insulin at wholesale prices by retail, food stores and chains, mass merchandisers, independent pharmacies, mail services, nonfederal and federal hospitals and clinics, closed-wall HMOs, long-term care pharmacies, home health care, and prisons/universities. Excludes comarketing agreements. Joint-ventures assigned to product owner. Data run by custom redesign to include completed mergers and acquisitions.

Source: IMS Health (2005), *IMS National Sales Perspective.*™ February. Fairfield, CT: IMS Health. Reprinted with permission from IMS Health.

Data from Verispan, another pharmaceutical market research firm, reveal that in 2004, 18 percent of the $173 billion in prescription drug sales in retail (community) pharmacies were for generic drugs. Interestingly, generic drugs represent less than 20 percent of retail pharmacy prescription sales, yet nearly half (48 percent) of the 3.1 billion prescriptions sold were dispensed as the generic versions of drugs. In addition, when ranked by number of dispensed prescriptions, four of the top five corporations are generic

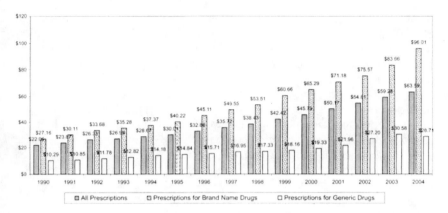

FIGURE 4.1. Average retail prescription prices, 1990-2004. *Source:* IMS Health (2005), *IMS National Prescription Audit Plus*™ (NPA Plus). Fairfield, CT: IMS Health. Reprinted with permission from IMS Health.

firms (including Sandoz).[1] The disproportionate sales and dispensed prescription volume for generic drugs is related to the differences in prices of prescriptions for brand name and generic drugs, shown in Figure 4.1. The proportion of prescriptions dispensed as generic drugs increased through the 1990s from about one in three in 1991 to roughly half of all prescriptions in 2004, but since the average price of a brand name prescription grew faster than the average price of a generic prescription during that time, the proportion of retail prescription sales dollars for generic drugs has remained small.

Distributors: Drug Wholesalers

Drug wholesalers serve as the middleman/middlewoman link between drug manufacturers and pharmacies. They perform what marketers refer to as the logistics function in the channel of distribution for pharmaceuticals: they assemble, sort, and disperse drug products. Although the role of distributor that wholesalers play is essential, as an intermediary in the channel with a somewhat limited scope of function and value added they less often are a policy focus. Generally, pharmaceutical policy related to drug wholesalers tends to be relevant regulations and requirements to ensure the integrity of the drug distribution system. For example, strict requirements exist for distribution of prescription drugs only to pharmacies and practitioners licensed to prescribe or dispense drugs, and special handling procedures and controls are in place for narcotics and controlled substances. In addition, drugs distributed in the United States must be approved for use and sale in the United States, raising issues about drug imports and possible counterfeit drug products.

The drug wholesaling industry tends to be very competitive. Since competing wholesalers generally sell the same products, price has been a primary competition variable, and they have focused on efficiency in their operations to ensure they can price competitively. Drug wholesalers compete with one another for market share, but also face corporate (chain store) distribution centers as additional competitors. According to the Healthcare Distribution Management Association (HDMA), wholesalers earned an average gross margin of 3.74 percent and net profit after taxes averaging 0.75 percent of total sales in 2004.

There has been consolidation in the drug wholesaling industry with a few large, national major wholesalers dominant in the market. These traditional, "full service" wholesalers, such as McKesson, Cardinal, and AmerisourceBergen are joined by smaller local or regional specialty wholesalers that may focus on special products or limited product lines. In addition, secondary wholesalers have served redistributive functions in the market between buyers, sellers, and other middleperson distributors. In addition to their main role in distributing pharmaceuticals, wholesalers also provide services to support pharmacies in providing patient care, such as financial and management consulting services to improve hospital and retail pharmacy operations and efficiency.

The HDMA (formerly the National Wholesale Druggists Association) reports forty-six distribution companies as members, and these companies operate 224 distribution centers in the United States. HDMA also reports that 63 percent of pharmaceutical manufacturers' sales are distributed through wholesalers, with most of the remaining sales being to chain warehouses and mail service pharmacies and a small percent of sales direct to other pharmacies. Typically, a pharmacy will select and use one wholesaler as a primary supplier, to maximize their purchase volume and obtain favorable purchasing terms; they turn to their secondary supply sources (other wholesalers, direct purchasing, etc.) as backup suppliers or for alternate sources of products not available through the primary wholesaler.

Retailers: Pharmacies

Pharmacies comprise the "retail sector" or terminal seller in the channel of pharmaceutical distribution. Pharmacies engage in the final transfer of title to consumers for pharmaceutical products. This sector of the market for pharmaceuticals is the most diverse; it encompasses different types of pharmacies (including institutional hospital and long-term-care pharmacies, community independent and chain pharmacies, mail-service pharmacies, etc.) and a variety of ownership structures (government and military, not-for-profit and for profit private organizations, independent entrepreneurs, and publicly traded corporate businesses). The sales of pharmaceutical manufacturers to different types of pharmacies that is summarized in Figure 4.2 provides a sense of the diversity of pharmacies and their relative sizes in the market.

The diversity in types of pharmacies in the market provides complexity to the context for policy related to the "retail" sector of the pharmaceutical market. A classic distinction for types of pharmacies has been by the kind of patient served, with institutional pharmacies (hospital and long-term-care pharmacies) serving patients confined to beds with professional or technical staff administering doses, contrasted with community pharmacies serving ambulatory, self-dosing patients. This kind of a distinction is useful because it reflects the relevant competitors and business units in the market. Such a simple distinction is less useful currently, since hospitals have

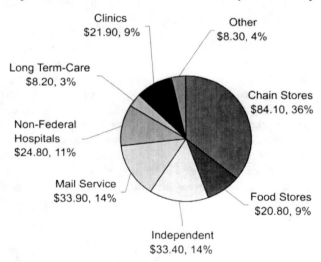

FIGURE 4.2. Sales of manufacturers to different classes of customers, 2004. *Note:* Data represent sales from manufacturers at the wholesale level (ex-factory) in $ billions; percent of total $235.4 billion market sales for 2004. *Source:* IMS Health (2005), *IMS National Sales Perspective.*™ Fairfield, CT: IMS Health. Reprinted with permission from IMS Health.

morphed into health systems with inpatient and outpatient services. As hospitals have evolved into health systems, a type of "corporatization" of ownership has occurred along with encroachment into community pharmacy care through clinic-affiliated or freestanding outpatient pharmacies as part of these health systems. In addition, some community pharmacies have developed home health care services to provide medications for homebound patients that may be self-administered or dosed by visiting nurses.

Distinction between a traditional chain versus independent ownership for community pharmacies remains, although independent pharmacies commonly belong to buying groups and others are part of franchise organizations, giving them some similarity to chain pharmacies. In addition, corporate (chain) pharmacies themselves can be quite diverse, including pharmacies in mass merchandiser stores and food stores. Some have suggested that operational characteristics, such as daily prescription volume, may be better classifying variables for community pharmacies instead of independent and chain ownership. The distinction between mail service and community pharmacies also becomes blurred when independent and chain community pharmacies offer extended-day-supplies or mail delivery service for prescription patrons.

Important market trends within the community pharmacy sector have been: (1) growth in the number of chain pharmacies and a decrease (albeit slowed in recent years) in the proportion of pharmacies that are independently owned, and (2) growth in the proportion of prescriptions dispensed by mail service pharmacies. Trends in the distribution of types of pharmacies are shown in Figure 4.3. The total number of community retail pharmacies has remained relatively stable in recent years, but some redistribution of outlets has occurred between corporate (including chain, mass merchandiser, and supermarket) pharmacies and independent pharmacies. Trends in the number of prescriptions dispensed by type of community retail pharmacy are shown in Figure 4.4. The amount of prescriptions dispensed from mail service pharmacies has grown in recent years. Some of this growth is a reflection of policies by insurers and drug coverage plans requiring or encouraging patients to obtain prescriptions from mail service pharmacies.

Other, Peripheral Market Parties

An additional aspect of the market for pharmaceuticals that adds to its complexity is a variety of other organizations that play a role with firms and transactions in the channel of pharmaceutical distribution. These other parties typically are not involved with the physical distribution of pharmaceuticals and thus never hold title to the drug products as they move through

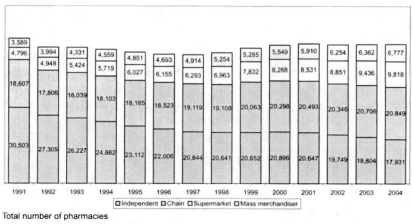

Total number of pharmacies

1991	1992	1993	1994	1995	1996	1997	1998	1999	2000	2001	2002	2003	2004
57,495	54,053	54,021	53,243	52,155	51,377	51,170	51,966	53,832	55,011	55,581	55,200	55,308	55,314

FIGURE 4.3. Trends in the distribution of pharmacy types, 1991-2004. *Source: MS Health, DDD™, 2005.* Reprinted with permission from IMS Health.

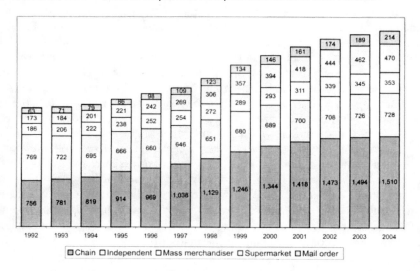

FIGURE 4.4. Trends in prescriptions dispensed in community pharmacies, 1992-2004 (millions of prescriptions). *Source:* National Association of Chain Drug Stores (NACDS) (2005). Available at www.nacds.org/wmspage.cfm? parm1=506. Based on data from IMS Health, *IMS National Prescription Audit™.* Reprinted with permission from NACDS.

the channel of distribution, but they can affect the flow of goods or the actions of channel members who do take and transfer title to the goods.

Physicians are central to the sale and use of pharmaceuticals, especially prescription drugs. They write orders for prescriptions that provide consumers with access to prescription drugs. They also make recommendations for use of nonprescription drugs. However, physicians (or, generically, prescribers) neither use nor pay for the drugs that consumers use. The government, via the Food and Drug Administration, determines which drugs will be available and whether a prescription is required for obtaining the drug.[2]

The financial aspects of pharmaceuticals and consumer purchase of drugs within the realm of private insurance connects employers, insurers, and insurance-related organizations such as claims processors or pharmaceutical benefits managers (PBMs) to the market for pharmaceuticals. Consumers of prescription drugs can purchase insurance coverage for prescription drugs or acquire coverage through their employment as a fringe benefit and part of their overall compensation (as an alternate form of income). Employers offer coverage to employees through selected insurers (that may take the form of traditional insurers, or managed care organizations, etc.). Insurers or managed care organizations may utilize PBMs to process claims and administer the specialized drug coverage aspects of the benefit. PBMs are connected to pharmaceutical manufacturers through rebate arrangements related to formularies and drug use policies. Publicly funded coverage for drugs, such as state Medicaid programs, may involve insurers and insurance-related organizations similar or parallel to the private insurance scenario, or they may undertake some or all of the roles or functions themselves. Ultimately, citizens are connected to publicly funded programs because their tax payments fund the coverage.

An important trend related to these other parties involved in the market has been an increase in the percent of prescriptions that are covered by public or private insurance. This trend is shown in Figure 4.5. The proportion of prescriptions that are covered by a private or public (Medicaid) insurance program, and thus have a third-party involved in the financing or payment of the prescription, has increased, especially since 1992. Private insurance coverage has become dominant in the market for prescriptions, at least in aggregate, and although a single private third-party program might not represent as large a proportion of an individual pharmacy's business as Medicaid, the private third-party business combined dwarfs the public programs. The proportion of prescriptions funded by public, government programs changed after January 2006 when Medicare Part D was implemented, but since Part D is administered by private insurers offering

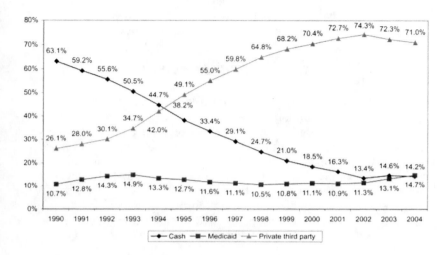

FIGURE 4.5. Prescriptions dispensed in community pharmacies by payor type, 1990-2004. *Source:* IMS Health (2005). IMS *National Prescription Audit™*, Method of Payment, 1990-2004. Fairfield, CT: IMS Health. Reprinted with permission from IMS Health.

prescription drug programs, the recent and current trend of private plans leading the way with policies and programs likely will continue.

Increased private and public coverage for prescriptions has had a large impact on retail/community pharmacies, because the insurance programs have established reimbursement systems that set the prices they will pay for prescriptions. The reimbursement levels set by insurers have reflected a "large purchaser" philosophy, extracting volume discounts from pharmacies as sellers. Insurers make payment to pharmacies for dispensed prescriptions, thus reimbursement cuts to pharmacies initially seemed the only way they could respond to increased costs. More recently, insurers have devised other methods in attempt to contain costs, and thus manufacturers also have been affected by policies related to coverage such as formularies and rebates.

The dominance of private insurance coverage plans for prescriptions raises the question of whether private third parties are more important than the public, government programs. Early in the evolution of drug coverage programs (i.e., through the 1970s and early 1980s), the trend was for private plans to adopt public policies (e.g., the federal maximum allowable cost, MAC, program). More recently, private plans seem to be leading the way with changes, including seeking deeper discounted payment rates to pharmacies and implementing more aggressive drug use policies or restrictions.

EXPENDITURES FOR DRUGS

Prescription drugs play an essential role in primary health care. They represent the most common therapeutic intervention in both community-based and hospital-based medical care. However, prescription drugs are a relatively small part of health care expenditures. As shown in Figure 4.6, prescription drugs have comprised a much smaller proportion of personal health care spending than hospital care or physician and clinical services. Through the 1970s to 1990s, less than 10 percent of personal health care expenditures was attributable to prescription drugs.[3] Recent changes in expenditures for prescription drugs, relative to changes in other health care expenditure components, especially since 1990, have heightened awareness

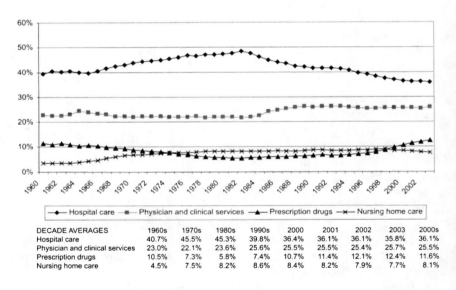

DECADE AVERAGES	1960s	1970s	1980s	1990s	2000	2001	2002	2003	2000s
Hospital care	40.7%	45.5%	45.3%	39.8%	36.4%	36.1%	36.1%	35.8%	36.1%
Physician and clinical services	23.0%	22.1%	23.6%	25.6%	25.5%	25.5%	25.4%	25.7%	25.5%
Prescription drugs	10.5%	7.3%	5.8%	7.4%	10.7%	11.4%	12.1%	12.4%	11.6%
Nursing home care	4.5%	7.5%	8.2%	8.6%	8.4%	8.2%	7.9%	7.7%	8.1%

FIGURE 4.6. Percent of spending for personal health care expenditures: Hospital care, physician and clinical services, prescription drugs, and nursing home care, 1960-2003. *Source:* National Health Statistics Group (2005). Baltimore, MD: Centers for Medicare and Medicaid Services. Compiled from data available at: http://www.cms.hhs.gov/NationalHealthExpendData/02_NationalHealthAccountsHistorical.asp#TopOfPage.

and concerns about spending for prescription drugs. Except for 1992, the annual percent change in expenditures for prescription drugs exceeded the percent change in hospital care or physician and clinical services (or both) since 1990; prior to 1990, the annual growth in prescription spending exceeded the change in these other components only six times after 1960. As shown in Figure 4.7, growth in prescription expenditures was considerably higher than the growth in other major health care components for several years since 1990, including nearly a 20 percent increase between 1998 and 1999. These increases in prescription spending have been a primary reason why policymakers have focused on drugs and policies aimed at curbing this growth in expenditures.

From an economic perspective, expenditures or spending for prescription drugs can be considered simply the product of price (P) and quantity (Q) of drugs consumed or alternatively price and utilization. However, growth or change in expenditures includes changes in prices of pharmaceuticals, and changes in utilization, where utilization has both a quantitative (how much) and qualitative (of what) aspect.

The quantitative aspect of changes in utilization captures increased intensity of use, either from more prescriptions dispensed and used or more doses per day, or both. The commonality of prescription drugs as a part of

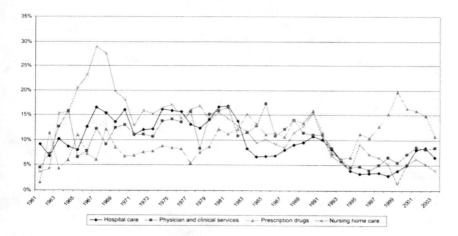

FIGURE 4.7. Percent change in national health expenditures, 1961-2003. *Source:* National Health Statistics Group (2005). Baltimore, MD: Centers for Medicare and Medicaid Services. Compiled from data available at: http://www.cms.hhs.gov/NationalHealthExpendData/02_NationalHealthAccountsHistorical.asp#TopOfPage.

primary care is fundamental to the quantitative utilization component as a contributor to expenditures and changes in expenditures. In the vast majority of instances, a patient visit or contact with a physician results in an order for a prescription drug. According to the 2002 National Ambulatory Medical Care Survey (NAMCS), 64.8 percent of physician visits by ambulatory patients in the United States resulted in a drug being prescribed.[4] For patients with chronic conditions requiring drug therapy, one physician visit generates multiple pharmacy visits for an original dispensing and refills of any prescription drug(s) being taken by the patient.

Table 4.2 summarizes utilization based on the numbers of prescriptions dispensed to consumers from community pharmacies and includes the total number of dispensed prescriptions and these prescriptions expressed on a per capita basis. Between 1992 and 2004, increased intensity of prescription utilization is evident; the total number of prescriptions dispensed grew at an average annual rate of 5.4 percent compared to a 1.1 percent population growth rate.

The qualitative aspect of changes in utilization can be considered change in the composition or mix of products used. As the mix of drug products used changes, it drives change in the average price of a prescription in an aggregate sense. The effect of a change in product mix on the average price

TABLE 4.2. Utilization of Prescription Drugs

	Total Prescriptions (million)	U.S. Population (million)	Per capita prescriptions
1992	1,873.4	256.9	7.29
1993	2,020.2	260.3	7.76
1994	2,088.3	263.4	7.93
1995	2,216.2	266.6	8.31
1996	2,315.6	269.7	8.59
1997	2,423.2	272.9	8.88
1998	2,587.6	276.1	9.37
1999	2,822.6	279.3	10.11
2000	3,031.0	282.4	10.73
2001	3,200.0	285.3	11.22
2002	3,343.5	288.2	11.60
2003	3,438.4	291.0	11.81
2004	3,519.4	292.8	12.02

Source: Prescriptions from IMS Health (2005), *IMS National Prescription Audit*™ (NPA) 1992-2004; population from *Statistical Abstract 2005/2006.* Fairfield, CT: IMS Health. Reprinted with permission from IMS Health.

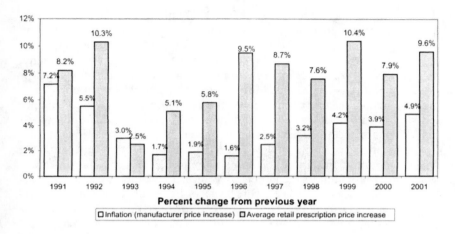

FIGURE 4.8. Changes in average prescription prices and manufacturer price increases, 1991-2001. *Source:* Manufacturer product price increases from IMS Health (2002). *Pharmaceutical Pricing UPDATE.* Prescription prices from IMS Health (2002). *IMS National Prescription Audit Plus™* (NPA Plus). Fairfield, CT: IMS Health. Reprinted with permission from IMS Health.

of a prescription is independent of and in addition to the effect of inflationary changes in the prices of pharmaceuticals; both product mix and inflation contribute to the price component of the price (P) times quantity (Q) determination of expenditures and changes in expenditures for prescription drugs.

The relative impacts of changes in qualitative utilization due to variation in the mix of products dispensed and price inflation are shown in Figure 4.8. If the same mix of products was dispensed from year to year, the average prescription price would change only due to inflationary changes in the prices set by manufacturers. Differences in the magnitudes of average prescription price changes and amount of inflationary price changes each year reflect the impact of product mix changes. Product mix has contributed to increased expenditures for prescription drugs as newer, higher-cost drugs are used to replace older, lower-cost (brand and/or generic) drug products. The total changes in expenditures for prescription drugs reflect the combination of quantitative utilization, price inflation, and product mix changes that occur.

A variety of phenomena can be considered underlying factors that contribute to expenditures and changes in expenditures for prescription drugs. Some of the factors affect price and/or utilization aspects of prescription expenditures, and some of these underlying factors may have synergistic effects in driving expenditure growth. The aging of our populace is one overall contributor to prescription expenditures and expansion in prescription spending as well as other health care spending. As the average population age increases, more age-related morbidity is present, and, correspondingly, more drugs are consumed. Increased prevalence of insurance coverage for prescription drugs has reduced price barriers to use of prescription drugs, creating a moral hazard or insurance effect that affects the quantity and potentially quality of drugs used. Promotion of drug products has been a hallmark of pharmaceutical manufacturers, and changed interpretations of marketing regulations in the mid-1990s led to increased consumer-directed advertising, in addition to the continued emphasis on physicians as traditional promotional message targets. Advances in technology and emphasis on those advances have been core aspects of health care, and pharmaceuticals are no exception. The imperative to constantly increase technology has contributed to higher costs for developing new pharmaceutical products, which are reflected in product prices. Advances in technology also have led to different mechanisms for treating conditions (e.g., biotechnology), new diagnostic procedures, and therapeutic agents for previously untreatable conditions or additional complementary treatments to enhance outcomes.

Although the previously mentioned factors are contributing to increasing expenditures for pharmaceuticals, some recent phenomena can possibly decrease expenditures or attenuate expenditure growth. Several prior blockbuster drugs have lost or soon will lose patent protection (e.g., Prozac, Prilosec, Zocor), opening the door for lower-cost generic versions of those drugs to be available in the market. Cost-sharing requirements and benefit structures in insurance drug coverage programs have changed to increase consumers' contributions to their drug spending and to sensitize them to the cost of their drug use. Many states have allowed increased technician-to-pharmacist staffing ratios for dispensing activities in pharmacies; this substitution of labor and/or adoption of automated systems in pharmacies has garnered some economies in dispensing prescriptions. Wholesalers continue to refine technologies and automation, reducing their operating costs (and margins) in distributing pharmaceuticals. These changes have not yet eliminated or reversed the factors contributing to expenditure growth, but they deserve mention.

UNIQUE CHARACTERISTICS OF PHARMACEUTICALS

Compared to other consumer goods, a number of characteristics of pharmaceuticals and the market for pharmaceuticals are unique, which can make policy interesting and/or challenging. Some of these characteristics have been mentioned or alluded to earlier in this chapter. Many of the aspects that make pharmaceuticals and the market for pharmaceuticals unique relate to the demand for pharmaceuticals, both in terms of the quantity of drugs demanded and what drugs are demanded.

Derived/Directed Demand

The demand for pharmaceuticals is considered a derived demand, derived from the demand for health, because pharmaceuticals can contribute to producing health. Some economists consider health as a durable good, and the demand for health care by individuals reflects their desire to increase their health capital. Another view takes a human capital approach, with the notion that individuals begin their life with an initial stock of health and they allocate resources to health care in an attempt to maintain their health capital or return to or retain their initial health stock. Consequently, it is not pharmaceuticals they necessarily demand, but they consume pharmaceuticals for the role they can play in affecting their health.

The demand for prescription drugs also is directed by physicians and others authorized to prescribe. Consumers may have varying degrees of input in prescription decisions, but they do not have the ability to access prescription drugs without a prescription order. Physicians are granted the authority to choose drugs and prescribe them for patients in their role as "learned intermediaries," helping consumers with decisions too involved or complex for them to make on their own. Individual patients are considered to be lacking in knowledge or information about diagnoses, drugs, and drug effects to be able to make decisions about use. This traditional, somewhat paternalistic view of the role of physicians and prescribers is being challenged or questioned by a perspective with more emphasis on self-care, and is based more on concordance as a way of thinking about medical decisions that includes the patient and their input as being important, useful, and even equal in the decision-making process. Concordance does not remove the prescriber from the process or alter the directed-demand aspect of prescription drugs, but instead expands or accentuates the role that consumers, as patients, play in having input about choices. Broader access to information, for example using the Internet, also can contribute to an increased role of consumers in medical decisions.

With the demand for prescription drugs directed by physicians, physicians act as agents for patients in making decisions. A physician acting as a perfect agent for the patient will act in the patient's best interest, presumably with full and accurate information about the patient's or principal's resources and preferences. However, the physician may not have full information, and this asymmetry between the principal and agent can yield erroneous decisions or imperfect agency. Imperfect agency also can result if the prescriber has different motivations and violates their agency role, such as attempting to influence their revenues or preserve consumer resources for themselves by selecting lower-cost treatments. Dual agency situations can also exist, in which the physician may be required or requested to engage in cost-control measures by an employer or managed care program, or to save resources either for themselves or others; this can put the prescriber in a dilemma about which agent is sovereign. These agency phenomena are common in medical care and typically absent in other transactions in which consumers select and purchase goods and services on their own.

Information Issues

Several aspects or issues related to information are characteristic of pharmaceuticals and prescription drugs. Some of these information issues relate particularly to the directed demand and agency situations described previously, and to the idea of information asymmetry.

In their role as agents and directing demand for prescription drugs, prescribers must rely on available information on which to base their decisions. Manufacturers or producers serve as primary information sources about products in practically all markets for goods and services, including pharmaceuticals, and promotion is the means by which information is communicated. This places manufacturers of pharmaceuticals in a position to control the amount and type of information available, and, as mentioned previously, this information role is an important aspect of the business of pharmaceutical companies.

Studies have shown that industry-provided materials are one of the primary sources that physicians rely on for information about drugs, and that physicians often are not knowledgeable about costs or relative costs of drugs. Sometimes it seems too much information is available; it can be difficult for prescribers to keep up with the volume of journal articles and other information available. In other cases not enough medical evidence may be available about what is appropriate. Reliance on industry sources is understandable, because promotion is active dissemination of information; information about drugs typically is most available and accessible via manufacturer's promotional efforts. Alternate sources of information about drug actions and effects, such as the FDA, do not take as much of an active, visible role as do the manufacturers. Journal articles or information from colleagues about drugs may be based on clinical studies about drugs in development, and the authors or individuals tend to be researchers involved in studies sponsored by the manufacturer ultimately interested in marketing the drugs; the information provided will be related to the objectives of the research, proving the worthiness of the drug for use. It could be argued that testing of new drugs and the benefits or outcomes from the drug focus on differentiating aspects of the drug that ultimately will stimulate market success. The information about benefits of new drugs from clinical studies is used, in part, to justify approval and indications for use; it also can provide the foundation for promotional campaigns.

Criticisms have been raised about a paucity of cost-effectiveness information or evidence of the comparative value of drugs. Such information is not required as part of the FDA approval process to market drugs, nor is it necessary or used to ensure coverage in public or private insurance plans. In clinical trials for safety and effectiveness, the tested drug may be compared with placebo only or typically with comparative agents in a narrow therapeutic subclass, restricted to agents within a basic molecular structure group. Comparisons of drugs across a broader range of therapeutic class agents are becoming more available as such examinations or clinical studies are being performed and evidence-based evaluations of existing available data are occurring (see Chapters 18 and 22). However, an accepted compilation or "gold standard" evaluation mechanism for drugs has not been set. In addition, placebo effects and idiosyncratic reactions or effects of drugs in individual patients make it difficult to make broad, sweeping generalizations about the "one best" drug in a therapeutic class or for a given condition.

Tacit development of information asymmetry about drugs by what is emphasized in clinical trials and approvals (benefits), by which drugs are promoted and what is emphasized in promotions (new drugs and differentiating aspects/advantages), and by limited objective, comparative evaluations of drugs and their relative values. This puts pharmaceutical manufacturers (especially) and prescribers in critical positions relative to the role and use of information in decision making about drugs. Prescribers use industry sources for information, directly and indirectly. Prescribers also lack cost information and/or awareness. Promotion generally occurs only for newer, patented drugs; generics are not promoted and promotional efforts are reduced on brand-name drugs as patent expiration nears. When prescribers choose the drugs to prescribe for consumers, this information asymmetry is actualized.

Demand Elasticity

Generally, the demand for pharmaceuticals (prescription drugs) is considered to be inelastic with respect to price; quantities demanded for drugs do not change to the same degree as any price changes. Several factors contribute to this price inelasticity. First, morbidity, or nonhealth is the reason individuals seek to purchase drugs, consistent with the notion of derived demand discussed previously. Individuals generally have a high preference for health, thus price becomes a secondary issue, and they will seek medical care in spite of the price of that care. Second, since demand is directed and physicians as prescribers seek first to do no harm (as part of their Hippocratic oath) and they neither consume nor pay for the drugs they select for patients, price is relegated to a more secondary role in selecting therapeutic agents. A lack of available comparative value information and a low awareness of drug cost levels by physicians also contribute to reduce the role that price plays in physician prescribing decisions. Patients cannot access prescription drugs without a physician's order, thus, consistent with their high preference for health (and risk aversion to avoid nonhealth), they follow through with purchasing prescribed medicines and minimize thoughts of substitute drugs or alternate courses of action. It even is possible to think that when elderly patients purchase prescribed drugs they are purchasing "hope" for extending their life or improving the quality of their life. Rational thinking about purchases may be replaced with emotion, reducing the role of price in decision making. Priorities, perspectives, and preferences can change with age.

Insurance coverage also can contribute to price inelasticity of demand. Coverage shields individuals from the true cost of care, particularly if no cost-sharing or copayment cost-sharing is included in which the cost of resources used is not reflected in the out-of-pocket cost that consumers experience. The shielding of costs by insurance can lead to increased use or the use of more expensive drugs (moral hazard or insurance effects). The trends of increased insurance coverage for prescriptions over time and the prevalence of copayment cost-sharing in drug coverage programs likely have exacerbated the price inelasticity of demand for pharmaceuticals.

Finally, a kind of "incrementalism" can be thought of as contributing to the demand and the inelasticity of demand for pharmaceuticals. New drugs are introduced to the market with potential benefits and advantages that represent incremental advances. The new drugs are tried and adopted to gain from the incremental advances; it is a part of the innovation adoption process. However, unless failure or major problems with trial of a new therapeutic agent occur, we rarely, if ever, apply recursive thinking or analysis and question whether a gain really occurred or whether returning to an older agent would yield outcomes similar (equivalent or even better, clinically) to the adopted innovation. Information asymmetry issues such as the type of information available about drugs, and especially a lack of comparative value information contribute to this "incrementalism" adoption imperative and reduce or avoid consideration of price. Since newer drugs typically cost more than the older drugs they replace within a therapeutic category, this adoption process of newer, more costly drugs reflects a kind of demand inelasticity for new drugs.

One Other Unique Aspect

As retailers, community pharmacies are an anomaly when it comes to pricing. Although community pharmacies appropriately are considered merchandising entities, a dispensed prescription is thought of as a combination of a physical good and a service. Prescription pricing techniques used by pharmacists vary from customary retailing approaches that establish selling prices via markups in the form of percentages applied to the cost of the product. Instead, pharmacists incorporate service enterprise pricing methods, in which fees are assessed for services rendered. Typically, the price of a prescription will somehow include a professional services dispensing fee amount added to the cost of the dispensed drug. As a result, the prices of prescriptions for different quantities of a given drug do not vary in straight line extrapolation based on quantity. The "mixed pricing" approach makes analyses of prescription price and expenditure trends and factors contributing to trends complex. It also presents challenges in projecting or determining the implications of policy changes. For example, a policy that would limit or increase the quantities of drugs dispensed in prescriptions would not correspondingly decrease or increase the prices or expenditures proportionately.

SUMMARY

Compared to other consumer goods, aspects of the market for pharmaceuticals are unique. The manufacturing sector of the market for pharmaceuticals includes brand and generic manufacturers that are interrelated in important ways, but also distinct and separate. Consumers obtain pharmaceuticals from a diverse array of pharmacies and third parties such as insurers have a financial stake in consumer use of pharmaceuticals. The demand for pharmaceuticals is inelastic with respect to price and demand is not determined by the consumer, but directed by prescribers. These unique aspects and characteristics can make policies related to pharmaceuticals interesting and/or challenging.

NOTES

1. Sandoz, a subsidiary of Novartis, is considered a generic firm by GPhA. Since Sandoz's sales are included with Novartis in Table 4.1, the number of generic firms in the top twenty manufacturers by sales could be increased to three.

2. Other countries have agencies similar to the FDA in the United States, making the determination whether a drug requires a prescription or not for sales.

3. Of note, expenditures for prescription drugs are ambulatory expenditures; the total proportion is higher if drugs dispensed to hospitalized patients are included. However, expenditures for drugs are not itemized as part of hospital expenditures, and thus the total amount of expenditures cannot be derived from these expenditure data.

4. See Woodwell, DA and Cherry, DK (2004). *National Ambulatory Medical Care Survey: 2002 Summary.* Advance Data for Vital and Health Statistics No. 346, August 26.

RESOURCES FOR MORE INFORMATION

Kaiser Family Foundation (2000). *Prescription Drug Trends: A Chartbook.* July. Menlo Park, CD: The Kaiser Family Foundation. Available at: http://www.kff .org/rxdrugs/loader.cfm?url=/commonspot/security/getfile.cfm&PageID=13504.
www.IMS Health.com
www.NACDS.org
www.GPhAonline.org

Chapter 5

Medicare's Prescription Drug Benefit

David J. Gross

INTRODUCTIONS

President Bush's December 2003 signing of the Medicare Prescription Drug, Improvement, and Modernization Act (also known as the MMA) set in motion the implementation of the largest social insurance program in the United States since the passage of Medicare nearly forty years earlier. After years of debate and at least one substantial false start at providing prescription drug benefits to this population, the new law fills one of the biggest gaps in Medicare—the lack of reliable and available prescription drug coverage. In doing so, however, Congress and the administration developed a system that is entirely new to Medicare beneficiaries, complete with a novel and complex benefit structure, an insurance framework administered by numerous private plans rather than through a centralized government agency, a nationally based framework for providing extra help for lower-income beneficiaries, and additional subsidies to induce employers, unions, and managed care plans to continue to offer (or to expand) drug benefits to Medicare beneficiaries. All of this had to be in place within twenty-four months of the bill being signed so that beneficiaries could be enrolled, and the first benefits paid out, by January 1, 2006.

Prior to the passage of this bill, Medicare did not offer coverage for most prescription drugs.[1] Since its passage in 1965, Medicare has consisted of two parts. Part A, which primarily is financed by a 1.45 percent payroll tax on both employers and employees, covers inpatient hospital care, some postacute care, some inpatient psychiatric care, and hospice care.[2] Part B, largely financed by a combination of beneficiary premiums ($88.50 per month in 2006) and general revenues from the federal government, covers outpatient medical services such as doctor visits, lab tests, durable medical equipment, some preventive services, and some home health services not covered under Part A.[3] (A Medicare Part C, currently known as Medicare

---

The views expressed in this chapter are solely those of the author, and do not necessarily represent the views of AARP.

Advantage, also exists, under which private health plans such as health maintenance organizations or HMOs contract with Medicare to provide all Part A and Part B services. This plan may offer additional benefits that Medicare does not cover, e.g., dental care, vision care, or some prescription drug coverage.) Medicare traditionally has not covered the costs of long-term care, vision care, dental care, or outpatient prescription drugs (except those that can't be self administered by the patient, such as injectable drugs).

Although Medicare itself did not cover prescription drugs, most Medicare beneficiaries received drug coverage from other sources. In 2001, the most recent year for which data are available, about three of every four Medicare beneficiaries had some form of prescription drug coverage at some point in the year. By far the largest source of coverage was employer-sponsored coverage, which provided drug coverage for about one-third of beneficiaries who had drug coverage. Other sources of coverage included Medicare+Choice plans, private supplemental insurance (i.e., Medigap), state Medicaid programs for low income persons, and other public programs such as state pharmaceutical assistance programs, CHAMPUS, and veterans' health programs (see Figure 5.1).[4]

However, this coverage was not necessarily secure. Employer-sponsored coverage has been dropping precipitously—35 percent of large employers offered retiree health coverage (which typically includes coverage for prescription drugs) to retirees in 2006 compared to 46 percent in 1991 and 40 percent in 1999.[5] Although many beneficiaries received drug coverage from Medicare+Choice plans, the number of plans and the generosity of plans dropped substantially after 1999.[6] And although Medicaid programs were not yet discussing elimination of drug benefits—coverage of prescription drugs is optional in state Medicaid programs, but all programs do provide it—some states were imposing cuts in the generosity of the coverage, including increasing cost sharing or imposing caps on the number of prescriptions that could be filled.

The original implementation of Medicare did not include a prescription drug benefit; prescription drug costs were viewed as less in need of insurance for individuals (when compared to hospital expenditures). However, efforts to include a prescription drug benefit date as early as 1967, when the Secretary of the U.S Department of Health, Education and Welfare (HEW) appointed a Task Force on Prescription Drugs to study whether such a benefit should be included.[7] Over time prescription drugs have become both a more important and a more costly form of health care. Some of the prescription drugs most widely used by older Americans today are used for conditions such as osteoporosis, lowering cholesterol, preventing acid reflux, and lowering blood pressure—that is, they are used to extend life or to prevent

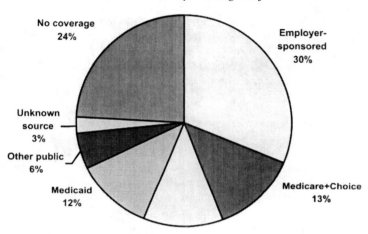

FIGURE 5.1. Sources of prescription drug coverage among medicare beneficiaries, 2001.Data are for noninstitutionalized Medicare beneficiaries from Cost and Use File of Medicare Current Beneficiary Survey. M+C refers to Medicare+ Choice coverage. Other Public includes state pharmaceutical assistance programs, CHAMPUS, and veterans health programs. *Source:* Adapted from Becky Briesacher, Bruce Stuart, John Poisal, Jalpa Doshi, and Puneet Singhal (2006). *Methodological Issues in Estimating Prescription Drug Coverage with the Medicare Current Beneficiary Survey.* AARP Public Policy Institute Issue Paper No. 2006-21. Washington, DC: AARP. Available at: http://assets.aarp.org/rgcenter/health/2006_21_coverage.pdf

the need for more costly medical treatments. Costs of drug treatment have also become substantial. Medicare beneficiaries age sixty-five and over were estimated to spend an average of $830 out-of-pocket for prescription drugs in 2003. Older beneficiaries with no drug coverage were estimated to spend an average of $1,190,[8] yet these beneficiaries often use fewer drugs than do beneficiaries with drug coverage, including for drugs used to treat important medical conditions.[9]

Although efforts to improve Medicare's coverage for prescription drugs date back to the Department of Health, Education, and Welfare's Task Force on Prescription Drugs in the late 1960s, the issue remained on the back burner of public policy until shortly before the passage of the Medicare Catastrophic Coverage Act of 1988, which, among other things, provided coverage for 80 percent of a beneficiary's drug coverage once out-of-pocket drug spending reached $600 in a single year. However, the negative public response to the financing mechanism—a mandatory, income-related premium imposed on all Medicare beneficiaries, many of whom would not receive any benefit (and who may already have had outpatient prescription drug coverage)—led to the bill's repeal the following year. The most recent wave began with proposals for prescription drug coverage made by President Clinton in 1999. Several years of congressional debate and one presidential election took place before the current bill was passed in November 2003 and signed into law early the next month.

BASIC ELEMENTS OF DRUG COVERAGE UNDER MEDICARE PART D

The basic elements of the new Medicare benefit are as follows. First, the benefit is available to all Medicare beneficiaries, regardless of income, health status, geographic location, or choice of health plan (that is, it is available to beneficiaries who continue in traditional fee-for-service Medicare as well as to those who opt for a Medicare Advantage plan). Second, the benefit is voluntary—no beneficiary is required to enroll. Third, beneficiaries receive coverage by enrolling in a private plan—either a Medicare Advantage plan that offers drug coverage or, for those beneficiaries who remain in fee-for-service Medicare, a private, Medicare-approved prescription drug plan (PDP), not through Medicare itself. Although each plan must be at least actuarially equivalent to a standard plan that is defined in law, in practice plans' benefit structures—and their accompanying premiums—can, and do, vary from one another substantially. Fourth, the benefit offers extra assistance to many lower-income beneficiaries who otherwise might not be able to afford the coverage. Finally, the law creating the benefit provides tax-free subsidies to employers that offer drug coverage that is at least as good as that offered under Medicare.[10]

Access to the Benefit

The Medicare prescription drug benefit is available to any of the 43 million Americans who are enrolled in either Part A or Part B of Medicare. All beneficiaries have the opportunity to enroll in the benefit, regardless of their income, health status, or choice of health plan (i.e., traditional fee-for-service Medicare versus Medicare Advantage). In addition, the program is voluntary; as with Medicare Part B, beneficiaries need to choose to enroll, but (also like Part B) may incur a penalty for not enrolling when first eligible.

Beneficiaries get prescription drug coverage by enrolling in a private plan that is offered in their area. Two types of plans may be offered: a prescription drug plan (PDP) that offers stand-alone drug coverage, or a benefit that is offered by a Medicare Advantage (MA) plan, such as an HMO or other type of private health plan.[11] By law, every Medicare beneficiary must have access to at least two drug plans in any given geographic area, at least one of which must be a stand-alone PDP. If an insufficient number of Medicare drug plans operate in any geographic area, the federal government is required to contract with private entities to offer a "fallback" plan.[12]

The initial enrollment period for the drug benefit runs from November 15, 2005, through May 15, 2006. In general, beneficiaries must choose a plan within a seven month period—three months before and three months after the month in which they become eligible for Medicare, otherwise they can enroll only during an open enrollment period (between November 15 and December 31 of every year), and will incur a penalty of at least 1 percent of the cost of the average national monthly premium for each month that they delayed enrollment (i.e., a twelve-month delay would result in an additional premium of 12 percent of the regional average monthly premium ad infinitum). A notable exception to this is if the beneficiary previously had *creditable coverage,* that is, drug coverage from another source (such as a former employer) that was at least as good as the coverage offered by Medicare. Beneficiaries who lose creditable coverage have sixty-three days to enroll after losing that coverage before incurring any financial penalty.[13]

Benefit Structure in Theory

In addition to having many plans to choose from, beneficiaries also have many benefit structures from which to choose. Medicare drug plans are required to offer a benefit that is *actuarially equivalent* to a standard benefit defined in law, but this can vary from that benefit.

In order to understand the different types of drug benefit structures that are available to Medicare beneficiaries, it is useful to first understand the standard benefit. The *standard benefit* for 2006 is defined as the following. First, a $250 annual deductible is set. Then, for the next $2,000 in drug spending, the cost is split—25 percent to be paid by the beneficiary and 75 percent by the Medicare plan. After this, the beneficiary receives no benefit until total *out-of-pocket* drug spending reaches $3,600.[14] Under the standard benefit, once this out-of-pocket coverage is reached, the beneficiary becomes eligible for a "catastrophic benefit," which covers up to 95 percent of the cost of any additional drug expenditure (see Table 5.1). For years after 2006, the deductible and benefit limits are pegged to the growth in prescription drug spending by Medicare beneficiaries; i.e., a 10 percent increase in beneficiaries' drug spending would result in a 2007 deductible of $275 (110 percent of $250) (see Figure 5.2).

The concept of a coverage gap (donut hole) and out-of-pocket spending limits both are unique to the Medicare drug benefit. In general, health insur-

TABLE 5.1. Medicare standard prescription drug benefit, 2006.

Prescription drug spending—(for beneficiaries who have no drug coverage other than Medicare)	Medicare-approved plan pays	Beneficiary pays (if he or she has no drug coverage other than Medicare; excludes premiums)
$0-$250	$0	Up to $250 deductible
$250-$2,250	75% of drug costs—Up to $1,500	25% of drug costs—Up to $500
$2,250-$5,100 coverage gap/donut hole	0% of drug costs—$0	100% of drug costs—Up to $2,850
Subtotal:	Up to $1,500	Up to $3,600 out-of-pocket
Over $5,100 (catastrophic benefit)	95%	5% or $2 copay/generic $5 copay/brand name

Source: American Association of Retired Persons (2005). *The New Medicare Prescription Drug Coverage: What You Need to Know.* Washington, DC: AARP.

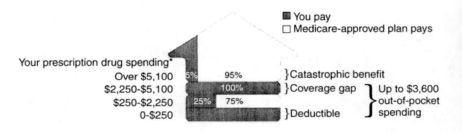

FIGURE 5.2. Illustration of medicare standard prescription drug benefit, 2006. *Source:* American Association of Retired Persons (2005). *The New Medicare Prescription Drug Coverage: What You Need to Know.* Washington, DC: AARP.

ance either provides continuous coverage (sometimes once a deductible has been met) or has a coverage limit after which no coverage is available. In the standard Medicare benefit, however, a gap in coverage exists. If beneficiaries with high drug costs are able to fill the gap out of their own resources (or those of family members or state pharmacy assistance programs) then Medicare will again cover, paying up to 95 percent of costs (with a minimum of $2 for generic drugs and $5 for brand name drugs); these figures will rise each year in proportion to the growth of per capita drug spending by Medicare beneficiaries.

For the purposes of the Medicare prescription drug benefit, out-of-pocket spending is defined as "true out-of-pocket spending," or TrOOP. TrOOP specifically excludes cost-sharing paid by employer-provided plans, but does include spending by state pharmaceutical assistance programs on behalf of Medicare beneficiaries.

Benefit Structure in Practice

Because the MMA was designed to promote innovation among plans in program design and benefit structure, plans were not required to offer benefits that were similar to the standard benefit; rather, they had to be at least *actuarially equivalent* to the standard benefit in order to be a Medicare-approved plan. However, since the idea of stand-alone drug plans was a new one, it was not known whether private insurance companies would bid to be a Medicare-approved drug plan, how many plans would be offered, whether plans would be available in all regions of the country, and what the plans would look like. Indeed, once the set of Medicare-approved plans was released by the Centers for Medicare and Medicaid Services (CMS) in late 2005, it turned out that few, if any, plans looked exactly like the standard benefit. This section describes the landscape of Medicare-approved drug plans in the first year of operation; whether the pattern described here will continue has yet to be seen.

Number of Available Plans

Despite the concerns shared by some observers of the Medicare drug benefit, it was apparent that beneficiaries would, indeed, have a choice from among many plans (at least during the first year of implementation). In 2006, every Medicare beneficiary had the choice of numerous stand-alone Medicare plans, ranging from a low of twenty-seven plans offered by eleven different companies (in Alaska) to a high of fifty-two plans offered by twenty-one different companies (in Pennsylvania and West Virginia). Most—although not all—beneficiaries also had a choice of MA plans that offer prescription drug coverage, although this choice was not as broad as with stand-alone PDPs. Beneficiaries in twenty-seven states had the choice of between four and nine MA drug plans; beneficiaries in another twelve states could choose from ten or more MA drug plans (including a high of thirty-seven MA drug plans in the District of Columbia). No MA plans with drug coverage existed in Alaska and Vermont, and five other states (Delaware, Maine, Mississippi, New Hampshire, and Wyoming) had three or fewer MA drug plans offered in 2006.

Benefit Package

As previously noted, when plan designs were released in the fall of 2005, most (if not all) of the plans were substantially different from the standard plan as well as from one another. For example, the standard plan has a $250 deductible. But relatively few of the plans had a $250 deductible. For example, of the fifty-two PDPs offered in Pennsylvania in 2006, only seventeen had a $250 deductible (the others had no deductible). Also, every state had at least six (and as many as nine) plans that offered coverage in the coverage gap (also known as the donut hole).

Premiums

At the time that the MMA was passed by Congress, it was estimated that the average premium for the standard drug benefit would be about $32 per month. Similar to the benefit structure, however, this premium is not mandated by law but rather is determined by the plan. Monthly drug premiums varied widely in the first year of the benefit, and the average premium was substantially lower than the originally estimated level of $32. The lowest monthly premium among PDPs in a state ranges from $1.87 (in Iowa, Minnesota, Nebraska, North Dakota, South Dakota, and Wyoming) to $20.05 in Alaska. The highest premiums in each state range from $61.93 in Alaska to $104.89 in Florida. Part of this variation reflects the many plans offering supplemental coverage, such as coverage in the donut hole. This, however, does not explain all of the variation, which could be due to factors such as different marketing strategies (a plan with a low premium may be trying to grasp a large market share), tighter formularies (a plan with a tighter formulary may be able to offer a lower premium), or higher cost-sharing requirements.

Table 5.2 gives a more detailed sense of the magnitude of choices facing beneficiaries. For beneficiaries residing in Maryland, Medicare beneficiaries can choose from among forty-eight stand-alone PDPs offered by twenty-one different insurers (as well as twenty MA plans offered by three different insurers).

The forty-eight stand-alone PDPs vary in several ways:

- Monthly premiums range from $6.44 to $68.64; nearly half have monthly premiums between $20 and $40.
- Slightly more than half the plans (26) have no deductibles, and three have annual deductibles of $100. The remaining plans have annual deductibles of $250.

- All but five of the plans have tiered copayments.
- Most of the plans have no coverage during the donut hole, or coverage gap. However, five plans provide continued coverage for generic drugs in the donut hole, and one offers continued coverage for both generic and brand name drugs.
- Plans generally have a formulary, but most plan formularies included more than 90 percent of the top 100 drugs. Eleven plans included all 100, and another eleven covered either 99 or 98 of the top drugs. The other six plans include between 78 and 88 of the top 100 drugs on their formularies.[15]

Extra Help for Lower-Income Beneficiaries

The Medicare Modernization Act includes special provisions to help lower-income beneficiaries pay the premiums and cost-sharing associated with the drug benefit. To be eligible for these subsidies, beneficiaries must have both low income (in 2006, about $15,000 for individuals and about $20,000 for couples) and low assets (in 2006, about $10,000 for individuals and $20,000 for couples; calculation of assets excludes a home, personal possessions, and—to a limited extent—the face value of life insurance and burial policies).[16] Beneficiaries at the lowest income levels have no premiums (as long as they choose a plan with a premium below the national weighted average premium) or deductibles, pay $1 or $2 for generics and $3 or $5 for brand-name drugs, and have no coverage gap. Others with slightly higher incomes have sliding scale premiums, a deductible of no more than $50 per year, and a maximum 15 percent copayment.

Lower-income beneficiaries must choose a plan that is priced at or below the regional average premium to be eligible for a full premium subsidy, otherwise they must pay the difference between the plan's premium and the monthly average premium. In every state, lower-income beneficiaries who are eligible for extra help with premiums can find a plan that is priced at or below the regional average premium. Lower-income beneficiaries in forty-two states and the District of Columbia have at least ten of these plans form which to choose; the lowest number is six (in Arizona and Florida).

Cost Control Under MMA

The MMA relies on competition between prescription drug plans to restrain the cost of the benefit. According to advocates of the approach used to offer benefits under the MMA, the private companies have an incentive to offer the best benefit at the lowest cost because they must compete for bene-

TABLE 5.2. Key characteristics of stand-alone PDPs available in Maryland, 2006.

Monthly drug premium	Annual deductible	Cost sharing	Coverage in the gap	Formulary (% of drugs covered)
$6.44	$250	25%	No gap	100
$12.58	$0	$7 - $60 25%	No gap	100
$19.80	$0	$0 - $66 31%	No gap	88
$21.21	$0	$10 - $42	No gap	78
$21.30	$0	$7.50 - $52.70 33%	No gap	97
$22.91	$250	25%	No gap	100
$23.16	$250	25%	No gap	90
$26.52	$250	$5 - $25 25%	No gap	93
$28.61	$0	$5 - $55 25%	No gap	100
$28.61	$0	$5 - $55 25%	No gap	100
$28.92	$250	$9 25%	No gap	93
$29.40	$250	$5 - $28 25%	No gap	91
$30.85	$0	$10 - $53 25%	No gap	100
$31.59	$250	25%	No gap	93
$31.93	$250	$0 25% - 45%	No gap	96
$31.95	$250	$2 25%	No gap	88
$32.07	$250	$4 - $17 25% - 75%	No gap	98
$32.13	$250	$5 - $25	No gap	86
$32.30	$0	$5 - $57	No gap	100
$33.87	$0	$10 - $30 25%	No gap	93
$34.10	$0	$7.50 - $65.30 33%	No gap	97
$34.64	$250	25%	No gap	100
$34.78	$250	$5 - $40 25%	No gap	100
$35.04	$0	$5 - $64 25%	No gap	100
$35.12	$0	$9 - $60 33%	No gap	99
$36.75	$250	$4 - $40	No gap	100
$38.16	$0	$7.50 - $52.60 33%	Generic Only	97
$39.83	$0	$0 - $50 30%	No gap	85

TABLE 5.2 *(continued)*

Monthly drug premium	Annual deductible	Cost sharing	Coverage in the gap	Formulary (% of drugs covered)
$40.02	$250	$4 - $40	No gap	96
$40.85	$250	$6 - $27 25%	No gap	93
$40.89	$250	$5 - $28 25%	No gap	93
$40.97	$250	$4 - $29 25%	No gap	93
$41.98	$0	$5 - $50	No gap	100
$42.67	$0	$0 - $60 30%	No gap	85
$42.82	$0	$7 - $35	Generic Only	86
$43.88	$100	$4 - $50	No gap	96
$44.16	$0	$0 - $6 20%	No gap	100
$45.18	$0	$10 - $60 30%	Generic Only	99
$50.95	$0	$5 - $50	Generic Only	100
$51.99	$0	$6 - $27 25%	No gap	93
$52.00	$0	$5 - $28 25%	No gap	93
$52.07	$0	$4 - $29 25%	No gap	93
$52.88	$0	$7 - $60 25%	Generic and Brand	100
$56.07	$100	$10 - $25 25% - 50%	No gap	98
$57.03	$100	$7 - $60 25%	No gap	98
$58.36	$0	$2 - $40	Generic Only	100
$68.64	$0	$4 - $42 25%	No gap	100
$68.91	$0	$6 - $40 25%	No gap	100

Source: Centers for Medicare and Medicaid Services (2006). *Medicare Rx Prescription Drug Coverage— Stand-Alone Prescription Drug Plans: Landscape of Plan Options in Maryland.* January 4. Available at: http://www.medicare.gov/medicarereform/mapdpdocs/PDPLandscapemd.pdf.

ficiaries. This should give them an incentive to promote the use of the most cost-effective products and to negotiate discounts and rebates from pharmacies and drug manufacturers. According to this view, drug plans should not rely on national negotiation for drug prices; indeed, Medicare is specifically banned from negotiating drug prices for the Medicare drug benefit.

Medicare-approved drug plans—both PDPs and MA plans—are allowed to use most of the tools that private plans use to restrain costs. These help to lower the costs of the benefit but, if applied too strictly, risk reducing access for beneficiaries. For example, they are allowed to establish pharmacy networks. This allows them to negotiate discounts from pharmacies that participate in their plans, but may limit access for some beneficiaries, particularly those in rural areas who do not have a choice of many pharmacies. One requirement of the MMA is that drug plans must allow beneficiaries to fill prescriptions at non-network pharmacies when the beneficiary cannot be reasonably expected to fill a prescription at a network pharmacy (for example, when traveling), but they can charge a higher fee for doing so. CMS does have regulations intended to guarantee adequate pharmacy access; for example, 90 percent of beneficiaries in urban areas must live within two miles of a network pharmacy, and 70 percent of beneficiaries in rural areas must live within 15 miles of a network pharmacy.

Plans can also limit which drugs they will cover, and can establish differential payments for different types of drugs. Specifically, plans can establish drug *formularies,* or lists of drugs that the plan will cover. CMS has established various standards for drug formularies in Medicare drug plans; for example, formularies must be established by a pharmacy and therapeutics committee that is largely composed of health care providers, they may not be designed to discourage enrollment by certain types of beneficiaries (such as those with high medical costs), and they must include coverage for at least two (and sometimes more, if deemed necessary by CMS) drugs in each therapeutic category. Plans can also implement *tiered cost-sharing* arrangements, whereby beneficiaries face lower cost-sharing for certain types of drugs. A typical tiered cost-sharing arrangement might feature a relatively low cost-sharing level for generic drugs, a slightly higher amount for "preferred" brand-name drugs, and a still higher cost-sharing level of "non-preferred" brand-name drugs. (Plans could have more or fewer than three tiers.) The main requirement on tiers is that the average benefit under the tiers must be at least as good as the standard Medicare drug benefit. In addition, plans can apply drug cost management tools, such as mandatory generic substitution, prior authorization, and therapeutic interchange. [17]

However, plans are also required to have certain consumer protections that may or may not exist among private sector plans. Some previously mentioned examples include the requirement that formularies must offer at least two drugs in every therapeutic category and that cost-containment mechanisms cannot be designed to exclude certain populations. In addition, Medicare beneficiaries have specified rights to appeal formulary coverage decisions, and even to grant a copayment associated with a lower-tiered drug when a high-tiered drug is determined to be medically appropriate. [18]

HOW THE MEDICARE DRUG BENEFIT
AFFECTS BENEFICIARIES

Medicare Part D will change the way that many people who received coverage will get it now. For many of these beneficiaries, the Medicare drug coverage is the first time that they will be able to obtain benefits. For the low-income beneficiaries who are eligible for extra help, this coverage provides access to prescription drugs at very low cost. For others, it offers a chance to save money, albeit not at levels as generous as for many employer-provided plans.

Dual Eligibles

An estimated 6.3 million (15 percent) of Medicare beneficiaries in 2006 are "dual eligibles"; that is, they are dually eligible for both Medicare and state Medicaid programs. Prior to 2006, dual eligibles typically received drug benefits through Medicaid, since Medicaid "wraps around" Medicare, providing benefits that are not covered by Medicare.[19] Since Medicaid is jointly funded by state and federal revenues, the federal government was paying part of these beneficiaries' drug costs through matching federal revenues.

However, the MMA mandates that, as of January 1, 2006, dual eligibles would be able to receive drug coverage through Medicare-approved drug plans—either PDPs or MA plans—and that state Medicaid programs could no longer receive federal matching funds for prescription drug costs incurred by dual eligibles. In order to ensure that these beneficiaries are enrolled in a plan, CMS automatically enrolls dual eligibles in a plan that has a premium below the regional average premium; these beneficiaries are also automatically enrolled to receive extra help. Beneficiaries can change their plan if they so choose.[20]

Moving dual eligibles' drug coverage from Medicaid to Medicare has both advantages and disadvantages for the beneficiary. Among the advantages is that enrolling dual eligibles in a Medicare plan ensures that they receive the same benefits to which other Medicare beneficiaries are entitled. In addition, it means that these beneficiaries are not subject to restrictions that some states are currently placing on Medicaid drug coverage, such as limits on the number of prescriptions that can be filled in a month.[21] However, many dual eligible beneficiaries may be overwhelmed by the complexity of Medicare Part D. Many may also lose some protections associated with Medicaid. For example, some state Medicaid programs have no cost sharing for drugs, and in those states with cost sharing, pharmacists are prohibited by federal law from not dispensing a drug because of a Medicaid beneficiary's inability to pay. By contrast, the Medicare drug benefit will have cost sharing. Although these costs are low relative to what other beneficiaries pay ($1 to $2 for generic drugs; $3 to $5 for brand name drugs), they may still be a barrier to access, particularly for beneficiaries with high utilization. Although some states are covering these costs for their dual eligibles, others are not, and no limit is placed on how much these low-income beneficiaries would have to pay out-of-pocket. In addition, the plan in which a dual eligible is auto-enrolled may not cover all of the beneficiary's drugs in its formulary, and some dual eligibles may lack the resources or cognitive abilities to easily switch plans.[22] Furthermore, dual eligibles lose coverage for some drugs (such as benzodiazepines) that were typically covered by Medicaid but that, by statute, are not covered under Medicare.

Beneficiaries with Private Supplemental Coverage

About 12 percent of Medicare beneficiaries receive coverage from privately purchased supplemental insurance policies ("Medigap"). As a result of legislation passed in 1990, these types of policies have been subject to federal standards that establish ten different policies, of which only three offer prescription drug coverage. Two of these policies (known as plans H and I) have a $250 annual deductible, and then cover 50 percent of the next $2,500 in prescription drug costs. Plan J also has a $250 deductible, but covers up to 50 percent of the next $6,000 in prescription drug costs. In addition to these plans, some people may have prestandardized plans (plans sold before 1990) that have different benefit structures.

Under the MMA, beneficiaries with Medigap prescription drug coverage can either keep that coverage or enroll in a Medicare drug plan—but they cannot do both. Furthermore, no Medigap plans with drug coverage can be sold after January 1, 2006. In general, beneficiaries who previously received drug coverage through Medigap plans will get more coverage at a lower cost under the Medicare drug benefit than under Medigap. This is because part of the cost of the Medicare drug coverage is subsidized, whereas the enrollees pay the entire cost of their Medigap policy. Medigap enrollees are able to keep drug coverage purchased prior to January 1, 2006, but will pay a late enrollment penalty if they later choose to enroll in the Medicare benefit, because Medigap drug coverage is not actuarially equivalent to Medicare's standard drug benefit. This penalty is equal to at least 1 percent additional premium per month that the person did not enroll when initially eligible.

Beneficiaries with Employer-Sponsored Coverage

By far, the greatest source of prescription drug coverage has been through employer-sponsored coverage, either from a current employer, a former employer (i.e., retiree coverage), or from a spouse's current or former employer. One of the concerns of the long-standing Medicare drug debate regarded whether the new drug benefit would induce employers to reduce retiree drug coverage, however employers had, as noted earlier, been reducing retiree drug coverage for several years prior to the bill's passage. To help keep employers offering drug benefits to retirees, the MMA contained provisions to subsidize employers that offer coverage that is at least as good as that offered under the standard Medicare drug benefit. Employers offering such coverage are entitled to tax-free subsidies of 28 percent of drug costs between $250 and $5,000 per retiree, so long as the employer's drug benefit is actuarially equivalent to the standard Medicaid drug benefit.[23] (Note that employers don't need to maintain drug coverage at pre–MMA levels—they only need to offer coverage that is actuarially equivalent to the Medicare standard drug benefit in order to provide the coverage.)

Beneficiaries with employer-sponsored drug coverage may not both keep that coverage and enroll in a Medicare drug plan. Whether or not beneficiaries are likely benefit from the Medicare drug benefit will depend on whether or not their coverage is *creditable*—that is, at least as good as the benefit offered by Medicare (on an average, or actuarial, basis). Employers that offer coverage to current employees or retirees are required by law to inform enrollees who are Medicare beneficiaries if the coverage is creditable. Beneficiaries who have creditable drug coverage can enroll in the Medicare benefit at a later date, without penalty, if the employer drops that coverage or reduces it to a level that is no longer creditable. Beneficiaries without creditable coverage, or who have no drug coverage under an employer-sponsored plan, must enroll during their initial enrollment period to avoid a late enrollment penalty.[24]

Medicare Advantage Enrollees

About six million Medicare beneficiaries were enrolled in a Medicare health plan (or Medicare Advantage plan)—that is, a health maintenance organization (HMO), preferred provider organization (PPO), point-of-service (POS) plan, or a private fee-for-service (PFFS) plan—in 2006. As of January 1, 2006, all MA plans (except for PFFS plans) must offer at least one option that includes prescription drug coverage. All of these plans must, by law, be at least as good as the standard Medicare drug benefit.[25] [The MMA increased payments to MA plans to increase the drug coverage offered by these plans.] Beneficiaries who were enrolled in MA plans prior to 2006 are likely to find that their coverage now includes substantially enhanced drug benefits, sometimes at a lower premium than they had paid in 2005. Other beneficiaries may be attracted to these plans because the premiums are often lower than for PDP plans, but they may face limitations on physician choice.

Enrollees in State Pharmaceutical Assistance Programs (SPAPs)

About 1.8 million people—mostly Medicare beneficiaries—receive drug coverage through SPAPs, which are state programs that have traditionally provided some prescription drug coverage to lower income Medicare beneficiaries who do not qualify for drug coverage under Medicaid. More than half the states have SPAPs, many of which have been more generous than the benefits offered under Medicare Part D, and passage of the MMA initially created confusion about whether and how SPAPs would coordinate with Part D, and whether SPAP enrollees would have to face a reduction in coverage as a result of Part D. However, as federal MMA regulations were being promulgated, many states with SPAPs passed measures under which the SPAP would "wrap around" Part D, that is, paying or all part of an enrollee's Part D premium, cost-sharing (including deductible), and coverage in the donut hole. This wraparound is particularly important for beneficiaries in states where beneficiaries who are not eligible for low-income assistance under Part D (i.e., with incomes above 150 percent of poverty or whose assets are too high to qualify for this assistance) are still eligible for their state's SPAP. This coordination allows the low-income beneficiary to continue receiving generous coverage and for states to save money by having Medicare Part D cover some of the costs that they were paying from state-only revenues.

POLICY CONCERNS

At this writing, it is too early to gauge the success of Medicare Part D's revolutionary approaches toward providing prescription drug benefits and to using market mechanisms to restrain the growth of prescription drug spending. Regarding providing benefits, several potential issues exist, including the following:

- How well do beneficiaries understand the benefit?
- Do Medicare beneficiaries feel that the benefit is worth their money?
- Do enough enroll to make the benefit sustainable?
- Does the benefit help—or, at least, not make worse off—the most vulnerable beneficiaries—both those with the lowest incomes and those who are the sickest?
- What is the effect of the benefit on employer-sponsored coverage?
- Are plans able to restrain costs?
- Are beneficiaries able to get access to the prescription drugs that they need?

Beneficiary Understanding of the Benefit

By almost any definition, the Medicare benefit is a complex one. It requires beneficiaries to choose from numerous plans, all of which could have different benefit packages. Consumers could also have difficulty determining drug prices and formularies. According to a poll conducted by the Henry J. Kaiser Family Foundation (KFF) and the Harvard School of Public Health shortly before beneficiaries were able to start enrolling in the benefit suggested mixed understanding, at best, of the drug benefit. Fewer than half (47 percent) of beneficiaries stated that they understand the benefit "very" or "somewhat" well. Nearly two-thirds knew that they would have to sign up for a plan (i.e., that enrollment was not automatic), and more than half thought that beneficiaries would or might face a penalty for late enrollment. Only 40 percent knew that they could get coverage without enrolling in a MA plan, and nearly one-third thought that they didn't have to sign up with a private plan to get the benefit. At the time the survey was taken, only 20 percent said they would enroll, 37 percent said they would *not* enroll, and 43 percent didn't know. Beneficiaries also felt that having more than 40 plans to choose from in most areas made it confusing and difficult to pick the best plan.[26]

CMS and state Senior Health Insurance Assistance Programs (SHIPs) have put in massive efforts to inform consumers, but reaching individual consumers is difficult under any circumstances. Their efforts have been assisted by various consumer and senior citizen organizations. In addition, CMS has established various Web sites to provide information to consumers. For example, CMS's Medicare Drug Plan finder allows consumers to choose a plan online. This online tool allows beneficiaries to view main characteristics of all the Medicare-approved drug plans—PDPs and MAs— offered in their geographic area. Consumers can compare the premium and benefit structures of plans, find out which plans cover their drugs, find out which include their preferred pharmacy in their network, and can estimate the total annual cost of each plan based on the prescriptions that they currently take.

Enrollment in the Benefit

In January 2005, the U.S. Department of Health and Human Services estimated that 29 million beneficiaries would be enrolled in Medicare Part D plans by the end of 2006. However, the jury is still out as to whether this goal will be achieved. Beneficiaries who were enrolled in Medicare when the benefit started had until May 15, 2006, to enroll in the benefit without a penalty. In the first four months of open enrollment (from mid-November 2005 through mid-February 2006), nearly 18 million beneficiaries had enrolled in the drug benefit. This figure included nearly 6 million dual eligibles who were automatically enrolled in Part D, about 5.7 million Medicare Advantage enrollees, and about 6.4 million enrollees in stand-alone PDPs. Another 10 million Medicare beneficiaries had creditable coverage, mostly through employer-sponsored plans. The mid-March enrollment level reflects an increase of two million from mid-February, which itself reflects an increase of 1.5 million from mid-January. However, 15.5 million beneficiaries—about 35 percent of all beneficiaries—did not have creditable drug coverage by mid-March, suggesting that HHS' still has a long way to go to meet their original enrollment target.

How the Benefit Affects the Most Vulnerable Beneficiaries

One way that this benefit will likely be evaluated is in whether it makes poorest and sickest beneficiaries better off. The benefit will no doubt be helpful to the substantial number of beneficiaries who qualify for the low-income assistance but do not qualify for state Medicaid programs. These beneficiaries, who are the most likely to lack prescription drug coverage, will have access to low-cost drugs. Whether or not outreach to these beneficiaries results in their enrollment remains to be seen. As of late February 2006, only 1.5 million beneficiaries who are not dual eligibles qualified for the low-income assistance. By contrast, HHS had estimated that 8.2 million beneficiaries would be eligible for the low-income subsidy and 4.6 million would actually receive the subsidy by the end of the year.[27]

The impact on other vulnerable beneficiaries is also not yet known. As stated previously, beneficiaries who already qualified for Medicaid benefits are likely to face higher out-of-pocket drug costs than they did under Medicaid, even with the substantial government subsidies. This could adversely affect utilization, particularly among those with high utilization. However, as also noted, some states have been placing limits on the number of prescriptions that Medicaid beneficiaries can fill in any one month; that Medicare does not have these limits may help these beneficiaries.

A third group that could be affected is those beneficiaries who reside in nursing homes. Many of these beneficiaries are dual eligibles, and are automatically enrolled in a Medicare drug plan. However, no guarantee exists that the plan to which a nursing home resident is assigned will cover all of the resident's needed drugs; for those who are not dual eligible, concerns exist about how these people will enroll if a family member or guardian is not available to make the choices for them. Although nursing home residents, unlike other beneficiaries, are allowed to switch plans every month in case their plan does not meet their needs, the limited abilities of these people may make such changes quite difficult.[28]

Effect of the Benefit on Employer Coverage

The employer subsidy is intended to help stanch the flow of employers from the retiree drug market. Some critics contended that the Medicare drug benefit would enhance the incentives for employers to drop coverage, and substantial anxiety existed among Medicare beneficiaries who had employer-sponsored drug coverage that they would lose coverage which, typically, was better than what Medicare offered.

It is too early to tell what employers will eventually do, and difficult at best to ascertain what effect the employer subsidy has on any actions. What is known is that, at least for the first year of the benefit, an estimated ten million beneficiaries—most of whom likely have coverage from employers—have creditable coverage outside of Medicare Part D.

Effect of the Benefit on Restraining Pharmaceutical Costs

With the benefit hardly haven taken effect, it is far too early to measure whether the competitive structure of the benefit will lead to slower growth in pharmaceutical costs. Certainly, if such restraint does not happen, the higher costs will be passed along to beneficiaries in the form of higher premiums and cost sharing levels. These higher costs, particularly to the extent that they outstrip increases in Social Security benefit, could create political pressure to enhance the benefit or to impose additional cost controls, such as allowing HHS to negotiate drug prices or to allow importation from Canada and/or the European Union.

Are Beneficiaries Able to Access the Drugs They Need?

It will be important to monitor whether the formularies and other utilization management tools used by drug plans result in more cost-effective pharmaceutical use or if they reduce access to medically appropriate drugs. The former can help promote tools for the private sector, whereas the latter will reduce confidence in the drug benefit and may lead to pressures to repeal the benefit.

Other issues will also be important, such as how stable the plans are; whether an adverse selection among plans will exist; and how people react to the donut hole. The bottom line, however, is that this is a new venture, and that only the passage of time will reveal how well it meets its goals.

NOTES

1. Medicare Part B does cover a limited number of prescription drugs—typically those that cannot be administered at home but that require administration in a physician's office or other outpatient setting.

2. Craig Caplan (2005). *The Medicare Program: A Brief Overview*. AARP Public Policy Institute FS103. Washington, DC: AARP.

3. Caplan (2005).

4. Becky Briesacher, Bruce Stuart, John Poisal, Jalpa Doshi, and Puneet Singhal (2006). *Methodological Issues in Estimating Prescription Drug Coverage with the Medicare Current Beneficiary Survey*. AARP Public Policy Institute Issue Paper No. 2006-21. Washington, DC: AARP. Available at: http://assets.aarp.org/rgcenter/health/2006_21_coverage.pdf.

5. Kaiser Family Foundation (2005). *Employer Health Benefit: 2005 Annual Survey*. Menlo Park, CA: Henry J. Kaiser Family Foundation. September 14, 2005. Available at: http://www.kff.org/insurance/7315/index.cfm.

6. Thomas Oliver, Philip R. Lee, and Helene L. Lipton (2004). A Political History of Medicare and Prescription Drug Coverage. The Milbank Quarterly 82(2): 283-354; Marsha Gold et al. (2004). *Monitoring Medicare+Choice: What Have We Learned? Findings and Operational Lessons for Medicare Advantage*, Mathematica Policy Research Report #8846-200, August. Available at: http://www.mathematica-mpr.com/publications/pdfs/monitor.pdf.

7. Oliver et al. (2004).

8. Craig Caplan and Normandy Brangan (2004). *Out-of-Pocket Spending on Health Care by Medicare Beneficiaries Age 65 and Older in 2003*. AARP Public Policy Institute Data Digest #DD101. Washington, DC: AARP). September 2004. Available at: http://assets.aarp.orgrgcenter/health/dd101_spending.pdf.

9. See, for example, John A. Poisal and Lauren Murray (2001).Growing Differences Between Medicare Beneficiaries With and Without Drug Coverage. *Health Affairs* (March/April): 74-85; Jan Blustein (2000). Drug Coverage and

Drug Purchases by Medicare Beneficiaries with Hypertension. *Health Affairs* 19(2): 219-230.

10. Kaiser Family Foundation (2005). *The Medicare Prescription Drug Benefit.* Washington, DC: The Henry J. Kaiser Family Foundation. September. Availble at: http://www.kff.org/medicare/upload/7044-02.pdf.

11. Henry J. Kaiser Family Foundation (2005). *Medicare: Medicare Advantage.* September. Available at: http://www.kff.org.

12. Juliette Cubanski (2004). *Continuing Policy Issues in Medicare Prescription Drug Coverage.* Washington, DC: Henry J. Kaiser Family Foundation. November.

13. American Association of Retired Persons (2005). *The New Medicare Prescription Drug Coverage: What You Need to Know.* Washington, DC: AARP.

14. Note that this figure does not include payments for Part D premiums.

15. Centers for Medicare and Medicaid Services (2006). *Medicare Rx Prescription Drug Coverage—Stand-Alone Prescription Drug Plans: Landscape of Plan Options in Maryland.* January 4. Available at: http://www.medicare.gov/medicare reform/mapdpdocs/PDPLandscapemd.pdf.

16. Kaiser Family Foundation (2005). *Low-Income Assistance Under the Medicare Drug Benefit.* Washington, DC: Henry J. Kaiser Family Foundation. September. Available at: http://www.kff.org/medicare/upload/Low-Income-Assistance-Under-the-Medicare-Drug-Benefit-Fact-Sheet.pdf.

17. For a discussion of issues relating to formularies, tiered cost-sharing, and cost control mechanisms that can be used by Medicare-approved drug plans, see Jack Hoadley (2005). *The Effect of Formularies and Other cost management Tools on Access to Medications: An Analysis of the MMA and the Final Rule.* Washington, DC: Henry J. Kaiser Family Foundation. March. Available at http://www.kff.org.

18. Hoadley (2005).

19. Although prescription drug coverage is an optional benefit for state Medicaid programs, all such programs do provide prescription drug benefits.

20. Although the reduced drug expenditures will reduce expenditures by state Medicaid programs, much of those savings are relayed back to the federal government through a "clawback" mechanism that was adopted as part of the MMA.

21. For a description of prescription drug benefits in state Medicaid programs, see National Pharmaceutical Council, Pharmaceutical Benefits Under State Medical Assistance Programs (2004). Available at: http://www.npcnow.org/resources/PharmBenefitsMedicaid.asp.

22. Jocelyn Guyer and Andy Schneider (2004). *Implications of the New Medicare Law for Dual Eligibles: 10 Key Questions and Answers.* Washington, DC: Henry J. Kaiser Family Foundation. January. Availible at http://www.kff.org/medicaid/upload/Implications-of-th-New-Medicare-Law-for-Dual-Eligibles-10-Key-Questions-and-Answers.pdf.

23. Kaiser Family Foundation (2005). *Medicare: The Medicare Prescriptions Drug Benefit.* September. Available at: http://www.kff.org.

24. People who have noncreditible employer-sponsored drug coverage should not automatically enroll in a benefit. Some plans require a retiree to drop *all* of their health insurance coverage if they choose not to participate in the employer's drug coverage. In such an event, a beneficiary must weigh the value of that coverage

against the late enrollment penalties associated with enrolling in a Medicare drug benefit after the initial enrollment period.

25. AARP (2005). *The New Medicare Prescription Drug Coverage: What You Need to Know.* Washington, DC: AARP.

26. The Henry J. Kaiser Family Foundation/Harvard School of Public Health (2005). *The Medicare Drug Benefit: Beneficiary Perspecties Just Before Implementation.* November. Available at: http://www.kff.org.

27. Kaiser Family Foundation (2006). *Tracking Prescription Drug Coverage Under Medicare: Five Ways to Look at the New Enrollment Numbers*, February. Available at http://www.kff.org/kaiserpolls/med111005pkg.cfm

28. National Citizens' Coalition for Nursing Home Reform (2005). *Medicare Prescription Drug Coverage: Q&A for Nursing Home Residents, Their Families and Friends.* Washington, DC: National Citizens' Coalition for Nursing Home Reform.

Chapter 6

Prescription Drugs Under Medicaid

Linda Elam

INTRODUCTION

Medicaid, Title XIX of the Social Security Act, is the nation's public health insurance program for individuals with low income. Medicaid is jointly financed by the federal and state governments, and administered by the fifty states, the District of Columbia, and the Territories (American Samoa, Guam, the Northern Mariana Islands, Puerto Rico, and the Virgin Islands), with federal oversight through the Centers for Medicare and Medicaid Services (CMS) in the U.S. Department of Health and Human Services (HHS). Although federal participation is tied to certain programmatic standards, each state sets eligibility rules, determines some of the services it covers, and sets payment rates, resulting in considerable variation between state Medicaid programs.

Medicaid is a means-tested, entitlement program that originally focused on recipients of cash assistance through welfare programs, but it has expanded over time to cover other low-income groups. Some forty years after it was enacted in 1965, Medicaid covers more than 52 million low-income children and parents, people with disabilities, and elderly Americans at an annual cost of over $300 billion, making it the largest health and long-term care program in the United States. Roughly one in seven Americans (and one in four children) is covered by Medicaid, and many of these people are members of vulnerable populations (see Figure 6.1).

Medicaid's Role in the Health Care System

Medicaid, as the source of nearly 20 percent of health care dollars and half of nursing home dollars, is a significant contributor to the health care economy. In 2004, Medicaid accounted for 17 percent of spending on both personal health care and hospital care, 46 percent of spending on nursing

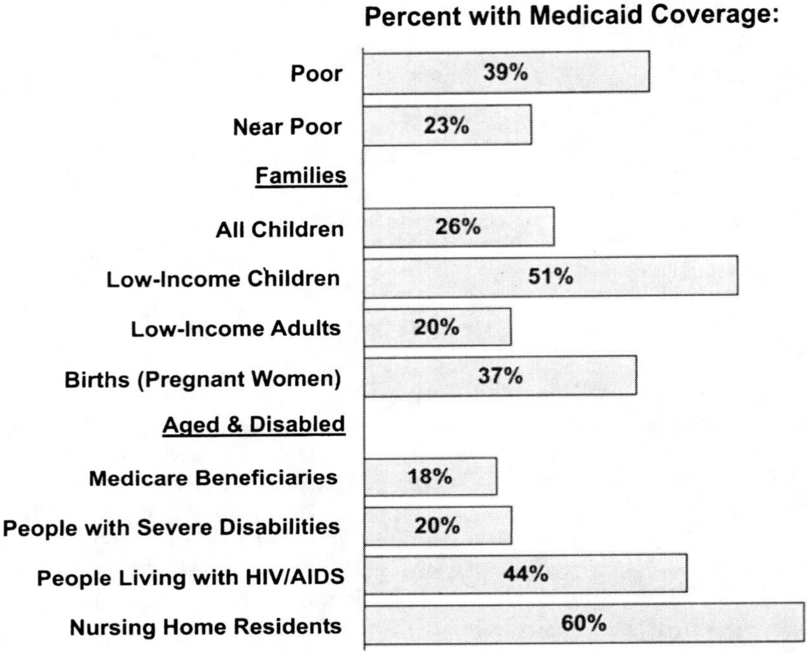

Percent with Medicaid Coverage:

Poor	39%
Near Poor	23%
Families	
All Children	26%
Low-Income Children	51%
Low-Income Adults	20%
Births (Pregnant Women)	37%
Aged & Disabled	
Medicare Beneficiaries	18%
People with Severe Disabilities	20%
People Living with HIV/AIDS	44%
Nursing Home Residents	60%

FIGURE 6.1. Medicaid's role for selected populations. *Note:* "Poor" is defined as living below the federal poverty level, which was $19,307 for a family of four in 2004. *Sources:* Kaiser Comission on Medicaid and the Uninsured, Kaiser Family Ffoundation, and Urban Institute estimates; Birth data: National Governor's Association, Maternal and Child Health Update.

home care, 19 percent of prescription drug spending, and 44 percent of public mental health spending. States spend about 17 percent of their own funds on Medicaid, making the program a significant component of state budgets, second only to education, and in turn, federal matching payments for eligible Medicaid benefits and services are the single largest source of federal grants to states.

Medicaid moderates the number of people without health insurance and helps other health insurance programs function. Compared to low-income individuals covered by private insurance, Medicaid beneficiaries are two and a half times as likely to live below the poverty line, four times as likely to have health conditions that limit their ability to work, and three times as likely to be in fair or poor health. Because of their high health care utilization and expenses and their preexisting health conditions, many of the people covered by Medicaid are unable to participate in the private insurance market. Medicaid, by insuring people and services that are not adequately covered through other financing options, helps to support the U.S. health system and allows private insurance to function. In addition, Medicaid picks up many of those who may have lost coverage through economic downturns, job losses, and the erosion of employer-based insurance. Medicaid also fills in the gaps in care provided by Medicare—the federal program designed to serve the elderly and disabled—providing assistance for premiums and cost sharing and covering services that Medicare does not, such as dental and vision care, and most notably, long-term care.

Medicaid's size and spending growth have prompted significant activity at the state and federal levels to control it, efforts sometimes known as Medicaid reforms. In particular, the increased spending for prescription drugs experienced broadly across the health care sector, coupled with increased budgetary pressures in the states between the mid-1990s through the middle of the first decade of the 2000s made Medicaid drug spending a target.

ELIGIBILITY

Although Medicaid is an important source of health financing for people with low incomes, not all low-income people qualify for coverage. States determine eligibility for Medicaid using financial criteria such as income and assets and nonfinancial criteria such as disability status or age. Medicaid law defines almost fifty groups of people that states must cover (mandatory groups) or may cover and receive federal matching payments for (optional groups). Mandatory beneficiaries include families who meet standards states had in effect in 1996 for Aid to Families with Dependent Children, the old welfare program: pregnant women and children under age six at or below 133 percent of the federal poverty level (FPL), children six to nineteen years of age with family income up to 100 percent of the FPL, and most people receiving cash assistance through the federal Supplemental Security Income (SSI) program serving the low-income aged, blind, and disabled populations.[1]

Optional groups include medically needy beneficiaries whose incomes are low but above thresholds set for categorically needy groups. Some individuals qualify as medically needy by incurring high medical expenses, a process known as spending-down. Once their spending for health care has surpassed a threshold, these beneficiaries are eligible for Medicaid coverage. Other optional groups include individuals with incomes under the federal poverty level. In 2001, although 29 percent of Medicaid beneficiaries fell into optional coverage categories, they accounted for more than 42 percent of program spending for services.[2]

Some low-income Medicare beneficiaries are served by the Medicare Savings Program, in which they receive assistance with their Medicare premiums and cost sharing from Medicaid. These beneficiaries are known as specified low-income Medicare beneficiaries (SLMBs), qualified low-income Medicare beneficiaries (QMBs), and qualifying individuals (QIs), receive varying levels of assistance and are not eligible for full Medicaid benefits. States are not required to provide the same benefits that categorically eligible beneficiaries are eligible to receive to the beneficiaries qualifying as medically needy or members of special groups.

BENEFITS

As previously mentioned, Medicaid law requires programs to cover some services (mandatory services) and permits federal matching payments for other services that states are not required to provide (optional services). Examples of mandatory services include physician care; inpatient hospitalization; nursing facility care for adults; early and periodic screening, diagnosis, and treatment (EPSDT) services for children; and pregnancy-related services. For medically needy beneficiaries, prenatal and delivery services and some postpartum and home health services are mandatory. States may provide other services at their option, including prescription drugs, dental coverage, and ambulance services. States are allowed the discretion to provide services to only certain groups of medically needy beneficiaries; however, all members of a group must have access to those services.

States must observe four basic federal guidelines in the provision of Medicaid benefits:

- *Amount, duration, and scope:* Services must be sufficient in amount, duration, and scope to achieve their intended purpose. The state may not arbitrarily deny or limit services to a beneficiary based on diagnosis or condition; however, the state may limit service delivery based on medical necessity or through the use of appropriate utilization controls.
- *Comparability:* Services available to those within the categorically needy group must be comparable, and services available to those within the medically needy group must be comparable; in addition, services available to the categorically needy must not be less in amount, duration, or scope than services available to the medically needy.

- *Statewideness:* The amount, duration, and scope of coverage must be the same statewide
- *Freedom-of-choice:* A state must allow beneficiaries to exercise freedom of choice among providers or plans, with certain exceptions.

The federal government may waive the general rules regarding services and populations that Medicaid covers. The Secretary of Health and Human Services may grant exceptions to rules on a state-by-state basis, making federal matching funds available for services or populations not mandated by Medicaid statute. States have also received waivers to limit the services provided to certain groups of beneficiaries. In applying for a waiver, states must demonstrate that the actions they are proposing will be budget neutral and will not cost the federal government any more than it would have paid without a waiver.

Even though the elderly and disabled populations constitute only about a quarter of Medicaid beneficiaries, about 70 percent of Medicaid spending on benefits is for individuals in those two groups (see Figure 6.2). A major component of this spending is for long term care. Medicaid is a primary payer for long term care in the United States, accounting for roughly half of

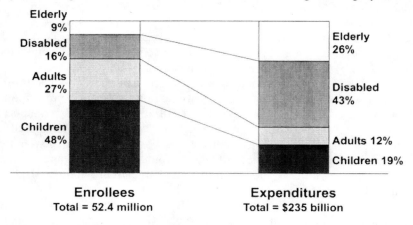

Enrollees
Total = 52.4 million

Expenditures
Total = $235 billion

FIGURE 6.2. Medicaid enrollees and expenditures by enrollment group, 2003. Expenditure distribution based on Congressional Budget Office (CBO) data that include only federal spending on services and excludes disproportionate share hospital, supplemental provider payments, vaccines for children, administration, and the temporary federal medical assistance percentage (FMAP) increase. Total expenditures assume a state share of 43 percent of total program spending. *Source:* Kaiser Commission estimates based on CBO and Office of Management and Budget data, 2004.

all national spending. Prior to January 2006 and the implementation of the Medicare drug program known as Medicare Part D, another significant component of spending for the elderly and people with disabilities was for prescription drugs.

Prescription drugs are an optional Medicaid benefit, but all states cover them. Historically, the prescription drug benefit has been one of the fastest growing components of Medicaid spending and one of the most widely used services; by 2003, Medicaid had spent over $26 billion, which accounted for 19 percent of national prescription drug purchases and made the program the single largest purchaser of prescription drugs in the United States.

Recent Federal Policy Changes Affecting Medicaid

Medicaid has provided access to prescription drugs for economically vulnerable persons without any other form of coverage, including aged and disabled beneficiaries—populations that were historically responsible for about 80 percent of Medicaid outpatient prescription drug expenditures. Many of these people are eligible for both Medicaid and Medicare (the "dual eligibles"), and, effective January 1, 2006, their drug coverage switched from Medicaid to Medicare Part D prescription drug plans. Enacted as part of the Medicare Prescription Drug, Improvement, and Modernization Act of 2003 (Pub. L. 108-173), Medicare Part D changes the Medicaid prescription drug picture considerably as it assumes drug payments for dual eligibles who accounted for almost half of Medicaid drug spending. Although Medicaid programs no longer finance prescription drug coverage for dual eligibles, states are still responsible for payments to the federal government to finance Part D. These payments are described in statute as "phased-down state contributions," or, more commonly, as the "clawback." States also may elect to wrap around Part D coverage for dual eligibles, paying for drugs not covered under Part D or providing assistance with cost sharing.

States have the option to charge nominal cost sharing (deductibles, copayments, or coinsurance) under Medicaid, however, not all benefits or all beneficiaries are subject to cost sharing. Children under eighteen years of age, pregnancy-related services for pregnant women, terminally ill patients receiving hospice care, or inpatients are generally exempt from Medicaid cost sharing. In addition, federal Medicaid law does not permit cost sharing for emergency services (although nonemergency services provided in a hospital emergency department are eligible for cost sharing) or for family planning services and supplies. The passage of the Deficit Reduction Act of 2005 (DRA), which was signed into law on February 8, 2006, enacted several federal changes to Medicaid policy, including permission to states to increase and enforce beneficiary cost sharing for services. The DRA permits states to charge cost sharing on a sliding scale up to 20 percent of the cost of nonpreferred drugs for Medicaid beneficiaries with incomes over 150 percent of the federal poverty level. The DRA also allows providers to withhold services or care from Medicaid beneficiaries who do not pay cost sharing, a practice that was previously prohibited by Medicaid law.

ADMINISTRATION AND FINANCING

States have the responsibility for day-to-day operations of their Medicaid programs and for determining covered services, provider payment rates, and eligibility standards; for overseeing program operations and compliance with laws; and enrolling eligible beneficiaries. Federal administration of the program is provided by the Center for Medicaid and State Operations (CMSO) within CMS. CMSO engages in a number of regulatory, financing, and administrative functions, including collecting program data from the states, ensuring that states get federal matching funds, and overseeing program compliance by states, providers, and plans. Medicaid administrative costs are historically lower than those for private health insurance plans. Roughly 5 percent of Medicaid spending is for administrative costs, compared to the nearly 7 percent average administrative costs found in private plans.

As part of the joint nature of the Medicaid program, each state receives matching funds for Medicaid expenditures from the federal government according to a formula known as the Federal Medical Assistance Percentage (FMAP). The FMAP, which is recalculated every year, ranges from 50 percent to 77 percent, depending upon the per capita income of the state, and averages 57 percent nationally. Federal matching funds for Medicaid covered services are provided on an open-ended basis, meaning that no limit is set to the federal share available to match eligible state spending. Federal matching payments through Medicaid are the largest single source of grant funds received by states, representing 44 percent of all federal grants to states.

States have the flexibility to cover services on a fee-for-service basis or through managed care programs. These include commercial managed care organizations (MCOs), Medicaid-only MCOs, and primary care case management (PCCM). MCOs receive capitated payments (fixed payments per beneficiary) for all covered services. Although enrollment in managed care varies considerably by state, in 2003, 62 percent of Medicaid beneficiaries were enrolled in managed care. States often require parents and children to enroll in Medicaid MCOs, however many states do not require the enrollment of the aged and persons with disabilities, although enrollment of these groups has grown in recent years. Medicaid programs have considerable flexibility to determine which benefits and populations are "carved out" or excluded from MCOs, meaning that these groups or services remain in fee-for-service Medicaid. PCCMs, entities that contract with the state to monitor beneficiaries' use of covered primary care services, are less risk-based than MCOs.

MEDICAID OUTPATIENT DRUG BENEFIT

Medicaid law defines prescribed drugs as "simple or compound substances or mixtures of substances prescribed for the cure, mitigation, or prevention of disease, or for health maintenance that are (1) prescribed by a physician or other licensed practitioner of the healing arts within the scope of this professional practice as defined and limited by federal and state law; (2) dispensed by licensed pharmacists and licensed authorized practitioners in accordance with the State Medical Practice Act; and (3) dispensed by the licensed pharmacist or practitioner on a written prescription that is recorded and maintained in the pharmacist's or practitioner's records."[3] This definition includes over-the-counter products ordered by a licensed practitioner, and most states provide at least limited coverage of products such as over-the-counter cough and cold preparations or digestive products.

People with low incomes who need prescription drugs but who do not have drug coverage are serially disadvantaged in that they do not benefit from volume discounts negotiated by insurers, and they must pay the full cost for their medications out of pocket. Medication costs can take up large proportions of household incomes and can cause some to forego filling their prescriptions. Medicaid has been vitally important to the provision of drugs for the low-income population that qualifies for coverage, particularly important given the greater burden of illness borne by this population.

DRUG EXPENDITURE AND UTILIZATION TRENDS

Pharmaceutical spending growth has been an important contributor to increased health care costs in all sectors, including Medicaid. At $33.9 billion, spending for Medicaid outpatient prescription drugs (including estimates of managed care spending) represented about 13.4 percent of Medicaid expenditures in 2003. Medicaid drug spending has grown in recent years by about 18 percent annually, but has moderated recently due in part to increased state efforts to control cost growth (see Figure 6.3).

ADMINISTRATION OF THE DRUG BENEFIT

Although states have wide latitude to design their Medicaid drug benefits, some federal guidelines exist to which they must adhere, including limits on the utilization and cost control measures that may be applied. Medicaid law has not allowed states unfettered use of these controls primarily to protect the vulnerable population served by the program. Some options (e.g., utilization review, federally allowed exclusions or generic substitution) have the potential to curb spending growth while also improving or maintaining quality of care. However, limits on the drug benefit such as increased cost sharing or prescription caps, often presented as strategies to increase patient accountability or reduce fraud, may instead unduly burden the poor, sick population served by Medicaid.

A key component of the Medicaid drug benefit is the formulary, or list of drugs that Medicaid covers. Medicaid is required to cover all drugs (with a few allowable exclusions, listed in the following section) manufactured by companies that have entered into a rebate agreement with the secretary of HHS. Medicaid's comprehensive coverage has provided access to drug therapies that would otherwise be beyond the reach of its beneficiaries, but this comprehensiveness makes controlling utilization more challenging

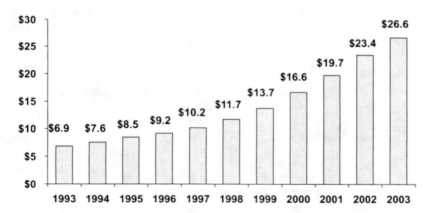

FIGURE 6.3. Estimated medicaid expenditures for prescription drugs, 1993-2003. *Note:* Expenditures are fee-for-service, net of rebates. *Source:* Urban Institute estimates based on HCFA-2082 and HCFA-64 reports.

than in most private plans, which have the option to simply not cover any particular drug. However, Medicaid allows states significant flexibility to control utilization through the following commonly used mechanisms (see Exhibit 6.1).

Drug Exclusions

Medicaid law allows states to exclude the following categories of drugs (subject to updates from the secretary of HHS) from their Medicaid formularies:

- Agents when used for anorexia, weight loss, or weight gain
- Agents when used to promote fertility
- Agents when used for cosmetic purposes or hair growth
- Agents when used for the symptomatic relief of cough and colds
- Agents when used to promote smoking cessation
- Prescription vitamins and mineral products, except prenatal vitamins and fluoride preparations
- Nonprescription (OTC) drugs
- Covered outpatient drugs that the manufacturer seeks to require as a condition of sale that associated tests or monitoring services be purchased exclusively from the manufacturer or its designee
- Barbiturates
- Benzodiazepines

These drugs are also excluded from Medicare Part D coverage, but states that elect to cover these drugs can continue to do so for their dually eligible population and still receive federal matching payments.

EXHIBIT 6.1. Strategies to influence utilization and prescribing patterns

Exclude certain drugs
Require or encourage the use of generics
Institute prior authorization
Establish formularies or preferred drug lists (PDLs)
Require fail-first or step therapy
Limit prescriptions
Impose or increase cost sharing
Utilization review

Requiring or Encouraging Generic Substitution

Many brand-name drugs have generic counterparts that provide therapeutic equivalence at lower cost. States can mandate generic substitution at the pharmacy level, although many allow generic substitution to be overridden through prior authorization, or they can provide incentives for pharmacists to dispense generics through additional fees or favorable reimbursement rates. In addition, some states conduct provider education programs promoting the value of generics. States also may set cost sharing for generic drugs lower than that established for brand name products.

Prior Authorization

States may require that prior approval (or prior authorization) be obtained from Medicaid before a pharmacist can dispense selected drugs. States have the option to subject any drug on the Medicaid formulary to prior authorization, and they are required to respond within twenty-four hours of a request for prior approval and make a seventy-two-hour supply of the drug available in emergencies. Whereas prior authorization can reduce access to unnecessary or dangerous drugs, when it is used to control costs it is unclear how patients' access to needed drugs is affected or how appropriate the mandated substitutions are.[4] On the provider side, the willingness and ability of physicians and pharmacists to navigate prior authorization can hinge upon how busy they are and their level of familiarity with Medicaid procedures. In addition, physicians and pharmacists may not be compensated for the administrative burden posed by prior authorization, which creates an incentive for them to limit Medicaid beneficiaries in their patient populations. Prior authorization is a major tool in the implementation of other initiatives such as formularies or preferred drug lists.

Preferred Drug Lists

In most cases, a preferred drug list (PDL) is a list of drugs that can be prescribed without prior authorization. In order to institute a PDL, federal regulations require states to: (1) set up a committee of physicians, pharmacists, and others to create the list; (2) exclude only those drugs that do not have a clinically meaningful therapeutic advantage over other drugs on the list; and (3) have a prior authorization program for excluded drugs. States use several criteria to compile their PDLs, including safety and therapeutic outcomes, manufacturer price concessions or rebates above the federal rebate (known as supplemental rebates), value-added programs such as disease or case management, and burden on certain patient populations (e.g., people with HIV/AIDS or mental illness). The first state to develop a PDL was California, in 1991. Some ten years later, PDLs were developed in several more states, and by January 2004 more than thirty states had implemented or planned to implement a PDL. Some states that were early adopters of PDLs, including Florida, Maine, and Michigan, were targets of unsuccessful pharmaceutical industry lawsuits, with the industry contending that both mandatory supplemental rebates and the process by which some states developed their PDLs violate federal Medicaid law.

Both patient advocacy groups and the pharmaceutical industry have attacked PDLs as threats to prescription drug access. In the case of beneficiaries as well as providers, the overarching philosophy and strategy employed by states to create PDLs may have implications for how well they are received; for example, in Florida, the exclusion of HIV/AIDS and psychotropic drugs from the prior authorization requirement deflected some criticism, although some critics expressed concern that the process used to compile the PDL was excessively cost-driven. On the other hand, Oregon's systematic, evidence-based process for developing its PDL was widely praised.[5] (See Chapter 22.)

Implementing "Fail-First" Policies

Fail-first or step therapy policies require that a prescriber demonstrate that an older, less expensive drug within a therapeutic class is inappropriate for a patient before a newer, more expensive medication may be prescribed. Fail-first policies are most commonly used for classes of drugs that have several less expensive alternatives, such as antiulcer drugs or antihistamines. Under some circumstances, requiring patients to fail first-line medications may cause unnecessary delays in access and subsequent compromises to care. For example, if a beneficiary taking a particular nonpreferred medication changes providers, he or she may have to fail the standard first-line therapy for the current prescriber, even if the previous prescriber demonstrated a need for the current medication.

Prescription Limits

States may limit the amount of medication dispensed to a patient through capping the drug quantity permitted per prescription, the number of refills allowed per prescription, the number of prescriptions per month or year, or expenditure per prescription. Some states apply caps to brand medications only. Also, some states have "soft caps," which means that beneficiaries may still get the drug in question through prior authorization, in contrast to "hard caps," which are firmer limits on dispensing. For the patient, limits on the quantity of medication dispensed or on the number of refills permitted can mean more trips to the pharmacy or the doctor, a particular problem for disabled beneficiaries or those with transportation difficulties. Moreover, a quantity limit translates into a greater number of refills, which, if co-payments are imposed, compounds the logistical burden with a financial one. Prescription limits can deny people with multiple illnesses access to necessary medications and have been linked to both increased institution-alization[6] and abrupt changes in drug regimens.[7]

Beneficiary Cost Sharing

States can require beneficiaries to pay "nominal" copayments for their medications. Federal regulations limit copayments to nominal amounts ($.50 to $3.00 per prescription). The DRA allows for those amounts to be indexed to inflation for the first time, as well as making copayments en-forceable. Part of the rationale for this provision was to increase beneficiary sensitivity to health care spending and to discourage wasteful consumption of prescription drugs and other services. Cost sharing does decrease utiliza-tion, but is a blunt tool, particularly for low-income individuals.

Research repeatedly raises concerns that cost sharing and caps have the potential to discourage beneficiaries from obtaining needed drugs. Benefi-ciaries may believe they cannot obtain drugs if they cannot afford co-payments, or people with multiple chronic illnesses might have needs that exceed prescription limits. Caps shift the full cost of prescriptions that ex-ceed the limit to the beneficiary, creating a severe form of cost sharing for people who receive multiple drugs. Prescription limits or caps in Medicaid programs have been associated with increased nursing home admissions and increased program costs,[8] as well as abrupt changes in drug regimens, particularly for elderly patients.[9] Not surprisingly, Medicaid patients fill fewer prescriptions in states that impose prescription copayments than in states that do not, but beneficiaries in worse health—a group that includes many patients who have the greatest need for drug therapy—appear to be most sensitive to copayments.[10]

Reviewing Drug Utilization

Federal rules require states to have drug utilization review (DUR) pro-grams for outpatient drugs that ensure that prescriptions are appropriate, medically necessary, and unlikely to result in adverse medical outcomes. Prospective DUR (PRODUR) programs target inappropriate drug access at the point of sale. Retrospective DUR (RetroDUR) programs generally track individual providers' prescribing practices as well as overall use of and expenditures for drugs, with many states tracking use of specific drugs. PRODUR and RetroDUR are designed to catch problems such as drug interactions, duplicative prescriptions, and improper prescribing practices. In addition to addressing patient safety and prescribing practices, DUR programs can help contain costs. (See Chapter 27.)

MANAGED CARE PLANS
AND PRESCRIPTION DRUG COVERAGE

A fundamental decision for states enrolling beneficiaries into capitated MCOs is whether to include payments for outpatient prescription drugs in capitation rates or to carve out the drug benefit and maintain it in the fee-for-service system. When medications are part of Medicaid MCOs' capitation rates, drug coverage is governed by the plans' contracts with the states. States' specific contractual requirements vary substantially.[11] Under federal regulations, states are charged with ensuring that plan enrollees have access to all prescription drugs covered by the state Medicaid plan, even if the MCO formularies do not normally include them. Oversight of managed care plans' formularies and utilization management strategies varies considerably by state. Because they are not reimbursed directly by the state and are instead a component of the capitation rate paid by states to plans, drugs that are purchased through MCOs are not currently subject to the federal rebate program.

Some issues related to drug coverage through managed care for Medicaid beneficiaries center around plans being at risk for drug payments and therefore have incentives to reduce access to care. Plans could achieve this through various means, including using narrow definitions of medical necessity or using restrictive drug formularies. Another area of concern is plan coordination, such as in the case of coordinating drug regimens between primary care providers and areas of care that may have been carved out, for example, mental health. In addition, plans may have incentives to rely more heavily on drug therapy rather than using other, effective but more expensive treatment modalities, such as psychotherapy in the case of mental health.

REBATES, REIMBURSEMENTS, AND PAYMENTS

States have two primary sets of financial controls over their expenditures for outpatient prescription drugs—payments to pharmacists and rebates from manufacturers—and they are using these and scrutinizing manufacturers' prices as they try to control drug costs. Under the federal rebate program, manufacturers return a portion of federal and state expenditures on drugs to the federal and state governments in return for the state including the manufacturer's drugs on its Medicaid formulary. All states participate in the federal rebate program, although in 2004, twenty-two states had enacted or implemented legislation to receive supplemental rebates from manufacturers (see Exhibit 6.2).

Payments to Pharmacies

Payments to pharmacies have two parts: reimbursements of acquisition costs and dispensing fees. Acquisition costs are the costs to pharmacists of obtaining the drugs that they distribute to Medicaid beneficiaries. In addition to those costs, Medicaid allows the payment of "reasonable" dispensing fees to reimburse pharmacies for their other costs associated with distributing the drugs, such as storage and patient counseling.

Ingredient Costs

States typically reimburse ingredient costs at a discount off of a list price such as the average wholesale price (AWP). The AWP is a price determined by manufacturers that is often much higher than what pharmacies actually pay for drugs. As a result, the use of AWP, even when discounted (in 2003, brand drug reimbursements ranged from AWP–5 percent in Alaska to AWP–17 percent in California[12]) has come under increased scrutiny amid

EXHIBIT 6.2. Strategies to influence the amount paid for drugs

Reduce pharmacy reimbursement
Seek supplemental rebates
Pursue legal action over alleged overpayment

charges that Medicaid is overpaying for drugs. For example, The Office of Inspector General of the U.S. Department of Health and Human Services (HHS-OIG) estimated that the actual acquisition costs for pharmacies were 21.84 percent below AWP in 1999.[13] Studies such as these prompted calls for reforms to Medicaid drug reimbursements.

The federal government has two ceilings on the amounts it will match for specific drugs paid for by state Medicaid programs. The first ceiling is the lower of (1) the estimated acquisition cost (EAC) of a drug plus a dispensing fee or (2) the usual or customary charges to the public. This ceiling applies to brand-name drugs and to those drugs with fewer than three therapeutically equivalent generic drugs. Pharmacies retain the difference between Medicaid reimbursement for acquisition costs and the price they pay to wholesalers. The second ceiling—the federal upper limit (FUL)—applies to drugs with at least two generic, therapeutically equivalent versions and was set at 250 percent of the average manufacturers price (AMP) as specified by the DRA. The AMP is the average price that wholesalers pay to manufacturers for the drugs they purchase for resale to retailers; the AMP is almost always lower than the AWP, which approximates the retail price of drugs. The DRA also included provisions to increase reporting of AMP and to allow greater transparency of reported prices.

Many contend that the biggest winners regarding inflated AWPs are the pharmacies and not the manufacturers, because the pharmacies benefit from the "spread"—the difference between payment and reimbursement. In the case of generics, those with the most inflated AWPs result in more profit for the pharmacy. Manufacturers with products that have the greatest spread are going to be at an advantage because of the profit potential to the pharmacy.

Critics of lowering pharmacy reimbursements contend that this strategy does not factor in all costs to pharmacies of acquiring and dispensing drugs for Medicaid enrollees, that pharmacists bear the brunt of cost containment initiatives for the Medicaid prescription drug program, and that cuts in reimbursement threaten to reduce access to and quality of prescription drugs for Medicaid beneficiaries. Early in 2002, several retail drug stores and pharmacists' representatives responded to states' planned or implemented reimbursement rate cuts by threatening to either curtail service or drop Medicaid participation altogether.[14]

Dispensing Fees

Medicaid is permitted to pay reasonable dispensing fees to compensate pharmacies for product handling and storage and patient counseling. As with other provider payments, dispensing fees are a frequent cost-cutting target. However, pharmacies maintain that they are not adequately compensated for serving the Medicaid population, and they tend to resist any decreases in ingredient reimbursement unless they are compensated through higher fees.

Manufacturer Rebates

Although states can control pharmacists' fees and acquisition costs, until fairly recently they have exerted less control over the rebates they receive from pharmaceutical manufacturers. In accordance with the Omnibus Budget Reconciliation Act (OBRA) 1990, federal and state governments receive rebates from manufacturers based on the amount of drugs Medicaid programs buy. The rebate program has been an important source of cost savings to Medicaid, returning $19.8 billion to state and federal governments between 1991 and 2000, and reducing fee-for-service drug spending by about 17 percent each year since 1996.[15] In 2000 alone, states received $4 billion in rebates, resulting in nearly 20 percent lower total drug spending compared to the prerebate total. In exchange for agreeing to give rebates, pharmaceutical manufacturers receive a guarantee that state Medicaid programs will cover their products, except for federally allowable exclusions. In addition to the federal rebate, many states are now assessing or implementing supplemental rebates that are negotiated and collected at the state level.

Two formulae determine the federal rebate amount, based on the average manufacturers price (AMP) that manufacturers report quarterly to the federal government. Rebates for brand-name drugs are the larger of: (1) 15.5 percent of the AMP or (2) the difference between the AMP and the lowest price the manufacturer offers to most other purchasers (known as the "best price"). The rebates for generics are calculated by multiplying the AMP by 11 percent. Proposals to increase the amount of the rebate have been floated as strategies to address drug costs, either through changing the formula by picking a different base number (e.g., AWP rather than AMP), increasing the percentage of the price used to establish the rebate, or by the institution of a flat rebate. Collecting the full amounts of rebates due is another consideration; in reviewing the rebate program the Government Accountability Office (GAO) found weaknesses in reporting and oversight at both the federal and state levels.

Many states have negotiated rebates, known as supplemental rebates, in addition to those received through the federal rebate program,. These rebates are frequently mediated through the use of PDLs, in which manufacturers may have their products added to the preferred list through payment of rebates to the states. The effectiveness of individual states' efforts to negotiate with manufacturers may vary considerably as small states do not have the leverage of larger states. State successes in securing supplemental rebate agreements may indicate the timeliness of possible changes to the federal rebate formula, ensuring that savings accrue to all states and the federal government.

Challenges to Manufacturers' Prices

States, consumers, and the federal government have all taken action against pharmaceutical companies, alleging unfair or illegal marketing and pricing strategies for both generic and brand-name drugs.[16] Several states have sued manufacturers, alleging that the companies misrepresented their AWPs, inflating both inpatient and outpatient drug costs. Class action antitrust lawsuits have also been filed on behalf of consumers against pharmaceutical companies, charging that drug companies have overpriced their drugs by stifling generic competition, price fixing, and other illegal and unfair practices.[17]

Action at the federal level regarding fraudulent pricing practices is based upon the federal False Claims Act that levies significant fines against contractors that submit false or fraudulent claims to the federal government. Two notable pharmaceutical False Claims Act cases involved AWP inflation by the Bayer Corporation and TAP Pharmaceutical Products. Settlement of these claims in 2001 resulted in payments of $31.7 million to states for Medicaid losses, and $567.3 million to the federal government for Medicaid and Medicare losses.

Given these activities and the proliferation of PDLs and formularies that use reference pricing or supplemental rebates as criteria for inclusion, containing costs by addressing pricing and rebates appears to be an expanding area for states trying to control Medicaid drug expenditures. However, these efforts' effects on beneficiary access and health and their long-term financial consequences remain to be seen.

Many states expect Medicare Part D to have an impact on their ability to negotiate prices and to secure supplemental rebates. Some states have seen roughly half of their prescription drug spending shift to Medicare drug plans. In the first year of Part D implementation, significant impacts on negotiations between states and drug manufacturers may not occur, but this may change with more experience with the program.

Discounts, Expansions, and Pools

The current policy and economic environment has pushed states to develop new strategies to maintain or expand Medicaid drug benefits and to address gaps in other coverage. Some states, notably Maine, Ohio, and California have advanced legislation requiring drug manufacturers to provide discounted drugs to low-income or uninsured residents or face limitations on their products' use in Medicaid, effectively expanding the Medicaid drug discount beyond Medicaid. These proposals have been vigorously attacked by the pharmaceutical industry.

Some states are trying to increase their bargaining power by pooling drug purchases, both between states ("multistate purchasing," e.g., Medicaid programs in several states) and within a state (e.g., Medicaid, state employees, corrections, etc.). Multistate purchasing may increase in prevalence across states, particularly since CMS provided guidance to states in 2004 and as they adjust to lower Medicaid drug volume after Part D implementation. The first multistate Medicaid pool approved by CMS in April 2004 is the National Medicaid Pooling Initiative, which includes Michigan, New Hampshire, Alaska, and Nevada as original states. The pool later expanded to include Hawaii, Minnesota, Montana, Kentucky, New York, and Tennessee. (Original member Vermont left the pool to create another with Iowa, Maine, and Utah.) (See Chapter 10.)

INSTITUTIONAL DRUG BENEFIT

Roughly two-thirds of residents in long-term care facilities are dually eligible for Medicaid and Medicare, making Medicaid the primary payer for nursing home care and, until implementation of Part D, prescription drugs dispensed to residents of nursing homes. People residing in nursing homes are some of the sickest beneficiaries with the highest drug utilization, receiving an average of more than six routine prescription drugs a day. To serve this population, nursing homes typically contract with institutional pharmacies, organizations that are tailored to fill special needs, such as twenty-four-hour drug delivery or unit dose packaging. Medicaid reimburses drugs dispensed in nursing homes using a formula that is similar to what is used in fee-for-service—an ingredient cost that is typically a discount off of AWP plus a dispensing fee. (An exception to this design is in New York, where daily reimbursements for nursing home services and payments for drugs are bundled into one payment, essentially putting nursing homes at risk for Medicaid drug spending.) Institutional pharmacies may get an additional payment in recognition of these extra services, whether an increased ingredient cost payment or an LTC add-on.

How the shift of dually eligible beneficiaries from Medicaid drug coverage to Medicare Part D will affect nursing home operations and the consultant or institutional pharmacy industry—which has received about 65 percent of its revenue from Medicaid—is yet to be determined. What is clearer is that states must decide upon their roles in supplementing or "wrapping around" Medicare covered drugs. Medicare drug plans are not permitted to cover drugs that are excludable in Medicaid, but some of these drugs (e.g., benzodiazepines) are commonly used in long-term care settings. States are allowed to cover such drugs and still receive federal matching funds, but only if they provide access to these drugs to all Medicaid beneficiaries.

WHAT'S AHEAD

As a major component of state budgets, Medicaid will continue to face pressures to constrain cost growth, even as it continues to serve the poorest and sickest Americans. Medicaid reform discussions are occurring in the context of pressures faced by all payers: increased prices, the introduction of new health care technologies, and changing U.S. demographics, in particular, the aging of the population. However, Medicaid's countercyclical nature—meaning that enrollment and expenditures grow during periods of economic downturn as workers lose jobs and health coverage—also leaves it perhaps more vulnerable to increased scrutiny by cash-strapped states because the program costs more when states have fewer resources to expend.

Although a large portion of prescription drug spending has switched to Medicare Part D, Medicaid still is an essential payer for prescribed drugs for the populations it serves, including people with serious mental illness or HIV/AIDS, and low-income families. Medicaid's responsibility to provide prescription drugs to dual eligibles was supposed to have ended with the advent of Part D; however, the difficulties encountered in early implementation of the program prodded states to step in and provide emergency coverage through at least the first quarter of 2006. Thirty-seven states provided drug coverage through Medicaid after January 1, 2006, for dual eligibles who were not able to access drugs through Part D,[18] an example of Medicaid's responsiveness to health care crises. States will continue to evaluate the appropriateness of wrapping around the Medicare drug benefit, including paying for drugs not covered by Medicare and providing assistance to beneficiaries with cost sharing.

Significant changes have taken place within Medicaid, and many more are being contemplated at federal and state levels. What remains the same is that Medicaid fills gaps in other forms of coverage, covers populations that cannot otherwise receive coverage, and pays for services such as long-term care that are inadequately provided through other sources. Unless these other critical coverage needs can be addressed through other avenues, Medicaid will remain the workhorse of the U.S. health care system.

NOTES

1. The 2006 Federal poverty levels are $9,800 per year for an individual and $13,200 for a two-person household in the forty-eight contiguous states and the District of Columbia.

2. Sommers A, Ghosh A, Rousseau D (2005). *Medicaid Enrollment and Spending by "Mandatory" and "Optional Eligibility and Benefit Categories.* June. Washington, DC: The Kaiser Commission on Medicaid and the Uninsured.

3. 42 CFR 440.120

4. Smalley WE, Griffin MR, Fought RL, Sullivan L, Ray WA (1995). Effect of a prior-authorization requirement on the use of nonsteroidal antiinflammatory drugs by Medicaid patients. *New England Journal of Medicine* 332(24): 1612-1617.

5. Bernasek C, Mendelson D, Padrez R, Harrington C (2004). Oregon's Medicaid PDL: *Will An Evidence-Based Formulary with Voluntary Compliance Set a Precedent for Medicaid?* January. Washington, DC: The Kaiser Commission on Medicaid and the Uninsured.

6. Soumerai S, Ross-Degnan D, Avorn J, McLaughlin T, Choodnovskiy I (1991). Effects of Medicaid drug-payment limits on admission to hospitals and nursing homes. *The New England Journal of Medicine* 325(15): 1072-1077.

7. Martin BC, McMillan JA (1996). The impact of implementing a more restrictive prescription limit on Medicaid recipients: effects on cost, therapy and out of pocket expenditures. *Medical Care* 34: 686-701.

8. Soumerai et al. (1991).

9. Martin and McMillan (1996).

10. Stuart B, Zacker C (1999). Who bears the burden of Medicaid drug co-payment policies? *Health Affairs* 18(2): 201-212.

11. Stuart B, Zacker C (1999).

12. National Pharmaceutical Council (2004). *Pharmaceutical Benefits under State Medical Assistance Programs.* Reston, VA: National Pharmaceutical Council.

13. Office of Inspector General (2001). *Medicaid Pharmacy: Actual Acquisition Cost of Brand Name Prescription Drug Products.* August 10. A-06-00-00023. Washington, DC: U.S. Department of Health and Human Services. Available at: http://oig.hhs.gov/oas/reports/ region6/60000023.htm.

14. Drugstores threaten to end Medicaid service (2002). *New York Times.* March 12.

15. Bruen B (2002). *States Strive to Limit Medicaid Expenditures for Prescribed Drugs.* February. Washington, DC: The Kaiser Commission on Medicaid and the Uninsured.

16. Office of Inspector General (2002).*Medicaid Pharmacy: Actual Acquisition Cost of Generic Prescription Drug Products.* March 14. A-06-00-00053. Washington, DC: U.S. Department of Health and Human Services. Available at: http://oig.hhs.gov/oas/reports/region6/ 60100053.htm

17. For more information, see http://www.prescriptionaccesslitigation.org/index.htm

18. Smith V, Gifford K, Kramer S, Elam L (2006). *The Transition of Dual Eligibles to Medicare Part D Prescription Drug Coverage: State Actions during Implementation.* February. Washington, DC: The Kaiser Commission on Medicaid and the Uninsured.

Chapter 7

Public Health Pharmacy

Theodore P. Chiappelli

Pharmacists sit on a hidden treasure in the practice of public health in America. The involvement of public health pharmacists is part of an invisible link to the health status of our nation provided by uniformed members of the United States Public Health Service (PHS) in particular, and public health, in general. This chapter will address the contributions pharmacists make to the broader goals of public health and the specific roles of pharmacists who serve in uniform as members of the PHS as well as those who work as civil servants in public health delivery.

Although no group or profession is formally known as "public health pharmacists," the sobriquet occasionally appears in job titles and increasingly has been cited as a need in public health delivery. Literature from both the United Kingdom[1] and Canada[2] call for the use of specialists in pharmaceutical public health as a key strategy in improving the health of their nations. The role of public health pharmacy in the United States, as Moore notes, is less clear.

> In the private sector, activities such as patient counseling, patient education and screening are often viewed as peripheral activities that are provided only when resources allow. The activities do not produce revenue and are cut back when in competition with other revenue producing activities. Even when undertaken, the activities are often ill-planned and without support linkages to other facilities that may be needed.[3]

Public health is "what we, as a society, do collectively to assure the conditions in which people can be healthy."[4] Certainly in compliance with this definition the case can be made that all pharmacists already are involved in the delivery of public health. Spencer lists the following activities to detail the role of pharmacists in public health:

- Knowing disease patterns prevalent in neighborhoods
- Reporting accidental poisonings
- Referring patients to physicians
- Monitoring communicable disease patterns
- Assisting international travelers on medications
- Supporting chronic disease prevention
- Participating in community health education programs
- Participating in health planning activities
- Becoming acquainted with local public health department personnel
- Participating in family planning activities
- Becoming acquainted with local organizations helping people to lose weight
- Becoming alert to environmental conditions prevalent in the community
- Detecting potential suicides and seeking appropriate aid
- Advising local agencies about drug and alcohol abuse
- Participating in public health research[5]

Despite their continuous involvement in this list of activities, pharmacists do not envision themselves as public health pharmacists; they see themselves as providers of health to individual customers. As an example of this lack of empathy with public health, in the 30,000 plus membership ranks of the American Public Health Association (APHA), only 120 members are pharmacists.[6] The APHA categorizes the activities that pharmacists can provide to the public health arena as follows:

- Participate in health planning activities
- Contribute to personal health services delivery
- Counsel, educate, and screen patients
- Participate in legislative and regulatory processes
- Encourage formal education and training in public health[7]

A public health professional is a person educated in public health or a related discipline who is employed to improve health through a population focus.[8] The National Academy of Sciences recommends that this education be based upon an ecological model of health that assumes that health and well-being are affected by interaction among multiple determinants of health. Public health education traditionally has had five core components: epidemiology, biostatistics, environmental health, health services administration, and social and behavioral sciences. New areas of study that increasingly are becoming critical to public health practice include informatics, genomics, communication, cultural competency, community-based participatory research, policy and law, global health, and ethics.

Public health problems are not considered on an individual basis but rather in the context of a community as a whole. Bush and Johnson (1979) explain that medical education traditionally has been disease oriented; likewise, pharmacy education has focused on drugs that respond to the disease in question.

> Usually, health professionals study basic sciences and then learn by "practicing" those skills . . . under the guidance of role models. For pharmacy students, this traditionally has meant learning about the drug...as well as how to translate a doctor's order into a therapeutic product. When pharmacy students "practiced," there was not necessarily any interaction between the pharmacy student and patients. . . . As pharmacy education became more patient-oriented, students began to "practice" in clinical settings. . . . In this respect, pharmaceutical education began to resemble that of medicine, nursing, and dentistry. . . . However, medicine and nursing educators long ago recognized that the health education model . . . failed in public health, because of its inherent inability to take a population perspective.[9]

The pharmacist who actively practices as a public health provider is rare. As a result, relatively few public health pharmacists are available as role models. Unfortunately, this lack of focus on public health is not limited to the pharmaceutical profession. Nationally, it has been estimated that 80 percent of public health workers lack specific public health training and only 22 percent of chief executives of local health departments have graduate degrees in public health.[10] Most people who receive formal education in public health are graduates of one of the thirty-two accredited schools of public health or one of forty-five accredited master of public health programs. Although it is unclear exactly how many public health workers exist in the United States, it is estimated that about 450,000 people are employed in salaried positions in public health and an additional 2,850,000 volunteer their services.[11]

As health care continues to evolve from an orientation on diseases to an orientation on an informed patient, the delivery of that care continues to move from behind the forbidding walls of a fixed facility (i.e., hospital or clinic) to the community setting. Pharmacists are uniquely sited in the community to provide public health services and thus are uniquely positioned in their communities to be the focal point for health information.

In broad terms the role of the pharmacist in public health can be defined in micro terms of individual one-on-one relationships with patients and in macro terms of population care. Examples of the microlevel relationships include patient education, patient counseling, screening, and referral. Macrolevel activities include formulating policy, setting health priorities, identifying community health problems, management and administration, community education, and research and evaluation activities.[12]

At a microlevel, public health service usually involves a direct relationship with consumers; for example, a community pharmacist might speak to community groups about drug abuse, provide hypertension screening at the community pharmacy, or advise a customer on the selection of a prescription drug plan. Pharmacists increasingly are finding their customers more willing to accept counseling services on prescribed medications. At least one study concluded that pharmacists see as very important the health objectives of Healthy People 2010 that directly links the role of pharmacists to the prevention, detection, and control of hypertension, heart disease, stroke, cancer, diabetes, and disability conditions.[13] Pharmacists can be even more hands-on, with forty-one states now granting pharmacists the authority to administer immunizations.[14] Pharmacists can provide a community service by explaining to their customers how to apply for benefits and social services they are entitled to under federal, state, and local legislation.

Pharmacists who deliver public health services at the community (micro) level retain their professional identity as a pharmacist in the eyes of the public. At the macrolevel of health planning, evaluation, and administration, the identity of a pharmacist often is lost; this could be one reason why the practice of public health is overlooked as a career track for pharmacists. Pharmacy educators recognize, however, that it is at the macrolevel that financial incentives are introduced that influence the practice of pharmacy and public health. Pharmacists who are skilled at the macrolevel can plan systemic changes that influence the training of pharmacists, nurture interprofessional relationships, impact health economics, and assess consumer needs.

According to a 2000 report from National Pharmacist Workforce Survey, demand for pharmacists has greatly outstripped the supply, leading to drastic increases in wages and competition for the available pharmaceutical workers.[15] A mailing list from a national medical marketing database used in the survey contained 216,982 names of licensed pharmacists in the United States. The survey found that only 73.3 percent of pharmacist work full time (greater than thirty hours per week), with 14.9 percent working part time, and nearly 12 percent of licensed pharmacists not actively engaged in pharmacy practice. Those not actively engaged included 6.2 percent who were retired and 2.6 percent who were not working at all. More than half, 55.4 percent, of pharmacists practice in a community pharmacy setting, with most of the remainder serving in institutional settings. In the survey, public health was not identified as a work setting. No valid information is available to accurately assess the number of pharmacists engaged in public health; the information that is available leads to the conclusion that the number is miniscule.

Social pharmacology is emerging as a concept that provides significant compatibility with practice as a public health pharmacist. Social pharmacology is the study of drug product use in a modern society and of understanding how society actually uses medicines. It also is an operative system that integrates the interrelationships among health professionals. It strives to integrate the findings of different health professionals in order to maximize public health goals.[16]

This discipline builds on the foundation of clinical research, bringing together a broad collection of disciplines engaged in the evaluation, efficacy, safety, effectiveness, compliance, and consumption of resources associated with the use of pharmaceutical products. This moves pharmacy from the micro to the macro. Patients who are better informed about their health can make informed decisions about their health care needs, including their drugs. Placing this in context with public health provides a particular advantage for public health pharmacists who study all variables that affect drug use from a population perspective rather than on an individual basis. Venulet (1985) states that social pharmacology is "the ultimate step in the natural history of pharmacology in which the properties of a drug, its availability, doctor's prescribing patterns, patient's compliance, etc., combine and interact in a manner which determines the final effects of the therapeutic efforts."[17]

Through social pharmacology, pharmacists acknowledge that consumers have many different ways of thinking about health and hygiene, with different levels of understanding and different attitudes on the use of drugs in the recovery process from disease or injury. This discipline further helps pharmacists recognize that patient compliance with prescribed drug use is influenced by cultural and environmental factors, and indeed, use of a drug often is influenced by a consumer's ability to pay for the prescription. Alloza (2004) notes that "even though established regulations regarding the product have been observed and it has been prescribed and dispensed correctly, when a drug is used in the marketplace, its benefits and risks are very diverse. The conditions associated with this setting are completely different from those of the controlled drug development setting where rigorous scientific protocols are employed."[18]

Social pharmacology responds to the challenges bearing forth from a society whose customs, health, and education are changing daily through increased access to medical knowledge via electronic information flows, as well as an increased understanding of this knowledge. The call to the mission of public health is easier said then done. The definition—fulfilling society's interest in assuring conditions in which people can be healthy—encompasses all insults on the health of a population, ranging from global environment conditions to singular microcosmic attacks.[19] The enormity of this challenge contributes in large part to the disarray in which public health is organized and practiced in the United States. In a report to the nation on the future of public health, an Institute of Medicine committee reported:

> An impossible responsibility has been placed on America's public health agencies: to serve as stewards of the basic health needs of entire populations, but at the same time avert impending disasters and provide personal health care to those rejected by the rest of the health system. The wonder is not that American public health has problems, but that so much has been done so well, and with so little.[20]

The events of 9/11 and 10/15 have called public health to the forefront of our nation's preparedness and ability to respond to man-made attacks on our social structure. The response to Hurricane Katrina, or lack thereof, made even more vivid the need for a role for public health in responding to natural disasters. All Americans remember the 9/11 attacks on the World Trade Center and the mobilization of the public health infrastructure to deal with the crisis. Less visible in our collective memories are the 10/15 anthrax attacks at a U.S. Senate office building, which further highlighted the importance as well as the limitations of our public health system.

Anthrax may only be the tip of a bioterrorist iceberg. Even before the events of 10/15, bioterrorism was a concern, as evidenced by the sarin chemical attack in the Tokyo subway. The World Health Organization has called smallpox of the most devastating diseases known to humanity, and even though a vaccine can prevent or delay the development of symptoms, smallpox has no cure.[21]

Factors that facilitate the spread of infectious disease include population growth and urbanization; economic development, which brings humans closer to animal and insect carriers of disease; climate change; and a worldwide collapse of public health systems.[22] The global movement of goods and services also play a role.[23] With growing numbers of U.S. citizens traveling abroad and citizens of other countries entering the United States, the likelihood of exposure to infectious disease is increasing. The growth of imports, including food, adds to this problem.

Another factor is microbial resistance. Microbes develop an ability to resist drugs commonly used to treat them, a problem exacerbated by the widespread dissemination and indiscriminate use of antibiotics throughout the world.[24] International travelers might be exposed to resistant microbes in one country and carry them to other countries where resistance can spread. In the case of tuberculosis, failure to treat new cases facilitated the development of multidrug-resistant forms of the disease. [25]

The aging of the population also contributes the public health problem of infectious diseases. As Garrett (2000) noted, aging results in a natural reduction in immunity, which explains why influenza and pneumonia often are lethal infections in elders while the identical microbes may produce little more than a few days discomfort in young adults. [26]

The intentional use of biological or other dangerous pathogens represents a distinct threat to our society. The federal Department of Health and Human Services has been assigned a pivotal role in protecting our homeland from a bioterrorist attack, and even more important role in responding to health consequences of such an attack. Bioterrorism could take the form of biological attacks from smallpox, anthrax, or plague; or a bio attack on the nation's food or water infrastructure, such as with salmonella or cryptosporidium distributed via those systems; or chemical attacks from agents such as sarin or mustard gas. The challenge is to build upon the existing surveillance in order to effectively identify, prevent, mitigate, or control any attacks that impact the public health infrastructure. The Centers for Disease Control and Prevention (CDC) has developed a critical biological agents list so that plans can be made to respond to threats. During the 1990s, 120 cities were provided with federal funds to form a Metropolitan Medical Response System with the goal of implementing a coordinating system at the local level that would allow cities to respond immediately to any terrorist threat. In part, this system is an acknowledgement that in the case of bioterrorism medical personnel at the local level will be the first responders.

A key component of the public health infrastructure is the National Pharmaceutical Stockpile program. Through this program, drugs and medical supplies can be moved anywhere in the country within 12 hours. The Stockpile is jointly managed by the Centers for Disease Control and Prevention and the Department of Homeland Security. The stockpile program was created in 1999 to help states and cities respond to public health emergencies resulting from terrorist attacks or natural disasters. Under the program, prepackaged shipments of pharmaceuticals, medical supplies, and medical equipment are located throughout the United States for immediate deployment. These prepackaged shipments are organized into "push packs." Each push pack contains fifty tons of supplies and equipment, including eighty-four separate items ranging from antibiotics, to needles and IVs, to a tablet counting machine, to nerve agent antidotes. The twelve-hour push pack is designed to provide a range of support in the early hours of an emergency when the threat many not be well understood. In addition to the push packs, the stockpile includes additional supplies or drugs, such as smallpox vaccine, that can be distributed when a specific threat is identified. The push packs are further complemented by large quantities of pharmaceuticals stored in manufacturers' warehouses. This is called the vendor managed inventory (VMI). The VMI and push packs combined have enough drugs to treat two million people for inhalation anthrax following exposure.

States must be prepared with a cadre of health professionals who can break down the 130 containers that arrive in every push pack and then distribute the drugs and supplies. The also need adequate, climate-controlled facilities to store the drugs and supplies. A mass casualty event conceivably could require hundreds of nurses and pharmacists working around the clock to screen, vaccinate, or treat victims of a biological or chemical attack, and then provide follow-up care.

Within the Commissioned Corps of the United States Public Health Service (PHS), a cadre of 150 pharmacists is assigned to response rosters in readiness for deployment wherever needed. These pharmacists are trained on a wide variety of missions and have received intense training on every aspect of the National Pharmaceutical Stockpile.

Approximately 15.6 percent of the 6,000 member Commissioned Corps of the PHS are pharmacists. Many of these 930 pharmacists serve in traditional (micro) roles in providing pharmaceutical services to Indian tribes, prison clinics, and community health centers, but they also are found in large numbers in policy, planning, and evaluating (macro) roles within the Food and Drug Administration (FDA) and National Institutes of Health.

The USPHS originated with the passage of the Marine Hospital Act signed by President John Adams on July 16, 1798, that established hospitals to provide for "the temporary relief and maintenance of sick or disabled Seaman." This law provided for a tax on sailor's salaries to be used by the Secretary of the Treasury to construct locally controlled Marine hospitals to provide medical services to merchant seaman in American ports. The earliest marine hospitals were located along the East Coast, with Boston being the first site; later hospitals were established along inland waterways, the Great Lakes, and the Gulf and Pacific Coasts. In 1870 additional legislation reorganized these locally controlled hospitals into the centrally controlled Marine Hospital Service with its headquarters in Washington, DC.

The position of Supervising Surgeon was created to administer the Service; this position eventually became the Surgeon General of the United States. A military model was adopted, and officers were required to wear uniforms. The Commissioned Corps of the Marine Hospital Service, comprised of medical officers appointed by the president with the advice and consent of the Senate, was established by an act signed by President Grover Cleveland on January 4, 1889. At first open only to physicians, the Commissioned Corps has since expanded to include eleven categories of health professionals, including pharmacists. Other health professional categories include dentists, veterinarians, dietitians, scientists, nurses, sanitarians, engineers, and a "catch-all" category of health service professionals.

The scope of activities of the Marine Hospital Service began to expand well beyond the care of merchant seamen in the closing decades of the nineteenth century, beginning with control of infectious disease. Responsibility for quarantine originally was a function of the states rather than the federal government, but the National Quarantine Act of 1878 conferred quarantine authority on the Marine Hospital Service.

Responding to a dramatic increase in immigration, the federal government also took over from the states the processing of immigrants, beginning in 1891. The Marine Hospital Service was assigned the responsibility for medical inspection of arriving immigrants at sites such as Ellis Island in New York. Commissioned Officers played a major role in fulfilling the service's commitment to prevent disease from entering the country.

The name of the service was enlarged in 1902 to the Public Health and Marine Hospital Service. In 1912 Congress passed a law that changed the name of the service to the United States Public Health Service (PHS) and extended its authority to include investigation of all illnesses of man and his environment. PHS Commissioned Officers served their country by controlling the spread of contagious diseases such as smallpox and yellow fever, conducting important biomedical research, regulating food and drug supplies, providing health to underserved groups, supplying medical assistance in the aftermath of disasters, and numerous other public health interventions.

The functions and responsibilities of the PHS expanded rapidly during the 1940s. Beginning in 1944 with the passage of the Public Health Service Act, a series of laws were passed that affected the nation's medical research and training efforts significantly. The legislation included the National Mental Health Act (1946) and the National Heart Act (1948). The name of the National Institute of Health, established in 1930, was changed to the National Institutes of Health (NIH) to accommodate both the newly established National Heart Institute and the National Cancer Institute, established in 1937. In 1955 the Indian Health Service was transferred from the Department of the Interior to PHS.

The PHS is commanded by the Surgeon General of the United States. The Surgeon General reports to the Assistant Secretary for Health, and together they advise the secretary of the federal Department of Health and Human Services on health and health-related matters. The PHS has about 6,000 Commissioned Corps officers and approximately 51,000 civil service employees.

The PHS is comprised of eight major agencies—the Centers for Disease Control and Prevention (CDC), the Agency for Toxic Substances and Disease Registry (ATSDR), the National Institutes of Health (NIH), the Food and Drug Administration (FDA), the Substance Abuse and Mental Health Services Administration (SAMHSA), the Health Resources and Services Administration (HRSA), the Agency for Healthcare Research and Quality (AHRQ) (formerly the Agency for Health Care Policy and Research [AHCPR]), and the Indian Health Service (IHS).

About half of all PHS pharmacists, numbering 438, serve with the Indian Health Service; 242 PHS pharmacists have assignments with the FDA; and 133 serve in clinics of the Federal Bureau of Prisons. Those PHS pharmacists who provided clinical support, as well as other pharmacists serving within the federal government, obtain their pharmaceutical supplies from a centralized source that also is supported by PHS pharmacists.

The U.S. Department of Health and Human Services Supply Service Center (HHS SSC) located at Perry Point, Maryland, serves as the worldwide source for federal health care facilities for pharmaceutical, medical, and dental supplies. The mission of the HHS Supply Service Center is to implement and manage a quality, timely, reliable, and cost-effective supply system. The HHS SSC is the only FDA-licensed pharmaceutical repackaging facility operated by the federal government that distributes products to several different federal agencies.

The HHS Service Supply Center came about through an executive order issued by President Warren G. Harding on April 29, 1922, that turned over a number of PHS hospitals to the newly created Veterans Administration. Buildings and supplies at the USPHS Purveying Depots were allocated between the Public Health Service and VA, based upon their future needs. As a result of this action, all PHS supply operations were consolidated into several buildings on the grounds of the Veterans Administration in Perry Point and renamed the PHS Supply Station. This has evolved into the HHS Supply Service Center which provides a full service supply, warehouse, and distribution center for pharmaceutical, hospital, medical, and dental supplies and special program needs. Logistical support is offered worldwide in concert with technical assistance and material management support.

The HHS Service Supply Center provides more than two hundred different solid and oral dosage unit-of-use pharmaceutical prepacks to a variety of federal customers including NIH, Department of Defense, Indian Health Service, Veterans Affairs, Peace Corps, and State Department embassies. Federal facilities that purchase over-the-counter medications repackaged by the HHS SSC dispense these medications only on receipt of a valid order from a licensed health care practitioner. The products are convenient, prescription size, patient-ready units labeled for direct distribution to patient by health care providers. All packaging is accomplished using state-of-the-art equipment operated by experienced personnel who follow standard industry and FDA approved methods for receiving, sampling, testing, accepting, and repackaging of all supplies. More than 9.3 million unit-of-use prepacks were produced in fiscal year 2004.

The HHS Supply Service Center also provides a comprehensive program for supporting clinical trials. The center provides technical assistance, inventory management, and logistical support to meet the packaging and distribution requirements of clinical drug trials. All services are provided in cooperation and sponsorship with the National Institutes of Health and other federal agencies.

Satisfying the public health challenges of the twenty-first century will require close cooperation of all disciplines within the medical, scientific, and public health communities. The primary focus of U.S. health efforts in the last century was on scientific advances tailored to the individual, and particularly to manifest diseases. As a result, most investments in capacity building had paralleled the dominance of this biomedical model, with public (mostly federal) dollars directed at capital investments in hospitals and medical schools, and on research activities on these issues in academic medical centers. Investments in population-based or public health capacity building have lagged behind.

Increasingly the prevalent crisis impacting the health care agenda are population based. Health problems are vast and costly. Scientific and methodological updates arrive daily. Health information flows freely to providers and consumers alike and expands exponentially. Consequently, the traditional distinctions between medicine and public health are disappearing. All health care providers need to become more aware of the impact of the population health upon individual practices from threats of bioterrorism, cost constraints, and the rising interest in health promotion and disease prevention among the population at large. In response to these changes, it is essential that the core curriculum of pharmacy education includes basic public health practices. Public health pharmacists must emerge from this mist.

NOTES

1. Asghar, M.N, Jackson, C., and Corbett, J. (2002). Specialist pharmacists in public health: Are they the missing link in England? *The Pharmaceutical Journal* 268: 22-25.

2. Canadian Conference on Counter-Terrorism and Public Health: Final Report (2004). *Canadian Journal of Public Health* 95(2): C1. Ottawa: March/April.

3. Moore, S.R. (1998). Pharmacy in the public health arena. *The Carolina Journal of Pharmacy* Available at: http://www.hhs.gov/pharmacy/phpharm/pub4.html.

4. Institute of Medicine (1998). *The Future of Public Health*. Washington, DC: Institute of Medicine, p. 8.

5. Spencer, F.J. (1980). The pharmacist and public health. In Osul, A (ed.), *Remington's Pharmaceutical Sciences,* 16th edition (pp. 1667-1676). Easton, PA: Mack Publishing Company.

6. American Public Health Association, membership division, telephone call (202-777-2491). January 26, 2006.

7. The role of the pharmacist in public health (1981). *American Journal of Public Health* 71: 213-216.

8. National Academy of Sciences (2003). Who will keep the public healthy? *Educating Public Health Professionals for the 21st century.* Washington, DC: NAS.

9. Bush. P.J. and Johnson, K.W. (1979). Where is the public health pharmacist? *Am J. Pharm Educ* 43: 249-252, p. 250.

10. National Academy of Sciences (2003), p. 51.

11. Center for Health Policy (2000). *The Public Health Workforce: Enumeration 2000.* New York: Columbia University School of Nursing.

12. Bush and Johnson (1979).

13. Suh, D. et al. (2002). Pharmacists' perceptions of healthy people goals in economically stressed cities. *Journal of Community Health* 27(2): 133. New York: April.

14. American Pharmacists Association (n.d.) Fact sheet. Available at: http://www.aphanet.org/pharmcare/immunofact.html.

15. Pedersen, C.A., Doucette, W.R., Gaither, C.A., Mott, D.A., and Schommer J.C. (2000). Final Report of the National Pharmacist Workforce: 2000. Midwest Pharmacy Workforce Research Consortium. Alexandria, VA: American Association of Colleges of Pharmacy.

16. Alloza, J.L. (2004). Social pharmacology: Conceptual remarks. *Drug Information Journal* 38(4): 321-330.

17. Venulet, J. (1985). Towards social pharmacology. In Alloza J.L. (ed.), *Clinical and Social Pharmacology: Postmarketing Period* (pp. 129-139). Aulendorf, Germany: Editio Cantor.

18. Alloza (2004).

19. Institute of Medicine (1988), p. 8.

20. Institute of Medicine (1988), p. 2.

21. World Health Organization (2001). Small pox: Historical significance. Available at: http://www.who.int/mediacentre/factsheets/smallpox/en/.

22. National Intelligence Council (2000). The global infectious disease threat and its implications for the United States. Available at: www.odci.gov/nic/pubs/other_products/inf_diseases_paper.html.

23. Kassalow, J.S. (2001). *Why Health Is Important to U.S. Foreign Policy.* New York: Council on Foreign Relations and Milbank Memorial Fund.

24. Ryan, F. (1997). *Virus X: Tracking the New Killer Plagues.* Boston: Little, Brown.

25. Farmer, P. (1999). *Infections and Inequalities: The Modern Plagues.* Berkeley, CA: University of California Press.

26. Garrett, L. (2000). *Betrayal of Trust: The Collapse of Global Public Health.* New York: Hyperion.

Chapter 8

Department of Veterans Affairs Pharmacy Programs

Michael A. Valentino
Jonathan B. Perlin

DEPARTMENT OVERVIEW

The Department of Veterans Affairs (VA) was established on March 15, 1989, succeeding the Veterans Administration.[1] The Department is responsible for providing federal benefits to veterans and their families—meeting the challenge President Abraham Lincoln laid out for the nation in 1865 "to care for him who shall have borne the battle, and for his widow, and his orphan." VA is the second largest of the fifteen U.S. cabinet departments, and operates nationwide programs for health care, financial assistance, and burial benefits. Of the 24.8 million veterans alive in early 2006, nearly three-quarters served during a war or an official period of conflict. About a quarter of the nation's population, approximately 63 million people, are potentially eligible for VA benefits and services because they are veterans or family members or survivors of veterans.

The most visible of all VA benefits and services is health care. From fifty-four hospitals in 1930, VA's health care system, managed by the Veterans Health Administration (VHA) now includes 154 medical centers, with at least one in each state, Puerto Rico, and the District of Columbia. VA operates nearly 1,400 sites of care, including 887 ambulatory care and community-based outpatient clinics, 134 nursing homes, 42 residential rehabilitation treatment programs, and 206 vet centers. VA's health care facilities provide a broad spectrum of medical, surgical, and rehabilitative care. VHA's expenses exceed $30 billion annually, and it supports about 198,000 employees, about 10,000 fewer than in 1995.

In fiscal year 2005, more than 5.3 million people received care in VA health care facilities. In that same year, VHA inpatient facilities treated nearly 586,000 patients, and outpatient clinics registered 57.5 million visits. VHA manages the largest medical education and health professions training program in the United States. The agency's facilities are affiliated with 107 medical schools, 55 dental schools, and more than 1,200 other schools across the nation. In 2005, more than 92,000 health professionals were trained in VA medical centers. More than half of the physicians practicing in the United States received some of their professional education in VA's health care system.[2]

VA's medical system serves as a backup to the Department of Defense during national emergencies and as a federal support organization during major disasters, such as 2005's Hurricane Katrina.

To receive VA health care benefits, most veterans must enroll. VHA's health care system had 7.7 million enrollees as of October 2005. When they enroll, they are placed in priority groups or categories that help the agency manage health care services within budgetary constraints and ensure that those enrolled receive the highest quality care.

Since 1979, VHA has operated Vet Centers, which provide psychological counseling for war-related trauma, community outreach, case management and referral activities, and supportive social services to veterans and family members. Vet Centers are open to any veteran who served in the military in a combat theater during wartime, or anywhere during a period of armed hostilities.

While providing high quality health care to America's veterans, VHA also conducts an array of research on some of the most difficult challenges facing medical science today. VA is a world leader in such research areas as aging, women's health, AIDS, post-traumatic stress disorder, and other mental health issues. VA researchers played key roles in developing the cardiac pacemaker, the CT scan, radioimmunoassay, and in improvements in artificial limbs.

VHA receives most of its funding from Congress, through annual authorizing legislation that serves as the basis for operating the administration, and provides guidance to the House and Senate Appropriations Committees as to appropriate levels of funding for its services. Until the mid-1990s, VA operated largely as a hospital system providing general medical and surgical services, specialized care in mental health and spinal cord injury, and long-term care through directly operated or indirectly supported facilities. Medical centers and other facilities operated relatively independently of one another, even competitively duplicating services. Anachronistic laws required that virtually all of VA's health care services should be provided in hospitals—which ran counter to changes in the remainder of the health care industry, which had already begun to move most care into the ambulatory environment.

In 1996, the Veterans Health Care Eligibility Reform Act was passed, enabling the VA system to be restructured from a hospital system to a health care system. The changes that followed were predicated on the assumption that providing effective, efficient care required coordination among VA's facilities, and that resources should be used synergistically—including the requirement that care to veterans be provided in the most appropriate environment. To accomplish this task, VA created twenty-two (now twenty-one) geographically defined Veterans Integrated Service Networks (VISNs). These networks allowed VA to redirect its resources in two ways: first, to follow the veteran population, which was shifting from the Northeast and Midwest to the Sun Belt and elsewhere; and second, to allow resources to be allocated to networks instead of facilities. This allowed VHA to create financial incentives to coordinate care and resources among facilities that previously competed with one another.

Relief from the requirement to operate a hospital-based system and the new network system allowed the agency to shift care from hospitals to ambulatory-care facilities and the home environment, which in turn enabled the reduction of authorized hospital and long-term care beds from 92,000 to 53,000. As hospitalizations decreased (from 900,000 in 1995 to 586,000 in 2005), outpatient visits and home care services increased (from 26 million in 1995 to 57 million in 2005), and the number of patients treated annually nearly doubled, from 2.8 million to 5.3 million.

Despite this large increase in number of patients, the cost of care per patient actually decreased by 0.2 percent over the ten year period—or $10 per patient per year. In 1996, VHA spent about the same amount per patient as Medicare did, but by 2004 the unchanged rate of spending per patient was nearly 25 percent lower than Medicare's cost. The 64 percent increase in the number of patients seen came at the cost of only a 32 percent increase in the total budget—and the number of employees per 1,000 patients was reduced by 37 percent.

It should be noted that VA's patients are older (49 percent are over age sixty-five, with a rapidly increasing population of veterans eighty-five and above); sicker (with an average of three additional non-mental-health diagnoses and one additional mental-health diagnosis than other age-matched Americans); and poorer (70 percent have annual incomes below $26,000, and 40 percent below $16,000) than their fellow citizens. The demographics of VA's patient base are changing as well. Currently, about 4.5 percent of VHA's patients are women; however, with the increasing numbers of women in the military (about 14 percent of the total force), this percentage will increase rapidly in the years ahead. Yet the care VA patients receive in many ways outshines that provided by any other caregiver. A 2004 study by the Rand Corporation concluded that "overall, VHA patients receive better care than patients in other settings." VA sets the benchmark for eighteen of eighteen comparable indicators of care, including breast, cervical, and colorectal cancer screenings; pneumonia and influenza immunizations; and a host of diabetes examinations. And for the past six years, VA's scores on the American Customer Satisfaction Index have been significantly better than the private health sector average, with particularly high "customer loyalty" and "customer service" scores.

VHA's expectation is that every veteran will be offered safe, effective, efficient, and compassionate care, without the need to resort to a patient advocate. Safety is fundamental in VHA, but patients require more than safety in their health care—they expect their caregivers to be effective in maintaining and improving their health, in managing the course of their diseases, and in alleviating their pain and suffering. They expect VHA to be efficient in the use of taxpayers' funding, in reducing waste, and in using its resources for maximal benefit. Finally, they expect their care to be patient-centered, so that the patient or his or her caregiver is at the center of all decisions; coordinated, so that from the home to the clinic to the hospital, care is provided seamlessly; integrated among disease-specific, general health and social needs; and anticipatory, so that risks can be modified and avoided, even before traditional risk factors manifest themselves. VHA's goals are simple: to avoid making mistakes in patient care, to consistently make the right decisions in maintaining and improving the health of patients, to make the best possible use of its resources, and to provide care that is predictive and integrated, and delivered in the time, place, and manner that the patient prefers.

VHA operates with both formal external and internal accountability for performance. Measurements are developed by using an evidence-based approach for both medicine and administrative issues. Clinical performance measures generally determine compliance with evidence-based clinical guidelines or other recommendations in the areas of preventive medicine, disease treatment, and palliative care. VHA also reconciles data in the areas of patient satisfaction, access to care, and improvement of function, community health, and cost-effectiveness, which are called "domains of value." All help to care for veterans, and to help them move forward in a meaningful way.

A central strategy in accomplishing VHA's goals is the use of information technology. Automated information systems have provided extensive clinical and administrative capabilities in all medical facilities since 1985, when a decentralized hospital computer program began operating. VHA's computerized patient record system (CPRS) provides a single, highly graphical interface for health care providers to review and update patients' medical records and to place orders for various items including medications, procedures, X-rays and imaging, patient care nursing orders, diets, and laboratory tests. Today, this system is fully operational at all VA sites of care. Vista imaging now provides a multimedia, online patient record that integrates traditional medical chart information with medical images of all kinds, and it is now operational at all facilities.

CPRS has other capabilities to support improvements in performance, including computerized provider order entry, clinical alerts, the ability to view data remotely from other facilities, and a clinical reminder system that provides real-time decision support. In addition, VHA is currently (in 2006) transforming the architecture underlying its health information systems to more effectively serve the needs of patients, providers, and the health system. The new architectural strategy, known as HealtheVet, fully integrates a health data repository with registration systems, provider systems, management and financial systems, and information and education systems.

This data repository creates a true longitudinal health care record that includes data from VA and non–VA sources, supports research and population analyses, improves data quality and security, and facilitates patient access to data and health administration. Today, a secure patient portal known as My HealtheVet provides patients access to their personal health record, online health assessment tools, mechanisms for prescription refills and making appointments, and access to high-quality consumer health information. The consumer information is evidence-based, consistent with clinical practice guideline recommendations and, ideally, inspires patients to participate in their own health care.

As of this writing, testing is being done that will provide veterans with copies of key parts of their own VA health record. By sharing health information, patients will be activated and empowered as responsible partners with health care providers in achieving optimal health.

MyHealtheVet is part of VHA's effort to make the patient the locus of control of his or her own health care, and to make the experience of care seamless across the various environments in which it is provided, including not only the hospital and clinic, but also the patient's home, workplace, and community. Patient-centered care coordination extends the focus of disease management to better and more efficiently integrate every patient's disease-specific and general health needs with the resources of the health system.

VHA's approach to care coordination uses technology to support patients' ability to successfully age and manage disease in their own homes. Using electronic health records as a foundation, advanced technologies now enable patients to be seen just in time, instead of just in case. For example, a patient with heart failure can enter his daily weight from home for review by a care coordinator. Should his weight exceed a clinical threshold, he would then be called to visit a clinic, or even be visited at home. This enables him to be seen just as he begins to retain fluid, instead of on an arbitrary schedule that is likely to fail to identify an impending crisis.

PHARMACY PRACTICE

The Department of Veterans Affairs offers a broad scope of pharmacy services across all patient care settings. With the exception of some of its community based outpatient clinics (CBOCs), VA operates pharmacies and provides pharmacy services in all of its medical care facilities. In addition, VA operates seven large, highly automated consolidated mail outpatient pharmacies (CMOPs), where prescriptions originating at VA medical care facilities can be filled.

Approximately 5,200 pharmacists and 3,300 pharmacy technicians deliver cognitive and distributive pharmacy services to 4.3 million geographically dispersed veterans.[3] VA pharmacists practice in the inpatient, outpatient, extended care, and home care settings, and many are able to provide direct care under a scope of practice authorized by the medical staff. Specific activities authorized under these scopes of practice vary across the system, but can commonly include initiation of drug therapy, monitoring drug therapy via ordering and interpretation of laboratory tests, continuation of drug therapy (extending expired prescriptions), discontinuation of drug therapy, and dose titration and adjustment.

In the outpatient setting, VA pharmacists deliver care through both primary care and specialty care clinics. In primary care, VA pharmacists are fully integrated in VA's primary care delivery model, conducting prospective and concurrent pharmacy therapy reviews, making recommendations and/or implementing medication therapy changes under a scope of practice agreement. In addition, VA pharmacists have assumed very active and leadership roles in focused clinics, such as anticoagulation clinics, lipid clinics, and a variety of other clinics designed to deliver focused care for drug-therapy-intensive disease states. It is estimated that greater than 90 percent of VA's dedicated anticoagulation clinics are pharmacist managed, where the pharmacist assumes complete responsibility for achieving the primary care or specialty care physician's anticoagulation goals.

DRUG BENEFIT DESIGN

VA offers more than 1,250 molecular entities and a large number of medical/surgical supply items and prosthetic supplies through its National Formulary.[4] These molecular entities include legend drugs, over-the-counter drugs as well as biological products, and in some cases, drug-containing medical devices. VA's National Formulary (VANF) is a "core" formulary in that the drugs listed *must* be made available through all VA medical treatment facilities. Individual regional delivery systems (VISNs) may add additional drugs to their VISN formularies, except in classes that are closed through national standardization contracts (e.g., statins, angiotensin receptor blockers, etc.).

To provide an affordable and comprehensive prescription drug benefit, VA uses generic substitution, therapeutic substitution, mandatory national standardization for high-cost and high-volume branded drugs, and evidence-based utilization management. VA patients pay $8 for each thirty-day supply of medication, regardless of the cost of the drug, or its legend or over-the-counter status. Some veterans are exempt from copayments by virtue of their military service, income, or other factors. In 2005, VA dispensed more than 231 million thirty-day equivalent prescriptions (81 percent via VA's CMOP home delivery pharmacies) at a drug ingredient cost of $3.4 billion.

FORMULARY MANAGEMENT

Prescription drugs constitute a large percentage of the country's overall health care spending.[5] Many U.S. citizens receive pharmaceuticals through some form of pharmacy benefits management to help achieve cost-effective and high quality pharmaceutical care. By necessity, VA is a leader in the pharmaceutical benefit management (PBM) movement, having the responsibility to provide all "needed" care to enrolled patients under Public Law 104-262, the Veterans' Health Care Eligibility Reform Act of 1996.[6]

VA offers a broad array of pharmacy benefits to its patient population, and similar to many other health care organizations, has seen its pharmaceutical expenditures rise in recent years. Drug expenditures in fiscal year (FY) 2005 increased to $3.4 billion dollars from $1.6 billion in 1999, largely driven by rising enrollment of new patients. To cope with the increased use of pharmaceuticals, VA implemented a national pharmacy benefits management program in 1995 to (1) reduce geographic variability of access to pharmaceuticals across the system, (2) improve the distribution of pharmaceutical agents, (3) promote appropriate drug therapy, (4) reduce inventory carrying and drug acquisition costs, (5) promote improvements in drug-related patient safety issues, and (6) design and carry out drug outcomes assessment projects.

EVOLUTION OF THE VA FORMULARY PROCESS

Prior to 1995, each of VA's more than 170 individual VA facilities managed its own pharmaceutical coverage via local pharmacy and therapeutics (P & T) committees. The VA Headquarters Drug Product and Pharmaceuticals Management (DPPM) division, based in Hines, Illinois, managed and monitored drug usage and purchasing options for those facilities, but had no utilization oversight responsibilities. In September 1995, Dr. Kenneth Kizer, then VA's Under Secretary for Health, established the VA Pharmacy Benefits Management Strategic Healthcare Group (PBM), directing it to develop and implement a national formulary; manage pharmaceutical costs, utilization, and related outcomes; and oversee pharmacologic guideline development of common diseases within the VA system. To do so, clinical pharmacists employed at DPPM headquarters collaborated with a newly established consultative body of eleven field-based VA physicians and VA clinical pharmacist specialists, called the VA Medical Advisory Panel (MAP).

Formulary decisions fall under the purview of two groups: the MAP and the Veterans Integrated Service Network (VISN) Formulary Leaders (VFLs). The VFLs are pharmacy leaders that manage the pharmacy benefit for VA's twenty-one regional care systems. Each VISN includes a variety of health care centers, such as tertiary facilities, ambulatory care centers, and associated community clinics. Under the oversight of the VFLs, each VISN's formulary committee collaborates with the P & T committees of its health care centers to allow for integrated multilevel decision making. Thus, VISNs and local facilities can communicate and provide guidance to the PBM, and vice versa, on policies determining drug use within the VA system.

Implementing the Veterans Health Administration National Formulary (VANF) evoked considerable scrutiny from stakeholders, and a series of hearings at the congressional level ensued. In 1999 and 2000, the Senate and House Committees on Veteran Affairs each requested an outside review of the National Formulary from the Institute of Medicine (IOM), and the United States Government Accountability Office (GAO) respectively to assess the clinical and economic integrity of the VANF and the formulary management process.

The IOM report, released in 2001, concluded that the VANF was not "overly restrictive" with respect to "formulary size and quality, coverage of drugs in different classes, timeliness of new drug additions, fairness and responsiveness of the non-formulary exceptions process, and sensitivity of therapeutic interchange policies and procedures."[7] According to this report, within its first two years, the VANF saved approximately $100 million via its closed and preferred drug classes.[8] Per the IOM report, during July 1997 to July 1999, only 0.4 percent (2,385 out of 570,937) of all complaints to patient representatives about VA involved a pharmacy issue.[9] A second study, conducted by the GAO, noted that VANF drugs accounted for 90 percent of outpatient prescriptions dispensed between October 1999 and March 2000 and that the VANF met veterans' needs.[10,11]

Both reports had recommendations for improved processes in the areas of use of nonformulary drugs and therapeutic interchange policy. VA acknowledged that changes needed to be made to its rapidly evolving formulary management processes, and in many cases, efforts to make those changes predated the IOM and GAO reviews. These changes included eliminating local facility formularies, eliminating a one year moratorium on adding new molecular entities (NMEs) to the VA National Formulary, taking steps to reduce variation across the system regarding the addition of new products, and conducting timely system-wide reviews of all newly approved NMEs. Last, the PBM began to develop an expanded research/outcomes assessment agenda to measure the effects of the VANF on patient outcomes and safety.

STANDARDIZATION CONTRACTING

By competitively sourcing branded products within a given drug classes, VA achieved nearly $1.9 billion in drug acquisition costs savings from 1999 through 2004. Standardization contracts have a compelling effect on adherence in the VA. After awarding a national standardization contract, VISNs encourage providers to switch to the contracted agent if clinically appropriate. This, in turn, leads to significant drug acquisition cost savings. As an example, after competitive bidding for proton-pump inhibitors (PPI) in 2001, 95 percent of patients switched to the contracted agent within six months. Patients tolerated this switch well, with only 5 percent needing another PPI due to suboptimal response or intolerance. This therapeutic interchange generated over $45 million in cost savings in FY 2001.

Through careful competitive bidding and other cost effectiveness measures (such as promoting use of generic drugs and the most cost-effective branded drugs whenever clinically possible), according to internal VA data, the average acquisition cost per thirty-day fill for drugs and the average outpatient drug ingredient cost per patient have remained relatively stable for approximately seven years. (See Figures 8.1 and 8.2.)

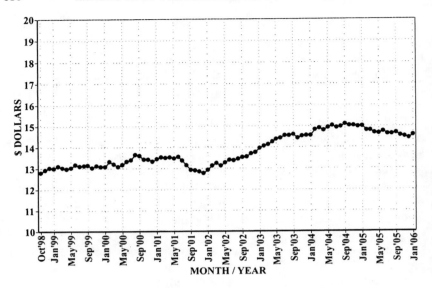

FIGURE 8.1. Average cost per thirty-day equivalent prescription in the Department of Veterans Affairs—October 1998 through January 2006.

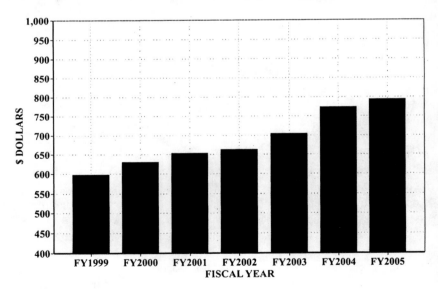

FIGURE 8.2. Average drug ingredient cost per pharmacy user per fiscal year—fiscal years 1999 through 2005.

Evidence-Based Reviews

One of the first issues addressed by PBM was to develop pharmacologic management guidelines for the most prevalent and most costly disease states observed in the VA population.[12] These clinical documents and algorithms of drug use initiated by the PBM rely on a process of peer review by the MAP, VFLs, and field-based experts (therapeutic advisory groups). The finalized drug and disease-state policies, together with utilization statistics from its national prescription utilization database, assist VA in advancing its national purchasing power to contract for quality drug products at competitive prices and to help assure equal access to specific drugs, for specific conditions. The PBM posts are available for general use and can be found on the PBM Web site.[13] PBM clinical pharmacists regularly monitor these drug-use documents, and updates occur according to PBM directors and advisors and VA health care system needs on an as-needed basis as new information become available in published, peer-reviewed literature.

OUTCOMES ASSESSMENT

Early in VA's formulary evolution process it became apparent that assessments of past formulary decisions were needed to (1) gain credibility among providers and oversight bodies for decision-making quality and (2) to make improvements in medication-related patient safety issues. It was further realized that using existing data to prospectively evaluate the likely impact of anticipated formulary decisions would be superior to retrospective analyses. By virtue of a relatively closed health care delivery model and the ubiquitous use of an advanced electronic medical record (EMR) system, VA was able to undertake formal assessmen·s of its past and future formulary initiatives.

Over time, PBM developed and improved its ability to conduct outcomes assessment and research to support and reinforce formulary and policy decisions in a variety of ways. Most outcomes assessment addresses quality improvement (QI) and patient safety initiatives using a pharmacy database developed by the PBM. This patient/provider-specific database includes information on all outpatient drugs dispensed from any VA pharmacy and provides a detailed profile of medications, dosing, quantities, and drug costs. Prescription use can be tracked on a macro (national, VISN, or facility) or micro (individual patient and provider) level. Furthermore, when required, merging this data with larger VA administrative and clinical databases can provide further information such as diagnosis, hospitalization, comorbidity, and laboratory data. In addition, the PBM utilizes data management software (ProClarity Professional, version 5.0) to create views of relational pharmacy databases, allowing quick queries of data on selected pharmaceuticals for questions requiring urgent responses.

Within VA, the PBM has spearheaded the nationwide monitoring and management of clinical pharmacy and pharmacy-related patient outcomes. The PBM's outcomes research group designs formal research evaluations looking at safety, appropriateness of use, effectiveness, and cost-effectiveness of prescription drugs in the veteran population for retrospective, real-time, and prospective analyses. PBM has published several quality improvement efforts in this regard.[14-26]

PATIENT SAFETY

VA is a recognized leader in patient safety, having undergone a transformational cultural change from punishment to prevention.[27] In addition to the medical error philosophical changes underway within VA and the careful data collection and analysis necessary for the reduction of medical errors, VA is also a leader in the deployment of technology to reduce the risk of medical errors. Through the ubiquitous use of its innovative electronic medical record (EMR), VA clinical and informatics staff have in many ways been the vanguard of EMR–based patient safety and clinical quality improvement efforts. Pace-setting improvements in drug-related safety is also occurring within VA pharmacy, where major system improvements have been achieved with the pioneering use of a system-wide bar-code medication administration (BCMA) system.[28] When used as designed, VA's BCMA system has the potential to virtually eliminate medication administration errors in the inpatient setting.

VA pharmacists also developed a highly automated home delivery pharmacy CMOP system in the early 1990s. Almost immediately and for several years after implementation, VA's CMOPs served as *the* home delivery system prototype in both the public and private sectors in the United States and abroad. VA CMOP continues to evolve in regard to efficiency and safety and is operating very near the six sigma threshold for accuracy. Additional improvements are currently being deployed that could further increase VA CMOP accuracy.

VA is in the third year of a five year $100 million project to update its computerized pharmacy software applications (Pharmacy Reengineering project or PRE). The PRE project is designed to take patient-specific information already available in the EMR and use it to guide drug therapy decision support at the point of prescribing. When PRE is fully deployed, prescribers will receive drug therapy recommendations based on information already on file, such as age, height, weight, gender, diagnoses, current drug therapy, laboratory data, etc.

EDUCATION AND TRAINING

VA's medical education program began in the post-war years of World War II. By forming affiliations with medical schools and universities, VA has become the largest provider of health care training in the United States. VA's graduate medical education (GME) is conducted through affiliations with university schools of medicine. Currently 130 VHA medical facilities are affiliated with 107 of the nation's 126 medical schools. Through these partnerships, almost 28,000 medical residents and 16,000 medical students receive some of their training in VA every year. Accounting for approximately 9 percent of U.S. GME, VA supports 8,800 physician resident positions in almost 2,000 residency programs accredited in the name of our university partners. VA physician faculty have joint appointments at the university and at VA, seeing patients at VA, supervising students and residents, and conducting research. It would be difficult for VA to deliver its high quality patient care without the physician staff and residents who are available through these affiliations.[29]

VA has been a leader in the training of associated health professionals as well. Through affiliations with individual health professions schools and colleges, clinical traineeships and fellowships are provided to students in more than 40 professions, including nurses, pharmacists, dentists, audiologists, dietitians, social workers, psychologists, physical therapists, optometrists, podiatrists, physician assistants, respiratory therapists, and nurse practitioners. More than 32,000 associated health students receive training in VA facilities each year, and provide a valuable recruitment source for new employees. The greatest majority (90 percent) of associated health trainees receive clinical experiences on a without-compensation (WOC) basis. Student funding support of approximately $38.8 million is provided each year to more than 3,000 trainees in the disciplines listed in Table 8.1. For additional information regarding without-compensation or funded trainee positions, contact the education office or the clinical discipline office at the desired VA facility.[30]

For 2007, VA will have a total of 343 pharmacy residency and fellowship positions and expects to train an additional 3,200 pharmacy students. Twenty seven of VA's 2007 residency positions will be funded through seventeen of its twenty-one Geriatric Research, Education and Clinical Centers (GRECC).[31] VA offers a small number of fellowships in the areas of pharmacoeconomics, palliative care, and patient safety. Additional pharmacy fellowships in pharmacy automation, pharmacy information technology, pharmacoepidemiology, pharmacy administration, and war-related illness and injury are being considered.

NOTES

1. Department of Veterans Affairs (2006). Facts About the Department of Veterans Affairs. Washington, DC: Department of Veterans Affairs. Available at: http://www1.va .gov/opa/fact/docs/vafacts.doc. Accessed March 27, 2006.

2. Department of Veterans Affairs (2006). Facts About the Department of Veterans Affairs. Washington, DC: Department of Veterans Affairs. Available at: http://www1.va .gov/opa/fact/docs/vafacts.doc. Accessed March 27, 2006.

3. Department of Veterans Affairs (2006). Facilities Locator Website. Washington, DC: Department of Veterans Affairs. Available at: http://www1.va.gov/directory/guide/ home.asp?isFlash=1. Accessed March 27, 2006.

4. Department of Veterans Affairs (2006). Pharmacy Benefits Management Strategic Healthcare Group. Washington, DC: Department of Veterans Affairs. Available at: http:// www.pbm.va.gov/PBM/menu.asp. Accessed March 27, 2006.

5. Emigh RC (ed.) (2002). *Novartis Pharmacy Benefit Report: Facts and Figures.* East Hanover, NJ: Novartis.

6. Department of Veterans Affairs (2006). Enrollment in VA's Healthcare System: Benefits. Washington, DC: Department of Veterans Affairs.   Available at: http://www.va.gov/elig/page.cfm?pg=3. Accessed March 27, 2006.

7. Blumenthal, D and Herdman R (eds.) (2000). *Description and Analysis of the VA National Formulary.* Institue of Medicine. Washington, DC: National Academies Press.

8. Blumenthal, D and Herdman R (eds.) (2000).

9. Blumenthal, D and Herdman R (eds.) (2000).

10. General Accounting Office (2001). VA Drug Formulary: Better Oversight is Required, but Veterans are Getting Needed Drugs (GAO-01-183). January. Available at: http://www.gao.gov/new.items/d01183.pdf. Accessed March 27, 2006.

11. General Accounting Office (2000). VA Health Care: VA's Management of Drugs on Its National Formulary (GAO/HEHS-00-34). Washington, DC. Available at: http://www.gao.gov/archive/2000/he00034.pdf. Accessed March 27, 2006.

12. Department of Veterans Affairs (2006). Pharmacy Benefits Management Strategic Healthcare Group.

13. Department of Veterans Affairs (2006). Pharmacy Benefits Management Strategic Healthcare Group.

14. Department of Veterans Affairs (2006). Pharmacy Benefits Management Strategic Healthcare Group.

15. Glassman PA, Good CB, Kelley ME, Bradley M, Valentino M, Ogden J, Kizer KW (2001). Physician Perceptions of a National Formulary. *Am J Manag Care* 7(3): 241-251.

16. Glassman PA, Good CB, Kelley ME, Bradley M, Valentino M (2004). Physician Satisfaction with Formulary Policies: Is It Access to Formulary or Nonformulary Drugs that Matters Most? *Am J Manag Care* 10(3): 209-216.

17. Burk M, Furmaga E, Dong D, Cunningham F (2004). Multicenter Drug Use Evaluation of Tamsulosin and Availability of Guidance Criteria for Nonformulary Use in the Veterans Affairs Health System. *J Manag Care Pharm.* 10(5): 423-432.

18. Burk M, Morreale AP, Cunningham F (2004). Conversion from Troglitazone to Rosiglitazone or Pioglitazone in the VA: A Multicenter DUE. *Formulary* 39(6): 310-317.

19. Siegel D, Lopez J, Meier J, Cunningham FE (2001). Changes in the Pharmacologic Treatment of Hypertension in the Department of Veterans Affairs 1997-1999: Decreased Use of Calcium Antagonists and Increased Use of Beta-Blockers and Thiazide Diuretics. *Am J Hypertens* 4(9 pt. 1): 957-962.

20. Ren XS, Kazis LE, Lee AF, Hamed A, Huang YH, Cunningham FE, Miller DR (2002). Patient Characteristics and Prescription Patterns of Atypical Antipsychotics Among Patients with Schizophrenia. *J Clin Pharm Ther.* 27(6): 441-451.

21. Siva C, Eisen S, Shepherd R, Cunningham FE, Fang MA, Finch , Salisbury D, Singh J, Stern R, Zarabadi A (2003). Leflunamide Use During the First 33 Months After FDA Approval: Experience with a National Cohort of 3325 Patients. *Arthritis Care and Research* 49(6): 745-751.

22. Hammed A, Lee A, Ren S, Miller DM, Cunningham FE, Kazis L (2004). Use of Antidepressant Medications: Are There Differences in Psychiatric Visits Among Patient Treatments in the Veterans Administration? *Med Care* 42(6): 551-559.

23. Charbonneau A, Berlowitz D, Kasiz L, Miller DM, Cunningham FE, Ren X (2004). Monitoring Depression Care: In Search of an Accurate Quality Indicator. *Med Care* 42(6): 522-531.

24. London MJ, Itani KMF, Perrino AC, Guarino PD, Schwarz GG, Cunningham FE, Gottlieb S, Henderson WG (2004). Perioperative Beta Blockade: A Survey of Physician Attitudes in the Department of Veterans Affairs. *J Cardiothorac Vasc Anesth.* 18(1): 14-24.

25. Huang J, Casebeer A, Plomondon M, Shroyer L, McDonald GO, Fullerton DF, Bell MR, Grover F, Cunningham FE (2004). Prescription-Filling Rates for Key Medications in Veterans Affairs Patients After Coronary Artery Bypass Grafting. *Am J Health Syst Pharm.* 61(12): 1248-1252.

26. Department of Veterans Affairs (2006). National Center for Patient Safety. Washington, DC. Available at: http://www.patientsaftey.gov/ vision.html. Accessed March 27, 2006.

27. Johnson, C, Carlson,R, Tucker, C, Willette, C (2002). Using BCMA Software to Improve Patient Safety in Veterans Administration Medical Centers. *Journal of Healthcare Information Management.* 16(1): 46-51

28. Johnson et al. (2002).

29. Department of Veterans Affairs (2006). Office of Academic Affiliations. Washington, DC: Department of Veterans Affairs. Accessed March 27, 2006. http://www.va.gov/oaa/GME_ default.asp.

30. Department of Veterans Affairs (2006). Office of Academic Affiliations.

31. Department of Veterans Affairs (2006). Geriatric Research Education and Clinical Center. Washington, DC: Department of Veterans Affairs. Available at: http://vaww1.va .gov/grecc. Accessed March 27, 2006.

SUGGESTED ADDITIONAL READING

Aspinall, SL, et al. The Evolving Use of Cost-Effectiveness Analysis in Formulary management Within the Department of Veterans Affairs. *Am J Manag Care.* 2005 Jul;43(7 suppl):Il20-6.

Business Relationships between VA staff and Pharmaceutical Industry Representatives. October 2003. Accessed March 27, 2006. http://www1.va.gov/vha publications/ViewPublication.asp?pub_ID=288.

Department of Veterans Affairs Home Page. Business relationships between vha staff and pharmaceutical industry representatives. October 2003. Accessed March 27, 2006. http://www1.va.gov/vhapublications/ViewPublication.asp? pub_ ID=288.

Principles of a Sound Formulary System. Formulary Principles Coalition. October 2000. http://www.pbm.va.gov/pbm/formularyprinciples.pdf. Accessed March 27, 2006.

Sales, MM, et.al. Pharmacy Benefits Management in the Veterans Health Administration: 1995 to 2003. *Am J Manag Care.* 2003 Feb;?(?):104-12.

Chapter 9

The Department of Defense Pharmacy Programs

W. Mike Heath

THE DEPARTMENT OF DEFENSE

In order to better understand pharmaceutical policy within the U.S. Department of Defense (DoD), it is first important to understand the basics about the delivery of health care and organizational structure of the Department of Defense Military Health System (MHS). This chapter will provide a general overview of DoD health care with specific emphasis on pharmaceutical policy and its application in the DoD as it pertains to pharmacy benefit management and the provision of pharmaceutical care for all patients served.

Organizational Structure and Governance

The primary mission of the Department of Defense military health system is to do the following:

- Create a healthy and fit force: When the Department of Defense puts a pair of muddy boots somewhere or deploys any war fighter he or she should be physically, mentally, and socially able to accomplish any mission our nation calls upon them to perform.
- Deploy with them to protect: The battlefield is the "office place" of the warrior, who deserves the best possible protection from risks that could prevent mission success.
- Restore health for service members deployed and at home: DoD is with them to deliver world-class care: treatment, stabilization, medical evacuation. At exactly the same time and level of importance, DoD delivers care to the families at home.

- TRICARE for life: America is a grateful nation that thanks its retired warriors by giving them and their families' health care for life.[1]

Health care within the DoD is an entitlement based on Title Ten of Federal Law specifically as contained in the Code of Federal Regulations (CFR) Section 32. The Military Health System is organizationally structured under the Department of Defense through the office of the Assistant Secretary of Defense for Health Affairs, a presidential appointee, who has historically been a physician. This individual is responsible to the Secretary of Defense for the oversight and management of the military health system and the department's heath plan. Currently, the Assistant Secretary of Defense for Health Affairs is also the Director of TRICARE Management Activity (TMA), which provides the day-to-day operational management of TRICARE. Each of the armed services (Army, Navy, and Air Force) is led by a senior physician, each of whom is the surgeon general of those services. These individuals are also appointed by the president and are directly responsible and report to their respective senior line officer (Chief of Staff of the U.S. Army, Chief of Staff of the U.S. Air Force, and Chief of Naval Operations). Although no direct command and control lines of authority exist from the Assistant Secretary of Defense for Health Affairs to each of the services' surgeons general, all four of these senior military health system leaders work closely together in providing the highest quality and most cost-effective health care to all patients eligible through the Department of Defense.

TRICARE is the health plan for all uniformed service members (active duty, family members of active duty, and retired service members and their families). Currently, approximately 9.1 million eligible beneficiaries (patient lives) are covered under TRICARE, which is provided through a combination of military treatment facilities and partnerships with three managed care support contractors. Patient enrollment and coverage options under TRICARE include the following:

Prime

- Similar to HMO (health maintenance organization) plan
- Patient care directed by a primary care manager (PCM)
- Enrollment fee only for age sixty-five retirees and family members
- No copays/cost shares, no deductible
- Penalties for out-of-network use

Extra

- Similar to PPO (preferred provider organization) plan
- Greater choice of network providers; however, access not guaranteed
- No enrollment fee
- Deductibles, copays/cost shares

Standard

- Similar to indemnity plan
- Greatest choice to include nonnetwork providers
- No enrollment fee
- Deductibles, higher copays/cost shares[2]

TRICARE is administered through three distinct regions within the United States, TRICARE North, TRICARE South, and TRICARE West. Figure 9.1 depicts the geographic areas of responsibility for each TRICARE region.[3]

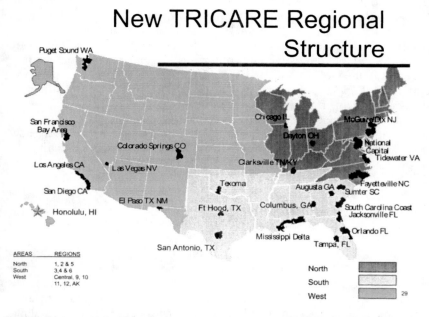

FIGURE 9.1. U.S. Department of Defense TRICARE Regions *Source:* TRICARE Management Activity (2005). Brief bulletin, unpublished. Washington, DC: U.S. Department of Defense.

Department of Defense Pharmacy Benefit, Organization, Structure, and Leadership

The strategic objective of the DoD pharmacy benefit is to "Uniformly, consistently, and equitably provide appropriate and safe drug therapy to meet patients' clinical needs in an effective, efficient, and fiscally responsible manner."[4] The pharmacy benefit within the department is provided to patients through multiple points of service, which include approximately 587 military treatment facility (MTF) pharmacies, one centralized TRICARE Mail Order Pharmacy (TMOP), and more than 55,000 retail network pharmacies and nonnetwork retail pharmacies.

Pharmacy leadership, who provide senior-level advice and recommendations to the Assistant Secretary of Defense for Health Affairs and the services' surgeons general, is provided through the DoD Pharmacy Board of Advisors,[5] which consists of the chief pharmacist/pharmacy consultant to each of the services' surgeons general, the pharmacy program director of TMA, the director of the DoD Pharmacoeconomic Center, and the pharmacy consultant for the Coast Guard. This group in collaboration with the DoD Pharmacy and Therapeutics Committee, the DoD Pharmacoeconomic Center, and others is responsible for monitoring and making recommendations to senior DoD health care leadership on opportunities to include potential policies to ensure a readily accessible, cost-effective pharmacy benefit. Similar to other civilian health plans, the expenditures on pharmaceuticals in the DoD has increased at a significant rate during the past several years. Figure 9.2 documents the growth of spending on pharmaceuticals within DoD from 1995 through 2004.

Several pharmaceutical cost drivers are responsible for the primary growth in the expenditures, which include actual drug cost inflation, new drug technologies introduced into the market, increased utilization of pharmaceuticals by patients, and the rise and mix of drugs.[6]

DEPARTMENT OF DEFENSE PHARMACY STANDARDS OF PRACTICE

With the focus on appropriate and safe drug therapy for all patients served by the DoD, the standards of practice and expectations for pharmacy and the provision of pharmaceutical care mirror those of national practice standards, which include compliance with applicable federal and state laws, Department of Defense and service-specific pharmacy regulations, and nationally accepted standards of practice as identified in the national policies and procedures of the American Pharmacists Association (APhA), the

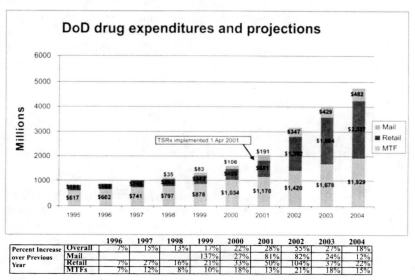

DoD drug expenditures and projections

		1996	1997	1998	1999	2000	2001	2002	2003	2004
Percent Increase over Previous Year	Overall	7%	15%	13%	17%	22%	28%	55%	27%	18%
	Mail				137%	27%	81%	82%	24%	12%
	Retail	7%	27%	16%	21%	33%	50%	104%	37%	22%
	MTFs	7%	12%	8%	10%	18%	13%	21%	18%	15%

* MTF costs do not include dispensing costs.

* Retail costs are contractor paid claims (HCSR Data); admin fees not included

* NMOP costs are net costs to government

Note: FY04 are contractor provided independent government cost estimates. These projections do not reflect pharmacy budget or funding per the POM.

FIGURE 9.2. U.S. Department of Defense pharmaceutical expenditures. *Source:* TRICARE Management Activity (2005). Brief bulletin, unpublished. Washington, DC: U.S. Department of Defense.

American Society of Health-System Pharmacists (ASHP), and other applicable federal or national organizations that are accepted as defining a national practice standard (e.g., The U.S. Pharmacopoeia [USP] as relates to the recently enacted federal standards pertaining to any sterile product preparation as contained in USP chapter 797).

COMPLIANCE WITH JCAHO MEDICATION MANAGEMENT STANDARDS

As with many civilian health care organizations and civilian hospitals, all DoD medical treatment facilities (hospitals, clinics, etc.) are accredited by the Joint Commission on Accreditation of Healthcare Organizations (JCAHO). Therefore, all aspects for the provision of pharmaceutical care within DoD healthcare facilities are expected to comply with the JCAHO medication management (MM) standards. Policies and procedures must meet the intent of these stringent standards, and it is expected that medication management within military health care facilities is patient-centered, multidisciplinary, and collaborative. The JCAHO coordinates the accreditation survey schedule, which now includes unannounced surveys.[7]

FORMULARY MANAGEMENT

During 2004, the Uniform Formulary (UF) rule was finalized and implemented for the Department of Defense. This final rule (a federal statute) directed the establishment of a Uniform Formulary to include three-tier copays (generic, formulary, nonformulary). The UF was mandated by Congress as part of the National Defense Authorization Act (NDAA) of 2000, but because of significant public comment it was some four years later (2004) when the UF became a final rule and was implemented. The UF was legislated one year prior to the TRICARE Senior Pharmacy Program, which was implemented on April 1, 2001, for all DoD beneficiaries over age sixty-five. The TRICARE pharmacy benefit access standards have become a national benchmark and in fact were utilized as the standard that was incorporated into the Medicare Advantage Prescription Drug (MAPD) program, which began implementation in January 2006. The TRICARE Senior Pharmacy Program, also known as TSRx, was legislated by the 2001 National Defense Authorization Act for DoD retirees and dependents over the age of sixty-five who meet eligibility requirements.[8] This program provided equal access for these DoD seniors to the TMOP, retail (network and nonnetwork) and retained their access to military medical facility pharmacies. The prescription copays for this program were the same as those DoD patients under age sixty-five. This revolutionary program, which was the first of its size in America to provide a comprehensive robust pharmacy benefit to the more than 1.6 million eligible patients was implemented on April 1, 2001.

The Uniform Formulary provides a standardized and centralized formulary management process for the department, which enhanced patient access to clinically appropriate, cost-effective medications. The UF also established the DoD Pharmacy and Therapeutics Committee and Beneficiary Advisory Panel (BAP). The DoD P&T committee is comprised of military and civilian health care professionals from each of the services. The primary responsibility of this committee is to evaluate drugs by review of the therapeutic class for consideration of inclusion on the Uniform Formulary. The DoD P & T committee is charged based on explicit provisions contained in the UF to evaluate drugs first based on their clinical effectiveness, and then based on their cost effectiveness. The Beneficiary Advisory Panel is comprised of civilian medical and professional lay personnel. This group meets after each DoD P & T committee during a public meeting held in Washington, DC, and reviews and comments on the formulary recommendations of the DoD P & T Committee. Both the DoD P & T and the BAP meet quarterly. Upon review and comment on the DoD P & T minutes and recommendations by the BAP, both the DoD P & T minutes (recommendations) and BAP comments are forwarded to the Assistant Secretary of Defense for Health Affairs for his or her consideration and review. Upon approval and signature by the Assistant Secretary, the minutes become final with the formulary recommendations fully implemented.

PATIENT SAFETY

The initial Institute of Medicine Report *To Err is Human* and subsequent follow-up publications opened America's eyes to the staggering problem of medical errors.[9] A significant subset of medical errors has been documented to be medication errors. Figure 9.3 documents and compares annual accident data cited as resulting in deaths. Interestingly, and perhaps of no surprise to health care providers, is that medication errors are believed to be one of the leading causes of deaths in the United States. The tragedy of course is that medication errors are most often preventable and the result of a series of breakdowns in the medication use process.

The Department of Defense has embraced the need to first do no harm in preventing and reducing medical and medication errors. To this end, the

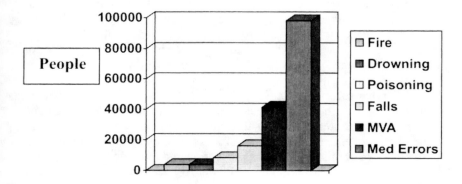

FIGURE 9.3. Estimated annual U.S. deaths from accidents. *Source:* Modified from National Safety Council (2006). What are the odds of dying? August 2. Available at: http://nsc.org/lrs/statinfo/odds.htm.

DoD implemented a patient safety center and a multidisciplinary patient safety committee. DoD has been a national leader in patient safety. Specifically, for decades DoD has included electronic physician order entry for medications as a component of the department's standardized medical information system, the Composite Health Care System (CHCS). The next generation of this system is currently being implemented and includes a commercial off-the-shelf software (COTS) pharmacy module that will revolutionize DoD's ability to better assure safe and appropriate drug therapy. From the medication management perspective, DoD's focus is the appropriate and safe use of medications. DoD has taken an integrated health care system focus in reporting, evaluating, and developing medication use process improvements based on data trend analysis. In 2001, DoD implemented the pharmacy data transaction service (PDTS). The primary purpose of this initiative was patient safety and facilitated DoD's ability to monitor its patients' medication use regardless of where the patient received their medication. PDTS connected the three primary points of service of the DoD Pharmacy benefit, which are either the medical treatment facility pharmacy, the TRICARE mail order pharmacy, or one of the 55,000 retail network pharmacies nationwide. Because PDTS electronically integrates all three points of service, this process includes provider (physician and pharmacist) warnings on dangerous drug-drug interactions or duplicate drug therapies. Once the system identifies a clinically significant level one drug-drug interaction or duplicate drug therapy, a review and hard-edit override by either the pharmacist or physician must occur in order for the prescription to be released from the system, allowing a label to then be printed and the prescription filled. As of 2004, the PDTS system had documented the identification of more than 50,000 level one drug-drug interactions. As a further commitment to improving patient medication safety, DoD procured the U.S. Pharmacopeia's Medmarx medication error reporting program as the DoD standard for reporting tracking and trending medication errors within the DoD.

As a service-specific example of the commitment within DoD to patient medication safety, the Army Medical Department in 2004 developed and implemented a strategic plan for the appropriate integration of pharmacy automation into the medication use process. The overriding goal and primary objective of this plan was the prevention and reduction in preventable medication errors in the outpatient (ambulatory) pharmacy work place. The Army fully funded this twenty-plus million dollar multiyear initiative to improve patient safety in Army medical facilities worldwide. The Air Force and Navy are equally committed to preventing medication errors and have implemented similar patient medication safety improvement initiatives.[10]

DEPLOYMENT OF MEDICATION MANAGEMENT POLICIES

As previously discussed in this chapter, pharmacy policies in the Department of Defense are often based on federal and state law and other applicable and nationally accepted standards of practice. Operational policies and procedures are typically service (Army, Air Force, Navy) based and are deployed and implemented at the local level. In addition, Department of Defense directives and regulations are applicable to pharmacy in DoD. Last, Health Affairs Policies exist that are signed under the authority of the Assistant Secretary of Defense for Health Affairs. These policies are primarily focused on the DoD pharmacy benefit to ensure standardization of procedures and the provision of a uniform and consistent benefit to all patients. These Health Affairs policies, once staffed through the services and approved by the Assistant Secretary of Defense for Health Affairs are routed to the service surgeons general for deployment and implementation.

EMERGENCY PREPAREDNESS AND HOMELAND DEFENSE

Readiness is always a number one priority of the Department of Defense, which also includes pharmacy. Much joint planning occurs among the services and other federal and state agencies, particularly post–September 11, 2001. Pharmaceuticals are widely used in the wartime environment during natural disaster and humanitarian relief efforts and in emergency preparedness and homeland defense. For example, data from the Army Medical Department for soldiers deployed to Iraq and Afghanistan post 9/11 document that approximately one out of every five mobilized and deployed soldiers is taking at least one medication for a chronic medical condition.[11] This led to development and implementation of policies and procedures by the Army to ensure that a deployment medication policy and process was in place to screen all soldiers for their medications, electronically record their medications necessary to treat any chronic medical conditions, dispense an initial six months supply of medications with a process in place to provide any refills during their deployment. This process is now referred to by Army pharmacists as the wartime provision of pharmaceutical care, which means appropriate and safe drug therapy for all deployment service members. Within the Department of Defense, which works closely with the Department of Homeland Defense and multiple other federal agencies, ongoing coordination and collaboration on the development of national policy applicable to the utilization of pharmaceuticals for various emergency preparedness scenarios is occurring. These include policies related to potential threats such as a chemical, biological, radiological, nuclear, or explosive attack as well as other potentially high-risk threats such as the avian flu. These policies are developed and coordinated at the agency secretary or assistant secretary level.

PARTNERSHIPS AND COLLABORATION WITH OTHER FEDERAL AGENCIES

Joint planning, coordination, and implementation focused on mission success is the norm within the DoD to include partnerships with other federal agencies. Such is the case of DoD pharmacy in partnership other federal agency pharmacists. These long-standing, mutually beneficial pharmacy partnerships by the Department of Defense with other federal agencies, which include the U.S. Department of Veterans Affairs (VA) and the Public Health Service (PHS). The DoD and VA have a long-standing partnership focused on maximizing joint pharmaceutical contracting, thus leveraging the drug purchasing power of two large federal agencies resulting in significant cost-avoidance savings. This program is managed and monitored through the Veterans Administration pharmaceutical benefits management (PBM) Office and the DoD Pharmacoeconomic Center (PEC). The DoD and VA have developed policies and procedures for this initiative, which is reported to the DoD/VA Federal Pharmacy Executive Steering Committee (FPESC), which is comprised of pharmacists from the DoD and VA. Another example of federal pharmacy collaboration is with DoD's use of the VA's consolidated mail outpatient pharmacy (CMOP) program. In 2002, this began in DoD as an initial "pilot test" at three sites, one each Army, Air Force, and Navy. Today this program continues at Naval Medical Center in San Diego and Kirtland Air Force Base, New Mexico, and provides a viable, cost-effective alternative for patients to receive their refill medications delivered directly to their home mailbox from the VA. The Army discontinued its CMOP program after the one-year initial pilot due to budgetary constraints, however it continues to consider reimplementing a partnership with the VA CMOP at an Army medical facility.

As another example of DoD and federal pharmacy collaboration, the surgeons' general of the Army and U.S. Public Health Service (PHS) signed a memorandum of understanding (MOU) policy that allowed for the utilization of PHS Individual Ready Reserve (IRR) medical professional personnel in Army medical treatment facilities as backfill for those Army medical personnel who were mobilized and deployed to Iraq, Afghanistan, or in support of other contingency operations. This MOU also included pharmacists and has proven to be a positive professional resource pool for the

Army, which continues to deploy pharmacists in support of the nation's global war on terrorism.

CONCLUSION

The Department of Defense and its dedicated pharmacists and pharmacy technicians have a proud tradition of selfless service performed with duty and honor in providing excellence in pharmaceutical care and service, never forgetting all of those who serve from the "soldier walking point" to the retiree at home. Future challenges faced by the DoD pharmacy community include the need to develop a right-sized, twenty-first century Department of Defense pharmacy work force that documents and validates the value of and need for pharmacists in the department and their having a significant impact in supporting the deployed soldier with relevance to the readiness mission of the Army, Air Force, and Navy. Development of enhanced organizational productivity policies with local business plans, consideration for manpower realignment, and ongoing monitoring with regional program oversight through the services in collaboration with TRICARE Management Activity level will also be challenges. To be successful in the future, DoD pharmacy and the DoD medical professionals must continue to gain a better understanding of effective formulary management strategies with the development and implementation of policies that improve patient access to needed medications. Development and implementation of business planning policies and tools will play a critical role in this future success. These include the development of a strategic business planning process that focuses on appropriately mitigating expenditures on pharmaceuticals and the appropriate utilization of pharmacy personnel resources with a focus on deploying pharmacists in more direct patient care roles. This should include the development of sound internal clinical business practice policies in compliance with JCAHO medication management standards that ensure all patient medication orders are reviewed by a pharmacist, and the involvement of the pharmacist at the beginning of the prescription order to provide drug expertise that results in the appropriate utilization of drug therapy. Prudent financial management policy development and monitoring will ensure improved utilization of resources. A renewed emphasis must be placed on the customer service component in the delivery of pharmaceutical care within the department, which includes medication error prevention strategies, appropriate resourcing of DoD pharmacies that results in improved pharmacy patient waiting times, and improvements to the DoD pharmacy benefit delivery processes. In addition, the paradigm must shift from taking drugs off the formulary to a focus on pharmaceutical cost drivers and ensuring that patients are first properly evaluated and placed on clinically appropriate medications. The focus for the future of DoD pharmacy and the effective management of the pharmacy benefit should be on best practices in managing pharmaceutical costs.

Additional information about DoD pharmacy and its associated policies may be obtained from the following Web-based sources:

- TRICARE Management Activity: http://www.tricare.osd.mil (select pharmacy)
- Pharmacoeconomic Center: http://www.pec.osd.mil

NOTES

1. U.S. Department of Defense (2004). DoD Military Health System Mission Statement. Washington, DC: Office of the Assistant Secretary of Defense for Health Affairs.

2. U.S. Department of Defense (2005). TRICARE Policy Manual. Title 32 Code of Federal Regulations. Washington, DC: U.S. Department of Defense.

3. TRICARE Management Activity, Pharmacy Operations Division 2005. Brief bulletin, unpublished. Washington, DC: U.S. Department of Defense.

4. U.S. Department of Defense (2004). DoD Pharmacy Board of Director's Mission/Vision Statement. Brief bulletin, unpublished. Washington, DC: U.S. Department of Defense.

5. U.S. Department of Defense (2005). DoD Pharmacy Transformation Plan. Office of the Assistant Secretary of Defense for Health Affairs and Director, TRICARE Management Activity. March 22. Brief bulletin, unpublished. Washington, DC: U.S. Department of Defense.

6. Hoffman J., Shah, D., Vermeulen, L., Scumock, G., Grim, P., Hunkler, R., Honitz, K. (2006). Projecting Future Drug Expenditures. *American Journal of Health-System Pharmacists* 63(2): 123-138.

7. Joint Commission on Accreditation of Healthcare Organizations (2005). JCAHO Accreditation Standards Manual (Medication Management), Oak Park, IL: JCAHO.

8. U.S. Congress (1999). National Defense Authorization Act of 2000, Subtitle A, Section 701. Public Law 106-65. October 5. 113 Stat. 677.

9. Kohn, L., Corrigan, J., Donaldson, M. (1999). *To Err is Human: Building a Safer Health System.* Institute of Medicine. Washington, DC: National Academy Press.

10. Army Medical Department Strategic Plan for Pharmacy Automation June 2004.

11. DoD Pharmacoeconomic Center, Predeployment Medication Analysis and Reporting Tool [PMART] 2004-2005.

Chapter 10

Outside the Pill Box: Innovative State Prescription Drug Program Practices

Brendan Krause
Kimberly Fox

INTRODUCTION

Prescription drugs, an increasingly important part of medical care, represent less of the health care dollar than other expenditures, such as those for inpatient hospital care and physician and clinical services.[1] They are, however, among the most rapidly growing health expenditures.[2] Although the vast majority of state spending on pharmaceuticals is associated with the Medicaid program, state governments purchase pharmaceutical and manage pharmaceutical benefits for various programs and populations. These include the State Children's Health Insurance Program (SCHIP), the employee and retiree coverage, state-only programs that provide adult health coverage, state employee benefit programs, state health departments, community health centers, and prisons. States now spend approximately thirty percent of their budgets on health care—more than elementary and secondary education combined.[3] Increased pharmaceutical expenditures have contributed to this shift in funding allocation.

Recent advances in pharmaceutical technology and the general trend toward an increased reliance on pharmaceuticals in medical care has driven utilization and cost of these benefits and programs, drawing the attention of state policymakers. The increased volume and variety of pharmaceuticals being prescribed—as well as the ever increasing cost—present care management, utilization management, and cost management challenges. States have responded by placing the pharmaceutical benefits under greater scrutiny. The new Medicare Prescription Drug Benefit provided through Medicare Part D in the Medicare Modernization Act of 2003 present further challenges and decision points for states as they maintain, add, or alter the benefits they provide.

State policymaking generally focuses on pharmaceutical coverage, purchasing, and utilization management.

STATE EMPLOYEE AND RETIREE BENEFITS

All states provide employee and retiree health benefits—compared to 62 percent of private firms.[4] Once a minor expense, these benefits now make up a growing portion of state spending.

In 2002, 3.4 million people were covered by state employee health benefits. Ninety-nine percent of these beneficiaries had prescription drug coverage. Although most employees who are offered coverage are full-time workers, states provide part-time and transitional workers health coverage far more often than their private-sector counterparts do. In fact, 74 percent of part-time state employees were offered health benefits, compared to 48 percent of part-time workers in the private sector.[5]

The type of health insurance plan that a state employee or retiree enrolls in varies greatly by region as well as whether they are retired or currently employed by the state. In general, most current state employees are enrolled in some sort of managed care organization (MCO). Whether the MCO is a strict health maintenance organization (HMO) or a more loosely controlled preferred provider organization (PPO) depends highly on where the beneficiary lives. For example, employees in the West and Midwest are more likely to be enrolled in and HMO, whereas those in the South are more likely to be enrolled in a PPO. In the Northeast, the mix of HMO and PPO is fairly even. Most state retirees are enrolled in traditional indemnity plans.[6]

Employers across the country are experiencing health insurance cost increases that are growing—particularly relative to their employees' wages. The cost of prescription drug coverage for a state employee was $1,288 in 2002.[7] Although the cost of annual claims paid for state employees and retirees were slightly higher than those for private sector employees, utilization was on average 6 percent lower for state employees.

In 2003, many employers reported that their health care costs were on average 15 percent of employee wages—and that that percentage will climb to 20 by 2008. For state employees, health care costs make up 16 percent of wages. Although prescription drug cost growth has slowed, they are still well outpacing wage inflation, contributing significantly to this trend. This means that although employees will enjoy the positive health benefits of improving pharmaceutical and bio technology, the cost of these technologies will take a bigger piece of their paychecks.[8]

STATE PHARMACEUTICAL ASSISTANCE PROGRAMS AND DISCOUNT CARDS

Prior to the enactment of the Medicare Prescription Drug, Improvement, and Modernization Act (MMA) in December 2003, many states were already providing some assistance to help low-income elderly or disabled residents who do not qualify for Medicaid purchase prescription drugs. Unlike Medicaid drug coverage, which has been an optional benefit offered by most states since the 1970s, the vast majority of State Pharmaceutical Assistance Programs (SPAPs) and discount card programs were initiated in the past five years, largely in response to federal inaction in passing a Medicare prescription drug benefit. Only ten states, including New York, Pennsylvania, and New Jersey, had programs in place prior to 1990. These older programs generally account for the vast majority of SPAP enrollment.[9]

States have pursued two strategies for filling the drug coverage gap for their lowest income or uninsured residents. States have either developed SPAPs that provide direct benefits or subsidies to pay for some portion of enrollees' prescription drug costs or initiated state-sponsored or state-supported discount card programs that allow participants to receive a reduced price for prescriptions at participating pharmacies at minimal or no cost to the state. The difference between SPAPs and discount card programs is significant in terms of the savings to the consumer. In an SPAP, depending on the benefit design, an enrollee may be required to pay a nominal copayment of only $5 to $10 for any covered drug, whereas a discount card program is likely to reduce the price of the drug by only 15 to 20 percent off the retail price, which may vary considerably from store to store.[10]

As of August 2004, forty-one states had authorized some type of prescription assistance program, with twenty states authorizing SPAP direct benefit programs only, eight authorizing discount programs only, and twelve authorizing both SPAP and discount programs. Of these, in 2004 only twenty-three SPAPs and nine state discount cards were operational.[11] Some states have multiple SPAP and/or discount card programs targeted to residents of different income levels.

Who Is Covered?

In 2003, SPAPs served more than 1.5 million elderly and disabled enrollees nationwide, most of whom were low-income Medicare beneficiaries.[12] In addition, approximately 575,000 persons were estimated to have enrolled in state-sponsored discount cards as of July 2002[13] All SPAPs offer benefits to older state residents that meet certain income requirements.

Eleven states also extend coverage to the disabled. Two states offer coverage to all residents who meet income and residency requirements of their programs regardless of age or disability.

SPAP income eligibility varies considerably by state, ranging from 100 percent to 500 percent of the federal poverty level (FPL), with the average falling around 220 percent FPL. This contrasts with the income eligibility levels required to qualify for "extra help" for Medicare Part D, which are defined in statute as below 135 percent FPL for full subsidies and below 150 percent FPL for partial subsidies. In addition, Part D subsidies have an asset test, which only two SPAPs (Maryland and Minnesota) currently require. Thus many enrollees in SPAPs are unlikely to qualify for the generous subsides available to low-income people through Part D and will only be eligible for the basic Part D benefit, which may be less generous than existing SPAP benefits.[14] (See Figure 10.1.)

Target populations for state discount card.programs also vary by state, with some limiting eligibility to only elderly residents and others to all Medicare beneficiaries and/or those below a certain income.[15]

SPAP benefit packages and cost sharing required varies considerably across states. Most states cover FDA-approved drugs for which manufacturers have agreed to offer a rebate, although five states (Illinois, Rhode Is-

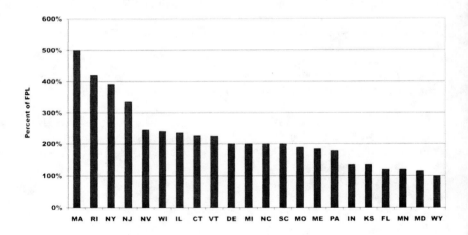

FIGURE 10.1. SPAP income eligibility requirements as a percent of federal poverty, 2003. *Source:* Rizzo J, Fox K, Trail T, and Crystal S (2007). State Pharmacy Assistance Programs: A Chartbook—Updated and Revised. January. New York: The Commonwealth Fund. Reprinted with permission.

land, Maine, and Vermont) cover only drugs/brand-name drugs for certain conditions. The level of coverage also varies, with eight states limiting coverage up to a set dollar amount or number of prescriptions per month (Delaware, Florida, Indiana, Kansas, Missouri, North Carolina, Nevada, and Wyoming).

All states require SPAP enrollees to contribute toward their drug costs. Some impose up-front costs, such as annual fees or premiums either through a flat fee (Connecticut and Michigan) or based on a sliding scale by income (Illinois, Massachusetts, Missouri, and New York). Six states have a deductible (ranging from $250 to $1,715), most commonly imposed in programs targeting moderate income persons and sometimes set on a sliding scale. All states require their enrollees to pay a percent of the discounted drug price (coinsurance), a flat copayment, or the higher of a flat copayment or coinsurance. The coinsurance and copayment requirements differ considerably across states, ranging from $1 to $40 per claim, or 20 percent to 85 percent of the price of the drug. [16]

Although all state discount cards seek to accomplish the same goal—to lower retail prescription drug prices charged to uninsured, cash-paying customers—they employ different approaches for achieving these lower prices, which directly affects the level of discount available, the drugs that are covered, and the pharmacies at which the discount card is honored. Generally, state discount programs either (1) extend all or a portion of Medicaid-level prices required under state and federal law to non-Medicaid eligible residents; (2) negotiate rebates from manufacturers for prices that are even lower than required by Medicaid, using prior authorization in Medicaid as leverage; or (3) employ private sector pharmacy benefit managers to negotiate pharmacy discounts on behalf of enrollees. Programs that seek only pharmacy-level Medicaid discounts have not been legally challenged, whereas those that seek manufacturer rebates have faced significant legal challenge. Programs that have attempted to get voluntary rebates from manufacturers have generally been unable to do so.

State discount cards provide discounts at participating pharmacies, which, depending on the state program, can include all pharmacies in the state that accept Medicaid or be limited to only those pharmacies for which the state has been able to negotiate discounts. Covered drugs may vary by the discount card program, depending on if the state seeks manufacturer rebates as well as pharmacy discounts. Precise estimates on discounts achieved through state discount cards are not available, but states estimate a savings of 10 to 24 percent off of retail price.

State Financing of SPAPs

SPAPs are supported by a combination of state tax revenues, pharmacy discounts, and manufacturer rebates and consumer cost sharing. In total, SPAPs paid approximately $2 billion of prescription drug claims in fiscal year (FY) 2003-2004. This contrasts with the estimated $39 billion that Medicare expects to spend on the Part D benefit in its first year of full implementation. New York, New Jersey, and Pennsylvania accounted for 75 percent of all SPAP drug expenditures. The cost to the state is directly related to the generosity of the benefit. Annual costs per enrollee in fiscal year 2003 averaged $1,332 in 2003 and ranged from $105 in North Carolina to $2,472 in New Jersey.

Although the source of funding varies by state, SPAPs are funded largely by either state general revenues or categorical funding sources such as lottery or casino revenues that have been earmarked for programs for the elderly. Six states (Illinois, South Carolina, Wisconsin, Vermont, Maryland, and Florida) receive Medicaid federal matching through Medicaid waivers to extend drug-only coverage to seniors or disabled persons who would not otherwise qualify for Medicaid in order to avert their spend down into the full Medicaid program. The future of these waiver programs is uncertain in light of the new Medicare drug benefit, which will assume responsibility for the drug coverage of all dually eligible persons for both Medicare and Medicaid.

In contrast to SPAPs, the reduction in price for state discount-card programs is largely absorbed through participating pharmacies, participating pharmaceutical manufacturers, or both. State-sponsored discount cards require minimal state funding, generally limited to covering administrative costs and/or outreach and education. In 2002, estimates of state discount card programs costs to the state ranged from $275,000 to $20 million in the state of Maine, which contributed a nominal amount per beneficiary toward the discount.

In addition to the state contributions, SPAPs are supported by consumer cost sharing and reduced prices paid to pharmacies and manufacturer rebates. Although several states contract with pharmaceutical benefit managers (PBMs) to negotiate these discounts, most states set pharmacy reimbursement rates and pharmaceutical manufacturer rebate rates in statute and require any pharmacy or manufacturer that wishes to participate to agree to these set payment rates. Although pharmacy reimbursement rates vary by state, generally SPAPs pay pharmacies a higher rate than the private sector. Manufacturer rebates, in contrast, are often higher than those believed to be achieved in the private sector, as many states require manufacturers to extend the "best price" to its SPAP.

Under the Part D benefit, the ability of states to control reimbursement rates and rebates as a secondary payer may be jeopardized. Although states may benefit from lower pharmacy reimbursement rates and dispensing fees negotiated in private pharmacy networks, Part D plans are unlikely to negotiate and/or pass on rebates as significant as they have obtained directly from manufacturers in the past.

Outlook for SPAPs and Discount Cards Post-MMA

With the enactment of the MMA and the new Part D prescription drug benefit, which will now be available to all Medicare beneficiaries who choose to voluntarily enroll, the future of state pharmacy assistance programs is somewhat uncertain. Many of the state programs, particularly those that have been enacted in the past five years, were initiated in response to the strong public outcry for some assistance with prescription drug costs among the most vulnerable disabled and elderly populations in absence of any drug coverage through Medicare. Now that prescription drug coverage will be available through Medicare, states are reassessing their roles and whether or not they should continue these programs at all, and if so, in what capacity.

The MMA explicitly acknowledged SPAPs and encouraged them to continue to supplement the Medicare Part D benefit as a secondary payer. SPAPs are allowed to either purchase supplemental insurance through Part D plans or wrap around Part D benefit plans by helping beneficiaries pay for premiums, cost sharing, or drugs not covered by the plans. In addition, under Medicare Part D, qualifying SPAPs are given the unique opportunity to count state expenditures made on behalf of a Medicare beneficiary to help pay for Part D cost sharing to count toward the enrollees' true out-of-pocket costs (TrOOP). This would allow the beneficiary to reach the more generous catastrophic coverage available under Part D sooner without having to pay the full price out of their own pocket. As a further encouragement to states, Congress also appropriated $125 million for grant funding to states with SPAPs to assist their current enrollees in enrolling in Part D plans and the low-income subsidies.

Nonetheless, although many states may wish to hold their enrollees' harmless, providing them with the same or similar coverage to what they currently receive through the SPAP, the administrative complexities may discourage states from maintaining coverage, particularly given significant state budget deficits. The Part D plans will be administered by private plans that are able to use a variety of cost-containment measures, including the use of closed formularies to minimize costs. States are prohibited from applying to be a Part D plan and thus must coordinate benefits with these plans, moving from being the primary insurer to being a secondary payer, wrapping around the Medicare benefit. To "qualify" as an SPAP, Medicare regulations require that states provide "wraparound" coverage for all Part D plans serving its region, regardless of how generous the benefit is relative to the state's plan.

Although states may see some savings from the basic Part D benefit, they stand to gain the greatest federal offsets from the low-income subsidies, for which many SPAP enrollees may be eligible. However, SPAPs were not given the same authority as state Medicaid agencies to determine eligibility for the low-income subsidy (LIS) along with the Social Security Administration. Thus, SPAP enrollees will need to apply to the SSA or Medicaid and provide asset information that they have not previously been required to provide to get drug coverage through their state program. These are significant barriers to getting current SPAP enrollees enrolled in the LIS. Even if the state mandates participation in Medicare, enforcement will be difficult.

Once their enrollees are enrolled in Part D plans, states will need to overlay their current eligibility and benefit designs with the basic Medicare Part D benefit and the benefit that will be available to low-income individuals to the degree that they apply. Coordinating the SPAP benefit with the new Medicare Part D benefit and the low-income subsidy benefit will be difficult, particularly given the variations in SPAP benefit designs and the equally complex benefit that will be provided through the new drug benefit. Cost sharing in many SPAPs is lower than what will be required for the basic Part D benefit and equivalent or higher than what will be available for those who qualify for the Part D low-income subsidies. Requirements that SPAPs overlay their current benefit design with each distinct Part D plan in the region multiplies the complexity of the task, particularly if the states elect to wrap around the Part D formularies, requiring the state to wrap around each plan's unique cost-sharing components. In the spring 2005, nearly a third of states that had SPAPs were proposing to drop their programs as of January 2006.[17]

State-sponsored discount cards are likely to continue particularly as a low-cost strategy to assist the nonelderly without drug coverage in paying for prescription drugs. During the interim eighteen month Medicare discount card program, existing state programs were excluded from Medicare endorsement since only private entities were eligible to apply. Nonetheless, even though they served similar target populations, most state discount cards remained in place, claiming that they were achieving better discounts than the private cards.

EMERGING STATE PURCHASING STRATEGIES

States also seek to become better pharmaceutical purchasers in order to protect access to benefits and to improve care quality for the people they cover.

Inter- and Intrastate Purchasing Pool Initiatives

Pooled purchasing offers the promise of cost savings and of quality improvement. However, the goals of pooled purchasing programs can be difficult to achieve given legal and political challenges. States consider purchasing pools for prescription drug benefits principally to achieve savings. But where do the savings come from, and how can purchasing coalitions improve the quality of care that patients receive? The benefits realized from purchasing pools generally fall into the following categories:

- *Market power.* Pooled purchasing can increase the market clout of buyers because manufacturers are more likely to negotiate favorable rebates with larger programs.
- *Efficiency.* Administrative costs—and therefore administrative fees—will decrease as the number of beneficiaries covered increases. Coalitions that allow a PBM to engage in rebate sharing might do so assuming that aligned economic incentives between the programs and the PBM will lead to greater program savings.
- *Benefits and care management.* Because most pools will utilize a pharmacy benefits manager, program savings and quality improvements result as states harness industry-best practices in disease and benefits management. Such practices could include state-of-the-art, evidence-based preferred drug lists and/or formularies. Furthermore, enhanced drug utilization review (DUR) capability could allow plans to more accurately analyze prescriber habits and monitor the treatment of patients with complex needs, assuring their care is appropriate. Clinical management and education programs for these high utilizers could also be included, presenting great potential for quality improvement and care integration in fragmented systems. This is particularly true for programs that rely on traditional fee-for-service arrangements with the health care delivery system.[18]

WHAT MAKES A SUCCESSFUL PURCHASING POOL
FOR PRESCRIPTION DRUGS?

Many states have discussed and pursued pooling programs to purchase prescription drugs. Purchasing pools generally involve agencies within a state or across multiple states that contract jointly with a PBM to negotiate manufacturer rebates and to manage benefits. The experiences of several states suggest design factors that make a pool successful. These include:

- *Volume.* The larger the number of pooled beneficiaries, the greater the potential to achieve discounts and rebates from manufacturers as well as realize administrative savings.
- *Technological capacity.* In order to maximize the benefits of enhanced pharmacy and disease management programs, coalitions must be capable of sophisticated analysis of beneficiary utilization and prescriber habits. This is true especially for coalitions trying to drive physician-prescribing habits toward a clinical standard.
- *Leadership, cooperation, and political will.* A strong motivating force is necessary to overcome the logistical challenges to pooling multiple programs, particularly across state lines. This force can come from either a person or a political mandate. States must cooperate with one another for multistate programs to be effective.
- *Similar preferred drug lists.* For coalitions to negotiate enhanced manufacturer rebates associated with a preferred drug list or formulary, savings are maximized when the specific drugs on each coalition member's list or formulary are similar across therapeutic classes.
- *Single negotiating entity.* When pooling for Medicaid programs, the pool also should use one entity to negotiate rebates with pharmaceutical manufacturers.
- *Similarity of plans and plan sizes.* PBMs dealing with commercial (non-Medicaid) groups such as employee benefit programs will have certain fixed costs—which are the same for a large group as for a small group. However, small groups will have fewer members across whom to disperse those costs. If all groups in a coalition of commercial (non-Medicaid) clients are charged the same fees, then the large groups will likely subsidize the smaller groups, making the arrangement less beneficial to the large group members.
- *Prioritized savings strategies.* Finally, pool members must determine how they will maximize savings from the group they form. States can choose to derive savings from among a lower administrative fee, rebate sharing, and state-of-the-art benefits administration and disease

management. Opting to derive the bulk of a pool's savings from decreased administrative fees and from a full pass-through of manufacturer rebates provides a high level of transparency,[19] but these choices decrease the aligned financial incentives between the coalition and the PBM. In other words, in this scenario a PBM does not enhance its own revenue by negotiating better rebates for its state clients. On the other hand, non-Medicaid coalitions that allow PBMs to share a percentage of the rebates negotiated from manufacturers in lieu of or along with a decreased administrative fee provide well-aligned financial incentives between the pool and the PBM, and provide less financial incentive for PBM interactions that result in a claim. (Pool members can also choose to pay either a per member per month fee or a per claim fee.) However, this option provides less public transparency regarding the way savings are derived. In any case, coalitions can employ state-of-the-art benefits administration including evidence-based preferred drug lists and prior authorization. Coalitions also can engage in clinical management for high utilizers or for patients in specific disease states.

INTRASTATE PURCHASING

States seeking to employ the concepts of collaborative purchasing and enhanced pharmacy benefits management can look within their borders to form purchasing pools. Rather than purchasing benefits separately by program, agency, or department, states can combine the market power of these purchasers by negotiating collectively.

Georgia

Georgia took the first step toward its intrastate coalition by creating the Department of Community Health (DCH) and giving the new department authority over the health benefits of the Board of Regents, state employee health plans, Medicaid, and the State Children's Health Insurance Program (SCHIP). The goals of the department include insuring two million state residents, maximizing the state's health care buying power, planning for coverage of uninsured state residents, and coordinating health planning for state agencies.

Specifically, DCH includes the State Health Benefit Plan, Office of General Counsel, Division of Medical Assistance, Managed Care, Office of the Inspector General, Composite State Board of Medical Examiners, Georgia Board for Physician Workforce, State Medical Education Board. The Board of Regents is technically not a DCH unit, but it does have a contractual relationship with DCH so that its University Health System health plan is included in DCH vendor contracts.[20]

The state used consultants, internal staff, and external interested parties (including CMS) to craft a Request for Proposals for a PBM contract. Express Scripts Inc. (ESI) was awarded the contract in July 2001. Services began for Medicaid on October 1, 2000; for the Board of Regents on January 1, 2001; and for the State Health Benefit Plan on July 1, 2001.

How Does it Work?

The state pays a preset administrative fee to the PBM and allows the PBM to share in the rebate, excluding Medicaid rebates. The PBM manages the Medicaid-contracted networks with rates specified by the state and maintains PBM-contracted custom networks for the employees plan.

Prior to this effort, Georgia's Medicaid program had no preferred drug list, limited prior authorization and quantity limits, a limited drug utilization review (DUR) program, limited paper claim submission, and imposed a 50-cent copayment on all prescriptions. The new program design includes features such as a preferred drug list, a maximum allowable cost expansion, tiered copayments for all programs, a provider generic substitution incentive program, and changes to its prior authorization system.

The system ensures that payment is made by the appropriate third-party payer, such as Medicare, before making a Medicaid payment. The PBM also negotiates expanded rebates in the Medicaid program, including those for items that fall outside of the federal Medicaid rebate program, such as diabetic supplies. The unique characteristics and rules of Medicaid have led to a separation between rebates negotiated for it and for the other pooled programs.

Clinical Programs

Georgia's contract includes some clinical programs that are managed by the PBM. Since it manages pharmaceutical benefits for all of the state-funded populations, the PBM has the data and the ability to intervene when clinically appropriate regarding patient safety and quality. Some of Georgia's clinical programs include:

- An expanded DUR program
- A long-term care intervention team

- Six disease management programs in which the PBM sends letters to patients and/or their doctors to provide advice regarding the patient's care management or to present problems regarding the patient's care

Results

This comprehensive approach saved the state $60 million between October 2000 and January 2003. Besides budget savings, the clinical initiatives launched as a part of the arrangement have enhanced quality of care and have educated physicians on standard treatment guidelines.[21] In Medicaid, on a per member per month (PMPM) basis, pharmaceutical expenditures were growing at a 22 percent rate in 2000. This growth rate dropped to 6 percent in 2002. Additional savings are anticipated due to the implementation of a Medicaid-specific preferred drug list program in 2004.

INTER- OR MULTISTATE PURCHASING

To date, the purchasing coalitions that have gained the most notice include those that reach across state lines.

The RxIS Coalition

The oldest of these is the Rx Issuing States (RxIS) coalition, an arrangement between four noncontiguous states—Delaware, Missouri, New Mexico, and West Virginia—to purchase prescription drugs for state employees and retirees. The coalition purchases drugs for 570,000 beneficiaries. Effective July 1, 2004, Ohio employees joined the coalition, adding another 106,000 beneficiaries.

The coalition grew out of the Pharmacy Work Group, a collection of twenty to twenty-five states sometimes referred to as the Southern States Coalition. Members of the coalition included officials from state employee health benefits and Medicaid programs, although only state employee programs ultimately joined due largely to the limitations associated with federal Medicaid statute. Of the working group's members, six states from the group decided to issue an RFP to select a single PBM to be purchaser and manager of the states' employee health benefit plans. Express Scripts was selected as the coalition's PBM in 2002. Some states—Delaware, for example—obtained legislative authority to join the coalition, whereas others already had the authority through existing procurement laws to join.

Ultimately, the PBM began purchasing prescription drugs for the four states that make up the current RxIS Coalition. The states receive 100 percent of manufacturer rebates. The PBM guarantees minimum rebates to RxIS states, and the states pay a per-prescription administration fee.

The success of the RxIS coalition demonstrates that logistical challenges to multistate pooling programs can be resolved to the benefit of participating states.

- The coalition meets periodically and the level of involvement is up to the individual RxIS state (although for maximum leverage and sharing of best practices, states should coordinate more rather than less). The states are permitted to include nonstate groups such as counties or other employers at their discretion, though none currently do so.[22]
- Each state can choose multiple options/packages for various populations and groups among their state employees and retirees. Individual states can choose from any program the PBM offers and can have any benefit design, formulary, or combination—or they can have one customized. The only limiting factor is that if a product is offered to one state, it must be offered to all participating states. Drugs are evaluated by an independent pharmacy and therapeutics committee.[23] Evaluations are made first on the basis of public information regarding efficacy and thereafter on cost.
- Each state has its own contract with the PBM to fit individual state requirements. The minimum rebate guarantee made by the PBM is based on the benefit design the state chooses. As the RxIS group grows, the administrative fee decreases. The benefit design chosen determines the minimum rebate guaranteed by the PBM.
- When selecting pharmacy networks, states must strike a balance between greater beneficiary access provided by broader networks and deeper discounts provided by tighter networks.
- Mail service is an option for additional savings, both for beneficiary and the health plan.

RxIS CLINICAL PROGRAMS

Participating states can establish various clinical programs to better manage or inform beneficiaries with particular health conditions. These include services such as retroactive DUR, step therapy, and prior authorization. States can choose the clinical programs best suited for their needs and can negotiate guaranteed savings for a package of these programs. Savings are calculated based on savings on prescription drug expenditures—not medical expenditures—with methodologies for calculating savings defined in advance. States can choose to pay by administrative fee, by sharing in the savings, or by a combination of both. Some clinical programs include:

- *Retroactive drug utilization review.* The PBM transmits safety alerts to pharmacies regarding drug-to-drug interactions, and screens claims data for potential oversights in safety, notifying physicians of potential problems via mail.
- *Step therapy.* Clients are encouraged or required at the point of service to try more common and less expensive alternatives to a medication before moving on to a newer, more expensive one.
- *Prior authorization.* Clients must receive prior authorization from a plan pharmacist before receiving the drug, either for clinical purposes or for directing product selection.

Results

All participating states have reported significant savings. The amount of savings depends on the specific components that each state implemented. For example, West Virginia estimates it has saved a total of $25 million.

Medicaid Prescription Drug Purchasing Groups

According to the Centers for Medicare and Medicaid Services (CMS) Office of the Actuary, Medicaid is projected to incur 18 percent of all U.S. prescription drug expenditures in 2004.[24] For years, states have considered ways to leverage this purchasing power by collaborating to negotiate supplemental rebates for Medicaid programs and to simplify benefits management.

In February 2003, Michigan and Vermont, who had contracts with First Health Services to manage their Medicaid pharmaceutical benefits, announced they would join forces to purchase prescription drugs for Medicaid and invited other states to participate. CMS has since approved state plan amendments for Alaska, Michigan, New Hampshire, Nevada, and Vermont that allow the five states to collectively purchase prescription drugs for their Medicaid programs—marking the first time a multistate purchasing pool for Medicaid prescription drugs has been implemented. Minnesota[25] and Hawaii[26] also have submitted a state plan amendment to join this pool, and Montana has expressed its intent to join, and have awarded competitively procured contracts to First Health Services.[27]

CMS issued guidance to states as to how they could join this existing pool or form a new one in September of 2004.[28] In June 2005, a second purchasing pool made up of Louisiana, Maryland, and West Virginia was announced. The pool is managed by Provider Synergies.[29]

HOW DOES IT WORK?

As with the RxIS model, the concept behind these coalitions is to allow participating states to maximize their bargaining power by using a single benefits manager to purchase and manage their prescription drugs. As more states join the pool program, discounts increase because of the "bidding model" used by the program. However, due to the unique rules of the Medicaid program, including the Medicaid "best price rule,"[30] only Medicaid programs or certain low-income, non-Medicaid programs approved by CMS can join this pool.

First Health Services is a pharmaceutical benefits administrator (PBA). PBAs vary from PBMs in that they derive no revenue from manufacturer rebates. (However, it should be noted that commercial PBM contracts can also be structured so that all revenues are passed on directly to the state by paying a per-claim administrative fee to the PBM, as in the RxIS contract.) In this case, Michigan and Vermont receive all rebates negotiated with manufacturers—and all rebate revenue is shared with CMS.

Although each participating state uses its own pharmacy and therapeutics committee to craft its preferred drug list, similarity between states yields greater savings and deeper discounts. The pooling program focuses on the "lowest net cost" of prescription drugs used in the benefits—the combined effect of compliance with low-cost therapeutically equivalent drugs and negotiated supplemental rebates.

Savings

All states estimate significant savings in their programs. In 2004, Michigan estimated it would save as much as $8 million; Vermont, $1 million; Alaska, $1 million; New Hampshire, $250,000; Nevada, $1.9 million;[31] and Minnesota, $11 million.[32] In 2006, Louisiana estimates that it will save $27 million; Maryland, $19 million; and West Virginia, $16 million.[33]

HOW DO STATES MANAGE THE PHARMACEUTICAL BENEFITS THAT THEY PROVIDE?

States have generally been less aggressive than the private sector in imposing utilization management and cost-containment strategies in state employee and retiree health benefits and state pharmaceutical assistance programs. Even states that have taken the lead in using preferred drug lists and other mechanisms to control utilization in Medicaid programs have been slower to impose similar benefit limitations in other state pharmacy programs.

However, in light of unsustainable double-digit increases in pharmacy costs driven in large part by increased utilization of higher cost drugs, states have begun to manage utilization both to achieve better value and higher quality outcomes and to control costs.

These strategies generally fall into utilization management, which may focus on reducing unnecessary or inappropriate utilization or on steering enrollees toward lower-cost; on therapeutically equivalent substitutes through administrative barriers or increased cost sharing or on efforts to reduce the purchase price, such as pursuing supplemental manufacturer rebates either individually or through pooled purchasing efforts; and lowering pharmacy reimbursement and dispensing fees.

Although states generally do not use closed formularies to manage utilization, many do a three-tier copayment model to encourage the use of generics or lower cost drugs in a similar drug class. A few states use deductibles and coinsurance as alternate mechanisms for benefits management.[34] And although some states maintain open formularies, the majority of states use some sort of prior authorization for high-cost drugs with therapeutic alternatives.[35]

Besides utilization controls such as prior authorization or cost sharing, many states are using prescription drug clinical intervention to steer beneficiaries toward cheaper, clinically equivalent therapies. This usually takes the form of a conversation between the pharmacist and a patient or the patient's physician.[36]

By far the most common utilization management strategy utilized by SPAPs is mandatory generic substitution policies that require participating pharmacists to dispense the generic substitute for a brand-name drug unless otherwise indicated by the physician. Although SPAPs previously allowed fairly liberal overrides by physicians if they indicated "dispense as written" on the prescription, an increasing trend exist toward proof of medical necessity, prior authorization, and even step therapy, in which an individual must fail first on a generic before being able to receive the brand-name drug.

In states where the SPAP is colocated within the Medicaid agency, many of the Medicaid-related management strategies including greater use of prior authorization by itself or in combination with a preferred drug list have also been used in the SPAP. In 2003, nearly half of SPAPs indicated that they had a preferred drug lists or prior authorization programs that require doctors or pharmacists to get prior approval prior to dispensing a nonpreferred drug.

Disease Management and Wellness Programs

State employee benefits programs have increasingly implemented disease management and wellness programs to prevent or manage chronic illness in their employees and retirees. These programs range from case management of diabetes, hypertension, and asthma, which can increase prescription drug utilization—and thus cost—while avoiding more expensive inpatient care or the development of comorbities. Some states have plans to link participation in such programs—or in wellness programs such as those for physical fitness or smoking cessation—with decreased premiums or cost sharing.

CONCLUSION

States have been working to become better providers, purchasers, and managers of pharmaceutical benefits, in all state-funded programs. Although Medicaid remains the biggest cost driver of state spending on pharmaceuticals, state employee and retiree benefits and state pharmaceutical assistance programs and discount cards are other ways that states provide significant levels of pharmaceutical access—and incur significant costs. Inter- and intrastate purchasing and management of prescription drug benefits are tools that some states are using to negotiate better discounts and supplemental rebates and to more efficiently manage their programs and benefits. Using a single PBM or administrator potentially provides a real benefit to patient safety and care management, encouraging integration in a largely fragmented health care delivery system. By better managing these important benefits, states are better able to maintain them for the residents they serve and to improve the quality of care that patients receive.

NOTES

1. Janet Lundy et al. (2004). *Trends and Indicators in the Changing Health Care Marketplace, 2004 Update*. Washington, DC: Kaiser Family Foundation.
2. Janet Lundy et al. (2004).
3. National Association of State Budget Officers (2006). *State Expenditure Report.* Available at: http://www.nasbo.org/Publications/PDFs/2005%20State%20 Expenditure%20Report.pdf.

4. Kaiser Family Foundation (2003). *Kaiser/HRET Survey: 2002 State Employee Health Plans.* July 23. Publication No. 6100. Health Care Marketplace Project. Washington, DC: Kaiser Family Foundation.

5. Kaiser Family Foundation (2003).

6. The Segal Company (2003). *Segal State Health Benefits Survey: Medical Benefits for Employees and Retirees.* New York: The Segal Company. Available at: http://www.segalco.com/publications/surveysandstudies/2003statesurvey_medical benefits.pdf.

7. The Segal Company (2004). *Segal State Health Benefits Survey: Prescription Drug Coverage for Employees and Retirees.* New York: The Segal Company.

8. The Segal Company (2003).

9. Trail, T., Fox, K., Cantor, J., Silberberg, M., Crystal, S (2004). *State Pharmacy Assistance Programs: A Chartbook.* August. Rutgers Center for State Health Policy. New York: The Commonwealth Fund.

10. Trail, T. et al. (2004); Fox, K., Trail, T., Frankford, D., Crystal, S. (2004). State Pharmacy Discount Programs: A Viable Mechanism for Addressing Prescription Drug Affordability? *New York University Annual Survey of American Law* 60(2): 187-240. Available at: http://www.cshp.rutgers.edu/PDF/60NYUAnn SurvAmL187_2004.pdf.

11. National Conference of State Legislatures (2004). State Pharmaceutical Assistance Programs, 2003 Edition. Available at: http://www.ncsl.org/programs/ health/drugaid.htm. Accessed November 11, 2004.

12. Fox, K., Crystal, S. (2004). Testimony for Public Hearing of the State Pharmaceutical Transition Commission. July 7. New Brunswick, NJ: Rutgers Center for State Health Policy. Available at: http://www.cshp.rutgers.edu/PDF/Testimony/ KFox_SPSPtestimony070704.pdf.

13. Fox, K. et al. (2004). Based on enrollment in four state discount program in Iowa, West Virginia, Maine, and New Hampshire. Figures do not include California and Florida discount card programs that extend the Medicaid level discounts to any Medicare beneficiary who shows their Medicare card. Neither state tracks the number of Medicare beneficiaries who use the discount.

14. Sia, J., Fox, K., Trail T., Crystal, S. (2003). *State Pharmacy Assistance Programs, 2003: A Chartbook.* Rutgers Center for State Health Policy. New York: Commonwealth Fund.

15. Fox, K. et al. (2004).

16. Sia, J. et al. (2003).

17. Based on informal discussions with state officials in spring 2005. States that had either passed or were proposing budgets tto pass legislation to terminate their SPAP benefit included Wyoming, Kansas, Minnesota, North Carolina, Florida, Indiana, and Michigan.

18. Although not necessarily an exact model for state purchasing pools for prescription drugs, the U.S. Department of Defense (DoD) and U.S. Department of Veterans Affairs (VA) have lowered prescription drug expenditures through partnership. It should first be noted that both the DoD and VA are direct purchasers of pharmaceuticals, whereas Medicaid and state employee health plans are not. Furthermore, the VA has established a national formulary that is far more restrictive

than Medicaid preferred drug lists. However, lessons learned from these two purchasers' market power suggest policy options for states. The federal government requires that manufacturers participating in the Medicaid rebate program offer the VA a minimum discount of 24 percent (discounts offered below this minimum amount are not considered in the best price calculation for the Medicaid program). However, partnering to purchase prescription drugs provided both agencies better discounts than they were already receiving.

In FY 2000, the VA and DoD joined together to negotiate eighteen joint manufacturer contracts and saved $40 million. Current and future planned joint contracting save the departments approximately $170 million per year on their combined prescription drug expenditures. *Source:* Ventimiglia, S, (2001). *Pharmaceutical Purchasing Pools*. October. Washington, DC: National Governors Association.

19. Medicaid rebates automatically pass through in totality.

20. Redding, G.B. (2002). Managing Prescription Drug Benefits. Presentation at the National Academy for State Health Policy Annual Health Policy Conference, August 4-6, Philadelphia, Pennsylvania.

21. Express Scripts (2003). *Express Scripts and State Government Programs Overview*. St. Louis, MO: Express Scripts.

22. Express Scripts (2003).

23. Express Scripts (2003). *Express Scripts: Making the use of Prescription Drugs Safer and Much More Affordable*. St. Louis, MO: Express Scripts.

24. Centers for Medicare and Medicaid Services (2002). Table 11: Prescription Drug Expenditures Aggregate and per Capita Amounts, Percent Distribution and Average Annual Percent Change by Source of Funds: Selected Calendar Years 1980-2011. Office of the Actuary. Baltimore, MD: CMS.

25. Office of the Governor (2004). Press Release: Minnesota Joins Multi-State Purchasing Pool to Negotiate Greater Prescription Drug Discounts. April 27. St. Paul, MN: Office of the Governor.

26. Hawaii Department of Human Services (2004). News Release: Hawaii Joins Medicaid Multi-State Pooling Program to Negotiate Greater Prescription Drug Discounts. April 18. Honolulu, HI: Hawaii Department of Human Services.

27. U.S. Department of Health and Human Services (2004). Press Release: HHS Approves First-Ever Multi-State Purchasing Pools For Medicaid Drug Programs. April 22. Washington, DC: HHS.

28. Center for Medicaid and State Operations (2004). SMDL #00-046. September 9. Baltimore, MD: Centers for Medicare and Medicaid Services.

29. U.S. Department of Health and Human Services (2004).

30. Much of the discussion about changes to Medicaid pharmacy benefits relates to the federal rebate agreement included in the Omnibus Budget Reconciliation Act of 1990 (OBRA 90). Under the arrangement, states choosing to participate agreed to cover almost all prescriptions in exchange for a rebate from participating manufacturers. The rebate agreement guarantees that the states receive the best or better than the *best price* available in the private sector. The law also provides for an additional rebate from manufacturers for any product for which the price increase exceeds the consumer price index.

31. Ibid.

32. Office of the Governor (Minnesota) (2004).
33. U.S. Department of Health and Human Services (2004).
34. The Segal Company (2003).
35. The Segal Company (2003).
36. The Segal Company (2003).

Chapter 11

State versus Federal Regulation of Pharmacy

Melissa Madigan
Ed Rickert

INTRODUCTION

Pharmacy is undoubtedly one of the most highly regulated of all health care professions. A variety of administrative divisions of the federal and state governments have been authorized to govern the many aspects of pharmacy practice.

The federal government regulates pharmacy through various laws, including the Controlled Substances Act, the Poison Prevention Packaging Act, the Omnibus Budget Reconciliation Act of 1990 (more commonly known as OBRA '90), and the Health Insurance Portability and Accountability Act (more commonly known as HIPAA), as well as through regulations promulgated by the administrative departments overseeing enforcement of these laws. In addition, Medicare and Medicaid laws and regulations regulate pharmacy to the extent that they direct the conditions of participation for health care providers and define the types of activities that result in program exclusion, fines, and imprisonment. State governments regulate pharmacy practice through such mechanisms as state pharmacy practice acts, controlled substance acts, needle and syringe acts, privacy laws, and other health care related statutes. The scope of each of these sets of laws and regulations is immense; therefore this chapter will focus only on those with the greatest impact on pharmacy practice.

The authority for state and federal governments to regulate drug distribution and pharmacy practice originates from the U.S. Constitution. Article 1, Section 8 of the Constitution, otherwise known as the "commerce clause," gives the U.S. Congress the authority to regulate the distribution of goods between and within the states. The states, on the other hand, get their authority to regulate pharmacy practice, as well other health care and professional practices, from the Tenth Amendment to the Constitution, which

171

says that the powers not specifically granted to the federal government are reserved for the states. Consequently, states have broad "police powers," the authority to pass legislation intended to protect the public health, safety, and welfare.

STATE REGULATION OF PHARMACY PRACTICE

Every state, through various statutes and regulations, has taken on the responsibility for regulating pharmacy practice. Through an enabling statute, usually a "pharmacy practice act," the state grants the authority to oversee and enforce pharmacy-related statutes to the state board of pharmacy. Practice acts define, among other things, board powers and responsibilities, board member qualifications, board appointment, terms of office, membership vacancies and removal, board organization, and rule-making authority. In addition, practice acts generally give boards the responsibility for licensing pharmacists, pharmacies and, in some states, pharmaceutical manufacturers, wholesale distributors, and pharmacy technicians; enforcing professional practice standards and disciplining licensees; and determining standards for recognition and approval of pharmacy schools and practical training of pharmacists. In sum, pharmacy boards have the authority to make rules or regulations that enable the state to enforce pharmacy-related statutes, including those that clarify such statutes or establish procedures by which pharmacy practice will be monitored and evaluated for compliance.

BOARD MEMBER QUALIFICATIONS

All states have specifications for those appointed to a board of pharmacy. Each state requires most, if not all, members to be licensed pharmacists, and most states require boards to have at least one public member or consumer representative.[1] A few states have made provisions for the inclusion of others, such as pharmacy technicians or other health care professionals, on their pharmacy boards. In the vast majority of states, it is the governor who makes appointments to the state board of pharmacy. Regardless of composition or method of appointment, a board's primary responsibility is to protect the public through its activities.

LICENSURE AND CREDENTIALING

One of a board's primary responsibilities is establishing qualifications for licensure of pharmacists. Generally most states require graduation from an accredited school of pharmacy, completion of practical experience, the passage of licensure examinations, and submission of required applications and payment of applicable fees.

All states require applicants for pharmacist licensure to have graduated from an accredited school of pharmacy. The Accreditation Council for Pharmacy Education (ACPE, formerly the American Council on Pharmaceutical Education) is the accrediting body for U.S. pharmacy schools. All boards of pharmacy recognize ACPE accreditation, thus avoiding the need for each board to approve each school individually. Each state also requires the completion of a certain number of hours of practical experience. Most states require 1,500 hours of experience, and some designate that experience be in certain practice settings, including community, institutional, and clinical settings.[2]

As part of each state's licensure process, candidates must pass a series of examinations intended to demonstrate minimum competence to practice pharmacy. All states require the passage of the North American Pharmacist Licensure Examination (NAPLEX), administered by the National Association of Boards of Pharmacy (NABP), and at least forty-three states require passage of the Multistate Pharmacy Jurisprudence Examination (MPJE), also administered by NABP. Some states require pharmacists to also pass other types of exams, such as a pharmacy dispensing exam, a patient counseling exam, or a pharmaceutical calculations exam.[3] Pharmacy candidates taking the NAPLEX, at the time of registration or soon after sitting for the exam, may elect to transfer their score to any number of states.

Most states have procedures for foreign pharmacy graduates to become licensed. Almost all of these states require foreign graduates to become credentialed by NABP's Foreign Pharmacy Graduate Examination Committee (FPGEC) Certification Program. Credentialing is received only after completion of a rigorous evaluation of educational equivalence by the FPGEC and the passage of the Foreign Pharmacy Graduate Equivalency Examination (FPGEE), the Test of Spoken English (TSE), and the Test of English as a Foreign Language (TOEFL). Once FPGEE certification is received, the foreign graduate may proceed to take the state licensure exams discussed previously. In response to the recent pharmacist shortage, a small number of states, including Vermont and New Hampshire, have made provisions for graduates of Canadian schools to avoid this process and proceed directly to the NAPLEX, MPJE, and other required pharmacy licensure exams.[4]

In addition, all states except California have provisions for pharmacists to transfer their license from one state to another, and require that the licensure transfer process be completed through NABP's Electronic Licensure Transfer Program (ELTP). Most states require that pharmacists at the time of initial licensure possess all the qualifications necessary to be eligible for licensure, and several require at least one year of practice. Almost all require licensure transfer candidates to take and pass state-specific exams, primarily the state's MPJE exam, and any other mandated exams.[5] In addition, as part of the licensure transfer process, the pharmacist must acknowledge any discipline of present or previously held pharmacist license or licenses. Florida, which only recently allowed for licensure transfer, has restrictions in place that limit transferees to those who apply for licensure transfer within twelve years of their original licensure.[6] This limitation will often work both ways since many states' eligibility for transfer of licensure is contingent upon the state in which the applicant was initially licensed, granting licensure transfer to that state's pharmacists under similar circumstances and conditions.

Every state requires its pharmacists to renew their licenses on a regular basis, usually every two years. Renewal in each state is contingent upon the pharmacist paying a license renewal fee and completing a certain designated number of continuing education (CE) hours, usually fifteen hours per year.[7] Pharmacists who are not practicing or who are practicing in another state may choose to place their license on "inactive status." Inactive status, in effect, places the license in limbo. A pharmacist does not have to demonstrate completion of CE hours, and usually pays a reduced fee, but he or she may not practice. The advantage of placing one's license on inactive status, as opposed to letting one's license lapse, is that if the pharmacist wants to practice again, he or she will only have to "restore" the license, usually by demonstrating completion of required CE and payment of a licensure activation fee, as opposed to retaking the state's required licensure exams.

DISCIPLINE OF LICENSURE

Of utmost importance to any board of pharmacy is its authority to discipline its licensees. Generally, states have the authority to revoke, suspend, place on probation, censure, reprimand, and issue warnings or cease and desist orders against licensees, as well as assess fines, penalties, and administrative costs. Prohibitions are vast, but primarily involve incapacity to practice, whether due to physical or mental disabilities or substance abuse, or violation of or failure to comply with pharmacy practice regulations established by the board, for example, improper or incorrect record keeping or dispensing. Other bases for discipline include conviction of a crime, disciplinary action in another jurisdiction, fraud, misrepresentation, cheating on a licensure exam, and the all-encompassing "unprofessional conduct."

Board actions may arise in many ways, but most are the result of deficiencies found during routine board inspections or complaints made against a licensee by a member of the profession or public. Action may be taken only in compliance with established "due process" procedures. Notice must be given to the licensee of the action and he or she must be given the opportunity to respond. Most boards proceed through informal disciplinary conferences in which both sides meet and attempt to come to a mutually agreeable outcome. Should an informal conference not result in an agreement, or if an informal conference is not called by the board, it may proceed to a formal hearing, in which evidence is presented to an administrative judge. Decisions made through these administrative proceedings may be appealed by either party to the state's court system.

PHARMACY PRACTICE STANDARDS

The great majority of pharmacy practice standards that have evolved over time are contained within state pharmacy practice acts and regulations. High on this list of standards are the responsibilities that pharmacists have with regard to the prescription filling process. Every state has given pharmacists the responsibility for such activities as interpreting prescription drug orders, drug product selection (generic substitution), the maintenance of patient profiles and drug utilization review (DUR), patient counseling, and all record keeping related to the receipt and dispensing of prescription drugs, including controlled substances. The following sections offer a short review of some of these activities as well as a review of prescription drug orders and their legality.

PRESCRIPTION DRUG ORDERS

State pharmacy practice acts and/or regulations generally lay out the specific requirements for prescription drug orders. Such requirements usually include the name and address of the patient; name, address, and, if the prescription is for a controlled substance, Drug Enforcement Administration (DEA) registration number of the prescriber; date of issuance; name, strength, dosage form, and quantity of drug prescribed; directions for use; refills authorized, if any; and the prescriber's written signature (unless it is a phone or electronically transmitted order).[8] The great majority of states have made provisions for the electronic transmission of prescription drug orders, including fax transmission and computer-to-computer transmission. These provisions generally are intended to limit fraudulent prescription transmission and maintain patient confidentiality by requiring such things as the identity of the sender on the electronic order, the pharmacist's exercise of professional judgment regarding the validity of such orders, and limiting the accessibility of orders to pharmacy personnel.[9,10] Although the computer-to-computer transmission of prescriptions is technologically feasible, several factors have contributed to its lack of implementation. The lack of uniformity of state laws and regulations addressing electronic prescriptions, computer equipment incompatibilities, and high expenses have put this practice on the back burner for now; however, DEA's efforts in this area, aimed at creating a secure, uniform system for transmitting controlled substance prescriptions (discussed later in this chapter), may bring it to the forefront in the near future.

The authority of a practitioner to prescribe is found in state law. All states give doctors of medicine (MD) and doctors of osteopathy (DO) unlimited, independent prescribing authority, and other health care providers, such as dentists, podiatrists, and veterinarians, independent prescribing authority limited to their scope of practice. The vast majority of states give advance practice nurses or nurse practitioners and physician assistants various levels of independent or dependent prescribing authority. Most states give optometrists the authority to independently prescribe from a limited formulary of medications related to certain treatment of the eye. Only a few states give homeopathic and naturopathic physicians independent or dependant prescribing authority.[11]

PHARMACY PRACTICE REGULATION

As was mentioned earlier, many pharmacy practice activities are specifically regulated. One of these activities is "drug product selection," also often termed "generic substitution." Drug product selection refers to the process by which a pharmacist legally dispenses a different product from the one prescribed that contains the same drug as the one prescribed. Over the past two decades, with medical costs spiraling out of control, states passed laws and regulations that made it easier for pharmacists to substitute a generic product for a brand name product. The differences in such laws and regulations among the states, however, are great. In the majority of states, drug product selection is "permissive," or voluntary, whereas in others, it is mandatory. Some states require drug product selection pursuant to a state formulary or the U.S. Food and Drug Administration (FDA)'s "Orange Book," whereas others have no guidelines as to the products that a pharmacist may use. Some states require prescribers to handwrite a certain phrase, such as "no substitution," "brand medically necessary," or "dispense as written," to prevent drug product selection, whereas others require less effort on the part of the prescriber, for example, checking a box or signing a certain line on the prescription form.[12] Regardless of the required procedure for avoiding drug product selection, if it is not followed by the prescriber, the pharmacist may presume substitution is allowed.

The requirements that pharmacists perform drug utilization review and patient counseling services and maintain pertinent patient information related to drug therapy are relatively recent and are, for the most part, in response to a federal mandate that directed states to require these services from pharmacists as a condition of receiving federal Medicaid funds. This federal mandate, also known as OBRA '90 (Omnibus Reconciliation Act of 1990), resulted in what has become a minimum national standard of pharmacy care. Specifically, OBRA '90 requires state Medicaid plans to require pharmacists to do the following for Medicaid recipients:

- Maintain patient records, including:
  —name, address, phone number, date of birth or age, and gender;
  —significant patient history, including disease state(s), allergies, adverse drug reactions, and medication use;
  —the pharmacist's comments relevant to the patient's drug therapy.[13]
- Drug utilization review. On this issue, OBRA '90 requires a "review of drug therapy before each prescription is filled . . ." The review "shall include screening for potential drug therapy problems due to therapeutic duplication, drug-disease contraindications, drug-drug interactions (including serious interactions with nonprescription or over-the-counter drugs), incorrect drug dosage or duration of treatment, drug-allergy interactions and clinical abuse/misuse."[14]
- Patient counseling. OBRA '90 directs that, as part of a prospective drug use review program, pharmacists must offer to discuss with patients or caregivers anything that the pharmacists in his or her professional judgment considers significant, including:
  —The name and description of the medication;
  —The route, dosage form, dosage, route of administration, and duration of drug therapy;
  —Special directions and precautions for preparation;
  —Administration and use by the patient;
  —Common severe side or adverse effects or interactions and therapeutic contraindications that may be encountered, including their avoidance, and the action required if they occur;
  —Techniques for self-monitoring drug therapy;
  —Proper storage;
  —Prescription refill information; and
  —Action to be taken in the event of a missed dose.[15]

The vast majority of states have expanded these requirements to all patients, not just those receiving Medicaid benefits. Of note, although OBRA '90 created a uniform national standard for these aspects of pharmacy care, state-by-state requirements still vary. For example, some states require the offer to counsel only on new prescriptions, while others require it for new and refilled prescriptions, and some require the pharmacist to make the offer to counsel, while others allow pharmacy technicians or other ancillary personnel to make the offer.[16]

EXPANDED PHARMACY PRACTICE

Numerous states have expanded pharmacy practice to activities beyond traditional dispensing. One such example is "collaborative pharmacy practice," in which pharmacists enter into agreements with legally authorized prescribers to initiate, modify, and/or discontinue drug therapy based on protocol. At least thirty-five states now allow pharmacists to enter into collaborative practice agreements.[17] Such agreements usually spell out the participants; each one's responsibilities regarding supervision by and reporting to the prescribing practitioner; the drug therapy protocol, including the medications to be used and dosing/monitoring parameters; and the effective dates of the agreement.

In addition, at least thirty-eight states allow pharmacists to administer immunizations.[18] Some states allow this within the context of collaborative practice agreements, whereas others have specifically carved out this activity in the pharmacy practice act or regulations. Some states limit the type of immunizations allowed (e.g., flu vaccines) and/or the patients allowed to receive such services (e.g., adults only). Others require pharmacists who participate in these activities to have undergone specialized training. Most recently, a few states have specifically granted pharmacists the authority to dispense emergency contraceptive medications without a prescription. Although some of these states require such dispensing to be via a collaborative practice protocol, others, including California, Maine, and New Mexico, have no such requirement, and pharmacists may provide such therapy independently.[19]

PHARMACIST IN CHARGE

All states have provisions for what is usually termed a "pharmacist in charge," the pharmacist with responsibility for all that takes place in a pharmacy. State requirements vary but, overall, pharmacists in charge have multiple and comprehensive responsibilities, including developing, maintaining, and complying with policies and procedures; addressing day-to-day pharmacy operations, including security provisions; licensure, training, and duties of pharmacy personnel, including pharmacy technicians; submission of any required reports or information; and, most recently, quality assurance. State boards of pharmacy require pharmacies to designate a pharmacist in charge and to be notified in a timely manner of any changes to that status.

PHARMACY TECHNICIANS

The use of pharmacy technicians has grown exponentially in recent years. Once not even recognized in most states, pharmacy technicians are now being given broader and more comprehensive responsibilities in light of increased prescription volume and a persistent shortage of pharmacists. This does not lessen the responsibility of the pharmacist for the final outcome of drug dispensing. In all states, pharmacists are responsible for ensuring that drugs are correctly dispensed and appropriate pharmaceutical care given. Expanded technician use, however, has, at least in theory, freed the pharmacist from technical prescription dispensing tasks to concentrate on patient care activities.

As is the case in other areas, state laws and regulations vary on such things as technician registration, training, and allowable tasks. Although technicians are not regulated in a significant number of states, at least thirty-five states either license, register, or certify technicians.[20] This type of regulation is necessary, because without it a state has little or no authority to discipline technicians and prevent them from working if it is in the best interest of the public.

Some states have gone further and required training programs and even the passage of an exam. At least twenty-eight states have some sort of training requirements for technicians and at least eleven require some sort of ongoing continuing education. In addition, at least fifteen states require passage of the Pharmacy Technician Certification Examination for, or as one way to qualify for, technician registration or licensure.[21]

In an effort to prevent overuse of technicians, at least thirty-three states have implemented a maximum technician-to-pharmacist ratio. Proponents of ratios argue that they prevent pharmacies from forcing pharmacists to supervise too many technical staff. Opponents of ratios, on the other hand, argue that pharmacies will not necessarily hire more pharmacists once the ratio is met and will operate with the minimal staff a ratio provides, resulting in overwork for all involved. Whether or not ratios work as intended remains to be seen.

QUALITY ASSURANCE/REGULATING FOR OUTCOMES

With the recent proliferation of reports of medication errors, an effort has been made on the part of regulators to institute requirements for quality improvement programs in pharmacy settings. At least fifteen states have instituted error reporting or quality improvement program requirements in some, if not all, pharmacy settings.[22] Some programs require pharmacies to document and report serious errors to the boards, whereas others require internal documentation and review of errors and subsequent system improvement to prevent further errors. This latter continuous quality improvement strategy, when required by regulatory boards, is a small part of a "regulating for outcomes" approach being tried by some boards in an effort to not only regulate the "structures and processes" of pharmacy practice, but to evaluate and improve patient outcomes as well. In pharmacy, outcomes regulation may evaluate compliance with "structural" requirements (e.g., the security of the pharmacy), and compliance with "process" requirements (e.g., patient counseling or DUR requirements), as well as the "outcomes" of pharmaceutical care (e.g., patient medication compliance, or even clinical outcomes such as blood pressure reduction in hypertensive patients). Outcomes regulation is still in its early stages within state pharmacy regulation, but is expected to gain ground in the future.

PHARMACY LICENSURE

Every state licenses pharmacies and maintains various requirements for such licensure. Such requirements address the structure of the pharmacy, such as the physical layout, unauthorized access, hours of operation, security, equipment, reference materials, and patient privacy, as well as responsibility for the operations, specifically the pharmacist in charge discussed earlier in this chapter.

Almost every state now requires "nonresident" pharmacies, those that ship medications to in-state patients from outside the state, to register with the board of pharmacy.[23] In addition, at least nine states require that at least one pharmacist, whether it be the pharmacist-in-charge or a staff pharmacist, to be licensed in the state where medications are shipped.[24] Generally, nonresident pharmacy laws and regulations require facilities to maintain current home state licensure, maintain readily retrievable records of the specific state's patients, and maintain a toll-free phone number for patients to call with questions. These requirements are in addition to completing any forms and paying any fees mandated by the board.

FEDERAL REGULATION OF CONTROLLED SUBSTANCES

As was stated early in this chapter, the federal government regulates pharmacy through various laws and regulations. The most prevalent in a pharmacist's practice is the federal Controlled Substances Act (CSA) and its accompanying regulations. The sections relevant to pharmacy practice lay out the requirements for the distribution of controlled substances, including the "scheduling" or classification of controlled substances; the registration of controlled substance manufacturers, researchers, wholesalers, dispensers, and prescribers; security requirements to guard against theft and/or diversion; requirements for controlled substance prescriptions; dispensing and record keeping requirements; enforcement and inspections; and penalties for violations.

CONTROLLED SUBSTANCE SCHEDULES

The CSA lays out five "schedules" or classes of controlled substances.[25] The schedules range from I to V, with each categorizing a drug's (1) potential for abuse, (2) level of currently accepted medical use, and (3) level of safety for use. Schedule I is the most stringent, with these drugs categorized as having a high potential for abuse, no currently accepted medical use, and lack of accepted information on safety for use. Schedule I drugs may not be prescribed or dispensed, and include such drugs as heroin, marijuana, lysergic acid diethylamide (LSD), and methaqualone. Drugs in schedule II may be prescribed and dispensed, but only with severe restrictions. Although such drugs have been determined to have a high potential for abuse, and such abuse may lead to severe physical or psychological dependence, they have currently accepted medical uses. Schedule II drugs include depressants, such as amobarbital, pentobarbital, and secobarbital; pain relievers such as codeine, methadone, meperidine, morphine, and oxycodone; and stimulants, such as amphetamine, methamphetamine, and methylphenidate. Schedule III drugs are those with a potential for abuse less than those in Schedules I and II. Although their abuse may lead to moderate or low physical dependence or high psychological dependence, they have currently accepted medical uses, and include combination pain relievers such as acetaminophen with codeine and aspirin with codeine; stimulants such as benzphetamine; and anabolic steroids. Schedule IV drugs are those with a potential for abuse less than those in schedule III, whose abuse may lead to limited physical and psychological dependence relative to those in schedule IV, and have a currently accepted medical use. Such drugs include depressants, such as chloral hydrate, phenobarbital, and the benzodiazepines (alprazolam, diazepam, flurazepam, lorazepam, and triazolam), as well as stimulants such as phentermine. Schedule V drugs have a low potential for abuse compared to those in schedule IV, and a limited potential for physical and psychological dependence relative to those in schedule IV, and, of course, a currently accepted medical use. Such drugs include codeine- or hydrocodone-containing products used for cough, and antidiarrheal products with an opium derivative, such as diphenoxylate.[26] The U.S. Attorney General has the authority to schedule, reschedule, or remove from a schedule drugs upon the recommendation of the Secretary of the Department of Health and Human Services.[27]

REGISTRATION

In an effort to control the theft and diversion of controlled substance and to maintain a system of accountability, each entity involved in the distribution process must register with the U.S. Attorney General.[28] Pharmacies and prescribers register as "dispensers" every three years. Pharmacists do not have to register individually since they serve as agents or employees of their registered employers.[29] Prescribers of controlled substances are determined by state law. All states allow doctors of medicine and doctors of osteopathy to prescribe controlled substances, and if a state allows midlevel health care practitioners, such as nurse practitioners, physician assistants, optometrists, or, in some states, pharmacists, to prescribe controlled substances, then such practitioners may apply for registration. As mentioned previously, although all prescribing registrants are registered as "dispensers," and they may provide controlled substances directly to their own patients if allowed by state law, they may not actually fill prescriptions for controlled substances. This right is reserved for pharmacists acting in the usual course of professional practice.[30]

Registration may be denied, suspended, or revoked by the Attorney General under certain circumstances, such as when an applicant falsifies an application; is convicted of a crime related to controlled substances; has had his or her state licensure suspended, revoked, or denied; is noncompliant with state or local laws; or participates in other conduct that threatens the public health.[31]

SECURITY REQUIREMENTS

"All applicants and registrants shall provide effective controls and procedures to guard against theft and diversion of controlled substances."[32] When evaluating for compliance with this requirement, the DEA may consider the following factors:

1. The type of activity conducted (e.g., processing of bulk chemicals, preparing dosage forms, packaging, labeling, cooperative buying, etc.)
2. The type and form of controlled substances handled (e.g., bulk liquids or dosage units, usable powders or nonusable powders)
3. The quantity of controlled substances handled;
4. The location of the premises and the relationship such location bears on security needs
5. The type of building construction comprising the facility and the general characteristics of the building or buildings
6. The type of vault, safe, and secure enclosures or other storage system (e.g., automatic storage and retrieval system) used
7. The type of closures on vaults, safes, and secure enclosures
8. The adequacy of key control systems and/or combination lock control systems
9. The adequacy of electric detection and alarm systems, if any including use of supervised transmittal lines and standby power sources
10. The extent of unsupervised public access to the facility, including the presence and characteristics of perimeter fencing, if any
11. The adequacy of supervision over employees having access to manufacturing and storage areas
12. The procedures for handling business guests, visitors, maintenance personnel, and nonemployee service personnel
13. The availability of local police protection or of the registrant's or applicant's security personnel
14. The adequacy of the registrant's or applicant's system for monitoring the receipt, manufacture, distribution, and disposition of controlled substances in its operations[33]

Specific security requirements for pharmacies are less stringent than those for manufacturers and distributors. In pharmacies, controlled substances listed in schedules II, III, IV, and V may be stored in a securely locked, substantially constructed cabinet, or they may be dispersed throughout the stock of noncontrolled substances in such a manner as to obstruct the theft or diversion of the controlled substances.[34]

PRESCRIPTION REQUIREMENTS

Under the CSA, prescriptions for controlled substances must be issued for a legitimate medical purpose by an individual practitioner acting in the usual course of his or her professional practice.[35] Although the responsibility for the proper prescribing and dispensing of controlled substances is upon the prescribing practitioner, a corresponding responsibility rests with the pharmacist who fills the prescription.[36] A prescription "issued not in the usual course of professional treatment or in legitimate and authorized research" is not a prescription. Any person knowingly filling such a purported prescription, as well as the person issuing it, shall be subject to the penalties provided for violations of the provisions of law relating to controlled substances.[37]

A controlled substance prescription must be dated and signed on the day of issuance. It must contain the full name and address of the patient; the name, strength, dosage form, quantity, and directions for use of the drug prescriber; and the name, address, and registration number (DEA number) of the prescribing practitioner. An agent or secretary of the practitioner may prepare the order for signature. Currently, the electronic transmission of such prescriptions is not allowed other than by facsimile in certain situations discussed below. For the past several years, however, the DEA has been working on developing regulations for the electronic transmission of controlled substance prescriptions from the prescriber to the pharmacy. Such regulations are anticipated to require the use of a public key infrastructure system, which provides for:

1. *Confidentiality.* Only authorized persons will be able to read the encrypted prescription order.
2. *Authentication.* The pharmacist will be able to ensure the prescription order was sent by the prescriber and not someone else.
3. *Integrity.* The pharmacist can be sure the message has not been altered.
4. *Nonrepudiation.* The sender will not be able to deny having sent the prescription.

An overview of the DEA's efforts with regard to electronic prescribing can be found at http://www.deadiversion.usdoj.gov/ecomme/e_ordrs/index .html. Interestingly, the DEA recently promulgated rules that allow for the electronic transmission of new controlled substance (schedule II-V) prescriptions for centralized prescription filling, and for centralized prescription refilling of schedule III to V prescriptions.[38]

SCHEDULE II PRESCRIPTIONS

Prescriptions for schedule II drugs must be written and bear the signature of the prescriber. Such prescriptions may be faxed to the pharmacy, but the original written, signed prescription must be presented to the pharmacy prior to dispensing. Exceptions to this rule exist for emergency schedule II prescriptions, for schedule II narcotic prescriptions that are compounded and administered parenterally (intravenous, intramuscular, subcutaneous, intraspinal), for schedule II prescriptions for patients in a long-term care facility, and for schedule II prescriptions for hospice patients. In these situations, oral or facsimile prescriptions are allowed.[39] Where oral orders are not allowed, the prescription must be written with ink or indelible pencil or typewriter and must be manually signed by the practitioner.[40]

Schedule II prescriptions must be labeled with the date of filling, the pharmacy name and address, the serial number of the prescription, the patient name, prescriber name, directions for use, and cautionary statements, if any.[41] If filled by a central fill pharmacy, the label must also identify such pharmacy.[42] Schedule II prescriptions may be partially filled in certain circumstances,[43] but in no case may schedule II prescriptions be refilled.[44]

SCHEDULE III, IV, AND V PRESCRIPTIONS

Prescriptions for schedule III to V drugs may be written, faxed, or transmitted orally by the prescriber or agent and reduced to writing by the pharmacist. Written and faxed prescriptions must be signed by the practitioner.[45] These prescriptions may be refilled up to five times in six months.[46]

Schedule III to V prescriptions must be labeled with the pharmacy name and address, the serial number of the prescription, date of initial filling, the patient name, prescriber name, directions for use, and cautionary statements, if any.[47] If filled by a central fill pharmacy, the label must also identify the pharmacy.[48] Schedule III to V prescriptions may be transferred between pharmacies on a one-time basis, except if the pharmacies electronically share a real-time, online database, they may transfer up to the maximum number of refills.[49]

RECORD KEEPING

The CSA mandates that registrants maintain controlled substance inventory records, and records of the receipt and sale of controlled substances.[50] These records must be maintained for at least two years.[51] Pharmacies must inventory their controlled substance stock every two years and maintain records of such.[52] Controlled substance dispensing records must be retrievable by prescription number and must contain the name and dosage form of the controlled substance, the date of filling or refilling, the quantity dispensed, initials of the dispensing pharmacist for each refill, and the total number of refills for that prescription. Automated data processing systems must allow for the retrieval of the original prescription number; date of issuance of the original prescription order by the practitioner; full name and address of the patient; name, address, and DEA registration number of the practitioner; the name, strength, dosage form, quantity of the controlled substance prescribed (and quantity dispensed if different from the quantity prescribed); and the total number of refills authorized by the prescribing practitioner.[53] Hard-copy prescriptions must be filed in one of several designated ways that allow easy retrieval of such prescriptions.[54] Also addressed by the rules are records of distributions from a pharmacy to another registered practitioner or reverse distributor[55] and records of destruction.[56]

STATE REGULATION OF CONTROLLED SUBSTANCES

Almost all the states have enacted their own laws and regulations addressing the distribution of controlled substances. Most of these laws and regulations expound upon the federal requirements and are more stringent. Sometimes such state laws may be in conflict with the federal law. In other words, it is impossible to comply with both laws, in which case the federal law prevails pursuant to the supremacy clause of the U.S. Constitution. This might happen if a state passed a law less stringent than a federal law on an issue. For example, if a state passed a law saying that schedule II controlled substance prescriptions may be refilled, this would conflict with the federal law, and thus the federal law prevails. If, however, a state passes a law that is more stringent than the federal law but is not conflicting, in other words it is possible to comply with both laws, then the more stringent state law must be followed. A good example of this is when states require that controlled substance records be kept for longer than the federally required two years. Other examples of state controlled substance laws and regulations include pharmacy and, in some states, pharmacist, controlled substance dispensing registration requirements; more stringent record keeping requirements;

controlled substance prescription monitoring program requirements (electronic or duplicate/triplicate prescription programs); and more stringent time limitations, for example, in some states schedule II prescriptions must be filled within a certain time (seventy-two hours, seven days, thirty days) of having been written, although no such federal requirement exists.

POISON PREVENTION PACKAGING ACT

Another federal law applicable to pharmacy practice is the Poison Prevention Packaging Act of 1970, which, in effect, requires all human oral prescription drugs to be dispensed in a child-resistant container unless the prescriber or patient requests a noncomplying container. Violators may face not more than one year imprisonment and/or a fine of up to $1,000.

PATIENT PRIVACY PROTECTIONS

One of the more recent federal enactments to impact pharmacy practice is the Health Insurance Portability and Accountability Act of 1996 (HIPAA) and its regulations addressing the privacy and security of patient health information. Prior to this law going into effect, patient health information and medical records were protected by various state laws, which left gaps in the protection of patient privacy and confidentiality. HIPAA set national standards intended to close these gaps, control the exchange of patient information, and set penalties for the misuse or wrongful disclosure of patient health information.

HIPAA regulations created protections for individually identifiable health information relating to the past, present, or future physical or mental health, the provision of health care, or payment for health care. "Covered entities," which include health care providers, hospitals, health plans and health insurers, and health care clearinghouses, are required to establish policies and procedures to protect the confidentiality of protected health information about their patients. According to the U.S. Department of Health and Human Services (HHS) Office for Civil Rights (OCR), the administrative agency charged with enforcing HIPAA, these requirements are flexible to allow different covered entities to implement them as appropriate for their businesses or practices.

With regard to their business practices, covered entities must:

- Maintain written privacy procedures, including a description of staff that has access to protected information, how it will be used, and when

it may be disclosed, and ensure that business associates with access to protected information agree to the same.
- Designate a "privacy officer" responsible for ensuring procedures are followed.
- Provide training for employees on privacy procedures.
- Ensure appropriate disciplinary action is taken against employees who fail to follow procedures.

With regard to their interactions with patients, covered entities must:

- Provide patients access to their medical records.
- Provide patients with a "notice of privacy practices" describing how they may use patients' personal medical information and their rights with regards to such uses.
- Generally limit the use of personal medical information to that related to treatment of the patient.
- Limit the amount of information shared with other health care providers to that necessary for a particular purpose.
- Obtain authorization from patients to release information to outside businesses not related to health care, including marketing purposes, but not including disease-state management programs.

The privacy regulations allow patients to file formal complaints regarding privacy practices, either to the covered entity directly or to the OCR.

Circumstances exist in which covered entities may, with safeguards and limitations, disclose protected health information. These include emergencies, identification of the body of a deceased person or the cause of death, public health needs, research that involves limited data or has been independently approved by an institutional review board or privacy board, oversight of the health care system, judicial and administrative proceedings, limited law enforcement activities, and activities related to national defense and security. In the cases in which a state has more stringent privacy protections than those offered by HIPAA, such protections remain in effect and are not preempted by the federal law.

Under HIPAA , for noncriminal violations, including disclosures made in error, civil monetary penalties exist of $100 per violation up to $25,000 per year, per standard. Criminal penalties for certain types of violations that are done knowingly include a fine of up to $50,000 and one year in prison for obtaining or disclosing protected health information, up to $100,000 and up to five years in prison for obtaining or disclosing protected health information under false pretenses, and up to $250,000 and up to ten years in prison for obtaining protected health information with the intent to sell, transfer, or use it for commercial advantage, personal gain, or malicious harm.

More information on HIPAA can be found on the HHS-OCR Web site at http://www.hhs.gov/ocr.

CONCLUSION

This chapter is by no means inclusive of all the laws and regulations that govern pharmacy. The U.S. Centers for Medicare and Medicaid Services, the agency overseeing the new federal prescription drug benefit, is making itself known in pharmacies throughout the country. New state laws are enacted and regulations promulgated on a continuous basis. It is important for pharmacists to remain abreast of any changes impacting their practice to protect their patients, their employers, and themselves.

NOTES

1. National Association of Boards of Pharmacy (2005). *Survey of Pharmacy Law.* Mount Prospect, IL: NABP, pp. 6-7.
2. National Association of Boards of Pharmacy (2005), pp. 12-14.
3. National Association of Boards of Pharmacy (2005), pp. 10-11.
4. National Association of Boards of Pharmacy (2005), pp. 18-20.
5. National Association of Boards of Pharmacy (2005), pp. 24-26.
6. Florida Department of Health (2004). Pharmacy: Overview. Available at: http://www.doh.state.fl.us/mqa/pharmacy/ph_home.html.
7. National Association of Boards of Pharmacy (2005), pp. 32-35.
8. National Association of Boards of Pharmacy. (2003). *Model State Pharmacy Act and Model Rules of the National Association of Boards of Pharmacy.* Mount Prospect, IL: NABP, pp. 80-81.
9. National Association of Boards of Pharmacy (2003), p. 83.
10. National Association of Boards of Pharmacy (2005), pp. 74-79.
11. National Association of Boards of Pharmacy (2005), pp. 82-88.
12. National Association of Boards of Pharmacy (2005), pp. 64-67.
13. 42 U.S.C. § 1396r-8(g)(2)(A)(ii)(II).
14. 42 U.S.C. § 1396r-8(g)(2)(A)(i).
15. 42 U.S.C. § 1396r-8(g)(2)(A)(ii)(I).
16. National Association of Boards of Pharmacy (2005), pp. 80-81.
17. National Association of Boards of Pharmacy (2005), pp. 102-108.
18. National Association of Boards of Pharmacy (2005), pp. 102-108.
19. National Association of Boards of Pharmacy (2005), pp. 102-108.
20. National Association of Boards of Pharmacy (2005), pp. 38-41.
21. National Association of Boards of Pharmacy (2005), pp. 38-41.
22. National Association of Boards of Pharmacy (2005), p. 23.

23. National Association of Boards of Pharmacy (2005), pp. 51-54.

24. National Association of Boards of Pharmacy (2005), pp. 51-54. These states include Arkansas, Michigan, Nebraska, North Carolina, North Dakota, Oklahoma, Oregon, Tennessee, and Vermont.

25. 21 U.S.C. §812.

26. 21 U.S.C. §812.

27. 21 U.S.C. §811.

28. 31 C.F.R. §1301.

29. 21 U.S.C. §822.

30. 21 C.F.R. §1306.06.

31. 21 U.S.C. §823(f), 824(a).

32. 21 C.F.R. §1301.71(a).

33. 21 C.F.R. §1301.71(b).

34. 21 C.F.R. §1301.75(b).

35. 21 C.F.R. §1306.04(a).

36. 21 C.F.R. §1306.04(a).

37. 21 C.F.R. §1306.04(a).

38. 21 C.F.R. §1306.15, §1306.27.

39. 21 C.F.R. §1306.11.

40. 21 C.F.R. §1306.05(a).

41. 21 C.F.R. §1306.14(a).

42. 21 C.F.R. §1306.14(b).

43. C.F.R. §1306.13.

44. 21 C.F.R. §1306.12.

45. 21 C.F.R. §1306.21.

46. 21 C.F.R. §1306.22.

47. 21 C.F.R. §1306.24(a).

48. 21 C.F.R. §1306.24(b).

49. 21 C.F.R. §1305.24.

50. 21 U.S.C. §827.

51. 21 C.F.R. §1304.04.

52. 21 C.F.R. §1304.11.

53. 21 C.F.R. §1306.22.

54. 21 C.F.R. §1304.04(h)(2).

55. 21 C.F.R. §1307.11.

56. 21 C.F.R. §1307.21.

Chapter 12

Evolution and Future Prospects of Pharmaceutical Industry Regulation

William Wardell
William Vodra
Judith K. Jones
Richard N. Spivey

INTRODUCTION

In this chapter the future course and prospects for regulation and drug development are discussed. Now is an opportune time to make these observations. Both the pharmaceutical industry and the Food and Drug Administration (FDA) are under special stresses, which are having negative effects on the discovery and testing of new drugs and on their availability to physicians and patients.[1-4] To start, the enormous changes since the Drug Amendments were enacted in 1962 are reviewed in order to understand what may (or should) happen in the future.

For purposes of drug research, development, and marketing, the Drug Amendments of 1962 (also called the Kefauver-Harris Amendments) constituted the most significant single piece of legislation. Congress mandated that drugs be proven effective for their intended uses through "adequate and well-controlled" clinical investigations. This deceptively simple requirement profoundly changed the pharmaceutical industry, the FDA, and the United States's—indeed, the whole world's—standards and expectations for therapeutic agents. The drug amendments also directed the FDA to become involved in the clinical research process, required companies to adhere to current good manufacturing practices in making pharmaceuticals,

This chapter was previously published in *The Textbook of Pharmaceutical Medicine,* Fifth edition, edited by John P. Griffin and John O'Grady, published by Blackwell Publishing, Oxford, England, 2006. Used with permission.

allowed FDA greater access to corporate records, and transferred regulatory control over the advertising of prescription drugs from the Federal Trade Commission.

Since 1962, the FDA and the pharmaceutical industry have achieved improvements in the effectiveness and safety of prescription drugs that are unparalleled in the history of medicine. Indeed, the methods of thinking about, analyzing, and implementing the steps needed to prove the effectiveness and safety of therapeutic drugs, and to guide their proper use in medicine and the marketplace, have led the field of evidence-based medicine and created its most extensive and well-defined example. The influence of drug regulation has extended to the use of all therapeutic or diagnostic interventions, including diet, exercise, watchful waiting, surgical procedures, and medical devices, and has set new standards that are still percolating through all branches of medicine and the related sciences. It is probably no exaggeration to say that these conceptual and operational advances in ensuring effectiveness and safety are among the most significant made in the field of therapeutic interventions since the Enlightenment.

In this chapter, sector by sector, the main components of this achievement are considered, as well as the corresponding problems that have arisen. Two other public policy changes since 1962 that have had enormous impacts on the pharmaceutical industry—the introduction of generic competition for pharmaceuticals and health care cost containment efforts—are also discussed. Last, we suggest how to overcome the problems and keep the field improving in the future.

THE EVOLUTION OF THE FDA AND THE PHARMACEUTICAL INDUSTRY FROM 1962 TO 2005

FDA and Effectiveness

The 1962 Act and the DESI Project

Before 1962, the FDA was legally empowered to evaluate evidence on safety of a proposed new pharmaceutical, but not evidence on effectiveness. In practice, however, the agency did consider efficacy, at least in the case of drugs with major side effects. It reasoned that the decision to approve a drug for marketing had necessarily to involve both safety and efficacy, because the amount of risk allowed had to take into account each drug's efficacy. Nevertheless, this approach was the exception, not the rule, and the agency rarely acknowledged any formal evaluation of effectiveness. By 1962, at least 13,000 New Drug Applications (NDAs), covering approximately

4,000 unique formulations of active ingredients and over 16,000 distinct therapeutic claims, became effective under the 1938 statute.

The 1962 legislation changed this situation in several respects. First, it required affirmative agency approval of the NDA. Under the old law, if the FDA failed to object in the first sixty days after an NDA was submitted, the drug could enter the market. Thus, Congress delayed the marketing until FDA had acted. Second, it insisted that a drug be effective for its declared use. Third, the legislation required that effectiveness be proved by adequate and well-controlled investigations, including clinical investigations. Finally, Congress directed the FDA to reassess all drugs that had entered the market under the prior law, to ensure their effectiveness.

This last provision had, in many respects, the most significant impact on the agency and the pharmaceutical industry over the next fifteen years. Initially, the agency contracted with the National Academy of Sciences (NAS)–National Research Council to conduct a review of the marketed products. The NAS–NRC in turn hired teams of physicians, pharmacologists, and clinical researchers to perform the actual reviews. At the end of 1968, NAS–NRC reported back that, for almost 15 percent of the claims, the products did not work; for another 24 percent, the claims were supported, but superior products were available for treating these conditions; and for another 42 percent, the evidence supporting efficacy was equivocal. In short, less than 20 percent of the efficacy claims were found to be supported without qualification. Moreover, the NAS–NRC found a large number of products ineffective as fixed combinations in that no substantial reason existed to believe that each ingredient added to the effectiveness of the combination.

The NAS–NRC report set the FDA and the pharmaceutical industry on a collision course. The agency was under orders from Congress to remove the ineffective products. The industry faced the choice of giving up products (and revenues) or investing in new research for old products. The Drug Efficacy Study Implementation (DESI) program resulted in protracted litigation and painful disputes between drug companies and the FDA over prescription drugs. In the process, both parties learned much more about the nuances and complexities of "adequate and well-controlled" clinical investigations in many diverse and previously inadequately studied diseases. The agency promulgated the first regulations defining the elements of such investigations and then, after much litigation, applied them to deny formal hearings to NDA holders in order to complete the DESI effort. Companies, physicians, and regulators grappled with how to design and interpret clinical trials in virtually all areas of pharmacotherapy. By the time DESI was over (1984), and partly in response to it, the science of drug development had taken an enormous leap forward. Moreover, academia, industry, and the

FDA had largely replaced disputes over the drug effectiveness requirement with a common understanding and acceptance of the methods and value of adequate and well-controlled studies. In sum, a complete paradigm shift had occurred.

The intensity and focus of the DESI program influenced the process of evaluating new NDAs. After 1962, the agency had greatly increased the number of physicians, pharmacologists, toxicologists, statisticians, and pharmacists to carry out both DESI and the review of pending NDAs. Many of these technical experts started their careers with skepticism about the merits of manufacturers' claims for drugs (vindicated by the DESI findings) and an intense course in the meaning of "adequate and well-controlled" studies needed to carry out the DESI project. The subsequent adverse effects on products in the pipeline gave rise to the drug lag and patient access debates, which will be discussed shortly.

Another collateral effect of the DESI project was the development of the "abbreviated NDA," by which a generic version of the innovator product could satisfy the statutory preconditions for entering the market without repeating the preclinical and clinical studies of the innovator. This administrative creation, designed to assure that generics were both pharmaceutically equivalent and bioequivalent to the pioneer product, was endorsed by Congress in 1984. As will be seen, this development had a staggering impact on the business model of the pharmaceutical industry.

FDA Organization and Attitudes Toward Industry

Implementation of the 1962 amendments, and subsequent challenges, led to a series of organizational changes within the agency. In the 1960s the FDA was organized along disciplinary lines (e.g., Bureaus of Medicine, Science, and Compliance). In 1970 it was reorganized along product lines (e.g., Bureau of Drugs and Bureau of Foods). Within the new Bureau of Drugs, the old separation between "new" drugs (NDA evaluation) and "marketed" drugs (evaluation of supplements and safety information) was eliminated by the creation of the Office of New Drugs. In 1972 a departmental reorganization resulted in the transfer of the Division of Biologic Standards from the National Institutes of Health to the FDA, which renamed it the Bureau of Biologics. For a brief period in the 1980s, the Bureau of Drugs was consolidated with that for Biologics into the National Center for Drugs and Biologics. The marriage failed, and by the late 1980s the agency created the Center for Drug Evaluation and Research (CDER) and the Center for Biologics Evaluation and Research (CBER). In 2002, jurisdiction for many therapeutic biologicals was reassigned from CBER to CDER.

Throughout this period, the agency has undergone a series of reorientations regarding its relationship with the regulated industry. In the 1960s and early 1970s, the attitude was frankly adversarial. The drug industry was characterized as unscrupulous seekers of profits. In a book called *Pills, Profits, and Politics,* Philip Lee (Assistant Secretary for Health in the Lyndon Johnson Administration) and Milton Silverman attacked the Pharmaceutical industry.[5] Even in the early to mid-1970s, Senators Ted Kennedy (D-MA), Gaylord Nelson (D-WI), and Congressman L.H. Fountain (D-NC) conducted hearings that regularly sought to expose problems with drug safety and alleged misconduct by the Pharmaceutical industry or the FDA (or often both). Although ignoring the obvious slowdown in new drug approvals, these well-publicized congressional investigations attempted to embarrass the FDA for failing to regulate the industry adequately. Among the outcomes of these investigations were greater agency attention both to post-approval adverse event monitoring and to rigorous enforcement of rules to assure the integrity of research data.

By the mid-1970s, however, attitudes within the agency were changing. Although some still viewed their role as finding industry errors, a new professional ethic emerged in which the FDA was to judge objectively the evidence presented. By the mid-1980s, the orientation shifted further, in light of the AIDS crisis. The picture changed to one in which new drug approval was no longer deemed to be a zero-sum game in which benefit for some was possible only at the expense of harm to others. Drug development was understood to be a process wherein approval could be speeded by efficient and timely review of relevant animal and human data so that every sector could benefit—the sick obviously, but also the medical profession, the FDA, and the industry. In the 1990s, the terminology became one of "stakeholders," in which the agency viewed itself as a neutral party mediating between divergent interests and serving all constituent groups, including industry. This "customer" focus became itself a target of criticism by those who felt the FDA could not serve both industry and the public at the same time.

The IND

Prior to 1962, the agency had played no role until the NDA was submitted. After learning, however, that pregnant women were given thalidomide (to prevent morning sickness) without being told what the drug was or that it was experimental, Congress demanded federal oversight and informed consent from all research subjects. The result was the Investigational New

Drug (IND) Application, and a new series of FDA regulations governing informed consent, protections of the rights and safety of human subjects, and good clinical practices (GCPs).

In response to demands to accelerate the drug review process, however, the FDA perceived opportunities to use the IND process to improve the chances that the subsequent NDA would answer the essential regulatory questions, or eliminate them by answering these questions before the NDA was submitted. Gradually, the chemistry, manufacturing, and controls segments of the IND application moved from merely being adequate, to assuring the safety and consistency of the investigational product, to being complete and acceptable for NDA purposes. Clinical reviewers provided more guidance on study design to avoid fundamental flaws that would render the final results scientifically invalid. Pharmacologists and toxicologists urged completion of all preclinical studies early in the IND process so that issues could be flagged in advance of NDA filing. Overall, the IND became burdened with regulatory requests that were unnecessary for subject protection but might shorten NDA review times and increase chances for ultimate drug approval.

The Drug Lag Debate and Its Consequences

By the early 1970s, many observers were questioning the impact and value of FDA review of NDAs for effectiveness. In particular, cardiologists could point to a period of almost five full years that the FDA had not approved a single new molecular entity (NME) in their field. The Pharmaceutical industry was keenly aware of the decline in approvals of NMEs via the NDA process, despite that many new products were available in Europe. William Wardell identified a "Drug Lag," showing that the United States had fallen behind other pharmaceutically advanced countries (as represented, for example, by the UK) in terms of the number of new drugs approved and the overall capabilities of the therapeutic armamentarium available. Work on the drug lag and the wider issues of pharmaceutical policy in government and industry led in 1974 to the founding of the Center for the Study of Drug Development (CSDD) by Louis Lasagna and William Wardell at the University of Rochester Medical Center. The CSDD moved to Tufts University in the 1980s.[6,7]

A few personal touches emerged to underline the drug lag issue, such as the FDA Commissioner's taking propranolol for hypertension at a time when it was not approved by the FDA for that purpose. Meanwhile, the more cautious parties cited the dangers of the perceived rapid and less stringent approvals in Europe and the example of practolol, a beta-blocker that was found to cause a severe "mucocutaneous syndrome" with sclerosis of eyes and internal organs that was severely debilitating and sometimes fatal. Its prodrome, "itchy eyes," had been noted and discounted in the clinical trials.

Although the charges of drug lag were greeted with hostility from Congress, the FDA, and the antidrug lobby, they were welcomed by the drug industry. In the end, the proponents had tremendous influence over the future of drug regulation in the United States.[8]

Interestingly, the debate went beyond the regulated parties. Economists and libertarians commenced a campaign to let the marketplace determine which drugs were effective. Advocates of laetrile (a purported cancer cure) fought in court for an exception to the effectiveness requirements for drugs intended for persons with terminal illnesses that could not be treated by any approved or recognized methods.

No one was officially declared the winner in the drug lag debate. The FDA, fearing for the survival of the effectiveness requirement, refused to admit that a lag existed, but pledged to eliminate it anyway. At the same time, the agency presented to Congress a legislative proposal that put the efficacy standard on the table, for ratification or repeal. Leaders in both houses made clear that repeal was out of the question. At about the same time, the Supreme Court rejected the arguments of the laetrile proponents, observing that the effectiveness requirement also protected patients with incurable diseases from quackery. Industry, moving past DESI and getting more and faster approvals of important new products, lost interest in attacking the efficacy provision and focused its attention on two new objectives. First, it sought restoration of patent life for time lost in the development and review process; this law was enacted in 1984. Second, it agreed to fund the FDA directly to provide more resources to shorten review times. The Prescription Drug User Fee Act (PDUFA) was enacted in 1992, and renewed in 1997 and again in 2002. Under PDUFA, each manufacturer of innovator prescription drugs pays an annual assessment based on the number of establishments it operates. In addition, for each original NDA or supplement that requires review of clinical data, the applicant pays a fee. The revenues are earmarked for drug review activities and may not be used by the agency to offset the funding it receives for these activities from the federal treasury.

By the mid-1990s, after two decades of attention, the drug lag had been eliminated; indeed, the pendulum had swung clearly in favor of the FDA. Whether due to the PDUFA resources, or to the advent of more bureaucracy overseas (e.g., the formation of the European Union's central drug approval authority), or to criticism of delays at the agency, today the United States is often the first country to approve new drugs.

The Patient Access Debate and Its Consequences

While the drug lag debate was waning, a new challenge emerged to the FDA standards for drug effectiveness. This time, it was patient advocates who led the charge.

Orphan diseases are those that affect such a small number of patients that the market cannot sustain the cost of research to find treatments. For some time, the agency, the industry, and patient support groups had recognized the problem. The FDA worked with various drug firms to find "homes" for potentially valuable orphan products. Nevertheless, the economics worked against those with rare diseases.

In 1979 Dr. Louis Lasagna wrote a seminal article, "Who will adopt the orphan drugs?"[9] which helped Abbey Meyers, the founder of NORD (the National Organization for Rare Disorders), to obtain enough congressional attention to start the move toward supportive legislation. Beginning in 1983, Congress responded to this situation by enacting (and in 1985 and 1986 strengthening) the Orphan Drug Act. This legislation allowed sponsors to seek FDA designation of pipeline products as "orphan drugs" for specific indications. Once designated, the sponsors could seek funding grants and could receive tax credits for research costs. Most significantly, if a sponsor was the first to get a particular product approved for an orphan indication, no other company could obtain FDA approval of an identical product for the same use for seven years. This exclusivity incentive proved powerful, and as a result many new drugs have reached the market.

In the mid-1980s, the AIDS crisis exploded. Activists behaved in ways no patient advocacy group had ever done, including picketing the agency's offices. Initially they demanded immediate access to any drug that might help the disease, and they objected to placebo-controlled trials as unethical. Libertarians and political conservatives (including in the White House) were also heard from, calling for a broader suspension of the effectiveness standard. In its first response, the agency rushed through the approval of the first diagnostics for HIV and the first therapies for AIDS and related opportunistic infections. It also adopted regulations (just before the 1988 presidential elections) to expedite the development, evaluation, and marketing of new treatments for life-threatening diseases. These so-called Subpart E rules allowed for early consultations between sponsors and the agency on study requirements, treatment protocols, active FDA monitoring of ongoing studies, Phase IV studies to delineate additional information after approval, and a risk-benefit analysis that explicitly recognized the severity of the disease and the absence of alternative therapies as factors to be considered.

The political pressures to expand early access for patients did not abate. Other policy changes occurred, such as the encouragement of community-based simple studies, and the initiation of fast-track review procedures (giving priority for important new drugs over those offering smaller contributions to patient health).

In 1992, the agency adopted another set of regulations to provide for the accelerated approval of new drugs for life-threatening illnesses. These rules, called Subpart H, were similar to the Subpart E policies (which remained in place), but now authorized the FDA to approve drugs based on surrogate endpoints rather than mortality effects, to restrict the distribution of drugs so approved to special settings, to preclear advertising, and to withdraw approval expeditiously if Phase IV trials failed to demonstrate a clinical benefit.

It is important to note that the majority of AIDS activists, after initially opposing controlled investigations, came around to recognize that improvements in HIV therapy could be identified only through such studies.

In 1997, Congress stepped in once again to tinker with the Federal Food, Drug, and Cosmetic Act. With regard to drug effectiveness, it directed the agency to develop guidelines on those situations in which a single satisfactory and well-controlled study would be adequate for approval of a new drug or a new indication for an approved product. The FDA issued the guidance the following year. To some observers, it offered little meaningful change from past practice.

Thus, by the end of the twentieth century, the effectiveness requirement, requiring proof through more than one adequate and well-controlled clinical investigation, remained the standard to which most new drugs were held. Important therapeutic breakthroughs, however, could reach patients earlier or faster through one or more administrative mechanisms created by the agency. As a result of the resources provided by PDUFA, the FDA has become the largest and best-staffed drug regulatory agency in the world, setting standards that influence all other countries.

Criticisms of slowness, rigidity, and authoritarianism are still heard from industry, but with less frequency. One can debate whether the decline is due to improvements within the FDA, or that industry now contains a large number of employees whose careers depend largely on satisfying FDA's demands, or to the reluctance of industry to express concerns publicly. The FDA has become a significant "sponsor" or "patron" of many diverse elements within the industry; its laws provide economic benefits to the industry (such as limiting parallel imports and generic competition), and it has the power to cripple or destroy individual companies. Thus for many reasons, regulatory decisions may be less vigorously challenged or resisted by industry today than they were forty years ago, at the height of DESI.

In 2003 then-commissioner Mark McClellan, who is both a physician and an economist, recognized the high and increasing cost of drug development and proposed, as part of a strategic plan, that the FDA should consider ways to reduce it. The following year, the agency announced its "Critical Path" initiative, to identify (and, one hopes, ultimately to solve) problems in drug development science that increase costs and add time to the process. A mutual commitment on the part of industry and FDA to boost efficiency and output represents a critical opportunity for drug developers.

EVOLUTION OF FDA'S APPROACH TO DRUG SAFETY

The concept of drug safety in 1938 focused on premarket testing and on postapproval adulteration. Adverse events emerging after a drug entered the marketplace were not really considered part of FDA's responsibility. When chloramphenicol was discovered (in the early 1950s) to cause aplastic anemia, the alarm was sounded to the American Medical Association (AMA). The AMA joined with hospital and pharmacy organizations to create a registry for reporting of these cases, and later, of adverse events associated with other drugs, thus forming the origins of what would ultimately be FDA's adverse reaction system. The registry was transferred to the FDA in 1969.[10,11]

Later,[12-14] the agency developed specific regulations for mandatory reporting of adverse events by holders of NDAs, but not by health care professionals who instead were encouraged to report voluntarily. Also, uniquely in the world, the agency accepted reports directly from consumers; and though attempts are made to get medical verification of such reports, this is one feature that has created skepticism over the value of the FDA adverse events data. This structure remains in place today. Voluntary reporting for all drugs tends to spike in the wake of publicity about safety issues requiring withdrawal of a product (after, for example, phenformin [1977], benoxaprofen and ticrynafen [1982], nomefensine [1987], and fenfluramine [1997]).[15]

These episodes also led to regulatory focus on recurring areas of drug toxicity, such as hepatic or renal injury and blood dyscrasias. With the advent of sudden cardiac death due to *torsades de pointes* associated with the antihistamine terfenadine and the gastrointestinal drug cisapride, drug safety entered a newer era. First, it was found that both drug problems were usually associated with drug interactions, specifically at the 3A4 cytochrome p450 metabolizing site. Thus, requirements for premarket testing for these and analogous interactions that might increase toxicity gradually became routine parts of the NDA requirements. Second, for these drugs and several others introduced in the 1990s, the discovery of preventable risks was rapidly followed by labeling changes and "Dear health care professional" letters, as had been the agency's routine practice for decades. But now, however, careful studies demonstrated that these warnings had little or no impact on physician prescribing behavior; the life-threatening risks due to drug interactions were still occurring. The FDA concluded that label changes had little or no impact. Third, an analysis of drug surveillance studies estimated that adverse events associated with drugs accounted for approximately 100,000 deaths per year, placing this event in the major public health problem arena.

In 1999, the FDA unveiled a new initiative on identifying and preventing risks from medical products, and in May 2004 the agency produced several specific proposed guidances on risk management, covering premarketing risk assessment, risk management programs, and pharmacovigilance programs, and it proposed the most comprehensive overhaul of the adverse event reporting regulations ever undertaken. In essence, the proposed guidances greatly extend the focus on drug safety from Phase I clinical studies right throughout the commercial life of a product. The FDA now expects detailed collection and analyses of clinical safety data in the NDA in addition to comprehensive pharmacovigilance programs that encompass not only passive spontaneous report surveillance but also proactive programs. The rigor of this examination is most recently reflected in extensive guidelines for the NDA safety review in February 2005. For drugs identified as posing significant risks, FDA will require risk minimization action plans (RiskMAPs) for specific interventions to minimize these risks and/or evaluate the effectiveness of the interventions; if the interventions do not work, additional steps may be necessary.

FDA has also formed a Drug Safety and Risk Management Advisory Committee during this time, provided specific training for the members, and subsequently placed selected members on advisory committee panels to consider various risks or to review existing risk management programs. Still more dramatic developments have emerged in the drug safety arena. In August 2004 the agency determined that at least some selective serotonin reuptake inhibitors (SSRIs) for depression may increase the risk of suicide in some patients, particularly children. The following month, the manufacturer of rofecoxib, a COX-2 inhibitor nonsteroidal anti-inflammatory drug (NSAID) for arthritis, suspended marketing worldwide because of cardiovascular risks. In both cases, the risks were identified (and only identifiable) through randomized controlled clinical trials, which traditionally have focused only on drug effectiveness. Some experts began suggesting the expanded use of such trials to assess safety. Meanwhile, congressional hearings unearthed scientific dissent within the agency and called for more effective safety monitoring. In February 2005, the agency announced a new Safety Oversight Board, comprised of experts from the FDA, other government agencies, and academia to provide oversight to the drug safety assessment process.

The FDA's approach to drug safety is thus in great flux. The final guidelines on risk management and the new regulations on adverse event reporting are expected soon. How the agency will incorporate the learning from the SSRI and COX-2 experiences, and will use the new Drug Safety Oversight Board, remains to be seen. Nevertheless, concern is growing that the FDA is becoming more risk-averse, resulting in more requirements for preapproval safety testing, more delays in drug approvals, and more restrictions on post-approval use of drugs.

The Changing Economics of the Pharmaceutical Industry

The business model for the pharmaceutical industry has also undergone important changes, especially in the past twenty years. Moreover, the pace of change seems to accelerate, challenging the managers who must guide their companies forward. Although many factors are at play, some that are unique to the pharmaceutical industry merit special recognition.

The Advent of Generic Drug Competition

Generic drugs have always been available in the U.S. market. When the DESI program was underway, the agency estimated that there were between five and thirteen products without NDAs that were identical, similar, or related to each of the 13,000 products that held NDAs under the 1938 act. These products might contain the same active ingredient in the same amount and dosage form; often, though, they claimed some unique characteristic: a different salt or ester, a different amount, a different dosage form, or an extra added ingredient. As part of the DESI project, the FDA sought to introduce uniformity and control over these products. First, the agency said that a copy had to be identical, unless the proponent got FDA permission to vary from the innovator. Second, the manufacturer had to obtain an "abbreviated" NDA (or ANDA) showing that the product was identical and could be made consistently. In essence, it was an application that contained all of the chemistry, manufacturing, and controls of a full NDA, but omitted any preclinical or clinical data. A number of generic firms opposed even these requirements, and significant litigation followed.

While the ANDA process was evolving, a new problem arose. Physicians were reporting that congestive heart failure patients who had been titrated carefully to a specific dose of digoxin went out of control upon getting prescriptions refilled. Investigation revealed that digoxin, a pre-1938 drug never subject to an NDA, varied from manufacturer to manufacturer, and from lot to lot: not in quantity of actual drug per tablet but in the amount of drug released from the tablet into the body. The consequences could be life threatening. The agency responded with an order that each manufacturer submit an ANDA that included bioavailability studies showing the rate and extent of absorption into the body. Thus was born the idea of bioequivalence: that competing products must not only be pharmaceutically identical but also show no significant difference in the rate or extent of absorption in controlled bioavailability studies.

The ANDA process and bioequivalence permitted the agency for the first time to declare individual generic products to be therapeutically equivalent to approved brand-name versions. The FDA began making such declarations in 1975 or 1976; by 1979, the agency began to publish them in the Orange Book. This step was critically important. Before this point generics did not pose a great competitive threat because state pharmacy laws did not permit the substitution of a generic for the innovator drug that had been prescribed. The premise of these laws was that pharmacists were not in a position to assure the equivalency of generic products. But once the FDA gave its imprimatur, the rationale for nonsubstitution disappeared. In 1979 the Federal Trade Commission unveiled a model state drug product selection law, which guided state legislatures on how to amend pharmacy laws to permit druggists to substitute equivalent generics for innovators without the permission of the prescribing physician.

Even this step did not have a profound effect, because the ANDA mechanism was only available to generic copies of drugs first approved before 1962. But in 1984, as part of the compromise to obtain restoration of patent life that was being lost during the drug development and review process, the Pharmaceutical industry agreed to extension of the ANDA requirement for copies of an approved product once the patent for the product had expired or was declared invalid. The impact of this change was first felt in the late 1980s, when important innovations went off patent. Whereas prior to the ANDA process an innovation could rely on retaining more than 80 percent of its market share for years after generic entry, now companies found themselves losing 90 percent of the market in three to six months.

The effect was staggering to the pharmaceutical business model. Henceforth, the only period during which a research-based drug sponsor could plan to profit from the sales of a new product was the time window from approval and launch to the date of patent expiration. Could things get worse? Within the 1984 law were seeds of further troubles for the pharmaceutical industry. One provision rewarded a generic manufacturer who challenged an innovator patent: if the patent were invalid or not infringed, the challenger would be rewarded with six months of exclusive marketing of the generic. During this window not only would the innovator lose its market share, but the generic could charge a premium price and make substantial profits. Moreover, experience began to reveal, after three or four generics entered the market, that their prices fell to pure competitive or commodity levels, with very low profit margins. The generic firm to survive and prosper would have to become aggressive in finding innovator patents to "break." By the end of the 1990s, it was increasingly common for generics to contest patents rather than wait for this expiration.

This foreshortening of the commercial life of a pharmaceutical would necessarily affect the projected return on investment for a pipeline product. The incentives were skewed in favor of "blockbuster" developments that would command both high prices and high demand despite the high prices.

The Accelerating Rate of Innovator Competition

The marketplace is indeed crowded, especially in the more traditional therapeutic areas. Furthermore, the time lag between when the first member of a class enters the market and a "me-too" follow-on product is approved is lessening. As a result, the ability of a company to maintain high prices before the entry of generic competition is also compromised.

The Emerging Demand for Cost-Effectiveness

Health care costs in the United States have become a major issue for government (which subsidizes health care for the poor, disabled, and elderly), business (which subsidizes health care for employees), labor unions (which are increasingly fighting to preserve benefits and jobs rather than to increase wages), and politicians (who recognize that a huge proportion of the population has no health insurance). Historically, drug costs were a trivial part of the health care budget. Indeed, in 1964, when Congress enacted the original Medicare program, prescription drugs were not covered. The political perception was that the products were inexpensive and not necessarily effective.

Beginning in the 1990s, prescription drug expenditures accelerated as a percentage of total health care costs. This shift should be viewed as a positive development, reflecting the discovery and introduction of agents to address a population whose life expectancy has been extended thanks to other medical advances. Unfortunately, but realistically, limits exist to the proportion of the economy that can be allocated to health. As a result, third party payers are searching for ways to reduce the total cost. At the same time, for the reasons just discussed, manufacturers introduced "value-based" pricing for new pharmaceuticals. The first drug to cost more than $10,000 per year for a single patient was AZT, the first AIDS drug. After initial complaints, the high price was accepted, and now products are launched at annual per person costs that are much higher. Thus, it is no surprise that the payers have focused on prescription drugs as a way to control costs.

"Newer" does not automatically mean "better," and today payers are insisting that innovations be more cost-effective than competitor products, in particular low-price generic competitors. It was once possible to launch profitably an eigth or twelfth beta-blocker or NSAID. But now, so-called "me-too" products must at least offer some cost-benefit advantage over the innovator. The prizes go to the first-in-class product (because it will have the greatest volume of use to support safety) and to the best in class (because it will have been shown to be superior in some way to the others). The rest fight over the crumbs.

Furthermore, some therapeutic areas are inelastic. For example, in the case of migraine, this market shows no sign of growth, despite that at least seven triptans available for patients, including four distinct dosage forms. New entrants employ large sales forces to launch new products, but often results are meager, until continued investment proves prohibitive to do even that. Meanwhile, managed care organizations decide that only one or two representatives of the class will be reimbursable, thus placing additional pressure on marketing organizations.

The economic implications should be clear. Today's drug development decisions must be made with a careful regard to the drug's place in the queue of likely competitors, and to the sponsor's ability to demonstrate therapeutic advantages. In the case of some drugs, such as proton pump inhibitors, the very mechanism of action limits the potential for significant improvements by later generations. In other areas, such as the calcium channel blockers diltiazem and verapamil, the chemistry may not permit a second-generation molecule.

The Declining Productivity of Research and Development

The productivity of research and development efforts within the pharmaceutical industry has declined significantly in the past decade. Although large numbers of INDs are submitted each year, only a small proportion of the pipeline emerges as NDA submissions or approvals. NDA submissions have fallen by half, from a high of fifty in 1995 to twenty-three and twenty-four in 2002 and 2003, respectively. Approvals have fallen from a high of fifty-three in 1996 to seventeen and nineteen in 2002 and 2003, respectively (although the 2004 result is considerably higher).[16] No clear reasons exist for this decline, especially in the face of record high levels of R & D investment. Speculation is that the "easy" targets have already been exploited, that profit potential for products cannot meet ever-increasing financial targets, and that safety concerns require inordinately clean safety profiles.

Research technology has advanced particularly rapidly over the past two decades, and techniques such as robotics, high-throughput screening, and computer-aided design and simulations have been instituted in discovery and early-development labs. Companies have established genomics departments to exploit the much-touted future benefits of pharmacogenomics. Given the declining level of NME NDA submissions, it appears that to date there has not been a high degree of payoff. With respect to genomics, arguments are made that it takes ten years to exploit such a fundamental technology, or that the industry had failed to adjust its business model to "personalized" medicine. Overall, however, the decline may be a symptom of a serious, long-term problem, which may necessitate more selective research investments in the future.

The Increasing Costs of Drug Development

The costs of bringing a new drug to market keep rising exponentially. This compounds the problems of persistently long development time (now averaging twelve years) and a remarkably high failure rate (75 percent) in the clinical research phase. The latest estimate from the Tufts Center for the Study of Drug Development puts large pharmaceutical's average out-of-pocket cost, including failures, of developing a new chemical entity to the point of NDA approval, at $403 million ($121 million preclinical plus $282 million clinical). When the cost of the capital, expended over the twelve-year average time of product development, is included, this figure rises to $802 million ($336 million preclinical plus $466 million clinical). Development speed and failure rates have a large effect on the cost of development: if development time could be cut in half, the $802 million would drop to $568 million. If the failure rate were reduced from 75 percent to 67 percent, total costs would be lowered by $217 million.[17-21] Some of the more potent causes of these increasing costs include the following:

- Chronic and complex indications demand longer, larger, and more complex studies.
- Comparative trials, needed to compete in the marketplace, may require larger populations and longer durations to have sufficient power to determine equivalency or superiority.
- Special preapproval studies are now expected, or required, to explore safety and effectiveness in special subpopulations. These groups in-

clude the elderly, children (which has four subsets: neonates and infants, toddlers, prepubescent, and postpuberty adolescents), women of child-bearing potential, persons with renal or hepatic impairment, and persons using foreseeable concomitant medications (looking for dangers such as QTc interval prolongation, a signal for possible *torsades de pointes*).

- More trials, with greater numbers of subjects, necessitate utilization of outside consultants and contract research organizations to manage sites, collect and verify data, and ensure protocol compliance and adherence to good clinical practice regulations. The number of outside companies who draw their livelihood from the growing size and complexity of the drug development process is itself an ominous portent.
- Competition for a limited pool of patients has led to recruitment and retention problems and to the need for direct payments to subjects for their participation.
- Increased use of information technology, such as remote electronic data entry and electronic diaries, creates the further need for additional data integrity controls and audit trails, plus the support of this whole industry infrastructure.
- More rigorous demands for the format of regulatory submissions. The FDA initiatives to eliminate unnecessary paperwork through electronic filings can lead to unnecessary technology and expense that, although perhaps leading to economy and efficiency in the long run, is far from that today. The agency's recent "refusal to file" Neurocrine's NDA—because the reviewer could not use the hyperlinked version that supposedly satisfied the FDA's own specifications—is a case in point.

Although any large R & D organization presents management challenges to overcome inefficiencies, every Pharmaceutical R & D organization has a special dimension: the number of tasks and people who are required to interact with the world's regulatory agencies. This requirement permeates far beyond the staff of the regulatory department itself. It extends to many other departments in which even an "expression of interest" by the FDA or another agency guarantees the jobs and careers of a large fraction of the department's employees, even if they have no direct participation in the drug development process or in the necessary development activities of the pipeline.

A representative example today is pharmacogenomics. Most would agree that in the future pharmacogenomics will contribute to drug discovery, development, and approval. But in the meantime, one of the stated justifications today for a pharmacogenomic department to be established in a pharmaceutical company is that "the FDA is very interested in the potential of this technology." In this way, the discipline is granted a place in the development pathway that may be independent of its actual current value to the process. Numerous other departments and functions in a pharmaceutical company enjoy similar privileges under the protection of real or putative FDA requirements or interest.

The compounding effect of so many added burdens from all directions—standards, size, quality, and speed—has itself produced new dimensions of complexity and costs not readily apparent to those outside, or even inside, the system. A real danger exists that the system will collapse of its own weight; growth at this pace cannot continue forever.

The Economic Effects on the Pharmaceutical Industry

Consolidation of the Industry

The steeply rising costs of R & D, combined with a foreshortened period of generic-free competition, has driven pharmaceuticals into maintaining large sales forces and an efficient supply chain. Its business model has further evolved to focus on blockbuster drugs, ones that today must generate at least $1 billion per year in order to make a profitable return on R & D investments before generics or "me-too" products enter the market. The declining productivity of R & D has forced the industry to cast a wider net to discover compounds and take them through the initial phases of development, but despite this, the lack of sufficient blockbuster products has forced the consolidation of the industry, in order to support the sales and manufacturing operations and ongoing R & D. Unprecedented consolidation has taken place over the past ten to fifteen years because of these economic pressures.

Even though these mergers may yield efficiencies in marketing and production, it is doubtful whether the same efficiencies hold in drug development. The search for blockbuster drugs has compelled research organizations to be more market-driven than science-driven. One result of consolidation has been the creation of mega–R & D organizations, some of which have 15,000 to 20,000 staff or more, with multiple research sites on several continents, creating the further challenge of managing these resources, and the need to hire yet more staff to administer these gigantic bureaucracies. Paradoxically, no evidence exists that consolidation has improved innovation, or that huge R & D organizations have useful economies of scale or efficiencies in discovery or development. Consolidation may have actually achieved the opposite of its intent in R & D, and discovery and innovation may have declined as a result.

The Rise of the Biotechnology Industry

A new drug discovery industry has emerged in parallel with the consolidation of the pharmaceutical industry. Beginning in the 1970s, boosted by the Bayh-Dole Act of 1980 (encouraging out-licensing of university-based discoveries made with NIH funds) and funded by venture capital, start-up biotechnology (biotech) companies, proliferated. The term *biotech* originally applied to the tools offered by recombinant DNA and monoclonal antibody technologies, but now loosely embraces start-up and small companies in general, using small molecule design and discovery, genomics and proteomics, bioinformatics, therapeutic vaccines, novel drug delivery systems, combinations of a medical device with a drug or biologic, nanotechnology, and other cutting edge biomedical research ideas and tools. Unfortunately, the great potential of these new technologies has not yet been fully realized. A staggering number of products and the start-up companies that spawned them have failed. Other great promises, such as interferon, endorphins, and gene therapy have proved so far to have limited clinical applications or unsuspected toxicity. The translation of new technologies to the hospital, pharmacy, and bedside is taking longer and costing more than was expected in the enthusiasm of the 1990s. Part of the reason is the enthusiastic hype that seems necessary to get new companies and industries started.

Nevertheless, biotechnology has made a very substantial contribution to the pharmaceutical pipeline and the therapeutic armamentarium, with approximately six to eight NME products reaching the market each year. The largest biotech companies (e.g., Amgen) are now indistinguishable, in the business sense, from traditional Pharmaceutical companies. The vibrant biotech small-company sector, particularly at the discovery and early-development level, is supplying candidates for licensing or acquisition by pharmaceutical companies to supplement their internal research operations. The relationship is mutually beneficial. Pharmaceuticals cannot afford to finance the scale of drug discovery operations needed to maintain a pipeline; companies funded by venture capital and stock offerings assume much of the risk of early failures. Both parties share in the rewards of success. As a result, every major pharmaceutical company scouts for new opportunities, and the most promising candidates become the subjects of intensive bidding competitions.

The rate of biotech discoveries reaching the market needs to increase rapidly if the overall pharmaceutical pipeline is to grow. At the very least, however, the advent of the biotech industry has greatly changed the face of pharmaceuticals worldwide, and may yet become—as has been touted for decades—the creative force that saves the pharmaceutical industry.

Outsourcing

The steady rise of outsourcing since the 1960s has greatly expanded the operating capacity and expertise base of the pharmaceutical industry. It began with the clinical contract research organizations (CROs) that handled the logistics of clinical trials, and with animal testing laboratories compliant with FDA's good laboratory practice regulations. Subsequently, the field expanded to include firms in the areas of formulation development, stability programs, pharmacokinetic studies, biostatistics, data management, clinical site management, auditing for compliance with good clinical practice requirements, and preparation of regulatory submissions. Even the duties of institutional review boards (IRBs) are undertaken for multicenter trials by freestanding, for-profit companies.

These diverse businesses have contributed to the rising standards of performance—and, unfortunately the costs—of drug development. Competition in individual areas has forced a "race to the top" in terms of quality, speed, and compliance. Pharmaceutical clients cannot risk obtaining data that will not be acceptable to the FDA. Thus, even more so than pharmaceutical companies themselves, the outsourcing industry shows a militant enthusiasm for complying with regulatory standards; rather than contesting the wisdom of an agency guidance or interpretation, contractors will embrace it to the letter and pass on the increased cost to the client companies. In addition to the general problem of high costs, this has a particularly dampening effect on the activities of the small, innovative start-ups from whom so much is expected: increasingly, they cannot afford to pay for a clinical program with the CRO help that they desperately need to proceed.

The future of outsourcing is clearly strong, but it also reveals a growing need for cheaper ways of satisfying the law's requirements for evidence of effectiveness and safety. One recent way that is growing steeply is to move activities out of the United States and other high-cost countries. Both pharmaceutical companies and CROs have invested in operations in Eastern Europe, India, and China. One CRO, for example, recently relocated its entire ECG (electrocardiogram) monitoring services to India and promises one-hour, 24/7 turnaround, in the same way that American hospitals have contracted for reading of X-rays in that country. Other specific functions, such as data management, analysis, and information technology, can also be performed elsewhere. The United States has thus forced a trend that could end its comfortable near-monopoly in pharmaceutical discovery and development.

Front-Loading the Drug Development Process

The potentially formidable power of the sciences of drug discovery and early development creates a plausible hope that candidate drugs can be screened earlier in the development process for potential problems, thereby reducing the failure rate at later stages. Although this argument is logically appealing, the results to date have disappointed. Moreover, the opportunity itself creates a new dilemma. By investing more in the numerous technologies available at the early stage of a drug's development, such a strategy "front loads" each compound's early development costs. Thus, if the compound still ultimately fails, the cost of failure is even higher than it was before the front-loading strategy. So far, that strategy has not worked well enough to reverse the pitifully low success rate of compounds that enter development. FDA's "critical path" initiative is a welcome new attempt to address the development-failure problem, but that it depends on further front-loading the activities and costs of the development pathway cannot be overlooked.[22]

The example of pharmacogenomics illustrates this dilemma, although one could equally well cite other new scientific techniques, such as extensive computer modeling and simulation, in this context. In the mid-1990s, in anticipation of the sequencing of the human genome, many new start-up pharmacogenomic companies were established, offering the vision of "individualized therapeutics," or "personalized medicine," based on the companies' claimed abilities to determine each patient's genomic variations (including single nucleotide polymorphism, SNPs) that they presumed must underlie interindividual differences in the patients' responses to drugs. It was asserted that this would enable the widespread prediction of responders and nonresponders to drug therapy as well as those at risk of adverse reactions, and that the result would be smaller, more powerful effectiveness trials, a cleaner safety profile, and the salvage of drugs that fail in development ("drug rehab").

With the exception of a few examples (e.g., Herceptin), the basic premise has not yet been widely demonstrated, though this area of tumor markers may well be the most promising in the long run. The prospects for more general applicability and cost-effective utility are still unclear at present. Many pharmacogenomic companies went public with stock offerings in the late 1990s boom, only to disappear in the crash of 2000. Nevertheless, the idea that much pharmacogenomics should be performed in the early development stage of drugs has been endorsed by the FDA, and as a result, has been taken up enthusiastically by pharmaceuticals, and is resulting in a very large amount of extra work being added to the early development of essentially all new drugs. For example, a new, more formal agency initiative for early pharmacogenomic work in early development has recently been announced.[23] It is still not clear whether these initiatives will turn out to be the salvation of the drug industry or yet another example of the unproven burdening of the front end of the drug development process.

In general, the front-loading of the development process by further use of any of the numerous modern available technologies would be attractive if one could be sure unequivocally that it would work. But to date it has not produced enough successful results to conclude that it is a superior strategy, and the success of clinical programs remains abysmal. The traditional approach of taking a new compound into human studies as early as possible so that human data can be obtained at an early stage has not yet been improved upon, despite the enormous frontloading of development across the whole industry.

Changing Public Attitudes Toward the Pharmaceutical Industry

In recent years, the drug industry has come under increasing criticism on a wide variety of fronts. The cumulative impact makes the industry look bad. Opinion polls place drug manufacturers among the least respected industries, near tobacco. Politicians score populist points by attacking drug companies. Prosecutors jump on the bandwagon, investigating and bringing actions for alleged violations of the Federal Food, Drug, and Cosmetic Act; the laws against fraud; abuse and kickbacks in the Medicare/Medicaid systems; prohibitions of deceptive and unfair advertising; securities statutes; and false claims against the government. And in the product liability arena, plaintiff lawyers are able to secure enormous amounts of punitive damages from juries angry with the pharmaceutical industry.

The number of books published in the United States in just the past few years attacking the pharmaceutical industry is sobering. A catalog of the public concerns and objections (real or imaginary) illustrates the complexity of the public relations challenge facing drug firms:

- *High prices for prescription drugs.* Americans are now convinced that they are paying more for drugs than residents in Canada and elsewhere. Moreover, those not covered by health insurance purportedly have to choose between food and their medicines.
- *Excessive total costs for prescription drugs.* Insurers and other third party payers see drugs as the fastest-rising component in total health care spending. For them, it is not merely the question of price per pill, but the aggregate utilization of drugs. With the advent of "lifestyle" drugs and later generation medicines that may offer no convincing advantages over those that are available as generics, real concerns exist regarding the diversion of limited resources to unnecessary products and the soaring costs for employee benefits that must be built into cost of goods sold.
- *Dubious practices in promoting prescription drugs.* Americans have long had a love-hate relationship with advertising, but the apparent excesses and misconduct linked to prescription drug marketing call it uniquely into question. Gifts, luxury trips, and consulting contracts for physicians smack of bribes. The ratio of sales representatives to prescribing physicians is stunning. The introduction of direct-to-consumer (DTC) advertising has led to charges that the public is lulled into ignoring the risks associated with prescription drugs and believing that pills are available for every ailment.
- *Disconnection between high industry profits and R & D spending.* For years the industry explanation for its prices and profits related to having sufficient money to carry out new research as well as sufficient profits to reward the inherent risks. Recent revelations that many companies spend more on promotion than on R&D, combined with the decline in the number of major new therapies, has made people skeptical of this claim. Even those who agree with it indicate to pollsters that they feel Americans are paying more than their fair share for the cost of drug development.
- *Fundamental distrust of the industry's ethics.* The public realization that research studies have been withheld from public view, or released in partial (and misleading) form, has created enormous pressures for industry to make information on all trials available via the Internet. The delays in relabeling products, the precipitous withdrawal of widely marketed drugs, and the failure to identify safety risks before approval (even when it was not scientifically possible to do so) gives support to the canard that companies put profits before people. And prosecutions of major companies for violations of myriad different laws seems to underscore the appearance of deficient basic ethics within the industry.

This catalog contains grossly overblown and unfair accusations. Unfortunately, sufficient numbers of isolated examples give the list credibility and tarnish the entire industry. Public sentiment no longer appears willing to recognize the high costs of new drug development and to meet, on a national basis, the challenge of paying for medical advances that improve the quality of life and the savings of health care money.

Changing Public Perception of Drug Safety

A tremendous increase has occurred over the years in the amount of knowledge available about a candidate drug at the time of NDA submission. The size of NDAs has grown enormously, and it is not uncommon for an NDA to contain data generated from scores of trials involving more than 10,000 patients, and sometimes several times that many. Much of this growth is in response to regulatory demands for a clearer delineation of the safety profile of a drug before approval.

Despite this record level of premarket risk information, new problems are invariably identified after approval. For many years, roughly 2 to 3 percent of the drugs approved by the FDA and by the United Kingdom regulators each year ultimately are removed from the market for safety reasons. This situation is understandable and expected; in fact, recognition that the postmarket experience inevitably reveals new adverse effects forms the basis for the requirement for postmarketing surveillance and other pharmacovigilance practices. It has always been a part of the tradeoff at the point of initial NDA approval, because the clinical trials cannot have realistically evaluated a drug in all the populations who may ultimately use it. Spontaneous reports from the entire population, plus Phase IV studies, usually provide the first signals of new adverse events. No matter how large the number of patients studied prior to marketing, discovery of new adverse events will always occur. Because of the very large size of the U.S. market, relatively rare events may have a better opportunity to be discovered here earlier and to be further examined in more formal studies.

Regrettably, the general public does not understand this. The layperson's view of drug risks might be summarized as follows:

- Drugs should generally not have any serious or life-threatening risks (except for lifesaving drugs; anticancer drugs have terrible toxicities, yet rarely provoke an outcry about side effects). Drugs for symptomatic relief or for lifestyle choices, especially for which alternatives exist, simply do not justify permanent injury or death.

- The devil you knew is safer than the one you've just heard about. In the rofecoxib debate, for example, the media rarely attempted to quantify the number of life-threatening gastrointestinal bleeds caused by first generation NSAIDs but avoided by rofecoxib. Instead, the discussion focused entirely on the newly identified cardiovascular risks.
- Science should be able to reveal all side effects during drug development. The failure to do so suggests concealment by industry and/or incompetence by the FDA.

When drugs are withdrawn for toxicity, the public debates whether the standards for drug approval should be increased. Sponsors and the FDA are pressured to identify as many risks as possible prior to NDA approval. A point of dispute is whether these events make the agency or the industry, or both, more risk-averse. Some industry members and observers believe so. They point to the natural caution of a regulatory agency that is subject to congressional criticism for appearing to have made a mistake. This problem is not new, of course, but new tools can aggravate it. For example, FDA reviewers now have access to electronic versions of the safety database in an NDA. Not surprisingly, this easier access has opened the door for ad hoc analyses and new safety concerns. The practice further raises the question whether any limits exist on the extent to which a sponsor must further explore potential risk signals derived from the clinical safety database.

In contrast, FDA officials have contended that the agency is more willing to admit (and leave) drugs on the market than are other national authorities. They assert that the FDA can do so because it has been proactive in developing programs to manage the known risks when a drug with a narrow benefit/risk ratio comes up for approval.

As we have described, the genesis of FDA's approach to risk management occurred after a string of withdrawals of such widely used drugs as terfenadine, cisapride, bromfenac, and troglitazone in the 1990s. Studies of the effects of new warnings and labeling changes demonstrated that they had done little to affect prescribing behavior. The agency recognized that it needed new tools to identify safety issues, to minimize preventable risks, and to inform physicians and patients about risks. The FDA's position paper on a framework for risk management issued in 1999, and the proposed guidances on risk management in 2003 and 2004, reveal some ongoing trends in FDA's philosophy on drug safety. In the proposed premarketing drug safety document, the desire for extensive information and analysis of the safety of a product is expressed. Carried to its logical extreme, it appears to request very extensive testing and evaluation beyond the customary practice. The risk minimization action plan (proposed guidance) contains an implication for interventions beyond labeling more often than has previously been the case. Such an approach could lead to limitations on access to many novel products, at least in the early period after approval.

If risk management activities are used to permit the marketing of drugs that otherwise would be kept off because of serious safety concerns, and the activities are effective, the public will be better off. On the other hand, if risk minimization tools are routinely applied to drugs that could be marketed without them, they could serve to deny access of physicians and patients to valuable and acceptably safe medicines. How the FDA will strike this balance remains to be seen.

IMPROVEMENTS NEEDED FOR THE FUTURE

From our discussion in the first part of this chapter, it is obvious that some of the industry's most serious problems could be solved if the development and approval processes were streamlined and facilitated so that unsuccessful drug candidates could be eliminated earlier, and successful candidates could, with appropriate safety, reach the market faster and at lower cost.

Despite numerous attempts in the past to streamline it, the drug development and approval process still takes far too long, is too expensive, and is getting steadily more cumbersome. The process urgently needs to be sped up. Incremental improvements (e.g., defining the optimal size of an IND) have worked for a while in the past, but the tendency for the system to accrete and bog down has become so persistent that bolder initiatives are needed to have any impact on speed and cost. For thirty years it has been recognized that such fundamental reforms are needed. The answer, we believe, is to work within the legal and regulatory framework of the current system and to implement some of the best reforms that have already been proposed. It is the difficulty of implementation, rather than the lack of ideas, that has prevented progress and allowed the system itself to become an ever-larger impediment.

Our main proposals are the following:

1. Simplify the initial IND filing, in order to facilitate, by partial deregulation, early-stage exploratory clinical development from Phase I through proof of concept in patients.
2. At the NDA stage, make more use of the NDA's current conditional approval mechanisms, so that in a wider range of circumstances (including at the request of a sponsor) a drug may be approved for the market for limited indications considerably earlier than it would be at present, on condition that the development program continues and

that the conditions of initial approval are enforced. In this way, the law's ultimate effectiveness and safety standards for a full approval are safeguarded, not compromised.

3. In addition, we have a number of smaller proposals that, taken together, would further facilitate the process.

Simplifying the IND Process for Early Clinical Studies Through Proof of Concept

Contrary to what one would wish to see in an efficient clinical development process, the de facto requirements for an IND continue to rise to the point where, in complexity and size, an IND today exceeds the size of some NDAs in the past. We recommend simplifying the IND requirements so that key safety and early efficacy studies can be performed very early in humans with the same protections, but at less time and cost than they are today.

Although the formal filing of a new IND is still relatively simple in principle, the amount of work that is actually required (or at least performed) to support it at present is much larger than an NDA used to be long after the 1962 amendments. The bureaucratic overhead that goes into managing the submissions and amendments, in both large pharmaceuticals and small start-ups, is excessive. The cost of impediments at this early stage is magnified because they contribute greatly to the front-loading of the clinical development costs that we have already described.

The filing of a full IND, with a formal coordinated write-up of all the supporting data, although necessary forty years ago, is now an unnecessary requirement in the early-stage clinical programs of most large pharmaceuticals and CROs that do this work today. It is a barrier to the easy access to human studies that is needed for proof-of-concept studies (Phases I and IIa). Very little trouble has occurred in the past twenty years with early INDs filed by responsible individuals, corporations, and institutions. The system can now be safely adjusted to recognize this, by scaling back the IND requirements for responsible entities, based on what has been learned in the past forty years.

This is not a new idea. It was seriously considered twenty-five years ago in the hearings of the McMahon Commission in 1980.

It should be noted that our proposal goes considerably beyond the current proposal of FDA to create a looser "Phase 0" stage for first-in-man pharmacokinetic and similar activities. Our proposal would cover all early human studies through clinical proof-of-concept, which usually occurs in Phase IIa. Only in the large pivotal studies (Phases IIb-III), when there is more assurance that the drug candidate has a solid chance of getting to an NDA submission, would the full formal IND filing be necessary.

The streamlined system would work like this:

The IND filing step, and the oversight of proof-of-concept clinical research, would be safely implemented by cutting back the detail customarily required from Pharmaceutical sponsors and others (i.e., CROs, institutions, IRBs, and perhaps other entities) that have been formally qualified as "responsible" in this context. All such sponsors would have been previously screened by the agency, and accepted for the accelerated program if qualified, based on the applicant's historical record with the agency.

For sponsors that qualify for this new status, the IND and all studies under it would be allowed by simple notification to the FDA—rather than by FDA's scrutiny and formal allowance in each case. This system would be similar, in some respects, to the former German Hinterlegungsstelle ("Deposition"), whereby the sponsor made a simple deposition of the supporting data that the sponsor deemed sufficient, with no review or attention needed by the agency unless a problem arose. If a problem did arise, the data deposition package would be opened and reviewed by the agency, and the sponsor would be held liable (and, among other penalties, would lose its responsible status) if safety or other key deficiencies were found.

The rationale for this proposal is that first-in-man and other early studies are of small size and are relatively safe when performed by experienced investigators, and that entities and individuals with a good track record and a reputation to lose have a powerful incentive to keep their record spotlessly clean and so retain their "responsible" status privileges. For investigators and institutions that have not been qualified as "responsible," the present IND system would apply unchanged.

Reforming the NDA by Extending the Option of Provisional Approval

Although the standards of ultimate NDA approval based on effectiveness and safety should be carefully maintained, existing regulations already provide for attaining full approval in stages. Our proposal is that these options should be made available in a wider range of circumstances, including at the option of the sponsor. That is, the sponsor would have the option of requesting earlier approval under, for example, a restricted range of uses or other postmarket controls.

This proposal reflects the reality of many approvals today, in addition to the not yet fully recognized set of additional utilization controls of considerable power that have arisen in the past few decades outside the drug regulatory system that can further direct drug use in many ways. That is, over the past forty years, the marketplace has developed a powerful, expanding set of utilization controls (based on payment, marketing, managed care, and information feedback) that already function as a de facto, additional utilization-control system, which can—and in some cases already does—act as an added safeguard for the use of new drugs in the early post-marketing situation.

The conditional approval step could be integrated with the existing system of marketplace utilization controls and thus be used as an option to expedite approvals for earlier access to promising therapies. However, it would be important not to burden new drugs unnecessarily with conditional approval status if there is not a real reason to do so.

The agency's accession to a sponsor's request for an earlier approval, with conditions, would, in addition to helping patients, help those small sponsor companies and products for which approval in some form, even with extensive restrictions, is an increasingly necessary option. It would be particularly useful, for example, for patients who might benefit from orphan drugs and drugs developed by the numerous small biotechnology companies that have products in development for limited indications.

Improving Success Rates

As important as—or even more important than—speed of development is the success rate of the overall process, which must be increased. It has been estimated (J DiMasi, personal communication, June 1995) that increasing the success rate by 10 percent across a portfolio of drugs at all stages of clinical development would have the same effect on development costs as reducing the development time by more than 20 percent.

Other Opportunities for Improvement in Discovery and Early Development

Finally, we discuss a further set of potential areas for improvement across a wide area of the drug development process. Having better new molecular entity (NME) candidates and better ways of choosing which of them should enter into development would be an important step forward. Although the enormous increase in power of the biological and pharmaceutical sciences has increased the quality of development candidates over recent years, prediction of consistently successful development candidates still eludes us, and the overall success rate of drugs in clinical development has changed little over the past few decades. The overall success rate—from the Tufts CSDD data—remains at approximately 20 percent, despite other estimates that suggest an even lower range of 5 to 15 percent. Much hope is currently held out for the potential effects of biomarkers, including genomic and other molecular markers, in improving the quality of targets, drug candidates, and their progression through early development.

At present, as we have discussed, these promises are still somewhat hypothetical, but progress is being made. Although we all have high hopes that the increasing sophistication of drug development sciences will solve the problems, particularly of success rate, it should also be borne in mind that the increasing cost being built into the system requires a continuous increase in success rates just to break even; and thus, if the pharmaceutical industry fails to deliver, will further threaten the future of the pharmaceutical development enterprise. Given the enthusiasm and the clamor for front-loading the development process with more science, and despite the plausibility of this approach, this aspect needs to be carefully tracked and made to live up to its claims, to prevent the situation from collapsing.

FDA's Skills

Using the increased skills and talents of the greater number of qualified staff now at FDA (made possible in particular by the budget expansions of PDUFA, and now in more concrete form in the agency's "critical path" initiative) is another avenue. DiMasi and Manocchia (1997) have shown that early and continuing discussions between the regulators and the regulated, in the form of FDA-sponsored conferences, facilitate drug approval. This is what one would expect if, by the time of filing an NDA, all the important questions had been asked and answered. FDA's critical path initiative is an obvious way in which the agency's skills and resources can be brought to bear, and the results of this effort will be followed with particular interest. Again, however, the amount and effect of front-end loading of the process needs to be carefully compared against the results.

Animal Data

It may also be possible for time and money to be saved by eliminating requirements for animal toxicity data that are found to be no longer necessary. Excessive use of toxicity data has been criticized, reminiscent of the days when LD50 values in laboratory animals were routinely performed even when the precision sought in such studies was unnecessary for product development.

"Naturalistic" Studies

The inclusion/exclusion criteria needed in formal clinical trials inevitably produce experimental populations that are not typical of patient populations in routine medical practice. More attention therefore needs to be paid to the "naturalistic" study of drugs, after marketing, in general clinical practice. Such studies could lead to an increased understanding of both effectiveness and risk in the intended patient population. Benefits will almost certainly accrue by identifying empiric relations between genetic makeup and drug response, with the possibility of increasing benefit or decreasing harm. Progress in this area is unfortunately predicted too optimistically at present by scientists who should be aware of the length of time that will be required to achieve these goals, but nevertheless ultimate progress will be made if we apply ourselves to the task.

Direct-to-Consumer Advertising

At this time when DTC advertising is again coming under criticism, debate over its nature, effectiveness, and overall effects must continue. Whereas some patients do not wish to play an aggressive role in affecting their physicians' prescribing, others do. The latter, understandably, do not consider themselves naive innocents who are too ill informed to play a useful role. And many physicians (perhaps most?) do not feel that they will be inevitably forced to prescribe badly because of patient pressures. On the other hand, scope exists for abuse here, and a balance needs to be identified and sought, particularly in the disclosure of side effects.

Secondary Indications

The current restrictions by FDA on the advertising of secondary or tertiary indications (that is, unapproved by FDA) for drugs need to reevaluated. Experience has taught us that often not all the uses of a drug are known at the time of first marketing, and indeed it is not unusual for later approved uses to be more important medically than the original indication.

On the other hand, the recent abuses and allegations of fraud that have occurred in manipulation of off-label drug use, resulting in the creation of the anti-kickback legislation and regulations, demonstrate that this is a complex matter that needs to be carefully controlled and adjusted to achieve the optimal balance between benefit and risk.

Incentives for Obtaining New Data

Because some additional uses may be discovered late in a drug's patent life (or even after the patent has expired), a company may be reluctant to spend the time and money to obtain formal FDA approval of new uses that would primarily benefit generic manufacturers. Optimal medical practice, however, calls for access to sound and persuasive data on new indications. Some method needs to be found to encourage sponsors to seek new indications during more of a product's patent life and—if possible—beyond.

The success of the various special-case areas of drug development regulation and performance, such as orphan drugs, cancer, and AIDS drugs, and the pediatric exclusivity extension could be a guide to how to approach—and what to avoid—in creating larger facilitatory approaches in the future.

CONCLUSIONS

After a difficult decade following the 1962 amendments, the pharmaceutical industry and the FDA have in general worked well together, and the thirty-five years from 1970 to 2005 mark an era of unparalleled achievement in the modernization of drug development and approval. The present system has achieved much in its near half-century of operation. Nevertheless, it is becoming in part a victim of its own successes, as the finely balanced processes are now paradoxically coming closer to bogging down under the weight of continually increasing requirements from many directions.

In the past ten years, cracks have become obvious in the system, just when it should be flowering. The pharmaceutical industry's output of new drugs has slowed despite unprecedented investment in discovery and development; and at the same time the industry, and the drug development process itself, has acquired the most negative public image ever, mainly because of pricing, marketing, and safety issues. The FDA, too, has come under criticism over drug safety questions, in part due to communication problems.

The causes of this unfortunate state of affairs are numerous, and require a variety of solutions as we have described in this chapter. Defining the roles of industry and government in the pursuit of effective new therapies and their appropriate use is one of the areas where attention is needed in the future.

We may in part be a victim of our own successes. For example, pharmaceutical's well-honed coping skills, evolved to respond to the growing tendency for society to pile on regulatory requirements and for the industry to accept and cope with almost any challenge thrust upon it, have hindered the necessary streamlining and reform efforts, while the system daily accretes more obligations for industry and for the FDA.

International harmonization has also turned out to be another effort that went far beyond its original aims, extending now into creating new regulations and becoming an end and career niche in itself. Some international safety consortia developed similar expansionist activities. The autonomy of these groups is creating problems as they expand, with Europe and the United States seeking to develop separate policies and rules, which not only defeats the original purpose of the harmonization efforts, but could easily result in problems worse than the original harmonization program was designed to cure. Overall, the regulatory bodies have made considerable effort to support the spirit of harmonization, but in practice, continue to devolve interpretations of some of the policies to the individual countries. For example, the FDA's recently proposed safety regulations contain new definitions for periodic safety update reports (PSURs) that deviate from the generally expected formats already adopted in many countries.

More aggressive reforms are needed if pharmaceutical and regulatory agencies are to serve the public optimally. In this chapter we considered how some of these hindrances—in particular, regulation of early drug development and also the approval stage—could be addressed. As we have shown, steps of the early IND research exist that have become routine and could be deregulated, under appropriate controls, with beneficial effects. And at the NDA approval stage, a considerable benefit could be achieved by combining approval earlier in the development process with existing safeguards in drug utilization controls necessary to guarantee safe use until enough experience is obtained to relax the initial marketing restrictions. Many other areas need to be addressed in addition to those we discussed here.

In summary, the main reforms we have suggested, involving both the IND and NDA, are a start, but much more is needed to adjust Pharmaceutical's productivity to the needs of society.

Drug development and regulation promises to be an interesting ride through the twenty-first century.

NOTES

1. DiMasi JA (2001). Risks in new drug development: Approval success rates for investigational drugs. *Clin Pharmacol Ther* 69: 297-307.

2. DiMasi JA (2002). The value of improving the productivity of the drug development process: Faster times and better decisions. *PharmacoEcon* 20 (Suppl. 3): 1-10.

3. DiMasi JA, Hansen RW, and Grabowski HG (2003). The price of innovation: New estimates of drug development costs. *J Health Econ* 22: 151-85.

4. Spivey RN, Jones JK, Wardell W, and Vodra W. (2006). The US FDA in the drug development, evaluation and approval process. In J Griffin and J O'Grady (Eds.), *The Textbook of Pharmaceutical Medicine,* Fifth edition (Chapter 21). Oxford, UK: Blackwell Publishing.

5. Silverman M and Lee P (1974). *Pills, Profits, and Politics.* Berkeley, CA: University of California Press.

6. Wardell W (1972). The "Drug Lag" and American therapeutics: An international comparison. Presentation at the 22nd International Congress of Pharmacology, San Francisco, California.

7. Wardell W (1973). Therapeutic implications of the drug lag. *Clin Pharmacol Ther* 14: 1022-1034.

8. Wardell W and Lasagna L (1975). *Regulation and Drug Development.* Washington, DC: American Enterprise Institute for Public Policy Research.

9. Lasagna L (1979). Who will adopt the orphan drugs? *Regulation* 3(6): 27-32.

10. Jones JK (1981). National/international systems for postmarketing surveillance. In Velo G and Wardell W. (Eds.), *Drug Development, Regulatory Assessment and Post Marketing Surveillance* (pp. 233-240). New York: Plenum Press.

11. Jones JK (1981). Broader uses of post-marketing surveillance. In G Velo and W Wardell (Eds.), *Drug Development, Regulatory Assessment and Post Marketing Surveillance* (pp. 203-216).

12. Jones JK (1981). Joint commission on prescription drug use. In G Velo and W Wardell (Eds.), *Drug Development, Regulatory Assessment and Post Marketing Surveillance* (pp. 191-200). New York: Plenum Press.

13. Jones JK (1984). Regulatory use of adverse reactions. In H Bostrom and N Ljundstedt (Eds.), *Detection and Prevention of Adverse Drug Reactions* (pp. 203-214), a report of the 16th Skandia International Symposia. Stockholm: Almquist and Wiksall International.

14. Jones JK, Faich GA, and Anello C (1985). Post-marketing surveillance in the general population—The U.S.A. In William H. Inman (Ed.), *Monitoring for Drug Safety,* Second edition (pp. 153-163). Lancaster, UK: MTP Press Limited.

15. Jones JK and Idänpään-Heikkilä, JE (1993). Adverse reactions, postmarketing surveillance and pharmacoepidemiology. In DM Burley, JM Clarke, L Lasagna (Eds.), *Pharmaceutical Medicine* (pp. 145-180). London, UK: Edward Arnold.

16. U.S. FDA (2006). Drug approval reports. Available at: http://www.accessdata.fda.gov/SCRIPTS/CDER/DRUGSATFDA//index.cfm?fuseaction=Reports.ReportsMenu.

17. DiMasi JA, Hansen RW, and Grabowski HG (2003).

18. DiMasi JA, Grabowski HG, and Vernon J (2004). R&D costs and returns by therapeutic category. *Drug Information Journal* 38: 211-223.

19. DiMasi JA and Manocchia M (1997). Initiatives to speed new drug development and regulatory review: The impact of FDA-sponsor conferences. *Drug Info J* 31: 771-778.

20. DiMasi JA and Paquette C (2004). The economics of follow-on drug development: Trends in entry rates and the timing of development. *PharmacoEcon* 22 (Suppl 2): 1-14.

21. Kaitin K and Cairns C (2003). The new drug approvals of 1999, 2000, and 2001: Drug development trends a decade after passage of the prescription Drug User Fee Act of 1992. *Drug Information Journal* 4: 357-371.

22. U.S. Food and Drug Administration (2004). Innovation, stagnation: Challenge and opportunity on the Critical path to new medical products. March. White paper. Available at: http://www.fda.gov/oc/initiatives/criticalpath/whitepaper.html.
23. U.S Food and Drug Administration (2004).

FURTHER READING

Food and Drug Administration Modernization Act of 1997 (FDAMA).
Food and Drug Administration Web site: www.fda.gov. The History section of the FDA's Web site is particularly informative.
McMahon Commission Report. Commission on the Federal Drug Approval Process. Final Report 1982.
Reichert J (2004). Biopharmaceutical approvals in the US increase. *Regulatory Affairs Journal* July: 1-7.
Tufts Center for the Study of Drug Development (2004). *Outlook 2004.* Available at: http://csdd.tufts.edu/InfoServices/OutlookPDFs/Outlook2004.pdf, and other publications.
Wardell W (Ed.) (1978). *Controlling the Use of Therapeutic Drugs: An International Comparison.* Washington, DC: American Enterprise Institute for Public Policy Research.
Wardell W and Lasagna L (1975). *Regulation and Drug Development.* Washington, DC: American Enterprise Institute for Public Policy Research.

Chapter 13

Managed Care Pharmacy:
The Past and Present

John D. Jones

It has been more than two decades since the term *managed care* entered the lexicon of pharmaceutical benefits management. In that time, principles such as formularies, prior authorization, and controlled access networks have gone from being novelties viewed with skepticism and distrust to accepted and commonplace business practices for virtually all health care plans offering a prescription benefit.

As managed care continues to become even more prevalent, it is often difficult to distinguish comprehensive managed care programs from other, more traditional, approaches to providing pharmaceutical benefits. For example, it is estimated that more than 90 percent of health plans today now use formularies,[1] a threefold increase from the late 1980s. With virtually all types of pharmacy plans using one managed care tool or another, it is often difficult to define exactly what managed care pharmacy today is and what makes the approach unique.

WHAT IS MANAGED CARE PHARMACY?

Part of the challenge in addressing the complexities of managed care pharmacy is that the term *managed* is widely interpreted by various healthcare entities. For purposes of this discussion, we will define managed care as a discipline that incorporates the following strategies and techniques into the day-to-day management of the pharmaceutical benefits:

- Utilization management
- Treatment options
- Prior authorization of restricted or nonformulary drugs
- Structured cost sharing

- Networks of preferred providers
- A defined list (formulary or preferred drug list) of clinically selected prescription drugs
- Medication therapy management of patients at risk

These processes are intended to manage diseases, to lower overall health care costs and to improve health outcomes.

Although this definition covers the fundamental design, another approach to the definition of managed care pharmacy is to more thoroughly explore what it is *not*. Unlike traditional pharmaceutical benefits programs, managed care pharmacy does not simply process claims, nor does it simply contract with pharmaceutical manufacturers and networks of pharmacies. Managed care pharmacy specifically addresses cost, utilization, and outcomes. The most successful managed care pharmacy plans extend their definition to include a benefit design that is integrated with the medical benefit. Such an approach helps to ensure that neither benefit operates independently. It is the integration of these two benefits that helps contribute to lower *overall* healthcare costs.

Even though managed care pharmacy is now prevalent, it continues to have detractors. For example, the perception of many health care executives regarding managed care pharmacy has been shaped by Medicaid prescription drug programs, many of which have failed to perform to expectation. The majority of such programs have failed however, not because of inherent flaws in the managed care strategies employed, but because these programs were stifled in their attempts to effectively adopt managed care tools. The use of strong therapeutic formularies and aggressively negotiated discounts and rebates from manufactures would certainly have more effectively harnessed the programs' drug expenditures and resulted in a more positive outcome. Health care leaders must be cognizant of the competing and confounding variables when evaluating the efficacy of managed care pharmacy.

A BRIEF HISTORY OF MANAGED CARE PHARMACY

The use of the principles of managed care to control costs and utilization began as a strategy primarily used by health plans on the west coast in the mid-1970s (following the HMO Act of 1973). By the late-1980s, most large health plans had implemented some type of program to control pharmaceutical benefits costs due to double-digit increases in expenditures. The movement continued to gain momentum and importance as pharmaceutical benefits costs began to outpace other health care expenses. Use of managed care pharmacy techniques grew strongly and steadily through the mid-1990s. By the end of the decade most health plans used at least one managed care pharmacy tool in their drug benefit programs.[2]

The broad acceptance of managed care by the public didn't last, however. Beginning in the late 1990s, an overall managed care backlash occurred, which, along with high-profile lawsuits against the largest pharmaceutical benefits managers (PBM), significantly tarnished the industry's reputation, and led to intense scrutiny of the tactics of some managed care pharmacy programs. Patients began to view managed care pharmacy as an impediment to their direct relationship with physicians. Physicians viewed it as a threat to their autonomy. Legislators feared it was limiting freedom of choice and adding to the coffers of big business without significant reductions in cost or improvements in care. As a result, federal and state legislators began to introduce legislation that would curtail the utilization of mail-service pharmacy, formularies, prior authorization, and other principles integral to the practice of managed care.

The growth of the "empowered" consumer and consumer-driven or self-directed health care also presented challenges to managed care. One trend among some health care plans today appears to favor benefit designs that provide a set sum of dollars to plan members and allow them to make decisions as to how to spend their healthcare dollars. Such an approach would require managed care to retool and appeal to the individual consumer of pharmaceutical benefits to recognize the value of a managed benefit when making choices as to the use of their health plan dollars. Without consumer recognition of the value of managed care pharmacy programs, benefits constructed around defined contribution would lack the consumer support necessary to achieve the best outcomes at the lowest cost, the essence of managed care pharmacy programs.

WHY PLAN SPONSORS ARE RETURNING TO MANAGED CARE

Costs Down; But Concern Over the Return of Benefit Inflation Remains

Recently, industry analysts have noted a change in the provision of health care services. Payers have begun to recognize that benefit dollars are finite and therefore must be wisely utilized. Because prescription drug expenditures continue to absorb a significant portion of the health care budget, plan sponsors are concerned that without management, cost trends will again escalate. Of equal interest to analysts, consumers have become used to managed care techniques and appear willing to accept a managed prescription benefit. They would like more control over their benefit dollar, but they are also willing to exchange some of that control for guidance on how to more appropriately utilize their limited pharmaceutical benefits.

Recognition of Value

The conclusions of a landmark study conducted by the General Accounting Office and Department of Justice in 2004 appear to lay to rest concerns regarding the fundamental principles and practices used by managed care. The study found that when allowed to operate in a competitive market and to use principles such as closed networks, formularies, and mail service, PBMs can play a significant role in helping plan sponsors manage costs.[3] The Federal Trade Commission weighed in and stated that a competitive pharmaceutical benefits market place gives buyers of services a choice and a "strong hand" in achieving value. Finally, the federal government has used managed care tools for its own programs for decades in the form of the Veterans Administration drug benefit program. A study summarized in the *American Journal of Managed Care* notes that, "the VA PBM has made significant progress in efficiently managing the clinical, economic, and pharmacy-related outcomes of patients; evaluating and endorsing the appropriate use of pharmacotherapies; ensuring the availability of drug products and supplies; and controlling the cost of pharmaceuticals."[4]

Medicare

Although the previously mentioned factors contributed to the renewed interest in managed care pharmacy, it was arguably the passage of the Medicare Prescription Drug, Improvement, and Modernization Act (MMA) of 2003 that served as the primary catalyst for its renaissance. The legislation includes several key parameters that are based on the principles of managed care. In particular, the MMA will have significant influence on formulary development of participating sponsors—a key tenet of managed care pharmacy.

Commercial plan sponsors are closely watching what happens with Medicare, and indications are that they will adopt many of the principles used successfully in the new Medicare benefit for their own plans. In particular, interest exists in the Medicare drug benefit serving as a benchmark for pharmaceutical benefits plans for retirees. Indeed, many employers covering the prescription benefits of their retirees are considering Medicare for retiree coverage with some level of subsidization. To the extent that successful initiatives concerning quality and cost improvements exist, a strong interest from employers in either adopting those techniques or moving retirees into Medicare programs that use them will likely exist.

MANAGED CARE TOOLS

Managed care pharmacy plans utilize a number of tools—many of which have become staples of mainstream pharmaceutical benefits plans. Although some plans may offer a formulary, or use prior authorization on a limited basis, the key difference between highly managed and traditional PBMs is an emphasis on getting the right drug, to the right person, at the right time and at the right cost. Today, those decisions are often supported by intensive clinical research and outcomes studies, as well as by technology. To achieve the objectives of managed care pharmacy, and to manage the varied needs demanded by the health care market, a full range of tools is required.

Formularies

Formularies have been a mainstay of managed care pharmaceutical benefits programs for almost three decades. However, the use of formularies by health plans has often been contentious. The view held by many beneficiaries is that formularies are primarily used to lower cost, and that preference is given to the lowest cost therapeutic agents at the expense of quality. Yet most forward-thinking PBMs have consistently fielded therapeutically strong formularies. For those PBMs, a focus on using formularies to ensure positive outcomes has grown. The benefits of this approach include:

- Lowered costs in other areas of the health benefit
- Improved patient satisfaction
- Increased beneficiary compliance and retention
- Improved ability to attract and retain clients

With a focus on improving outcomes, less focus is placed in these benefit management companies on the cost of drug acquisition, and less reliance is placed on formularies as a tool to drive rebates.

Challenges remain regarding the effective development and utilization of formularies. Plan members often want unfettered access to the newest and most heavily marketed prescription drugs. In addition, drug manufacturers are creating new categories of drugs for conditions that, although troublesome to some patients, may not always require the use of high-cost prescription drugs. Examples of these drugs include medications for incontinence, nail fungus, simple heart burn, and eczema. Pharmaceuticals deemed to be "lifestyle drugs," including those for male pattern baldness and erectile dysfunction, also create challenges for plan sponsors. The difficulty arises because the payer must balance patient demands against limited benefit dollars.

Addressing these issues can best be accomplished by a recognition of the fundamental goal of an effective formulary program—to align the incentives of plan sponsors and plan members. In today's complex pharmaceutical benefits environment, pharmacy and therapeutics (P & T) committees can be essential to that effort. At some PBMs and health plans, the P & T committee members once consisted primarily of the medical director and employee pharmacists. Committee compositions of this nature fueled accusations that the formularies were actually "rubber stamps" for lists of drugs that were predominantly preferred for their ability to provide rebates, driven by the strength of manufacturer contracts and not for their clinical efficacy or the lowest net cost to the health plan.

However, many managed care PBMs did not operate in that manner, and most have taken significant steps to assure their process is focused on more than simply an ability to increase rebates. Toward that end, PBMs have taken measures to ensure that the composition of the P & T committee is diverse, clinically sound, functionally independent from pharmaceutical contracting, and focused on ensuring optimal health outcomes. An effective P & T committee should include internal resources, as well as nonemployee, practicing physicians from the community, and medical specialists (e.g., when reviewing the latest medication for diabetes, an endocrinologist, nephrologist, or other specialist would be included in the review). In addition, many PBMs today are including in the services of medical ethicists to help ensure that quality-of-life issues and potential conflicts of interest are considered when assessing the impact of P & T formulary decisions on beneficiaries.

The primary areas examined by the P & T committee are safety, efficacy, and cost. In addition, issues such as potential side effects, propensity for negative drug interactions, and ease-of-use of the drug (e.g., once-a-day dosing) are addressed. Review of the latest clinical literature and outcomes data by the P & T committee members is essential to making informed decisions concerning therapeutic agents and alternative treatment options. Some managed care entities opt not to include new drugs on formularies until significant post-marketing outcomes data are available. Although not often popular with members who want the "latest and greatest," it can play a significant role in ensuring that only proven drugs attain formulary status. In addition, it can decrease the likelihood of a dangerous situation some plans have faced. In those cases, in which an accelerated FDA approval process and rapid adoption on the formulary by the P & T committee occurred, the drug was later recalled or withdrawn from the market because of unforeseen complications when exposed to the general population in a "real world" setting.

Another strategy used by managed care PBMs is analysis of existing claims data in order to better customize a clients' formulary to the unique needs of its member population. For example, analysis may show that members within a certain plan have a high incidence of heart disease. In light of this insight, the plan will want to ensure that it has adequate coverage of medications within the therapeutic class for cardiovascular drugs, including lipid-lowering agents and drugs recognized by national guidelines as first-line to effectively treat patients' post–myocardial infarction. Conversely, drugs that are popular due to heavy marketing, but that are not recognized as the preferred treatment for heart disease, may be subject to restrictions or nonformulary status to ensure use of the preferred drug first.

Exceptions Process—Prior Authorization

Although a pharmaceutical benefits plan may encourage utilization of a preferred drug list, it must also include a means by which physicians can request nonformulary medications. Managed care pharmacy programs have traditionally used prior authorization to help review such requests. However, prior authorization has come under considerable scrutiny over the past several years. Some plan sponsors are turning away from the practice due to concerns that it is overly limiting or an obstacle to treating patients. Some PBMs view prior authorization negatively due to the cost of staffing a robust program. Still others question whether the financial and quality benefits to be gained from the method are worth the additional effort. Despite these concerns, many proponents of managed care pharmacy continue to believe that when properly structured, prior authorization can be an important component of a high quality, cost-effective, pharmaceutical benefits plan.

The key to a successful prior authorization program is to ensure that it does not become a mechanism to deny access. The prior authorization process must be based on the latest clinical guidelines, scientific literature, and outcomes data. When formularies are properly structured, and when they are supported by strong prescribing guidelines for physicians and education for patients, prior authorizations are rarely required. In fact, recent studies have found that in a population adapted to a benefit using the tool, fewer than 2 percent of all pharmacy claims required prior authorization. When this option is exercised by a prescribing physician, it must be a rapid and seamless process. In the event a request for a medication is denied, the physician should be supplied with detailed clinical and outcomes data supporting the rationale for the denial. The denial can them be challenged through an appeals process—the weight of scientific authority is required to prevail in such cases.

One of the primary concerns many in the industry have with prior authorization is that it will not provide adequate return on investment (ROI). The belief is that if physicians and plan members are educated about the formulary, and if the decision making behind the drug selection is sound, the prior authorization process should be unnecessary. Numerous reasons (including the provision of a significant return on investment to clients) exist for why many managed care plans continue to use prior authorization. For example, one large employer on the east coast saved 9 percent—$1.9 million— through their prior authorization program over one year. A well-known national retailer was able to save close to $350,000 simply by instituting prior authorization for two highly utilized therapeutic categories—nonsedating antihistamines and proton pump inhibitors.

Yet another benefit of prior authorization is that once the program is fully implemented, it often has a sentinel effect on physicians and patients. Although the physician's first exposure to the prior authorization program is typically patient-specific, that encounter can influence all future prescribing—if the physician has accepted the therapeutic rationale behind the treatment guidelines. In addition, prior authorization is especially important for patients who are prescribed multiple refills because it can serve as a mechanism used to check for adverse drug interactions and unintentional duplication of prescriptions. Finally, without prior authorization, plan members and physicians have little to balance the influence resulting from advertising, detailing, and other direct-to-consumer marketing techniques.

These are just a few examples as to the value of prior authorization, but for those plan sponsors considering eliminating the process, a review of successful programs is warranted before making a final decision.

Utilization Management

The goal of an effective pharmaceutical benefits program must be to encourage appropriate utilization, not to limit utilization. Effective utilization management (UM) programs begin with an understanding of current utilization patterns and plan-member needs. Analysis of existing pharmacy, lab, and medical claims data can help to indicate which therapeutic categories are widely utilized, the physician prescribing patterns, the areas of need, and other information necessary to the development of an effective UM program.

Once this information is gathered and analyzed, it is easier to identify areas that could benefit from interventions, to pinpoint potential problems, and from that to develop an action in order to provide a more "tailored" pharmaceutical benefits for clients. For example, if data analysis indicated high utilization of prescription antihistamines or allergy medications, the plan sponsor could implement one or more of the following:

- Education programs
- Formulary therapeutic category review
- Generic incentives (e.g., tiers, lower copays)
- Promotion of lower cost alternative prescription treatments (e.g., intranasal topical steroids or antihistamines for allergy patients)
- Coverage of over-the-counter medications.

All of these approaches can help to manage utilization of expensive and perhaps clinically unnecessary medications while ensuring that plan members have access to the therapies needed to provide relief for their ailments. Most important, this approach to UM is not generally perceived by plan members as restrictive. Through the incorporation of educational programs designed to answer questions and meet specific needs, and benefit design changes that allow low-cost coverage for generics and OTCs, UM programs are often seen as an enhancement to the existing benefit.

Quality Assurance

Quality assurance (QA) programs are key to managed care pharmacy for three reasons: (1) their focus on quality can improve health outcomes and facilitate cost containment efforts by ensuring prescribing within accepted guidelines and by improving dispensing accuracy, (2) they can minimize the perception that managed care is concerned only with cost cutting, and (3) they provide an opportunity to help improve member satisfaction. Quality assurance programs typically consist of a number of programs, including medication therapy management and drug safety. As these are also two of the key components of the Medicare Modernization Act, expect quality assurance to play an even larger role in managed care pharmaceutical plans in the future.

Quality assurance programs incorporated into managed care pharmaceutical plans also play a significant role in helping health plans meet Health Plan Employer and Data Information Set (HEDIS) measurement goals, and other private and public quality improvement initiatives. Quality assurance is partially dependent upon capture of accurate clinical data that in turn supports the HEDIS goals of health plans.

Therapeutic Interchange

Therapeutic interchange programs (TIP) are designed to transition members from one medication to another, ideally to one that is lower in cost and provides equal or superior outcomes. However, several years ago a few PBMs, under the guides of legitimate TIP programs, switched members to drugs that provide higher rebates or because they received reimbursement for conducting the program from manufacturers. Due to these practices, some states have taken legal and/or legislative actions against at least one of the large PBMs' TIP programs. If the programs are properly designed however, they can remain an important component of a successful managed care pharmacy program. Therapeutic Interchange programs must be designed, taking into account clinical efficacy, health outcomes, and quality of life. To foster support for TIP programs, health care organizations must ensure unbiased clinical literature is available, conflicts of interest are absent, and outcomes data exist to support the decision. In addition, decisions must be based on what is best for the patient, and not only on what generates the most revenue or savings for the plan. When these steps are taken, physicians, patients, and legislators may more readily accept TIP programs.

Promotion of Generics

One of the primary influences managed care pharmacy has had on the benefits' marketplace is to introduce payers and consumers to the value of generics. Although generic utilization is now at an all-time high—about 50 percent[5]—not all plans are using generics to the extent they could and should. In addition, little advertising or active promotion of generics is occurring, meaning that pharmacists, physicians, and PBMs must find innovative strategies to encourage generic utilization instead of the heavily marketed competing branded drugs. Even small increases in the utilization of generics can impact a sponsor's costs and bottom line. For example, one midsize employer instituted a more aggressive generic incentive program, increasing utilization to 51.9 from 47.5, and saved close to $300,000 in one year.[6] One caveat exists: many branded drugs are without an identical generic equivalent. In these cases, a number of generically available drugs are often present in the same therapeutic class. For example, statins (lipid-lowering agents), selective serotonin reuptake inhibitors (SSRIs), antidepressants, and nonsedating antihistamines all have both branded only, and branded with generic options that can be used to effectively treat the corresponding illnesses. Plans can work with their PBMs to identify generic alternatives within therapeutic classes so that they can ensure utilization of the most cost-effective agent.

The overall key to an effective generic program is therapeutic equivalence between the generic drug and the branded drug with comparable clinical outcomes at a lower cost.

Mail Service

Although currently under fire from some state legislators and special interest groups, mail-service pharmacy remains a popular benefit design for many plan members. It enables members on maintenance medications to secure their prescription drugs safely and conveniently via shipments to their home. It also provides significant cost savings. Most mail service programs offer a ninety-day supply of medications for two, thirty-day copays as an incentive to members. Many mail programs also often include other incentives, such as free shipping, discounts, and coupons that provide further value to plan members.

Mail service also offers significant savings to plan sponsors compared with retail pharmacy prices. Depending on the benefit design, plan savings can be upward of 15 to 20 percent.[7] Because of this, some plan sponsors have opted to mandate the use of mail for their members on maintenance medication. This move has proven highly controversial. In fact, some of the leading pharmacy retailers have sought to counter this action by refusing to accept the pharmacy network contracts of health plans that mandate mail service. This has resulted in legislative battles and caused confusion and animosity on both sides of the issue.

Although providing savings and convenience, a less controversial alternative to mandated mail service is to share some of the savings of mail service by providing incentives to encourage mail service utilization. For example, plans can structure beneficiary cost sharing to favor mail service over retail for the filling of maintenance prescriptions. This is accomplished by using the savings achieved by mail service to offset the copay. Allowing beneficiaries continued access to retail pharmacy but with a greater cost share than available by mail is usually adequate incentive to move a significant volume of prescriptions to mail. Again, programs that provide discounts, coupons for other products, and services and other incentives, often provide the encouragement needed for members to choose mail service on their own—without mandates.

Another key issue for plan sponsors to recognize is that in addition to being a highly accurate and efficient prescription delivery system, mail service can be an important tool to improve outcomes and lower overall costs. Some mail service programs provide highly targeted education on specific disease states. They also emphasize the importance of compliance, perform disease management, and provide case management as well as other services and information. In fact, studies have shown that patients who use mail service for certain therapeutic categories are often more persistent and compliant (they tend to adhere to the recommended dosage schedule and for the prescribed length of therapy) than those who use a retail pharmacy.[8] Such compliance rates are specifically important for members with high cholesterol or other diseases for which patients often forget to take or just quit taking their medications when they no longer "feel sick," thereby leading to minimal improvement in their health status. When patients are compliant, it means that both the patient and the plan sponsor are ensuring the best possible outcomes and the best value for their prescription dollar.

Controlled Pharmacy Networks

Another tool often associated with managed care pharmacy is the use of controlled, "closed," or "limited" networks of pharmacy providers. Utilization of a closed network of pharmacies can help to lower costs since PBMs can opt to work with pharmacies that have the clinical, managed care contracting and technological knowledge to meet their needs. Such arrangements also allow the PBM to negotiate the lowest price in exchange for market exclusivity and increased volume. However, closed networks in particular are among the most controversial practices of managed care pharmacy. They have been heavily fought by retail pharmacy through any willing provider laws and regulations. Recognizing provider concerns, as well appreciating the value of controlled networks, managed care PBMs have reached out to a wider array of retail pharmacy stores, including independent pharmacies. A few large pharmaceutical wholesalers are stepping up to the plate by helping to ensure that their contracted independents have the systems in place to work with managed care PBM contracts.

Most important, PBMs are creating their networks based on preference and convenience to members, not just on cost. Such moves allow the PBM to continue to contract for the competitive reimbursement rates, but also show plan sponsors and members that their convenience and satisfaction is a high priority.

THE USE OF MANAGED CARE TOOLS
FOR SPECIALTY PHARMACY

Traditional managed care tools are particularly important as specialty pharmacy utilization and costs increase. Specialty pharmacy drugs (most often high-cost biotechnical or injectable drugs), are among the most promising and costly of emerging prescription drug options. To ensure plan sponsors secure maximum value—managed care principles such as prior authorization, adherence to treatment guidelines, and utilization management will be critical. Strong case management and education programs will also be critical for an effective specialty pharmacy program. As with other prescription drugs, the emphasis must not be simply on limiting access but on ensuring appropriate access to needed therapies. Managed care must take its approach to specialty pharmacy even further. For example, in the event a patient is not responding to the prescribed medications, the program must include guidelines for therapeutic end points—such as alternative therapies and options—if the specialty pharmacy drug does not provide the desired outcomes. The program should also include guidelines for off-label usage where clinically appropriate. PBMs that have strong pharmacy and therapeutics committees to develop their treatment guidelines will be better able to identify those cases that warrant the use of a specialty pharmaceutical for off-label purposes. For instance, one managed care PBM approved the use of an injectable hepatitis medication for a patient that did not meet labeled indications. The prescribing physician did so because she believed that doing so would more quickly allow the patient to become a marrow donor for a sibling with leukemia. Strong case management and education programs will also be critical for an effective specialty pharmacy program.

MANAGED CARE FOR COMMERCIAL MEDICARE/MEDICAID

The specifics of Medicare Part D for pharmaceutical benefits are discussed in Chapter 5. However, several components of the MMA specifically relate to the area of managed care pharmacy.

Formularies and P &T Committees

The MMA rules states that every prescription drug plan must provide "adequate coverage of the types of drugs most commonly needed" by Medicare beneficiaries. These include drugs to treat high blood pressure, heart disease, cancer, osteoporosis, and Alzheimer's disease since these diseases are common among the elderly beneficiaries. The rules also state that a plan can establish a list of preferred drugs. The intent of the MMA legislation is to ensure that the formulary reflects the needs of the Medicare-eligible population to be served. However, some ambiguities exist within the MMA statute. For example, the regulations state that a plan can refuse to pay for other medicines not deemed medically necessary. Yet language also exists that can be interpreted to mean that the Center for Medicare and Medicaid Services (CMS) could require plan sponsors to cover specific drugs, or types of drugs, that will be "identified in the future." Although this ambiguous language concerns some in the industry, it is believed that pharmacy plans that have formulary development guidelines, supported by a strong P & T process, will be able to readily uphold and defend their decisions when challenged by regulators.

Managed Care and Medicaid

It is estimated that Medicaid programs, which are jointly funded by the federal government and the states, will see the most significant increase in prescription drug expenditures over the next decade. This will be mitigated somewhat after January 1, 2006, because as a result of MMA, Medicaid will no longer cover individuals who are enrolled in Medicaid and are eligible for the new Medicare drug benefit. CMS projects that by 2011, Medicaid will be paying for almost 20 percent of all U.S. prescriptions.[9] To help manage these costs, many states are turning to specialty Medicaid managed care PBMs. According to a 2004 study by Atlantic Information Services, a leading publisher of health care data, managed care PBMs could save some states up to 50 percent in Medicaid costs through strategies such as pharmacy networks, formularies and prior authorization.[10]

A particular challenge is the continued effort by interested parties to mandate inclusion of specific drugs on Medicaid formularies. Both pharmaceutical companies and patient advocacy groups have attempted to influence legislation that would force individual state Medicaid organizations to include certain drugs on the formulary. Although assuring patient access, such efforts would also destroy any incentive by a pharmaceutical manufacturer to negotiate aggressively to reduce pricing in exchange for formulary placement. The keys to the successful implementation of a managed care Medicaid program are:

- Education and case management
- Strong formulary development
- Prior authorization process to allow for formulary exceptions
- Efficient appeals process

LEGAL AND REGULATORY ISSUES IMPACTING MANAGED CARE PHARMACY

Despite the emphasis on managed care principles such as formularies, prior authorization, and controlled networks in federal programs for Medicare and Medicaid, some state legislatures are opposing these business practices. Most legal and regulatory issues of relevance involve three key aspects of managed care pharmacy.

1. Mail service. A number of states have introduced legislation that includes provisions to: (1) prohibit the use of mandatory mail service benefits, (2) to allow retail pharmacies to dispense up to a ninety-day supply of drugs, and (3) to provide parity in beneficiary cost sharing between retail and mail. Such an approach would benefit retail pharmacy, particularly smaller chains and independents, but could generate additional expenses for plan sponsors. Specifically, the cost savings and increased accuracy available through mail service pharmacies would be diminished by laws favoring the plan member using the retail network.

2. Formulary development. Some states have introduced legislation that would require coverage for any FDA–approved drug prescribed for a beneficiary of a health plan. Various stakeholders, including drug manufacturers, have tried to take an active role in the P & T process to attempt to force broader coverage of certain drugs. Both consumers and clinicians want to ensure access to the drugs they need. However, carefully developed formularies and clinically based prior authorization programs can help ensure adequate access to the drugs consumers and clinicians need, without adding unnecessary costs for open coverages.

3. Pharmacy network. Any willing provider laws have been an ongoing issue for managed care pharmacy. More than twenty-two states have these laws in place, which in effect limit a PBM's ability to contract exclusively with retail pharmacies that agree to competitive pricing terms and performance and service standards. Any willing provider status clearly benefits retail pharmacists, but it does so at the expense of the plan sponsor and member. The ultimate goal of the sponsor and the contracted PBM is to ensure that the network meets the needs of plan members in a satisfactory manner. Pharmacy access is typically negotiated between the plan sponsor and the PBM during the contracting process. Many believe that free-market forces can more readily address the issue of pharmacy networks than can access mandates achieved through legislation.

One of the most significant issues impacting managed care pharmacy are the efforts by some states to use the recent settlements state and federal governments have made with large PBMs and apply those to all PBMs. The settlements against these PBMs involve managed care tools—such as therapeutic interchange programs—and focus on the disclosure of financial and contractual terms to government offices and agencies. Sensitive issues surrounding disclosure, transparency, and fiducial responsibilities are all critical areas to an effective managed care pharmaceutical plan. Open disclosure of pharmaceutical pricing and rebates or networking pricing agreements would reduce the ability of the PBM to negotiate aggressively and increase the overall pricing to the purchaser. Although the specifics of disclosure vary, effective disclosure should remain between the two parties to the PBM services agreement. Plan sponsors should ensure that their PBM provides information about all revenue sources related to their business, how income is reported, types and amounts of administration fees, rebate accounting and allocation according to contract terms, and other pricing policies.

Legislation is the foundation for all PBM regulation. However, state regulatory agencies often extend their authority through their interpretation of laws, creating complexities and challenges for PBMs. For example, in one state, the Department of Insurance said that under their understanding of state law, only a physician could deny a request for a prescription drug. PBM prior authorization programs were therefore deemed to be illegal, unless every denial was signed by a physician. In another state, regulators held that PBMs had to cover any drug viewed as medically necessary, including those for lifestyle drugs such as Viagra and antiobesity prescriptions. Two of the state's largest health plans sued to block their regulator and won—the courts agreed that regulators had overstepped their authority. However, the regulators then introduced legislation specifically stating that "medically necessary" drugs were to be covered, thus trumping the court's decision. As of this writing, plans in this state must cover all "medically necessary" drugs, although drug benefit exclusions approved by the regulator are exempt.

BENEFIT DESIGN IN A MANAGED CARE PLAN

One of the critical factors to examine with regard to a managed care pharmaceutical benefits is the impact of pharmacy on medical benefits. For example, a focus on a low-cost medication might help to lower costs on the pharmacy side, but could impact the medical benefit in terms of increased physician visits and hospitalizations. An effective managed care pharmacy benefit will ensure that coordination and integration with the medical benefit occurs.

One of the most important steps that managed care pharmacy can take with regard to benefit design is to ensure that the benefit is tailored and not a one-size-fits-all approach. For example, instead of standard disease management programs, a strong managed care pharmacy program will analyze the needs of the member population and design programs that best meet those needs. This more targeted approach helps to manage utilization while improving quality. Examples of a targeted benefit could include programs designed to promote education and appropriate utilization of drug therapies for plan sponsors with large populations of members with diabetes, high blood pressure, or heart disease. Such programs can be intense—to include case management, physician education on the latest clinical guidelines and therapies, and targeted interventions—or more general and focused on formulary selection and general education.

PERCEPTIONS OF MANAGED CARE
AND IMPLICATIONS FOR BENEFIT DESIGN

Despite efforts to tailor benefits and focus on quality and outcomes a significant percentage of the population continues to have a negative impression regarding the tools of managed care pharmacy. Unfortunately, a few managed care organizations have contributed to this perception by placing too much emphasis on cost and not enough on quality, outcomes, and patient satisfaction. However, the opinions surrounding managed care are often based on perceptions and not real-world experiences. For example, most of the public strongly supports the use of generics and a growing number recognize the value of formularies.

Because of these perceptions, it is of critical importance that the managed care pharmacy industry ensures that benefit designs and tools are based on quantifiable evidence-based literature and solid outcomes data. Members and physicians will adopt and support tools such as controlled formularies and restricted networks, but only if a value proposition for them exists (e.g., better outcomes and lower overall costs), and only if they recognize that decisions are based on clinical evidence, not simply financial gain for a PBM or plan sponsor.

MANAGED CARE PHARMACY: TODAY AND TOMORROW

Of all the trends facing managed care pharmacy, one of the most significant and challenging is the aging of the baby boomer population. As this group ages, their utilization of pharmaceuticals will increase. However, unlike past generations, this population is familiar and somewhat comfortable with many of the principles of managed care pharmacy. They understand formularies and are more likely to tolerate some limitations on their utilization of prescription drugs when they are supported by their physician and clinical literature. However, this group will also demand accountability and quality. Customer service, strong education programs, flexibility, and benefit design options will be important to maintain member satisfaction.

WHAT MAKES MANAGED CARE PHARMACY TODAY UNIQUE

Although the lines between the various choices among pharmaceutical benefits plans of today often seem blurred, managed care remains unique in its use of tools and its overall concept. As when it was first introduced, managed care pharmacy remains focused on providing the best outcomes at the lowest cost. However, over time, managed care has come to recognize that to be successful in today's health care environment, it must also adopt new tools such as electronic prescribing, prospective and retrospective data analysis, pharmacoeconomics, and sophisticated predictive health and benefit modeling to better predict the impact of new drugs.

Through it all, managed care has remained true to the belief that by analyzing data, by using clinical guidelines and literature, and by controls including formularies and prior authorization, it can help its clients better meet their needs and those of members. Most important, those involved in managed care continue to believe that their approach to pharmacy programs is far better than programs that provide little guidance to plan sponsors or plan members or that simply process claims.

Managed care plans also dispute the allegation that they are simply middlepersons in the process. An examination of the tools utilized and programs developed supports this premise. Managed care pharmacy plans don't just process claims, and they don't just negotiate for lower-cost drugs and rebates. They also don't limit appropriate use of prescriptions through their use of formularies and controlled networks. Far from being a middleperson, managed care pharmacy organizations today strive to be the solution for escalating costs, growing demand, and the promising potential new drug therapies. They reach these goals through a team of dedicated clinical pharmacists and clinicians who use clinical literature, outcomes data, intensive analysis, and innovative member-centric programs to improve outcomes and lower costs. The focus is always on maximizing the benefit value. A high-value benefit means spending the health care dollar wisely while striving for healthier, better educated, and more satisfied patients. This will ultimately produce the highest quality with the lowest cost benefit design.

MANAGED CARE PHARMACY—THE SOLUTION

To meet the demands and fulfill its potential, managed care pharmacy will continue to grow and change. Legislation and regulations will continue to evolve and impact design and flexibility. The consumer empowerment movement will also influence both plan sponsors and PBMs by encouraging the adoption of pharmacy programs that provide flexibility, beneficiary cost, and choice, while providing the appropriate structure and guidance.

As health care becomes more complex and as pharmacy costs continue to remain a significant component of plan sponsors' budgets, two viable options for the payment and delivery of drug benefits—(1) government control and (2) private sector managed care. Although some in the industry believe that government-sponsored health care is likely, others recognize that if those sponsors of pharmaceutical benefits incorporate the principles of managed care that have proven to provide value, it will lower costs, expand access, and meet all the health care demands of our nation.

NOTES

1. Pharmacy Benefit Management Institute (2003). *The Prescription Drug Benefit Cost and Plan Design Survey Report, 2003.* Pharmacy Benefit Management Institute.

2. Mays G.P., Claxton G., White J. (2004). Managed Care Rebound? Recent Changes in Health Plan's Cost Containment Strategies. *Health Affairs* 11(August).

3. General Accounting Office (2003). Report to the Honorable Byron L. Dorgan, U.S. Senate, Federal Employees Health Benefits: Effects of Using Pharmacy Benefit Managers on Health Plans, Enrollees and Pharmacies. January. Washington, DC: GAO.

4. Sales M.M., Cunningham, F.E., Glassman P.A., et. al. (2005). Pharmacy Benefits Management in the Veterans Health Administration: 1995 to 2003. *American Journal of Managed Care* February: 104-112.

5. Continued Increases in Generic Utilization Mean Big Savings. (2004). *Drug Benefit News* October 15: 27.

6. Information on file with Prescription Solutions and available upon request.

7. Supporting data on file with Prescription Solutions and available upon request.

8. White T.J., Chang E., Leslie S., et al. (2002). Patient Adherence with HMG Reductase Inhibitor Therapy Among Users of Two Types of Prescription Services. *Journal of Managed Care Pharmacy* August: 186-191.

    9. PBM Medicaid Programs Show Promise. *Drug Cost Management Report* May.
    10. Medicaid Plan Programs Cited for Improving Care Quality While Controlling Rx Costs. (2003). *News and Strategies for Managed Care Medicare and Medicaid* May 12: 11,13.

Chapter 14

Pharmaceutical Benefits Managers

Kimberly P. McDonough

Pharmaceutical benefits managers (PBMs), or as they are sometimes classified, pharmaceutical benefits administrators (PBAs), represent a widely diverse business sector that serves as an operational intermediary to the health insurance industry for the processing of prescription drug claims in insurance benefits. Some PBMs offer a wide option of services, ranging from claim processing to clinical intervention programs, whereas others are more focused on limited services. PBMs offer services to insurance companies, as well as to governmental programs or directly to self-insured employers. Although they are widely unrecognized outside of the health insurance industry, as of 2004, approximately two-thirds of all U.S. prescriptions are processed by PBMs.[1] The implementation of a Medicare prescription drug benefit program in 2006 will likely increase that number.

The anticipated goal of a quality pharmaceutical benefits management program is to control cost of drug treatment and to increase the safety and quality of care beneficiaries to the program. To facilitate these services, employers, health plans, and government benefit programs will often contract with pharmaceutical benefits management (PBM) firms, organizations that specialize in pharmacy claim and distribution services. PBMs typically offer their potential clients a variety of clinical and administrative services, but the services offered and administration methods vary significantly across PBMs. Examples of services that are typically offered in the industry include:

- Claims processing and adjudication
- Point-of-service (POS) online edits, including concurrent and prospective drug utilization review
- Retail and mail-order pharmacy network management
- Pharmacy network auditing program
- Reporting tools, including standard and query tools

- Rebate program, consisting of monies obtained from pharmaceutical manufacturers and discounts negotiated with the network
- Clinical services provided by PBMs include formulary development and management and drug utilization management involving physician intervention, client initiated management initiatives, disease management programs, and treatment guidelines. Outcomes management and patient education are also provided by the more clinically focused and managed care experienced PBMs.

HISTORY OF THE PBM INDUSTRY

Although the PBM industry did not evolve until the early 1990s, predecessors to the industry have been in existence for many years. PBMs have their roots in one of three different areas: administrators of prescription drug cards, mail-service pharmacies, and prescription management groups within managed care organizations. In fact, the technology associated with prescription claim processing is comparable to technology used in credit card transactions for commercial sales. Several early claims transaction companies provided services to both industries.

Electronic transaction of pharmacy claims offered employers and health plans significant savings in operational costs. Prior to the advent of electronic claim adjudication capabilities, the processing of pharmacy claims was labor intensive and time consuming. Individuals would typically purchase their prescriptions, saving the receipts for submission to their insurance carrier. Considerable paperwork was necessary for the completion of these claims, and the complexity of this paperwork made completion of this function difficult for many individuals. Likewise, the level of paperwork for the processing of pharmacy claims created significant operational costs for health insurers. Paper claims were received by the health plan, and each claim was manually reviewed by a claim adjuster against individual's insurance benefit. Because of the extensive amount of manual intervention throughout the claim process, the potential for error was quite high, requiring follow-up or possibly even resubmission of the forms. However, after the claims were successfully competed and processed, individuals received reimbursement for a portion of their out-of-pocket costs, depending on their level of insurance coverage.

Pharmacy claim processing for Medicaid programs was equally labor intensive. When a pharmacy dispensed a medication to a Medicaid beneficiary, claims were typically submitted through a paper claim process. The pharmacist, or the pharmacist's assistant, completed a series of forms that provided information regarding the prescription, including the patient information, drug dispensed, quantity, and cost. Often, Medicaid forms were structured to permit the billing of multiple prescriptions on each form, often completed in duplicate or triplicate. As with the paper claims submitted by patients, Medicaid forms were completed manually and were subject to high potential for simple transcription errors or omissions, both by the individuals completing the forms as well as by the staff that were charged with processing of the forms within the Medicaid department. As a result of the manual process employed for the processing of claims, the turnaround time for compensation for Medicaid claims could take several months or more, creating cash-flow problems for pharmacies.

The advent of claim adjudication services, and the birth of what was to become the PBM industry, offered an efficient and consistent method to process pharmacy claims and facilitate the claim payment process. The industry emerged in the early 1980s as state Medicaid programs mandated electronic processing of prescriptions for improved efficiency and greater accountability. As electronic claim processing became more universally available in pharmacies, the industry evolved to provide pharmacy networks with negotiated discounts for drugs and dispensing fees.

In the early 1990s, the PBM industry experienced significant growth that was fueled by expanded adoption of prescription drug benefits as part of an insured health plan program. At this time, expansion of services to include claim processing, clinical interventions and mail-order prescription services resulted in what is now recognized as the PBM industry.

SERVICES PROVIDED BY THE PBM INDUSTRY

Claim Adjudication

The primary function of the PBM industry has historically been, and continues to be, the industry's ability to provide electronic claim processing services to clients. Claim processing functions are similar across the industry and provide the single greatest source of administrative efficiency to the health insurance industry with regard to pharmacy benefit administration. PBMs typically charge their clients a claim processing fee, ranging from $0.15 to $1.25 per claim for each claim that is adjudicated. Lower claim processing fees may be offered by the PBM, but this lower fee is typically offset by revenues that are retained in other services offered by the PBM. However, the claim processing fee charged by PBMs is more than offset by the savings generated through the elimination of the manual claim administration process.

Claim Processing Standards

Pharmacy claims are processed electronically in accordance with standards that have been established by the National Council for Prescription Drug Programs, Inc. (NCPDP). NCPDP is a not-for-profit ANSI–Accredited Standards Development Organization that creates and promotes standards for the transfer of data within the pharmacy sectors of the health care industry.[2] The organization is governed by its membership, which represents virtually every sector of the pharmacy services industry, including pharmacies, government, insurers, manufacturers, wholesalers, and telecommunication vendors.

NCPDP's claim transmission standards establish the requirements for the submission of electronic claims within the United States. Factors that are addressed within the claim standards include telecommunication procedures for claim submission, standards for fields that are maintained in the claim transaction process, and unit standards for quantities that are dispensed.[3] NCPDP claim transaction standards were adopted as the required format for pharmacy claim transactions under the Health Insurance Portability and Accountability Act of 1996.[4] NCPDP also provides guidelines to the processing of pharmaceutical rebates, the format of prescription cards that are issued to beneficiaries, enrollment processes, procedures for the implementation of prior authorization requirements, and professional services implementation.

Electronic Data Interchanges

The electronic processing of claims greatly improved the efficiency of the claim submission and payment process. However, in any given pharmacy, prescriptions and services may be provided to patients with a wide variety of third party coverage. If the number of patients with a particular level of coverage is great, the pharmacy may establish a direct transmission line, through a T1 or comparable interface, to the third party payer. However, the cost of these lines can be prohibitive, particularly if the volume of claims submitted to a single source is low. To facilitate the transfer of claims to the appropriate resource for payment, electronic data interchanges (EDI) are utilized.

Electronic data interchanges (EDI) serve to route the pharmacy claim from the pharmacy, where the claim is being generated, to the appropriate payer.[5,6] This process is completed in the same manner as many forms of electronic claim transmission for credit card and banking procedures through direct managed network connection options, frame relay, and virtual private networking (VPN) technology.[7] A list of organizations that provide EDI services is included in Exhibit 14.1.[8-13] These companies typically offer connectivity to more than 1,000 payers nationally, providing pharmacies with a single interface for all claim transactions. Services are provided twenty-four hours per day, seven days per week.

Pharmacy claims are submitted to the EDI electronically, where the claim is electronically routed to the appropriate payer. The claim adjudicates against the claim processing system of the payer, and is evaluated for a number of edits, including the eligibility status of the individual; coverage of the applicable drug; assignment of any prescription edits or messages; determination of the individual's copay, coinsurance, or deductible; and designation of the approved payment amount. These transactions are completed in nanoseconds, permitting point-of-sale transactions in the pharmacy.

In addition to claim routing services, EDI vendors offer a variety of services that are designed to improve efficiency in pharmacy operations and in the claim adjudication process. One example is electronic claim editing that uses client-determined edits to test claims prior to submission to the appropriate payer. This testing process is designed to reduce the number of claim transmission errors and to maximize reimbursement opportunities for the pharmacy. Other services that are offered by EDI vendors include electronic signature capture, integrated response voice (IVRU) systems for prescription renewal, refill reminder systems, as well as a variety of electronic systems designed to improve work flow and prescription processing within the pharmacy.

EXHIBIT 14.1.
Some major companies that provide
electronic data interface services

ERx Network
Freedom Data Services (FDS)
Per-Sé Technologies (formerly NDCHealth)
QS/1
Rx Linc
Emdeon (formerly WebMD)

NDC Codes

When prescriptions are submitted for adjudication, either in electronic or paper form, a national drug code (NDC) is used to identify the medication that is being dispensed. The NDC serves as a universal product identifier for prescription and selected over-the-counter, insulin, domestic, and foreign drug products that are in commercial distribution in the United States. The national drug code system was established by Congress under the Drug Listing Act of 1972, an amendment to the Federal Food, Drug, and Cosmetic Act.[14] The purpose of the development of this coding system was to facilitate out-of-hospital drug reimbursement under the Medicare program. The coding system provides the commissioner of the Food and Drug Administration (FDA) with a current list of all drugs manufactured, prepared, propagated, compounded, or processed by a drug establishment registered under the Federal Food, Drug, and Cosmetic Act.[15] The act requires submission of information on commercially marketed drugs and is used in the enforcement of the Federal Food, Drug, and Cosmetic Act.

Under the coding system, each drug product is assigned a unique ten-digit, three-segment number that identifies the labeler/vendor, product, and trade package size. Segments may be divided into one of three configurations: 4-4-2, 5-3-2, or 5-4-1. The first segment, the labeler code, is assigned by the FDA. A labeler is any firm that manufactures, repacks, or distributes a drug product. The second segment, the product code, identifies a specific strength, dosage form, and formulation for a particular firm. The third segment, the package code, identifies package sizes. Both the product and package codes are assigned by the firm.

The NDC directory is updated quarterly within five working days after the end of March, June, September, and December. Reasons why certain drug products may not be included in the NDC directory include the following: (1) the firm has not submitted the listing information to the FDA, (2) the product is no longer being marketed, or (3) the firm has not complied fully with the listing process. Commercial drug pricing sources such as First Databank or Medispan will frequently maintain discontinued NDC codes in their listing for a period of time to facilitate claim processing transactions.

The FDA publishes a Drug Registration and Listing System (DRLS) Instruction Booklet that describes in detail the registration and listing process and also contains the applicable code of federal regulations (CFR).

Government agencies other than the FDA may display the NDC in an eleven-digit format for purposes of consistency. For example, the Centers for Medicare and Medicaid Services (CMS) displays the labeler code as five digits with leading zeros, the product code as four digits with leading zeros, and the package size as two characters with leading zeros.

Provider and Pharmacy Identification

In addition to claim transmission standards, NCPDP develops provider and pharmacy identification systems. Working with the National Association of Boards of Pharmacy (NAPB), NCPDP established and maintains a unique, national identifying number that would assist pharmacies in their interactions with federal agencies and third party providers. The NCPDP Provider Identification Number, formerly the NCPDP/NABP numbering list, is assigned to every licensed pharmacy qualified Alternate Site Enumeration Program (ASEP) sites in the United States and contains over 70,000 pharmacies. It is a seven-digit numbering system NCPDP currently maintains and updates this database, and it is available for processing and reference purposes.

NCPDP has also established HCIdea, a provider identification system with unique coding for a wide variety of individual health care providers for the purpose of identification in claim transactions. Providers that are identified in the HCIdea database include physicians, pharmacists, and other health practitioners who are licensed to prescribe pharmaceuticals. The database uniquely identifies each individual prescriber with an HCIdea and provides information on practice addresses, DEA numbers, demographic information, specialty, and other identifiers.

PHARMACY NETWORK MANAGEMENT

One of the primary services that is provided by the PBM industry is the provision of a pharmacy network that will provide prescription services to designated beneficiaries. All major PBMs offer a wide variety of network options, including both chain and independent community pharmacy and mail service (home delivery) pharmacy. Increasingly, PBMs are able to offer specialized networks that include pharmacies that specialize in infusion or biotechnology therapies, long-term care services, and compounding services.

Contracted negotiation with pharmacy networks generates savings to the health care purchaser. In a 2003 report to Congress, the General Accounting Office evaluated the impact of PBM contract negotiations on pharmacy costs, compared to the fee-for-service prices that would have been paid by individuals. In this study, the average retail prescription price negotiated by the PBM was approximately 18 percent below the average cash prescription cash price for both brand and generic medications.[16]

A similar evaluation of savings associated with PBM–administered prescription drug discount cards in California, North Dakota, and Washington,

DC, showed variable savings when compared to cash prices paid by senior citizens for the top nine medications used by this population.[17] The variable level of savings obtained through PBM–sponsored discount cards is probably attributable to a variety of factors. Whereas the original GAO study evaluated all drug prices, the second study reviewed only a select group of drugs that excluded generic products that offer a greater potential for discounted prices. The second study also limited its review to pricing in three states, one of which was California. However, California Medicaid regulations already provided a clause that allowed senior citizens to purchase drugs at the Medicaid-negotiated rate. This regulation minimized the added value of a PBM–sponsored discount card in that state. Finally, it is reasonable to assume that pharmacies may be willing to accept a higher level of discount for an insured product that comprises a significant portion of their business, whereas a discount card does not offer the same level of volume increase and may reduce overall revenue from prescriptions. Regardless, these studies demonstrated that negotiation with pharmacy networks can generate modest savings in pharmaceutical costs when compared to the fee-for-service costs for prescriptions.

Community Pharmacy Networks

PBMs offer community pharmacy networks that are very broad or fairly restrictive, depending on the client's needs and the desired cost of the pharmacy services. Typically, PBMs offer a wide network that includes most community pharmacies nationwide. This offers a distinct advantage to beneficiaries who may have prescription needs while they are away from their primary residences. Examples include students who are attending colleges at a location that is not proximal to their home, individuals who maintain multiple residences in different parts of the country, or for individuals on vacation or business travel. In fact, pharmacy choice is a primary consideration for many employers, government plans, and insurers as they consider PBM options.

To obtain more favorable pricing terms, PBMs may contract with a limited number of pharmacies in a more restrictive pharmacy network. Usually restrictions affect the number of chain pharmacies that are included in a network, while preserving the availability of independent pharmacies. Not surprisingly, restrictive pharmacy networks are promoted aggressively by PBMs that are owned by retail pharmacy chains or by health maintenance organizations that own and operate in-house pharmacies.

Although restrictive networks decrease the pharmacy options that are available to the beneficiary, they theoretically offer the potential for both clinical and financial benefits. For example, pharmacies that participate in a small network may be willing to provide deeper discounts in exchange for a higher volume of prescription business. Likewise, clinical initiatives might be more easily implemented in a limited, localized pharmacy network as compared with a broad, diverse pharmacy network. In reality, very little objective information is published about the benefits or limitations of a restrictive pharmacy network.

Several states have enacted "any willing provider" regulations, which prevent PBMs or health plans from restricting access to pharmacies, provided that the pharmacy is willing to accept the reimbursement level that is offered to any other pharmacy. The Federal Trade Commission has expressed an opinion that any willing provider regulations may decrease the willingness of pharmacies to offer deep discounts to insurer and PBMs.[18] Considerable opposition is given by the health insurance and PBM industry to these regulations,[19-21] out of a concern that any willing provider regulations will increase pharmacy costs. However, the regulations appear to have little impact on the actual cost of pharmaceuticals that are negotiated by PBMs or health plans.[22]

Mail-Order Services

PBMs often offer mail pharmacy services as a convenience to the client's beneficiaries and to provide added savings to the pharmacy program. Typically the PBM will contract with a single mail-service vendor in an exclusive arrangement that offers deep discounts on the purchase of pharmaceuticals.

Mail-order pharmacies typically centralize their pharmacy distribution operations into a small number of locations that serve a wide geographic region. Prescriptions are received via mail, fax, or electronic transfer, and are delivered to the patient through mail or other courier services. Typically, patients obtain a ninety-day supply of medication, a convenience for patients who take maintenance medications. The mail-order pharmacy is also able to distribute prescriptions to varying locations for a single patient. This offers a tremendous advantage to patients who live in different locations throughout the year. By using the mail order pharmacy, the patient eliminates the need to obtain multiple prescriptions that are filled in different pharmacies.

By centralizing the location of the mail-order pharmacy, the volume of prescriptions within the pharmacy is increased, offering cost savings opportunities. Increased volume allows the pharmacy to negotiate aggressively for prescriptions drug purchase prices, particularly for generic medications.

Furthermore, the pharmacy is able to take advantage of automated systems for the fulfillment of prescriptions. In fact, in very sophisticated mail-order pharmacies, prescriptions are processed using robotic equipment with electronic record keeping. Finally, because prescriptions are filled for a ninety-day supply, dispensing fees and professional costs for handling of the prescription are minimized.

The focus of mail-order pharmacies varies based on the business model. Some pharmacies, such as AARP and Liberty Medical may offer discounted prescriptions to cash paying patients. More typically, mail pharmacies contract with PBMs to provide services to insured patients. Several major PBMs own mail-order pharmacy services, including CareMark, Express Scripts, and Medco. For these organizations, the mail pharmacy provides services for covered beneficiaries, but the pharmacies are also used by the PBMs for the purpose of enhanced patient management initiatives of the PBMs. All of these mail-order pharmacies just described essentially compete with community pharmacies for prescription volume.

Mail pharmacy services can also be used to enhance the efficiency of community service pharmacy. Kaiser Health Plan maintains two mail-order pharmacies in California.[23] The purpose of these pharmacies is to provide refills for maintenance prescriptions that have been originally filled in Kaiser's clinic pharmacies. The use of the centralized pharmacy for refills greatly enhances the efficiency of Kaiser's operation and reduces the number of pharmacists needed for prescription fulfillment. This enhanced efficiency has allowed Kaiser's pharmacists to engage in more clinically focused activities with patients and has eased concerns for pharmacist shortages in the region.

Mail-order pharmacies can also be used effectively for implementation of clinical services. In theory, targeted drug programs can be easily coordinated in a single pharmacy as opposed to across a large pharmacy network. For example, Medco maintains a targeted program that promotes conversion of prescriptions to generic when a product loses patent protection. In 2004, Medco reported a generic substitution rate of 93 percent within the first month following the introduction of new generic products.[24] Although generic penetration is high nationally following the introduction of a generic product, a rapid conversion process offers savings to clients.

Because mail-order processing is more profitable than claim processing, PBMs have a significant incentive to promote their own pharmacies' services. Although retail sales have increased steadily over the past decade, the percentage of prescriptions that have been filled in mail order pharmacies has grown at almost twice the retail rate.[25] Use of mail-order pharmacy is greater in the Medicare-eligible population,[26] which is consistent with the higher utilization of long-term maintenance medications in this population.

Furthermore, many self-insured employers promote mail pharmacy use, often through reductions in copay levels which offer savings to patients, particularly for branded medications that have higher copayment levels. For example, a patient may be able to obtain three months' supply of medication for only two months' copayment. Other plan sponsors may implement mandatory mail order programs by limiting benefit coverage in community pharmacies for maintenance medications, forcing the use of the mail-order pharmacy.

In contrast to the savings provided to patients, it is unclear if mail-order pharmacy actually generates substantial savings for health plans and self-insured plan sponsors. Mail-order pharmacies provide prescriptions at a greater discount than is typically provided in the retail pharmacy setting.[27] In addition, mail pharmacies often offer lower dispensing fees and, because the drug is dispensed less frequently throughout the year, dispensing fees are incurred at a lower rate than would be in the retail setting. These lower product costs are a significant factor in the adoption of mail incentives or mandates by plans' sponsors. However, some significant offsets to the product savings are offered by mail pharmacies. In order to promote mail-order pharmacy use, employers and health plans will often offer a lower copayment. The copayment reduction may exceed the savings associated with the drug, particularly as copayments have risen in recent years. Furthermore, the dispensing of prescriptions in large quantities may result in wasted medication, particularly when a drug is discontinued or the patient's eligibility for coverage ceases.

Specialty Pharmacy Services

Recently, several PBMs have focused significant efforts on the acquisition of specialty pharmacies as a product extension. Specialty pharmacies limit their drug dispensing activities to those medications that require unique handling or patient monitoring. These pharmacies may service a specific patient population, such as HIV patients or provide fertility services, or they may offer a broader range of products. Services tend to be provided over a larger geographic region than is common with community pharmacies.

Most specialty pharmaceuticals are injectable, and many are designed using biotechnology methods. Specialty pharmaceuticals are typically very high cost and are targeted treatments for diseases that are less prevalent in the population, but for which adequate treatment options do not otherwise exist. Examples of diseases for which specialty pharmaceuticals are available include multiple sclerosis, rheumatoid arthritis, growth hormone deficiency, and Crohn's disease. Specialty pharmaceuticals may be self-administered by the patient, but many of these medications are administered in clinic settings or by home health care agencies.

It is, as yet, unclear the extent of benefit that the PBM industry provides with regard to specialty pharmaceuticals when compared to a localized pharmacy network. PBMs do offer savings on these pharmaceuticals, particularly when compared the prices that have been paid for these drugs when they are submitted to the medical benefit program. In large part, the savings are due to the enhanced pricing accountability that can be achieved through the POS pharmacy claim system, as compared to medical billing systems that utilize HPCPS codes. However, billing of specialty products through the pharmacy benefit as opposed to the medical benefit may result in cost shifting that could result in higher costs to the plan sponsor. For example, a self-insured employer who provides pharmacy benefits to retirees may actually see costs increase if specialty medications are billed to the pharmacy program as opposed to Medicare Part B. In contrast, patients may benefit from pharmacy program coverage of these expensive medications because pharmacy copayment levels may be less than the deductible and coinsurance required under medical benefits.

PBMs that own specialty pharmacies tend to promote the use of these pharmacies by offering discounted prices on the products. However, it is unclear if the discounts offered exceed what is provided in the community pharmacy setting. Because the cost of specialty pharmaceuticals is far higher than typical medications, any added waste that might occur from a centralized distribution operation could very quickly offset any savings associated with product discounts.

Some operational considerations significantly impact the success of a PBM–managed specialty pharmacy program. Because many of these medications, including chemotherapy agents, are administered within a physician's office or clinic setting, the billing of the product raises concerns. Most physician office billing systems are unable to process claims in accordance with NCPDP standards. As a result, many physicians who purchase and administer pharmaceuticals will bill these products exclusively to the medical claim system of the patient's insurer. PBMs promote an alternative process through which the specialty pharmacy would supply the drug to the physician's office and bill directly to the PBM. This process has received only lukewarm reception from physicians out of concern for a lack of timeliness for receipt of the drug in relation to the patient's office visit and due to the loss of revenue to the office practice. However, Medicare reductions in physician payments for drugs administered in their office settings may result in increasing acceptance of these medications being supplied by specialty pharmacies.

Network Management As a Revenue Source

Pharmacy network management services are a prime source of revenue for the pharmacy benefit industry. Some of these revenues are fairly straightforward, whereas others are less easily identified and are a source of controversy within the industry. As is typical of all prominent industries, PBMs utilize the float of pharmacy revenues for investment purposes in short-term financial markets. PBMs typically batch pharmacy claims in a two-week cycle period. At the end of the prescription cycle, claims are summarized and plans sponsors are billed for the cost of the prescriptions. Typically payment is required, through electronic transfer of funds, within 24 to 72 hours of billing. Simultaneously, PBMs summarize pharmacy remittances in preparation for payment of the pharmacies. Pharmacy payments are often made using paper checks that are generated and mailed to pharmacies, typically five to seven days following the end of the pharmacy cycle. During the lag between the time that funds are received by the PBM and the time that a check is cashed by a pharmacy, the funds are maintained in an account that is used by the PBM to generate revenues. Use of this type of short-term financial investment is a sound practice that is universally accepted within the business industry.

Less commonly recognized as a source of revenues are funds that are retained by the PBM in the event that a pharmacy does not cash a check that it has received as remuneration for prescriptions dispensed. Although no studies have been documented to address the value of uncashed checks, privately, insurance companies have estimated the value at approximately one percent of prescription costs. PBMs may reasonably be reluctant to credit these amounts to their plan sponsors for several reasons, including that the check could be presented at a later date and the costs of stopping payment on any given check could be considerable. Although many organizations place limits on the amount of time a check is valid, systems for enforcing these limits in the banking community are not consistently reliable.

PBMs also generate significant revenues from the pharmacy network when the PBM has an ownership stake in the pharmacy. Many PBMs have some level of common corporate ownership with a pharmacy. When the PBM's benefit programs are structured to promote the use of their own pharmacy, additional profits are generated from the sale of the pharmaceutical.

Controversies Regarding Network Management

Because PBMs control the contracts and reimbursement levels to the network pharmacies, differing expectations exist regarding the role that the

PBM plays in providing this service. Although many drug benefit purchasers expect that the PBM is conducting network negotiations and payments on behalf of the purchaser, the PBM may actually be conducting services on their own behalf. Furthermore, when a PBM has an ownership relationship with a pharmacy, a potential exists for a conflict of interest that can arise in the services that are being provided.

One of the most common controversies related to pharmacy network management is in the payments that are made to the pharmacies on behalf of the client. Typically, a PBM will contract with a client for pharmaceuticals with a guaranteed discount for brand pharmaceuticals and a discounted rate or maximum allowable cost (MAC) price structure for generic products. However, when negotiating these contracts, the PBM may generate a differential, or network spread, in the pricing. In this case, the PBM is paying the pharmacy an amount that is different, and typically lower, than the amount that is billed to the client. The PBM retains the difference between the payment and billing rate as additional revenues. Although PBMs do not typically advertise this practice, some PBMs do provide some disclosure that, when contracting with pharmacies, they are acting on their own behalf, and not on behalf of the client. However, this is not a universal practice in the industry, and the scope of the spread is rarely disclosed.

Investigations into pharmacy network spreads have yielded some disturbing findings. In an investigation into PBM pricing practices, the *Wall Street Journal* reported excessive profits through network spreads on selected prescriptions for generic medications at Express Scripts and AdvancePCS.[28] The article cited a profits ranging from $18.00 to $200.00 on individual prescriptions for generic medications and an average profit margin of 22 percent related to network spreads at one PBM. (See Exhibit 14.2.)[29] Although focusing on individual prescriptions may inflate the extent of pharmacy network spreads, the presence of this practice and the extent to which it may occur remain a source of significant controversy and legal action.[30]

Ownership relationships between the PBM and a pharmacy have also created conflicts of interest. In 1998, Eagle Managed Care, a wholly owned subsidiary of Rite Aid Corporation, initiated new pharmacy contracts within the Philadelphia area. The rates, which were accepted by Rite Aid, but viewed as too low by many pharmacies, were essentially viewed as an attempt by the PBM to limit the pharmacy network to its own pharmacies.[31] The practice was eliminated under an investigation by the Pennsylvania Attorney General.

Likewise, the United States District Court in Massachusetts found PharmaCare and CVS guilty of colluding to circumvent that Massachusetts's Any Willing Provider regulation through its reimbursement prac-

EXHIBIT 14.2. Generic profits

How generic drugs yield big profits
Example: A thirty-day prescription of generic Prozac

Patient's copayment to pharmacy	$5.00
Pharmaceutical benefits manager's payment to pharmacy	$2.50
What the manufacturer charges pharmacy for the prescription	$1.50
Pharmacy's profit (Patient's copayment plus PBM's payment minus manufacturer's price)	**$6.00**
PBM bill to patient's employer	$13.00
PBM's profit (PBM bill to employer minus Payment to pharmacy)	**$10.50**

Source: Martinez, B. (2003). Hired to Cut Costs, Firms Find Profits in Generic Drugs. *Wall Street Journal,* March 31. Reprinted with permission from Dow Jones and Company, Inc.

tices.[32] PharmaCare, a wholly owned subsidiary of CVS Corporation, initiated a capitated reimbursement program for pharmacies that were providing services on behalf of Harvard Pilgrim Health Plan (HPHP). The capitation rate was considered to be too risky by the community pharmacies in the state, and most could not accept the contract, essentially creating an exclusive network for CVS. However, the amount that PharmaCare invoiced HPHP for services offset any financial risk to CVS Corporation associated with the capitated pharmacy reimbursement program. Essentially, CVS was being made whole, while community pharmacies were at significant financial risk. Because of the premeditated nature of the actions, the judge viewed the entire arrangement as fraudulent and awarded treble damages to the plaintiffs.

Similar ownership concerns have been raised regarding the relationship between a PBM and its own mail-service pharmacy.[33] When the PBM owns a mail-service pharmacy, it is effectively serving in a capacity in which it is policing its own services. Consequently, when engaging in product selection and pricing, a risk exists that the PBM will act in its own interest, in conflict to the interest of its client, when it comes to the oversight of the mail facility.

PBMs have been accused of engaging in a variety of practices with regard to the oversight of the PBM's own pharmacy. For example, it is possible that the mail pharmacy will use inflated AWPs, either through selective use of NDC codes for billing or through the use of repackaged products with inflated NDC price codes.[34] Because AWP has little or no correlation to the price actually paid by the pharmacy, inflation of the AWP raises the revenues and profitability of the PBM's mail pharmacy. PBM-owned pharmacies may also engage in drug-switching activities to profit the PBM. For example, when a PBM retains a portion of the rebates on medications, or is paid a drug-switch fee by a manufacturer, the pharmacy may engage in drug-switch activities. Upon receipt of a prescription for a target medication, the mail-pharmacy staff will contact the prescribing physician to obtain approval to make a change in drug therapy. Unfortunately, this drug switch may actually result in increased costs to the client, but higher manufacturer revenues to the PBM.[35]

Although an ownership relationship between a PBM and a pharmacy is not an absolute conflict, the potential will always exist for the PBM to provide preferential pricing arrangements to its own pharmacy. Diligent evaluation of pricing methodology and contracting practices is essential to assure that the client's needs are being met without a conflict of interest to the client or its beneficiaries.

PHARMACEUTICAL BENEFITS ADMINISTRATION

Because claim processing systems used by the PBM industry are highly automated, PBMs are able to administer a wide range of benefit designs on behalf of client. Benefit designs may include parameters surrounding patient copays or coinsurance rates, benefit exclusions and limitations, and clinical edits, depending on the population being served and the desires of the plan sponsor.

Out-of-Pocket Expenses

The level of out-of-pocket expense that a patient will incur when obtaining his or her pharmacy benefits is the primary focus of the pharmacy benefit. Patient expenses can range from no cost to 100 percent of the discounted cost of the medication, depending on the program focus. Furthermore, the level of discount may vary based on the type of drug that is being obtained and its formulary status. Out-of pocket expenses are typically divided into one of three categories: copays, coinsurance, and deductibles. Furthermore, pharmacy benefit may be limited to a maximum coverage level, or capitation. These programs are outlined in more detail in the following paragraphs.

Copayments

By far the most common pharmacy benefit design calls for the use of copayments. A copayment is a predetermined dollar amount that is applied to the purchase of each prescription, regardless of the prescription cost. Although originally copayments were a single amount for any prescription, throughout the 1990s two-tier copayment programs were most commonly used. In a two-tier program, the patient typically pays a low copay for a generic medication, with a higher copayment for brand prescriptions. Since the turn of the century, the use of three- and four-tier copayment programs has gained popularity as a method to promote the use of preferred medications and to address cost-sharing for very high-cost medications. In 2002, average copayments ranged from $8.33 for generic medications to $33.23 for third-tier medications.[36] These values are expected to grow, especially for branded medications, as prescription drug costs increase. Although a copayment program allows patients to know, in advance, their out-of pocket cost for prescriptions, it does minimize the patients' true understanding of drug costs. Many a patient has been shocked when, upon losing drug coverage, they learned that a medication for which they typically paid a low copay actually costs one hundred dollars or more.

Coinsurance

Of increasing interest to plan sponsors are programs that employ the use of coinsurance. In coinsurance benefits, patients pay a set percentage, typically 20 to 25 percent of the drug cost, regardless of drug type. The advantage of a coinsurance program is that patients are more aware of the true cost of their medications, and they save when they use less expensive medications. This knowledge of drug pricing may influence patients to seek lower cost therapies, when appropriate. Coinsurance also offers an advantage to plan sponsors in that the patient's contribution to their pharmaceutical costs remains current with inflation. The disadvantage of a coinsurance program is that the patient's cost for medications is not predictable, and may vary from month to month, or from pharmacy to pharmacy depending on the PBM's contract with that pharmacy. Nonetheless, coinsurance programs are gaining in popularity and the use as a component of benefits programs is predicted to increase.[37]

Deductibles

Deductibles are fixed amounts of expenditures that must be incurred by the patient, or the patient's representative, before the patient is eligible for insurance coverage. The use of deductibles has been a common feature in major medical benefits of health insurance programs for many years. The interest in using deductibles for pharmacy programs has increased in recent years as a way to increase patient awareness of drug prices. Deductibles are typically applied on an annual basis. As a result it is not uncommon to see patients stockpiling medication at the close of their annual period so as to defer the cost of the deductible for a period of time.

Capitation

Capitation, or maximum out-of-pocket programs, limit the total amount of drug coverage that is available in a set time period. These programs have been a common feature in Medicare Plus Choice programs over the past several years and a variation of a capitation program is included in the Medicare Prescription Drug Benefit program.[38] Capitation allows a plan sponsor to provide modest pharmacy benefits, but to reduce the financial exposure and thus maintain affordable premiums for the coverage.

Early drug capitation benefits were based on a maximum for each plan year. For example, a patient might have a maximum benefit of $1,000 beginning in January and extending for the year. If the patient submitted claims totaling $1,000 in only three months, additional resources were not applied until the next year. Under this type of plan, many plan sponsors experienced significant patient disenrollment as soon as the maximum was reached, resulting in adverse selection for the benefit. Consequently, many plan sponsors apply a smaller capitation on a quarterly basis. An example would be a benefit in which $250 of coverage is provided every quarter.

Prescription Limits

A key feature of pharmaceutical benefits programs implemented by the PBM industry is the availability and use of limits on the quantity of medications that can be obtained. Quantity limits serve a wide range of purposes from prevention of drug diversion to promotion of clinical appropriateness of drug use. Following are examples of commonly used quantity limits and examples of their uses.

Days Supply

Specifies the number of days supply of medication that can be obtained at any given time. Typically the number of days supply is thirty to thirty-four days at retail and ninety days at mail, although some programs permit up to ninety days at retail. This edit is used to prevent drug stockpiling and waste of pharmaceuticals.

Refill Too Soon

Establishes a time limit between the refill of prescriptions. Using the date of filling of the prescription and the number of days supply submitted by the pharmacist, an edit is applied requiring that a certain number of days of therapy must have elapsed prior to the payment for a subsequent supply of medication. This edit is commonly used to prevent drug misuse, particularly for those medications that are subject to abuse.

Quantity Limits

This restricts the quantity of medication that is covered under insurance benefit during a specified time period. Quantity limits often are applied to medications of a lifestyle or controversial nature. For example, many employers provide coverage for erectile dysfunction, but limit the number of courses of therapy to four to six doses per month. State mandates for coverage of fertility therapy may be restricted to a certain number of attempts per lifetime.[39] Quantity limits can also be used to promote appropriate clinical utilization. For example, many health plans limit triptan coverage to two courses of therapy per month, in accordance with guidelines for the use of migraine abortive therapy. Health plans may limit the cumulative doses of combination narcotic analgesics (Percocet, Vicodin, etc.) to prevent overuse of acetaminophen, a common component of these therapies.

Restrictions

A drug restriction is a benefit limitation that excludes the coverage of certain medications or classes of medications. Drug restrictions are applied to pharmacy benefits based on a wide variety of reasons that are typically unique to the concerns of the plan sponsor. Drugs that are often excluded from standard pharmaceutical benefits include products for cosmetic uses, over-the-counter agents, and investigational drugs. Drugs for uses that are lifestyle in nature may or may not be covered, depending on the plan sponsor. These may include drugs for weight control, erectile dysfunction, cough and cold therapies, and drugs for smoking cessation. Medicaid programs preclude coverage of many of these products, as well as drugs that have a DESI designations from the FDA and drugs that are used for fertility purposes.[40]

Drug restrictions can be controversial, particularly when they could be viewed by some groups as discriminatory. For many years, employers excluded coverage of contraceptives from prescription benefit programs, in part due to religious affiliations of the employer. In response to these restrictions, a majority of states have implemented mandates requiring the coverage of contraceptives when a pharmaceutical benefit is offered to employees.[41] However, many organizations oppose these regulations, and ongoing pressure exists to permit greater flexibility for drug coverage decisions by employers.[42,43]

CLINICAL PROGRAMS

Drug Utilization Review

Because of the vast amount of drug utilization information in their databases, PBMs are in a prime position to conduct drug utilization review, on behalf of an individual's drug plan sponsors as well as to review drug utilization trends regionally or even nationally. Drug utilization review programs help to manage costs as well as provide quality assurance and fraud prevention functions. (See also Chapter 27.)

Concurrent DUR

The first line for drug utilization review is the concurrent review edit. Concurrent drug utilization review (DUR) functions are provided at the point-of-service (POS) and include real-time system edits that can impact prescribing patterns. When a claim is submitted by the pharmacy, it is assessed against patient demographics and prior drug utilization that is maintained in the pharmacy claim database. Electronic messages are sent to the pharmacy, during the adjudication process, to inform the pharmacist of the potential drug problem.

In state Medicaid programs, concurrent DUR edits have been in place since the adoption of the Omnibus Budget Reconciliation Act (OBRA) of

1990.[44] (See Table 14.1.)[45] These edits are designed to prevent inappropriate drug utilization and to reduce drug interactions. (See Table 14.2.)[46] These same tools are also features of drug utilization management programs administered by private pharmaceutical benefits managers.

Unfortunately, the PBM and pharmacy claim database do not have critical items that would make these edits more valid, such as patient diagnosis and over-the-counter drug therapy (unless covered under the benefit). As a result, drugs are used as markers for disease, resulting in many false positive warnings. For example, prenatal vitamins are used as a marker indicating pregnancy. However, these vitamins are often prescribed for the elderly population because, unlike general multivitamins, prenatal products are provided as a covered benefit in most prescription programs. Thus an edit will be activated for any patient taking a prenatal vitamin in combination with a drug, such as an ACE inhibitor, that is contraindicated in pregnancy. This limitation is compounded by the criteria behind the data possibly identifying drug interactions or contraindications that are of little clinical significance in the majority of the patient population. Finally, when a pharmacist receives notice of a drug-related problem, he or she may not have access to all of the drug history of the patient, particularly if the patient uses more than one pharmacy for prescription needs. As a result, many electronic communications are viewed as "false" messages, and pharmacies have simply disabled these features in their computer system or they routinely override PBM messaging without review.

TABLE 14.1. Savings from a prior authorization program for selected drugs/ drug categories, 2000.

Drug category	Percent decrease in use**	Mean PMPM Costs (Range Across Plan Sponsors)		Mean PMPM savings***
		Prior authorization	Drug covered	
Erectile dysfunction	39	$0.10 ($0.01-$0.34)	$0.25 ($0.05-$0.76)	$0.15
Sporanox®/ Lamisil®*	54	$0.10 ($0.03-$0.20)	$.24 ($0.07-$0.78)	$0.14
Anti-obesity	59	$0.07 ($0.02-$0.20)	$0.15 ($0.01-$0.25)	$0.08
Smoking cessation	80	$0.01 ($0.00-$0.03)	$0.06 ($0.01- $0.15)	$0.05
Wellbutrin SR® 150mg	29	$0.13 ($0.06-$0.17)	$0.17 ($0.00-$0.67)	$0.04

* Includes oral formulations only
** = (Average utilization if covered— average utilization if on PA)/ average utilization if covered
*** Includes charge to plan sponsor for PA calls

Source: Express Scripts (2003). *Express Scripts Drug Benefit Guide 2003.* Maryland Heights, MO: Express Scripts, Inc.

TABLE 14.2. OBRA requirements for state Medicaid DUR.

Guidelines	Description
Concurrent (prospective) DUR elements	Establishment of screening mechanisms to identify the following: • Therapeutic duplication • Drug-disease contraindication to detect for potential undesirable or adverse events • Incorrect drug dosage • Incorrect duration of drug treatment • Drug-allergy interactions • Clinical abuse/misuse related to over or underutilization

Source: Code of Federal Register, 42 CFR456.7.

Retrospective DUR

Retrospective drug utilization programs involve an evaluation of drug utilization after the drug adjudication process is complete. This review can be focused on individuals' claims for patients or on the drug therapy trends over a large number of patients. When individual claims are reviewed, the DUR process is focused on identifying circumstances in which drug utilization patterns might be improved for a given patient or for a group of patients being seen by a specific provider. When an opportunity is identified, a letter or fax is sent to the provider, informing that individual of the opportunity. This type of retrospective DUR is common in state Medicaid programs and is used to a lesser degree in commercial drug benefit programs. Recognizing the inherent limitations of retrospective drug review, PBMs have expanded follow-on activities to increase this program's effectiveness. Some of these enhancements include telephone follow-up with providers, incorporating community pharmacists into the intervention process, the issuance of actionable and precisely written letters, and the addition of academic detailing programs.

Because of the extensive volume and history of drug utilization that is maintained in their databases, PBMs are in a prime position to evaluate and monitor drug utilization trends on a larger scale. Within the PBM industry, all three major PBMs produce a report of drug utilization that analyzes trends and cost drivers for prescription benefits nationally on an annual basis.[47-49] Researchers from these PBMs have also published findings from retrospective analysis of drug utilization of a variety of therapies, based on the utilization patterns of their entire populations. This information can be useful as a benchmark to plan sponsors and to provide guidance regarding future pharmaceutical benefits management initiatives. For example, results from a recent utilization study reported that, over a four year period, users of silfenadil were typically younger males and females, without an underlying etiologic reason for use of the drug.[50] This information could be used by PBMs and plan sponsors to quantify the cost of inappropriate drug utilization and to adjust coverage limitations to promote appropriate drug utilization.

Step Therapy Edits

Step therapy edits are employed by PBMs for the purpose of promoting the use of a certain drug or class of drugs prior to the use of a second drug. In many cases, the use of step therapy edits is designed to reduce overall drug expenditures in circumstances in which many drugs of similar efficacy, but with very different costs, exist. For example, a step-therapy edit may require a trial therapy with over-the-counter loratadine prior to the coverage of a prescription nonsedating antihistamine.

The step-therapy edit is implemented in the claim-processing system electronically. When a prescription is presented for a medication that is subject to a step therapy requirement (Drug A), the claim adjudication system searches the patient's recent drug history to determine if the prerequisite medication (Drug B) has been used. If a match is found for Drug B, the claim for Drug A will adjudicate at the patient's copay level. If a match for Drug B is not found, the claim will reject for coverage. The step-therapy edit can typically be appealed through a call to the PBM for patients with unique medical considerations (e.g., an allergy) that would preclude use of the prerequisite drug.

Prior Authorization

Prior authorization (PA) is a process of obtaining certification or authorization from the insurer or from the PBM acting on behalf of the insurer for the coverage of a specific drug or quantity of medication. Prior authorization is often utilized for high-cost medications, which may be indicated for very specific purposes and for which a potential exists for medication misuse. The request for coverage of the drug is assessed against predetermined criteria that have usually been approved by the pharmacy and therapeutics (P & T) committee or other physician practice committee. PBMs often offer a variety of PA programs for use by employers of health plans.

An example of a drug that often is subjected to prior authorization review is human growth hormone. Growth hormone is an effective therapy for the treatment of growth hormone deficiency, Turners Syndrome, and HIV-wasting. However, it is also used for sports enhancement or cosmetic purposes. Prior authorization is applied to growth hormone to assure that when the drug is covered under an insured program it is being used for approved medical purposes.

Prior authorization can also be used as a method to manage the formulary that is selected by the health plan in a closed formulary benefit. In a closed benefit, a formulary of preferred medications is covered under the prescription drug plan, whereas any nonformulary medications are covered, only when approved through a PA process. The approval is often based on clinical criteria that may be unique to the patient, such as an allergy to the formulary drug or excipient, or failure with a trial of therapy with the formulary agent. PA management of a closed formulary is very effective in moving medication use to preferred agents and in managing pharmaceutical benefit costs. However, widespread PA for formulary management purposes is disruptive to patients and providers, and for this reason is not often promoted or utilized by commercial pharmacy benefit programs.

A leading PBM reported significant savings in additional drug categories that featured prior authorization. The average percent decrease in usage among those drug categories surveyed was 52 percent and the mean per member per month (PMPM) savings, $0.09.

Dose Optimization

Similar to quantity limits, "dose optimization" edits, although not a typical industry practice, have been shown to reduce costs in targeted drug categories. Dose optimization edits target drug utilization that is suggestive of multiple daily dosing of a low dose of a medication when single daily dosing of a higher dose is clinically appropriate.[51] This circumstance occurs often as providers are adjusting medication doses in patients. For example, a patient taking 10 mg of Lipitor daily may be instructed by the physician to increase the dose to two tablets daily. If the cost of a 20 mg tablet is lower than that of two 10 mg tablets, a dose efficiency edit might encourage adoption of a 20 mg tablet taken once a day. Through the dose optimization process, the PBM will notify the pharmacy or provider of the opportunity to change therapy. In some cases, claim edits may be applied to these situations, prompting the pharmacist to consult with the prescriber regarding a change in therapy. Through this process, the patient's drug and daily dose are maintained, but at a lower cost to the plan sponsor.

FORMULARY MANAGEMENT

The PBM industry provides formulary management as a basic component of the services that it provides to its clientele. A formulary is a list of mediations that is preferred for use in a patient population. Based on recommendations used by hospitals and required by the Joint Commission for the Accreditation of Healthcare Organizations (JCAHO), PBMs utilize the service of pharmacy and therapeutics (P & T) committees for the development of the formulary.

The P & T committee of a PBM is comprised of experts in medical and drug therapy from throughout the Unites States. Depending on the PBM, the P & T committee may include representatives from their clientele as well as employees of the PBM, although PBM employees are often nonvoting members. The P & T committee evaluates new and existing drug therapies to select medications that offer superior drug therapy benefits for the populations. Depending on the needs of the PBM's clients, several formularies may be developed. For example, a PBM might develop a more restrictive formulary focused on generic medication for a Medicaid population, while offering a more extensive, but more costly, formulary for its commercial customers. The P & T committee bases its recommendations primarily of the clinical merits of a drug. A medication that is clearly superior to any existing therapies would be readily accepted onto a formulary, whereas a product that offers little benefit or is inferior to existing therapies would probably be excluded from the formulary. Cost of drugs, and rebate levels, are not typically considered by the P & T committee unless marginal differences between therapies exist and cost is the only clear distinguishing factor between medication options. In some PBMs, cost considerations are applied by a separate formulary committee, after the P & T has determined that two or more products offer comparable effects.

Although the PBM industry offers and maintains a formulary of preferred medications, clients are not obligated to use the PBM's formulary. Many health plans operate their own P & T committee that conducts formulary evaluations and makes independent decisions regarding formulary status of a product. However, the health plans' P & T committees often review the formulary recommendations of the PBM and tend to concur with the recommendations on many occasions. In contrast, self-insured employers often accept the decisions of the PBM's P & T committee without revision. Many employers do not have the internal medical expertise to independently assess drug therapies. In addition, many employers are hesitant to engage in clinical decisions that may be viewed as intrusive to their employees.

The PBM maintains a preferred formulary for all clients and encourages the client to adopt pharmacy benefit management techniques that promote utilization of the preferred drug items. Examples of such activities include the use of restrictive formularies or tiered formulary benefits. Restrictive formularies exclude coverage of nonformulary products, except for those cases in which the patient is unable to tolerate or does not respond to a formulary product. Tiered benefit programs establish higher copayments for nonformulary products, thus encouraging patients to discuss formulary alternatives with their physician. Furthermore, if the PBM maintains a mail pharmacy, this pharmacy may also engage in activities that are designed to promote utilization of the formulary agent.

REBATE ADMINISTRATION

Negotiation for and allocation of rebates is one the primary services that the PBM industry offers to its clients. Simply stated, a rebate is a discount on the cost of the drug, provided after the drug has been dispensed. The concept of rebates originated from drug discounting negotiations that were common in hospitals. Hospitals, as direct purchasers of medications, negotiated with manufacturers to obtain discounts on the medications that they provided to patients. To improve their negotiating leverage, many hospitals coordinated the management of their formulary in conjunction with rebate contracting, particularly for medications that offer similar therapeutic effects.

The concept of using a formulary and negotiating discounts for drugs was embraced by the managed care industry in the late 1980s. In 1990 the Omnibus Budget Reconciliation Act (OBRA) required payments of rebates for drugs provided to Medicaid beneficiaries. The use of these practices evolved first in health maintenance organizations where close working relationships existed between physicians and in-house pharmacy services. As with hospitals, these in-house pharmacies were able to negotiate purchase discounts in exchange for preferred utilization of certain medications.

As the concept of drug discounts expanded to the traditional insurance industry, the method for issuing the discount also required revision. Although a managed care organization (MCO) is the ultimately purchaser of the medications, most MCOs never take physical possession of a medication, but instead contract for a discount that is paid after the prescription has been adjudicated, essentially creating the rebate.

Historically rebate contracts were based on the formulary status of a drug. If the drug was maintained on a client's formulary, rebates were provided by the manufacturer. Rebates were paid on a fixed amount for each unit of medication that was dispensed. Additional discounts could be offered based on the volume of purchases that were made by the health plan or PBM. However, in 1995, a group of pharmacies banned together to raise concerns about rebate contracting activities as a possible violation of the Robinson-Patman Act. In this suit, the pharmacies alleged that the payment of rebates to some purchasers, such as a PBM with a mail pharmacy, but not to all purchasers, created unfair competition within the prescription drug sector. Manufacturer's countered that the mail pharmacies were working on behalf of health plans that had the ability to control drug utilization for their members. The case was ultimately settled by most manufacturers. As a function of that settlement, manufacturers have adopted performance-based contracting in which higher rebates are paid based on sales of their medications as a share of the market within a therapeutic category. Thus, if several drugs are in a market category, and the utilization of Drug A is 25 percent, a higher rebate will be paid to the PBM by the manufacturer of Drug A if utilization is increased to 35 percent of the market.

PBMs and Rebate Contracting Services

The PBM industry embraces rebate contracting as a method to provide additional services to their clients, and most PBMs engage in rebate contracting with the vast majority of pharmaceutical manufacturers. Although some HMOs and MCOs have sufficient staffing and expertise to engage in rebate contracting, many smaller health plans and self-insured employers do not have this level of expertise or are too small to justify the administration associated with rebate contracting functions. For these organizations, PBMs are able to provide rebate contracting that generates pharmaceutical cost reductions for their clients. The PBM can centralize this service for all clients, thus creating operation efficiencies for the service. The large patient populations served by a PBM can also provide leverage for pharmaceutical contracting, particularly if the PBM has proven successful in working with its clients to move market share to the preferred formulary products.

In the commercial market, rebates are paid to PBMs almost exclusively on branded products, with little or no rebate paid on generic products. Rebates or discounts for generic products are typically offered at the pharmacy level, including to those pharmacies that have an ownership relationship with a PBM.

PBMs typically submit for rebates on a quarterly basis at the end of each calendar quarter. Using the adjudicated claim files, the PBM identifies all prescriptions that are eligible for rebate and summarizes the utilization by the number of units dispensed. Certain claims may be excluded from the rebate submission based on manufacturer requirements. Examples include prescriptions that are filled for Medicaid-eligible individuals and prescriptions filled from hospital or military pharmacies. In these cases, the manufacturers may already be supplying a discount or rebate to the other entity. Manufacturers may also exclude 100 percent copay (discount-only) prescriptions that are not insured, or prescriptions from certain states for political reasons. Manufacturers review the rebate submissions and may adjust the rebate payment based on the manufacturer's internal criteria for data integrity. A rebate payment is made, typically 90 to 120 days following the receipt of the rebate invoice.

Once the PBM receives the rebate from the manufacturer, the PBM must review and validate any rebate adjustments that were made by the manufacturer. Rebates are then allocated to individual clients.

Rebate allocations are based on a wide variety of criteria, depending on the terms of the contract between the PBM and its clients. In some cases, the PBM may pay a basic guaranteed rebate amount on a per-claim basis. Other contracts call for a sharing of percentage of the rebates that are received, with the PBM retaining 10 percent to 20 percent of the rebate as an administrative fee. Express Scripts offers a "bid grid" system that provides a predetermined level of rebate, depending on formulary and benefit decisions that are chosen by the client. PBMs may use rebate revenues to lower administrative fees or other costs that are paid by the client. In some cases, PBMs use rebate revenues to buy down the cost of the medication or pharmacy dispensing fees that are charged to their clients.

In general, rebates can offer reductions equal to 2 to 8 percent of the total drug cost, depending on the benefit design and formulary utilization of the PBM's client. Higher levels of rebates are received by those plans that have higher utilization of selective brand medications within a therapeutic category. However, rebate revenues do not offset savings that could be achieved through the use of generic medications, where they are available. Consequently, PBM clients must balance the diversity of medications on their benefit programs with the financial impact of generic use and the revenues from rebates when making benefit design decisions.

CONTROVERSIES IN THE PBM INDUSTRY

The PBM industry has been under considerable scrutiny with regard to their business practices. Although many clients contract with PBMs under the expectation that the PBM is acting on behalf of the client, recent disclosures regarding the industry suggest that this may not always be the case. As a result, investigations into PBM business practices and litigation against the industry has been common in recent years.

Nowhere has this scrutiny been more evident than in the relationship between PBMs and pharmaceutical manufacturers. The concern regarding PBM business practices was originally fueled by the purchase of several large PBMs by pharmaceutical manufacturers. In 1993, Merck purchased Medco Containment Services, while SmithKline Beecham purchased Diversified Pharmacy Services (DPS). These acquisitions were followed very quickly by the purchase of PCS by Eli Lilly & Company. The appeal of a manufacturer owning a company that exerted significant influence on insurance benefit programs and drug-use patterns was apparent. Following the acquisition of Medco, distribution of Merck products by Medco increased approximately 50 percent.[52] However, these acquisitions very quickly raised concerns regarding the potential for anticompetitive activities within the industry. The Federal Trade Commission stepped in, forcing firewalls in business practices and ultimately entering into consent agreements with the manufacturers in question.[53]

Following the investigations by the FTC, both Eli Lilly and SmithKline Beecham divested their ownership in the PBM industry. Merck retained ownership of Medco until 2003. However, the influence of pharmaceutical manufacturers in PBM decisions was not necessary lost. In January 2002, David Halbert, Chairman of AdvancePCS, reported to stockholders that the majority of the company's profits would come from pharmaceutical manufacturers rather than from its clients.[54] These revenues were paid as administrative fees for rebate contracting, switch programs, academic detailing to physicians, and for other clinical interventions by the PBM.

The shifting of corporate revenues from plan sponsors to manufacturers has raised significant concerns regarding the intended focus of PBM business practices. These drug interventions may provide savings to a plan sponsor, but it is also quite possible that the interventions could result in decisions that are not in the interest of the health plan, particularly when the activities are a significant source of the PBM's profits. The inherent conflict of interest within the industry became apparent. Furthermore, many of these relationships were not disclosed by the PBM when contracting with a client.[55]

As early as 1997, business practices of the PBM industry were under scrutiny and litigation was filed, alleging that Medco engaged in a variety of practices that were undisclosed, and adverse to the interests of their clients. Alleged inappropriate practices included failure to pass on negotiated discounts on medications, side deals with manufacturers to promote use of certain medications, drug switching that resulted in higher costs to clients, and refusal to provide financial accounting of transactions.[56]

At the same time, James Sheehan, a U.S. assistant attorney in Philadelphia, identified irregularities in PBM and manufacturer relationships as part of his investigation into Medicaid pricing activities. He ultimately filed suit against Medco, alleging that "to enhance its revenue regardless of health plan costs, or of any potential adverse or life threatening clinical outcomes to patients," Medco engaged in drug switching to Merck products, for which Medco was paid $440 million in 2001.[57] A Merck regulatory filing in March of 2002 noted that Merck products' market share among Medco clients "exceeded" the national market share, but Merck declined to say by how much.[58]

Subsequent cases were filed by Mr. Sheehan against Express Scripts and AdvancePCS.

Not surprisingly, the litigation and corresponding publicity has generated a large interest by others regarding PBM practices. Additional litigation has been failed against the PBM industry. Medco ultimately settled several large cases, without admission of guilt. However, the settlements included agreements for changes in Medco's rebate contracting and drug switching activities. In addition, the agreements require disclosure of manufacturer revenues to clients on an annual basis.[59] Whether these agreements will improve that accountability of PBM industry to its health plan and employer clients is unknown. Concerns about drug dispensing and pricing practices in PBM-owned pharmacies and pharmacy network management activities remain unresolved.

LEGAL AND REGULATORY OVERSIGHT

Historically, the PBM industry has been largely free from regulatory oversight. Although a pharmacy operation is subject to state pharmacy laws and any publicly traded companies were subject to SEC regulations, the actual business practices of the PBM were not subject to regulation. Unlike a health insurance company that is subject to considerable regulatory oversight, the PBM industry, as a claim processor, was viewed as a service vendor, subject only to contractual obligations to its clients.

However, through the evolution of its services, the PBM industry evolved into a role that is viewed as more comprehensive than its roots as a claim processor. PBMs act on behalf of clients to negotiate drug prices and discounts, an activity that is viewed by some as a fiduciary role. Clinical activities, such a prior authorization, are viewed in some states as potentially subject to utilization review regulations.

In 2003, the Office of the Inspector General for the U.S. Department of Health and Human Services issued a guidance for pharmaceutical manufacturers that outlines their relationships in drug pricing and marketing activities.[60] Included in this guidance are requirements related to manufacturer relationships with PBMs. Failure to comply with the requirements of the guidance could leave a manufacturer open to allegations of fraud in government contracting and sales, with penalties of treble damages. Although not a direct regulation of the PBM industry, the implications to pharmaceutical manufacturers are sufficiently high as to influence their contracts and relationships with PBMs.

Individual states have also initiated legislation to address PBM activities.[61] Proposed regulations require a wide range of business practice oversight and disclosure, including licensure with a state, and disclosure of financial and business accounting practices. The regulations also mandate definitions of certain pricing and rebate terms, with disclosure to clients. The State of Maine was the first state to enact laws that oversee the PBM industry. These regulations were immediately challenged by the PBM industry as a threat to trade secrets. Although an attempt to enact a stay of implementation of these regulations was refused by the courts, the State of Maine has delayed implementation of the regulations, pending the outcome of the case.[62]

To address increasing concerns about the PBM industry practices, Congress included an investigation of the PBM industry as a portion of the Medicare Prescription Drug and Improvement Act. This investigation, which will be conducted by the Federal Trade Commission, will assess whether PBMs make decisions on a variety of matters that increase the PBM's profits while increasing expenses to their clients.

Average wholesale price (AWP) reform may also have a significant impact on the PBM industry. Currently, AWP is the basis of payments that are made to pharmacies as well as invoices to customers of the PBM industry. AWP is also the source of most Medicaid payments to pharmacies. In an evaluation of AWP pricing, the Office of the Inspector General for the U.S. Department of Health and Human Services determined that significant variations exist between AWP and the manufacturer sales price that is reported to Medicaid, the average manufacturer price (AMP) or the average sales price (ASP).[63] As a result, HHS recommends that methodology for reimbursing drug expenditures be changed from AWP to AMP/ASP. Because of the ambiguity associated with AWP prices, a considerable interest in the publication of AMP/ASP and its use as a basis of pharmaceutical pricing in the commercial section exists. This change could affect the PBM's ability to generate network spreads that represent a portion of their company profits. However, use of ASP/AMP would provide greater accountability to clients as they assess their PBM's performance and compare administrative costs of using different PBM vendors.

FUTURE OF THE PBM INDUSTRY

As with the entire health care industry, considerable change is occurring within the PBM industry. Changes in electronic capabilities, enhanced oversight, and industry competition will all play a role in the scope of services offered by the industry in the future. The implementation of prescription benefits for the Medicare populations will have an enormous effect on the industry as well. Finally, overriding concerns about prescription drug prices will lead to a revised emphasis in evaluating PBM performance.

Without a doubt, the electronic capabilities of the industry are essential for efficient adjudication and payment of claims in the health care industry. This capability will increase over the next decade. Technology that supports electronic transmission of prescriptions exists and will be implemented under the new Medicare prescription drug benefit program. By electronically transmitting prescriptions, physicians will be able to identify other medications that the patient is receiving, regardless of the source of this prescription. Feedback regarding cost-effective alternatives and clinical literature will be available to the prescriber when initiating the prescription. Information regarding patient compliance and potential drug interactions will also be made available. Clinical information and diagnosis can be captured during the prescription transmission, providing the dispensing pharmacist with valuable clinical information regarding the patient for the purpose of counseling patients regarding their drug therapy.

Technology improvements will also permit enhanced analysis of drug outcomes within a patient population. Rather than a focus of drug discounts and rebates, a savvy PBM will be able to demonstrate changes in patient outcomes over time compared to the cost of the drug therapy. This information will give all health care providers better information from which to make clinical and financial decisions regarding drug therapies. Ultimately, a PBM may not be evaluated based on the discounts that it offers, but on a global perspective, with costs associated with managing key diseases based on patient outcomes.

Regulation of the PBM industry is almost guaranteed given the significant controversies that have arisen over business practices. However, a desire for profitability and competition within the PBM industry will also have a profound effect on business operations. Over the past several years, a new generation of PBM has emerged in the market place. These companies offer complete transparency with regard to drug pricing and rebate management activities. Rather than retaining revenues through undisclosed revenues and margins in business practices, these newer PBMs offer flat-rate pricing of services, with a complete pass-through of all discounts and rebates. Whether these companies can offer better prices than existing PBMs remains to be seen, but the transparency that is offered has already forced changes toward greater disclosure in the existing industry.

The health care industry will also look toward having greater flexibility with regard to their prescription drug programs. Rather than centralizing all pharmacy benefit services with a single company, health plans and potentially employers will break up services into individual segments, possibly retaining some activities to be managed in-house. Already this trend is apparent in the health insurance industry. With very inexpensive access to claim processing capabilities, many health plans have in-sourced their rebate contracting and formulary activities to give a greater level of focus on the healths plan's individual needs.

Finally the introduction of the Medicare prescription drug program will have overwhelming impact on the industry. As a result of this program, millions of individuals will be added to the existing lives that are served by the PBM industry. With this program comes significant potential for oversight and enhanced level of services. Unlike the current commercial market, the Medicare program will require coordination of pharmacy benefits to other government programs as well as with commercial insurance programs. The Medicare program will also result in a higher level of scrutiny into services and comparative drug pricing within the program. Although the PBM industry remained free of significant oversight for many years, participation in this new government program will impart new expectations on the industry. Ultimately any expectation of the Medicare program is likely to be required for commercial insurance as well.

Whenever change occurs, the opportunity for growth and development exists. No greater example of this philosophy is the current PBM industry. Although long and sometimes turbulent history to this industry exists, components of the industry will continue to evolve and provide a valuable contribution to the health care system in the future.

NOTES

1. CareMark (2005). *2005 TrendsRx Report*. Northbrook, IL: CareMark, pg 5.
2. http://www.ncpdp.org.
3. National Council for Prescription Drug Programs (2005). *NCPDP Basic Guide To Standards*. May. Scottsdale, AZ: NCPDP.
4. 45 C.F.R. Parts 160-64.
5. Available at: http://www.webmdenvoy.com/pages/pharmacies/pharm.html.
6. Available at: http://www.ndchealth.com/pharmacy/pharmacy.htm.
7. Available at: http://www.erxnetwork.com/Connect.aspx.
8. Available at: http://www.qs1.com.
9. Available at: http://www.erxnetwork.com.

10. Available at: http://www.webmdenvoy.com.

11. Available at: http://www.ndchealth.com/pharmacy.

12. Available at: http://www.freedomdrugstores.com/products/z_eznet.htm.

13. Available at: http://www.rxlinc.com/site/index.htm.

14. 21 C.F.R. Part 207.

15. U.S. Food and Drug Administration, Center for Drug Evaluation and Research (2005). Federal Food, Drug, and Cosmetic Act. Bethesda, MD: U.S. Department of Health and Human Services.

16. General Accounting Office (1997). *Pharmacy Benefit Managers: FEHBP Plans Satisfied with Savings and Services, but Retail Pharmacies Have Concerns.* Report to congressional requesters. GAO/HEHS-97-47. February. Washington, DC: GAO.

17. General Accounting Office (2003). *Prescription Drug Discount Cards: Savings Depend on Pharmacy and Type of Card Used.* Report to congressional requesters. GAO 03-912. Washington, DC: GAO.

18. Federal Trade Commission (2004). Rhode Island Bills Would Raise Prices for Pharmaceuticals. FTC File V040013. Available at: http://www.ftc.gov/opa/2004/04/ribills.htm.

19. Academy of Managed Care Pharmacy (2003). Position Statement, Any Willing Provider Legislation: Revised. October 15. AMCP.

20. *Kentucky Association of Health Plans v. Miller,* 123 S. Ct. 1471 (2003).

21. *Texas Pharmacy Association v. Prudential Insurance Corporation of America,* 105.F.3d.1035 (5th Circ. 1997).

22. (2002). *Journal of Health Policies and Law* 27(6): 927-945.

23. (1997). *Am J Health-Syst Pharm* 54 (Mar 1): 520-523.

24. *Drug Trend Report* Vol. 7, Medco Health Solutions, Franklin Lakes, NJ, May 2005, p. 32.

25. Lawrence, J. (1998). Does Mail-Order Pharmacy Really Deliver the Goods? *Managed Care* June.

26. Novartis (2002). *Novartis Pharmacy Benefit Report: Facts and Figures,* 2002 edition. East Hanover, NJ: Novartis, pp. 15-16.

27. Takeda Pharmaceuticals (2003). The Prescription Drug Benefit Cost and Plan Design Survey Report. Takeda Pharmaceuticals, pp. 6-7.

28. Martinez, B. (2003). Hired to Cut Costs, Firms Find Profits in Generic Drugs. *Wall Street Journal,* March 31.

29. Martinez, B. (2003).

30. New York State Office of the Attorney General (2004). Express Scripts Accused of Defrauding State and Consumers Millions of Dollars. Available at: http://fairchild.oag.state.ny.us/rx/consumer_info/aud4a_04.html, August 2004.

31. Gelles, J. (1998). RiteAid's Role in Managed Care Riles Competitors. *Philadelphia Inquirer* August.

32. *J.E. Pierce Apothecary et al. v. Harvard Pilgrim.* CVS Corporation, PharmaCare Management Services, Inc. United State District Court, District of Massachusetts, Civil Action No. 98-12635-WGY. March 31, 2005.

33. Langenfeld, J. and Maness, R. (2003). The Cost of PBM "Self-Dealing" Under a Medicare Prescription Drug Benefit. Available at: http://www.mpaginc.com/news/pbmreport.pdf.

34. Langenfeld, J. and Maness, R. (2003).

35. Consumers Union. Disclosing Relationships Between Pharmacy Benefit managers and Drug Companies. Available at: http://www.consumersunion.org/campaigns/learn_more/001812indiv.html.

36. Takeda Pharmaceuticals (2003).

37. Takeda Pharmaceuticals (2003).

38. Medicare Prescription Drug, Improvement, and Modernizations Act of 2003, 108th Congress, H.R. 1, 2003.

39. The Family Building Act (A1862,S1076) State of New Jersey, 209th Legislature, 2001.

40. Colorado Medical Assistance Program (2003). *Pharmacy Requirements and Benefits.* December. Colorado Medical Assistance Program.

41. Center for Contraceptive Rights (2003). *Contraceptive Equality Laws in the United States.* July. Center for Contraceptive Rights.

42. Pennsylvania Catholic Conference (2005). Know the Facts About a Contraceptive Mandate. Harrisburg, PA: Pennsylvania Catholic Conference. Available at: www.pachatolic.org.

43. Illinois Right to Life Committee (2003). Invoke Conscience Act. July 7. Available at: http://www.illinoisrighttolife.org/InvokeConscienceAct.htm.

44. Code of Federal Register, 42 CFR456.7.

45. Express Scripts (2003). *Express Scripts Drug Benefit Guide 2003.* Maryland Heights, MO: Express Scripts, Inc.

46. Code of Federal Register, 42 CFR456.7.

47. Medco Health (2005). *DrugTrend Report,* Volume 7. May. Franklin Lakes, NJ: Medco Health.

48. Express Scripts (2005). *Express Scripts Drug Benefit Guide 2005.* Maryland Heights, MO: Express Scripts, Inc.

49. CareMark and Thompson Financial Services (2005). Benefits Barometer. New York: CareMark, Inc. and Thompson Financial Services.

50. Delate, T., Simmons, V.A., Motheral, B.R. (2004). Patterns of Use of Silfendail Among Commercially Insured Adults in the United States: 1998-2002. *Int J Impot Res* 16(4): 313-318.

51. Delate, T. et al. (2004). Randomized Controlled Trial of a Dose Consolidation Program. *J Manage Care Pharm* 10(6): 564-565.

52. McCarthy, R. (1999). Managed Care Matters—Vertical Integration from the Bottom. *Drug Benefit Trends* 11(1): 10.

53. Eli Lilly (1995). Press Release: FTC Gives Final Approval to Lilly Order: Pledges Continued Monitoring for Anticompetitive Practices. July 31. Available at http://www.ftc.gov/opa/1995/07/lilly22.htm.

54. AdvancePCS Tapping Into Rx Marketing Budgets For Revenues, *The Pink Sheet,* Jan 14, 2002, p. 25.

55. Consumers Union.

56. United States District Court, Southern District of New York, 97 Civ. 9167 (CLB).

57. Vardi, N. (2005). Rx for Fraud. *Forbes Magazine.* Available at: http://www.forbes.com/forbes/2005/0620124_2.html.

58. Available at: http://www.josmc.org/pipermail/mednews/2003-January/000 280.html.

59. Kaiser Network Daily Reports (2004). Medco reaches $29M Settlement with States Over Allegations of Unethical Drug Switching, Not Passing Along Savings. April 27. Available at: http:www.kaisernetwork.org/daily_reports/rep_index.cfm? hint=3&DR_ID=23411.

60. Federal Register, Vol. 68, No. 86, May 5, 2003, pp. 23731-23743.

61. South Carolina General Assembly, 116th Session, 2005-2006, Chapter 71, Title 38 of the 1976 Code, Article 16.

62. First Circuit Refuses to Stay Maine PBM Law's Implementation Pending Appeal (2005). *Pharmaceutical Law & Industry Report* 3(27).

63. Office of Inspector General (2005). *Medicaid Drug Price Comparisons: Average Manufacturer Price to Published Prices*. Publication OEI-05-05-00240. June. Washington, DC: U.S. Department of Health and Human Services.

Chapter 15

Risk Minimization:
A New Regulatory Directive

Louis A. Morris
Eva Lydick

THE NEW ERA OF RISK MANAGEMENT

Drugs are approved only if they are determined to be safe to use for the conditions described in their label. This basic tenet of the Food, Drug, and Cosmetic Act has not changed. What has changed in recent years is interpretation of the term *safe*. Modern concepts of pharmaceutical risk management are based on the premise that drug manufacturers, health care professionals, and patients have a responsibility to minimize the risks of using pharmaceutical products. It is not enough to make drugs minimally safe, they must be as safe as possible over the life cycle of the product's use.[1,2,3]

Historically, the Food and Drug Administration (FDA) has interpreted the requirement that a drug must be safe to mean that the benefits of a drug outweigh its risks. The determination was made on a categorical basis, on which the totality of risks was weighted against the totality of benefits when considered for the purposes outlined in the drug product's labeling. If a drug did not meet this criterion, it was not approved or its label was rewritten to narrow the conditions for use. This logic was endemic in the FDA for most of the twentieth century. On average, two to four drugs over each five-year period were withdrawn from the marketplace after postmarketing data uncovered new risks.[4] On occasion, the FDA would require some special tool or intervention to improve a product's safety profile. For example, patient package inserts were used to warn women about the risk of birth control pills, and a special distribution system was used to limit the dispensing of Clozaril (clozapine) to patients who undertook blood tests that demonstrated that they were not having a serious adverse reaction. However, starting in the early 1990s, this philosophy started to change as the FDA began to take a more active role in postmarketing surveillance and began instituting a more aggressive management process to assure greater safety in the use of marketed drugs. No longer do the manufacturer and the FDA provide passive oversight and labeling changes to control risks, now the manufacturer must actively monitor for suspected but unquantified risks and actively manage and minimize known risks.

PRECURSOR HISTORY

The FDA's new concepts for risk management amount to a cultural shift in the logic of drug approval and the FDA's role. The key events that led to this change can be traced to a series of reports that highlighted the need for improved medical safety. In 1999, the Institute of Medicine released a report titled, *To Err is Human*.[5] This report reviewed the nature and cause of medication errors, estimating that up to 98,000 people die each year due to these errors. The IOM included both adverse drug reactions and human errors in drug administration in their assessment. The report captured the attention of news reporters and the government. Headlines shouted alarm at the larger number of fatalities caused by medical errors. A government-wide initiative was started to develop methods and institute procedures to reduce medical errors.

For its part, the FDA was already concerned about medical safety and sought to increase its oversight and control of the safe use of marketed drugs. The IOM report provided both impetus and support for an already developing policy of increasingly active intervention. During the four-year period from 1998 to 2001, at least ten drugs were withdrawn from the market (see Table 15.1). For each preceding five-year period from 1979 to 1998, only two to four drugs were withdrawn.

In recent years, the impact of this new philosophy of risk management has continued with the withdrawal of Vioxx, Bextra, and Palladone and the initiation of risk management programs for NSAIDS, ED drugs, and SSRIs. Product liability cases for Vioxx and press reports have also demonstrated public the concerns for drug safety.

Statements made by FDA officials regarding some of these withdrawals suggested that the FDA no longer believed that passive oversight and relabeling drugs with new warnings was sufficient. Furthermore, the FDA no longer believed that it was sufficient to identify safe conditions of use in the label; health care professionals and patients had to comply with advocated directions for use for the drug to remain on the market.

As a summary of this new philosophy of risk management, FDA staff issued a report to the commissioner that highlighted processes for developing

TABLE 15.1. Drugs Withdrawn from 1998 to 2001.

Drug	Date withdrawn
Seldane (terfenadine)	2/98
Posicor (mibefradil)	6/98
Duract (bromphenac)	6/98
Hismanal (astemizole)	6/99
Roxar (grepafloxacin)	11/99
Propulsid (cisapride)	3/00
Rezulin (troglitazone)	3/00
Lotronex (alosetron HCl)	8/00
Raplon (rapacuronium)	3/01
Baycol (cerivaxtatin)	8/01

risk management systems and signaled new ideas for measuring risks and intervening to manage risk titled, "Managing the Risks of Medical Products,"[6] the FDA report borrowed heavily from risk management philosophies in other fields, such as environmental risk management and airline safety. It emphasized the process of developing risk management plans to control and manage drug safety.

The risk management revolution at the FDA continues today. Under FDA regulations and the Food and Drug Administration's Modernization Act, the FDA may approve new drugs with new restrictions that intended to assure safe use (Subpart H). These restrictions include limiting distribution to certain facilities or physicians with special training or experience or limiting distribution based on the condition of the performance of specified medical procedures. The regulations specify that the limitations must be commensurate with the specific safety concerns presented by the product. In addition, drugs continue to be approved with restrictions imposed by manufacturers seeking FDA approval.

In March 2004, the FDA released a series of draft concept papers focusing on premarketing risk assessment, risk management, and pharmacovigilance. These papers became guidances for the drug industry in May 2005. The risk management guidances described a new requirement for drug manufacturers. For certain new drug application, companies need to develop a risk management action plan (RiskMAP).

A RiskMAP is a strategic safety program designed to minimize known product risks while preserving its benefits. RiskMAPs target one or more safety goals and use one or more interventions or tools. These tools extend beyond the package insert and routine postmarketing surveillance. They are categorized into three areas: education and outreach, reminder systems, and performance-linked access systems. The FDA guidance also describes the conditions stimulating the need for a RiskMAP, the selection of tools, the format for RiskMAPs, and the evaluation processes necessary to develop and monitor the success of a risk minimization plan. The RiskMAP describes the background, research, rationale, and logic necessary to develop and implement the strategy and tactics for the risk management program.

The development of a RiskMAP requires pharmaceutical companies to think through not only how a drug is supposed to be used (the indications, contraindications, precautions, warnings, etc.) but how it may be used or misused by prescribers, dispensers, and patients using the medication. As a matter of best practices, some companies have begun to apply the RiskMAP development process to all drugs, not only to those that will require formal RiskMAPs, to more thoroughly apply the risk minimization process to improve drug safety. The role of the RiskMAP is to minimize risks throughout the life cycle of the drug. For the most part, the plan deals with the control of known or suspected risks, whereas other risk management activities concentrate on the discovery and quantification of suspected risks.

To fulfill the obligations of developing a competent RiskMAP, drafters must seek to influence the behavior of the parties responsible for drug safety, particularly patients, physicians, pharmacists, and allied medical staff. This is not an easy task. It requires understanding of the specific behaviors to be influenced, the environment in which the behaviors take place, the development of a set of strategies to influence behaviors, and an evaluation program to determine the impact (and source of failure) for intended interventions. Therefore, a reasonable RiskMAP must demonstrate that the company understands the system of drug prescribing, dispensing, monitoring, and use for their particular product, the impact (positive and negative) and limits of various tools or combination of tools selected for implementation, how to test tools before implementation and evaluate the implemented RiskMAP with sufficient specificity to understand the impact of the selected interventions, and how to improve outcomes if the original program does not reach reasonable effectiveness targets. In addition, the implemented RiskMAP should not detract from product sales. Developing risk minimization action programs that assure safe use while maintaining sales presents an added difficulty and series of concerns.

To comply with the guidance, drafters need to apply an appropriate analytical framework, along with insights from original research:

- to conceive of a rational approach for controlling risks,
- to justify the selection of tools or the development new tools,
- to justify why other tools that may be more "potent" (but cause patients or prescribers to reject the medication) are not selected,

- to evaluate the tools prior to implementation and the program after implementation, and
- to plan for quality improvements in the plan as it evolves and to plan for the ultimate withdrawal of the risk management program.

The purpose of this chapter is to describe the FDA's RiskMAP requirements and to suggest how to develop a RiskMAP.

WHEN IS A RISKMAP NEEDED?

To determine if a new drug will need a RiskMAP, the company must consider the risks posed by the product in light of its benefits. For drugs for serious or life-threatening illnesses, such as cancer and AIDS, a great deal more tolerance for personal risk exists than for drugs used for cosmetic purposes, such as for acne or head lice. However, even for serious drugs, when the risk posed may be prevented, a RiskMAP will need to be seriously considered.

The starting point for any RiskMAP is as complete knowledge as possible of the product's safety hazards. Some hazards may be suspected and subjected to continuing postmarketing surveillance. A debate regarding which signals denote real risks and which denote false positives always occur. Following the precautionary principle, it is likely that even suspected risks will be the subject of some risk intervention, even if it means only notifying prescribers of its possibility. The target product profile or proposed package insert is likely to serve as the best source of information about the known or suspected risks of the product and the best basis for risk minimization planning.

The FDA suggests three considerations for determining if a RiskMAP is needed: the nature of risks verses benefits (risk tolerance issues such as population affected, alternative therapy available, and reversibility of adverse events); preventability of the adverse event; and probability of benefit or success of the risk minimization intervention. Drugs that have serious or life-threatening contraindications, warnings, precautions, or adverse effects are the most likely candidates for a RiskMAP. Patient behaviors such as pregnancy prevention, blood tests, overdose/misuse avoidance, awareness, and action related to specific safety signals (e.g., a hypersensitivity reaction, depression, and suicide) that can mitigate risks make a RiskMAP more appealing. When people other than the patient may be at risk (e.g., a child may use the product inadvertently), a RiskMAP may also be required. FDA singles out Schedule II drugs, with concerns for misuse, abuse, addiction, diversion, and overdose as likely candidates for a RiskMAP.

RATIONALE AND JUSTIFICATION

The most important aspects of developing a RiskMAP is to understand the risks involved in using the product in question and the factors that might increase or mitigate those risks. The drug development program should provide information on safety and potential adverse reactions of the drug, as well as potential misadventures in using the drug. In addition, clues from similar medications and animal or mutagencity studies may also indicate potential risks. The sections of the drug label where the risk information is provided may provide a clue as to the overarching goals or objectives for the RiskMAP. Contraindications may be related to patient selection or testing that must occur before the drug is prescribed, precautions may relate to advice about how to use, or not use, the product, and adverse reactions may be related to warning signs that must be monitored by the patient and physician or risk/benefit decisions underlying use of the medication.

Companies must provide a logical rationale for the implementation of a risk management program. The RiskMAP developed must specify this rationale in the background section. Here, the company must enumerate each of the risks to be managed by the program. For each risk, the company must fully characterize the risk severity; the population (or subpopulation) at greatest risks; the extent to which the risk is predictable, preventable, or reversible; and the time course of the risk (if the risk is time-limited, continuous, or cumulative).

GOALS, OBJECTIVES, AND TOOLS

The guidance mandates that each plan must specify the overall goals of the risk minimization plan. These goals are the desired endpoints for safe product use. For example, if a drug causes birth defects, a reasonable goal would be that no women who are pregnant should be given the drug. A second goal might be that no women should become pregnant while taking the drug. It should be noted that some goals may never be fully met. However, making progress toward meeting the goal, rather than actually achieving the goal, may be an acceptable outcome.

Once the goals have been enumerated, the company must identify a series of objectives for each goal. The objectives must be specific and measurable. They specify the behaviors and processes necessary for the stated goals to be achieved. For example, if the goal is to prevent pregnancy, then an objective may be specified that all women must have a negative pregnancy test performed within seven days of initiating therapy. Objectives often identify particular people (i.e., patient, pharmacist, physician, allied health professional) responsible for the desired behavior. This aids in the development of a communications plan directed to that individual, which will likely be a core element of the risk management program.

Once goals and objectives are specified, the company must select a series of tools designed to intervene and mitigate risks. The FDA specifies three categories of tools. The first category is targeted education or outreach. These tools concentrate on the communication of information intended to minimize risk. They include a variety of media that carry messages to health care professionals (e.g., letters; training programs (including continuing education programs, courses, or materials); and public notifications (such as letters to the editor). In addition, promotional techniques can be used to publicize risk management concerns, including advertisements and sales representatives' distribution of risk minimization information. Similarly, communications to consumers such as medication guides and patient package inserts may be used. Interestingly, the FDA includes limitation on the use of promotional techniques such as product sampling or direct-to-consumer advertising as a risk minimization tool. However, these latter tools may do more to limit demand for the medication than directly communicate information on how to minimize product risks.

The second category of risk minimization tools is characterized by FDA as reminder systems. This is a broad category of tools that goes beyond mere information dissemination. Often, they solicit a commitment to engage in the dictates of the risk minimization program. For example, these tools include training or certification programs or physician attestation of capabilities to use the medication safely. They also include patient agreements or acknowledgment forms that seek the patient's commitment to follow dictates for safe drug use. They include specialized product packaging to enhance safety by influencing who may take a medication or providing reminder information at the point of product use. This category also includes distribution channel controls such as limiting the amount of medication in any single prescription or refill of product as well as specialized systems or records that limit dispensing unless certain measures having been satisfied (e.g., prescription stickers).

The third category of tools described in the FDA guidance is performance-linked access systems. These are tools intended to limit access to the medication based on the fulfillment of certain criteria. For example, the product may not be made available unless an acknowledgment, certification, enrollment, or appropriate test records are made available. This category of tools would also include limiting prescribing to specially certified health care practitioners, and limiting dispensing to specially certified pharmacies or practitioners or to patients with evidence of fulfilling certain conditions (e.g., negative laboratory test results).

The FDA tool characterization is helpful in providing a wide range of options for RiskMAP designers. However, it does not provide a mechanism for determining which tools (or combinations of tools) would be most appropriate in which circumstances. To be fair, even though some risk management interventions have been evaluated.[7] an inadequate knowledge base exists for objectively determining how these tools should be applied. However, a broad set of theoretical models exists that may be applied to characterize the behavioral aspects of product prescribing, dispensing, and utilization. These models may be applied to help determine what mix of tools makes the most sense in terms of influencing safe use behavior. However, acceptance of the tools must also be considered. It is clear, even at this early stage, that risk management tool implementation may have unintended consequences. Prescribers may find certain tools overly burdensome, offensive, or adverse, and may avoid use of the drug because of the risk minimization tools selected. Therefore, acceptance as well as effectiveness of any risk minimization plan must be considered when designing the RiskMAP.

DESIGNING THE RISKMAP

Companies must select and justify their choice of tools. In doing so, it behooves a company to develop a conceptual model for how their drugs are used and what system failures may lead to product misuse. In addition to relying on a systems analysis, using a behavioral model of product use (i.e., how beliefs, motives, and situational constraints influence how a drug is used) can help a company select a coordinated set of tools and specify core messages that must be communicated or systems that must be implemented to define the elements of their risk management program.

A good starting point for developing a model of drug use is to identify the various steps necessary to use a drug properly. Failure mode and effects analysis (FMEA) is a systematic analysis of how failures in any system may occur.[8] An FMEA is conducted before the system is implemented and delineates the steps in a system and identifies potential mistakes that may occur at each step (i.e., potential failure modes). It is a complement to root-cause analyses, which are aimed at identifying the source of a system failure once a mistake is identified. If a drug is already marketed, a root cause analysis should be used to identify problems or concerns based on existing information. If the drug has not been marketed, an FMEA is the best alternative. In addition to listing the steps in using a drug effectively, an effective FMEA identifies corrective actions required to prevent failures and to assure the highest possible system quality.

To undertake a FMEA, the system steps and potential failure modes are identified. Each step may be broken down into subprocesses with each substep in the system being considered as a separate element with the potential for failure. Each of the postulated steps in which failure might occur is assigned a severity value, a probability that a given effect might occur, and a likelihood value that user may detect (and correct) the problem. Recommended actions (i.e., tool interventions) are developed to reduce the probability and (most important) severity of harm, with priority given to the highest risk.

Although developed as a method to improve product quality, FMEA can only be as good as the quality of the system description. Specifying steps at too broad a level of specificity can miss important elements. For example, a system analysis for a medications error problem found that many physicians clearly wrote the drug name on the prescription and the pharmacist accurately dispensed what the physician had written. The problem was that physicians recalled the incorrect drug name from memory when they wrote the prescription. A FMEA that did not specify the need for the physician to recall the correct drug name from memory would have missed an important source of error.

In addition, to specify the subprocesses, it is necessary to understand the system from the perspective of the individuals performing the tasks involved. It is well established that the relationship between knowledge and behavior is not direct or simple. We often know what we should do but fail to behave in a fashion consistent with our knowledge. To develop a predictive model, it is necessary to understand (1) the full set of beliefs underlying behavioral intentions, (2) the motivations that support or stand in the way of exhibiting desired behavior, and (3) the environmental conditions that facilitate or place barriers to compliance.

A variety of psychological and health-behavior models can be used to organize these influences. Some models may help to improve the processing of presented information, for example, by improving participants' involvement (personal relevance) or competency (self-efficacy) with the information or advocated behavior. Some models may help to understand the processes underlying choice among alternative courses of behavior (behavioral decision making). Some models may help to structure advocated behavior into a series of stages, permitting a series of messages that seek to move respondents through a necessary series of stages in order to attain behavioral compliance (stage models or precaution adoption). Some models seek to motivate compliance through emotion (fear appeals or positive affect) or through highlighting desired outcomes (approach or avoidance goals).

Which model to use depends on the particular problem (objective) addressed. If we advocate complex behaviors, such as avoiding drug dependency, it may be necessary to move respondents through a series of stages in order to overcome situational barriers. If we advocate simpler behaviors, such as standing upright when taking tablets; providing a strong, even emotional, rationale for compliance; and developing a reminder system might provide the best model to influence behavior. Diagnosing the behavioral problem and selecting (or custom building) the correct behavioral model can provide a clear method for design of the risk management plan.

Because we are dealing with programs that are expected to reach and influence the vast majority of participants, it may be difficult to anticipate the full range of issues influencing the behavior of all of the patients and health care professionals. Identifying particular at-risk segments can also help to design program interventions targeted at particular failure modes for a specified group of individuals.

COMMUNICATION TOOLS:
MESSAGE, DESIGN, AND DISTRIBUTION

A variety of interventions may be used to influence patient behavior. For purposes of communication, these tools may be cataloged by the format and media to communicate information. In this chapter, the focus will be on communication tools used to deliver information to patients. Additional tools are used to communicate relevant information to physicians and as forcing functions that guide or direct behavioral compliance. These forcing functions include programs that certify prescribers, dispensers, or patients. They may also require patients to obtain certain tests prior to refill authorization; other systems may also be developed to help improve patient compliance or avoid noncompliance.

To develop an acceptable patient communications plan (i.e., selecting an optimal set of tools), it is important to consider the communications objective (CO) and the recommended behaviors necessary for safe use of the medication. The COs are the key messages included in a risk-communications document (such as a patient brochure) that outline what patients must know to use the drug safely. The recommended behaviors are actions the patient must undertake to use the medicine properly (such as avoid contraindicated drugs or monitor their bodily state for signs of possible side effects). Obviously, for simpler behaviors, brief communication tools may be indicated. For more complex behavior, where more explanation is needed, longer forms and multiple interventions may be necessary. Although all tools have a general purpose to inform, various tools have different advantages and disadvantages. Tools may have one or more purposes, with certain tools better suited for different functions. Table 15.2 shows a set of sample tools and their communications function.

Perhaps, even more important than form, the content of the patient communication requires careful planning and an understanding of the target audience. For prescription drugs, the product label (or package insert [PI] written for health professionals) summarizes the scientific basis of product approval and lists the conditions under which the drug may be used safely and effectively. Under the Food, Drug, and Cosmetic Act, virtually all communications about the product provided by the manufacturer are characterized as labeling and must be consistent with the PI to avoid misbranding charges. Thus, the PI serves as the basis for the content of all patient communications.

Based on the PI, one can draft a series of communicator goals describing the educational goals of patient information. By reviewing these objectives and the general purpose of the communication, a tool, or series of tools, to match the function can be selected. For example, if the purpose of a communication is to help a consumer decide whether to take a medicine or to select an alternative form of therapy, then the communication tool must function as a decision aid that provides the advantages and disadvantages of various therapy alternatives. However, if the function of the communication is to simply remind the patient of a particular behavior to avoid (e.g., not to use if pregnant) then a simple warning message may be placed on the pack-

TABLE 15.2. Patient Communications Vehicles

Tool	Distribution	Purpose
Brochure	Physician	General information
Patient package insert	Package or pharmacist	Risk communication
Medication guide	Package	Risk communication and methods of avoidance
Informed consent	Physician	Acknowledgement of risks
Warning stickers	Package	Risk "signal"
Wallet card	Starter kit	Reminder
Stickers for medication vial	Pharmacist on medication vial	Reminder
Patient agreement or contract	Physician	Behavioral commitment
Decision aid	Physician	Choice of therapy
Videotape or CD	Physician or starter kit	Persuasion or choice of therapy
Recurring interventions (telephone calls)	Telephone	Behavioral maintenance

age (perhaps backed up with a symbol that reminds the patient not to use if pregnant).

Moderate length patient communication tools (e.g., patient package inserts and medication guides) tend to follow a general format that (at least in theory) matches the general script (i.e., cognitive model) of how a patient would seek to learn about a new medication. Six topic headers are required for medication guides:

- What is the most important information I should know?
- What is the name of "Drug"?
- Who should not take "Drug"?
- How should I take "Drug"?
- What should I avoid while taking "Drug"?
- What are the possible or reasonably likely side effects of "Drug"?

Under the first heading (most important information), key risk management messages are provided. This placement and heading provide explicit emphasis to help patients recognize the most important information for them to learn about the medication. It also provides an intellectual scaffold for patients to store additional information about the drug, and it permits reinforcement and redundancy within the document. A variety of graphic (e.g., typeface, bolding) and language devices (e.g., headers, core concepts) can help structure the document to provide signals (i.e., methods to emphasize the importance of certain sections) that improve the communication of essential information to patients or health care providers.[9] At the same time, language can be simplified and extraneous information can be deleted (socalled seductive details that provide interesting but nonessential information regarding risk management). This combination of drafting techniques reduces the cognitive load and increases the ease of processing while focusing readers on the most important information.

In addition to content based on the drug product's risks, benefits, and usage directions, additional information can educate patients, and stimulate behavioral compliance. However, fully explaining every possible risk in terms of its causation (i.e., physiological pathway), significance (e.g., severity), likelihood (probability of occurrence), and means of control or avoidance would lead to a very long and arduous document. Such a document would be too long and complex for an average reader to use. Rather, explanatory language must be used selectively. It should be based on the readers' existing knowledge and beliefs and communicate information that is consistent with the COs for the document.

Morgan, Fischhoff, Bostron, and Atman (2002) advocate a mental-models approach to risk communication in which the mental schema of product experts is compared to the mental schema of laypersons.[10] Communications are drafted to correct misconceptions of laypersons and increase awareness of less obvious, but important, information. Using a mental-models approach may help us understand which aspects of the developed document are successful and which messages should be emphasized in further interventions. However, a drafting communications based on a mental-models approach must be guided by the COs for that particular product, because experts are likely to have much more complete schema for prescription medication and because much of their knowledge is irrelevant to patients' choices and product use.

THE NEED TO INFLUENCE BEHAVIOR

There is an old expression, "it's easier to sell soap than brotherhood." Selling soap requires both convincing people that one brand is superior to another and controlling the sales environment so that the promoted brand is widely available and well regarded. Selling brotherhood requires a more extensive selling process. For example, we must clearly define what we mean, convince the audience that a problem exists, suggest solutions perceived as acceptable, demonstrate that such solutions can be effective and implemented by the respondent, provide people with information and training necessary for implementing the proposed solution (e.g., use of the product), and convince the respondent that any perceived barriers or negative impacts can be overcome or negated.

This expression is meaningful in its application to prescription drug usage behavior because of the range in complexity in the type of behaviors necessary to comply with safe usage directions. For example, a patient may comply with dosing instructions by simply taking one tablet by mouth each day. Risk avoidance sometimes may be in the form of a fairly simple behavior. For instance, alendronate (Fosamax) patients are informed to stand upright for one half hour after ingestion in order to avoid side effects affecting the esophagus.

For other drugs, compliance may require a more complex set of behaviors. For example, for certain cholesterol-lowering drugs, patients are told to undertake liver function tests prior to treatment, after twelve weeks of treatment, following any elevation of dose, and periodically (e.g., semiannually) thereafter. Obtaining a liver function test may require complex problem solving for the patient. He or she may need to find a laboratory acceptable to the patient's medical insurance company and may need to fast for twelve hours before undertaking the test, depending on what specific tests the physician orders. The patient also may need to make an appointment and travel to the testing facility. Having to repeat this behavior over many years adds to the behavioral complexity as the patient's situation may change and new adaptations may be necessary.

For some drugs, patients should look for the warning signs of serious side effects. For example, some people who have taken metformin (Glucophage) for diabetes have developed a serious condition called lactic acidosis. Lactic acidosis is caused by a buildup of lactic acid in the blood and can be fatal. Patients are told to look for signs of lactic acidosis and report them immediately to their physician. Such signs include the following:

- Feeling very weak, tired, or uncomfortable
- Unusual muscle pain
- Trouble breathing
- Unusual or unexpected stomach discomfort
- Feeling cold
- Feeling dizzy or lightheaded
- Suddenly developing a slow or irregular heartbeat

Because these symptoms also occur frequently in people who are not taking the medication and who do not have lactic acidosis, detecting and interpreting these signs may be complicated. Patients must determine that (1) they have the indicated symptom, (2) the symptom is caused by a medical problem, and (3) the symptom (or constellation of symptoms) is a sign of lactic acidosis.

The particular set of skills and resources necessary to obtain a liver function test differ considerably from the problem-solving skills necessary to determine whether to ask the doctor about various common symptoms. Interventions to help patients comply with these varying instructions would similarly require a vastly different set of information.

DISTRIBUTION AND BEHAVIORAL CONTROL SYSTEMS

Although much of what we hope to accomplish in managing pharmaceutical risks may be realized through carefully designed communications, information dissemination may not be sufficient to lead to behavior change. Often, information is viewed as a weak intervention. For information to have an impact it must be received, read, understood, motivational, persuasive, remembered, and implemented for behavior change to be effective. Furthermore, behavior maintenance means that information must be effective over the long term, often for many years. Although voluntary adaptations are viewed as the most positive method of influencing health behavior, it may also be necessary to institute distribution or behavioral control systems that influence risk avoidance behavior.

A distribution system is necessary for a drug to be delivered to the patient. For all prescription drugs, it is necessary for the physician to order a prescription (in writing or orally) and a pharmacist to dispense the drug. Certain drugs, such as scheduled medicines, also require limits on refills and additional record keeping. For certain risk management programs, additional controls have been developed to minimize risky behaviors. For example, for Clozaril (clozapine) (where certain blood disorders may result from taking the drug), patients are required to obtain monthly blood tests that show the drug is not having an undesirable effect. This "no blood, no drug" policy has minimized the impact of these problems and permitted a useful drug to remain on the market. Another example of a distribution-control system is a verification sticker program as used by certain acne drugs (most notably Accutane [isotrentinoin]). In this instance, the drug may have important adverse consequences (such as causing birth defects if taken during pregnancy). A woman taking Accutane must have a monthly test to demonstrate that she is not pregnant. The test results are forwarded to a centralized system. The pharmacist must access this system to verify that the patient is not pregnant prior to dispensing the prescription.

Other distribution control systems, such as obtaining a prescription for the medication only from a physician who has been certified to prescribe the medicine or providing medication only to a patient who has been certified to receive the prescription have been suggested or implemented by various companies. The logic underpinning such designs is derived from systems theory, which has been used by various industries (such as the aircraft industry) to design safety into the systems used.

Systems theory relies on a number of design elements to force an individual to behave in a prescribed fashion. According to systems theory, any activity may be conceived as a system that requires actions to occur for the activity to be accomplished. For example, the issuance of a prescription requires the doctor's diagnosis of an illness (or prescribe a drug to prevent an illness), the choice of a medication (along with dosage and directions), the issuance of a prescription, the delivery of the prescription to a patient (or surrogate), the delivery of the prescription to a pharmacy, the review and checking of the prescription by pharmacy staff, the retrieval of the medication from storage, the counting of tablets, the labeling of the vial, the temporary storage of the prescription, and the dispensing of the prescription to the patient (or surrogate). There may (and should) be additional stages in this model, such as counseling of patients by physicians and pharmacists, information collection and retrieval, administrative activities for reimbursement, and compliance with various laws and regulations and additional risk management activities). However, even this simplified system requires many different activities, and mistakes may occur at many different points. To prevent such errors, we may institute various procedures, controls, or design changes. For example, to prevent taking the wrong bottle off the shelf, we may color code bottles, use bar codes that must be checked, or institute a mandatory checklist of actions to prevent dispensing the wrong medication. A number of forcing functions (design features that build in safety, such as having drug names be printed in a certain size or constitute a certain percentage of the front display panel) and redundancies (such as having the drug name on multiple places on the bottle of medicine) help design safety. At the heart of systems theory is the logic that such procedures must be followed every time an activity is undertaken, or the resulting action cannot take place.

EVALUATION

An important contribution of the FDA guidance on risk management that should not be overlooked is the need to fully evaluate the impact of both the entire risk management program and of the individual tools intended to control risks.

As in the drug development program itself, three levels of evaluation should occur. First is the test of individual tools, perhaps as a part of the development process. For example, implementing comprehension tests early may aid in the design of impactful communications. Second, a series of interventions may be instituted in a field test in the form of a clinical trial in which various distribution sites are randomized to deliver various combinations of interventions. By comparing results between the sites, the value of various interventions may be evaluated. However, care must be taken to ensure sufficient power to determine differences among sites and avoiding confounding site with intervention biases.

Third, the FDA proposed that all RiskMAPs be fully evaluated once implemented. The FDA proposes three broad ways to evaluate effects of the RiskMAP—analysis of spontaneously reported adverse drug events, analysis of administrative databases, and active surveillance, to include surveys. As each method has problems, FDA suggested the evaluation incorporate two different methods and use well-defined and validated measures for assessing the effect.

Ideally, intervention effectiveness should be evaluated based on ability to improve actual health outcomes, for example, decrease cases of jaundice, liver disease, and/or liver failures. However, these endpoints may be rare and would require following up large numbers of patients for a long period of time. A quicker assessment of the value of the RiskMAP could be obtained by monitoring surrogates (for example, changes in laboratory markers that are known to precede the actual health outcome, as, for example, in the previous case, increases in Alanine aminotranferease [ALT]/aspartate aminotransferase [AST]). A less optimum but useful evaluation could involve ascertainment of process measures (for example, the frequency of testing for liver enzyme elevations). A third evaluation criterion would be testing for comprehension, knowledge, and attitude among patients, prescribers, and pharmacists about the risks and consequences or the drug.

The first line of evaluation is the careful review of spontaneous reports of adverse drug events and changes of number and kind of such reports. However, multiple biases exist in the determination of which events are reported, so this analysis is merely the first step in the evaluation.

A strict risk management program can require all individuals receiving the drug to be followed for appropriateness of treatment and monitoring and/or specific outcomes under conditions of a registry. However, more broadly, the term *registry* means only a cohort formed on the basis of all individuals included possessing some attribute in common, for example, exposure to the drug in question. This could be a sample of individuals followed for specific monitoring and/or outcomes such as compliance with laboratory monitoring and/or the effectiveness of that monitoring in preventing one or more clinical adverse events. Although ideally one would wish to follow all individuals exposed, in all likelihood logistics will dictate that only a percentage of these individuals can be followed for the occurrence of health outcomes, surrogates, process measures, or comprehension. A registry is commonly composed of willing individuals who have received the drug or have the underlying disease for which the drug may be prescribed.

Large linked databases of health care claims, such as outpatient visits, inpatient visits, pharmacy fills, and laboratory tests and results have proven valuable in both the assessment of the magnitude of risks and for monitoring the effectiveness of specific interventions to decrease risk. These administrative databases can be used to answer routine queries on the occurrence of contraindicated coprescribing or overdosing, appropriate monitoring, and associations between prescribing of selected drugs and specific events.[11] Note that observed associations do not imply causality, but can add to the understanding of the effectiveness of the RiskMAP.

The third type of evaluation method involves active surveillance. This methodology would be very expensive for rare outcome events, but surveys of health care practitioners or patients could provide some information about the rate of more common events. In addition, the effectiveness of the

RiskMAP to change knowledge, attitudes, and practices could be ascertained through such surveys.

When it is not clear which intervention(s) would be most effective, it may be worthwhile to use an experimental design comparing different interventions. This interventional design could be followed either through administrative databases or actively with surveys.

Based on the evaluation of the RiskMAP, a consequent obligation exist to modify or increase interventions if not successful. Few interventions implemented in the past have been rigorously evaluated. Those that have been evaluated have too often shown that for all their good intentions, the effect was less than desired. For example, package insert requirements for liver-enzyme monitoring are not well followed, even in the face of major media coverage of the risks of hepatic failure.[12] Risk management programs must eventually be able to show that they decrease or mitigate the likelihood of adverse events.

Regardless of evaluation study, interventions need to be assessed not only on their effectiveness of preventing serious adverse events but also on their cost and burden on the health care system. Too rigorous an intervention may result in many additional visits, tests, and other forms of monitoring. This, in turn, may result in increased mistakes due to increased tasks. Increased costs may make the new therapy of less value than other, less-effective therapies and/or raise patient privacy concerns. Decreased benefits that follow from risk management interventions that are too stringent can result from decreased patient compliance and decreased drug access to patients that would benefit from that particular drug therapy.

CONCLUSION

In conclusion, risk management is a new and evolving discipline. It is difficult to argue that drugs should not be provided to patients in a manner that minimizes potential hazards. The FDA has advanced the public health by fostering greater attention over the discovery, quantification, and management of risks. However, any policy that results in new activities to control one set of hazards may result in creating new, unexpected hazards. Thus, continuing to evaluate not only the hazards of drugs but the interventions intended to control these hazards, is essential to assure that the benefits of a RiskMAP will, itself, outweigh its risks.

NOTES

1. U.S. Food and Drug Administration (2005). Guidance: Premarketing risk assessment. March. Available at: http://www.fda.gov/cder/guidance/6357fnl.htm.

2. U.S. Food and Drug Administration (2005). Guidance: Development and use of risk minimization action plans. March. Available at: http://www.fda.gov/cder/guidance/6358fnl.htm.

3. U.S. Food and Drug Administration (2005). Guidance: Good pharmaco-vigilance practices and pharmacoepidemiologic assessment. March. Available at: http://www.fda.gov/cder/guidance/6359OCC.htm. March 2005.

4. U.S. Food and Drug Administration (2002). Report to the Nation: Improving Public Health through Human Drugs. Washington, DC: Center for Drug Evaluation and Research. Available at: http://www.fda.gov/cder/reports/rtn/2002/Rtn2002.pdf.

5. Kohn, LT, Corrigan, JM, and Donaldson, MS. (eds.) (2000). *To Err is Human: Building a safer healthcare system.* Committee on Quality of Health Care in America, Institute of Medicine. Washington DC: National Academies Press.

6. U.S. Food and Drug Administration (1999). *Managing the Risks from Medical Product Use: Creating a Risk Management Framework.* Report to the FDA Commissioner from the Task Force on Risk Management. May. Washington, DC: U.S. Department of Health and Human Services. Available at: http://www.fda.gov/oc/tfrm/riskmanagement.pdf.

7. Goldman (2004). Communication of Medical Product Risk: How Effective is Effective Enough? *Drug Safety* 27(8): 519-534.

8. Stamatis, DH (1995). *Failure Mode and Effects Analysis.* Milwaukee, WI: American Society for Quality.

9. Morris, LA and Aikin, KJ (2001). The "pharmacokinetics" of patient communications. *Drug Information Journal* 36(2): 509-527.

10. Morgan, MG, Fischhoff, B, Bostrom, A, and Atman, CJ (2002). *Risk Communication: A Mental Models Approach.* Cambridge, UK: Cambridge University Press.

11. Chan KA, Daviss RL, Gunter MJ, et al. (2005). The HMO research network. In Strom, BL (Ed.) *Pharmacoepidemiology,* Fourth edition (pp. 261-269). New York: John Wiley & Sons.

12. Graham DJ, Drinkard CR, Shatin D, Tsong Y, Burgess MJ (2001). Liver enzyme monitoring in patients treated with troglitazone. *Journal of the American Medical Association* 286: 831-833.

Chapter 16

Drug Importation and Reimportation

Albert I. Wertheimer
Thomas Santella

INTRODUCTION

Due to the ever increasing prices of pharmaceuticals in the United States, compared to those in many other countries, consumers and innovative entrepreneurs have devised various means of obtaining cheaper pharmaceutical prices through purchases abroad where prices are lower. Purchases of this kind fit into one of several categories falling under the umbrella category of drug importation and drug reimporation.

Many seniors physically travel across the border to Mexico or Canada and purchase their drug needs from legitimate pharmacies. Others who are not so close to an international border utilize Internet pharmacies, whose location and legitimacy are often questionable. Some of the drugs imported into the United States are making their second international border crossing, having been originally made in the United States or a least under the auspices of an American pharmaceutical company. Many argue that these "reimported" drugs, because they have already met Food and Drug Administration (FDA) standards for safety and efficacy, should be eligible for sale within our borders.

The issue of drug importation/reimportation is both complex and important. The issue involves questions of safety, concerns about opportunities for counterfeiting, and worries about false advertising, bribery, and bad batches, as well as exposure to temperature extremes and changed labels disguising expiration dates. The issue also creates debate regarding the impact of drug prices, and particularly industry profits, on innovation and the development of new medicines. Separating serious political concerns from political or industry interests is a complex matter, which this chapter addresses. This chapter defines the terms involved in the debate, describes the scope of the problem, contextualizes the debate within its political context, searches abroad to see how other industrialized nations are dealing with the problem, explains the array of strategies being attempted to obtain lower prices from foreign drug sources, and looks into the future of drug importation.

DEFINITIONS

Before reaching a deeper understanding of the complexities of the drug importation debate, it is first crucial to understand precisely what we are talking about when we refer to imported drugs and reimported drugs. For the purposes of this chapter, we will utilize the definitions for imported and reimported drugs provided by the recently released report on drug importation from the U.S. Department of Health and Human Services (HHS).

Imported drugs: According to HHS, imported drugs are "drugs manufactured for sale inside and outside of the U.S., then brought into this country for use by U.S. consumers." The report also specifies that "importation" includes "a) *personal importation* (Internet sales, foot traffic across the border, mail order) where the drugs are purchased by those who consume them, and b) *commercial importation* where drugs are purchased by pharmacies and wholesalers for resale to the ultimate consumers."[1]

Reimported drugs: According to the same report, reimported drugs refer to "FDA-approved prescription drugs that were made in the U.S., sent abroad, and then brought back into the U.S." As of this writing, the only party legally able to reimport a prescription drug is the original manufacturer, and only when that manufacturer ensures the drug's authenticity.

Various types of imported drugs exist, each with its own level of associated risk. Among these, only two types of legally imported drugs exist, which include those manufactured in foreign but FDA–inspected facilities meeting U.S. standards and those that were manufactured in an FDA–approved U.S. facility, sent abroad, then reimported by the manufacturer under the requisite conditions.

Another type of imported drug is one manufactured in a foreign facility that also produces the FDA–approved U.S. version. In this case, the facility may have a separate production line for the non–FDA–approved version. As such, the FDA does not recognize the drug as safe and effective by American standards, although it is most likely exactly or at least very similar to the U.S.–approved version.

Finally, a drug may be imported from a facility that has not been inspected by the FDA and therefore is not recognized as a producer of safe and effective drugs. Importantly, this does not necessarily mean that the drugs produced at the facility are substandard, though they may be, only that the FDA has not actually witnessed and inspected the production facility or its production methods. Most of the debate concerning drug importation regards drug products obtained under this third scenario, from a manufacturer operating outside of FDA jurisdiction. In addition to these major definitions, this chapter will also address and describe parallel imports and their significance in examining the U.S. drug distribution system.

BRIEF HISTORY OF DRUG IMPORTATION/REIMPORTATION

Today, most Americans, when prescribed a medication by their doctor or when selecting an over-the-counter medication, believe that the selected drug will not only be safe but will also do what it says it is supposed to do. In this blind faith in pharmaceutical products Americans take for granted that the safety and efficacy of medicines were not always so guaranteed. In fact, for the majority of our nation's history, no regulation of drug products occurs. Drugs could be sold with extravagant claims, whether true or untrue, whether safe or unsafe. Over the past hundred years, with the development of the Food and Drug Administration (FDA, created in 1906), the laws regarding medicines sold in America have no doubt worked to all Americans' advantage. But the history of laws related to drug importation really begins in 1938, with the creation of the Food, Drug, and Cosmetic Act (FD&C Act).

Up until 1938, the manufacture and distribution of prescription and non-prescription drugs was still mostly unregulated in America. At the time little control over the claims drug makers made and no oversight over how the products were made existed. The FD&C Act, passed on June 25, 1938, was an important milestone in drug regulatory history for several reasons. For one, the act made it mandatory for drug manufacturers to prove that their products were safe for human use. The law also asserted that labels must be accurate and include instructions for proper use. Most important, however, the act formally allowed the FDA to inspect production facilities to ensure the accuracy and credibility of manufacturer-provided information.

Another critical legislative addition to the drug regulatory system came in 1962 with the Kefauver-Harris Amendments. In short, the amendment to the FD&C Act made it mandatory for drug manufacturers to prove not only their product's safety but also its effectiveness. It is the combination of these laws that allow consumers to place trust in the medicines they receive. The emerging debate surrounding drug importation/reimportation is quite similar to the debate about drugs produced in America that resulted in this new legislation.[2]

As a result of the FD&C Act, many regulations concern which drugs are allowed to enter the United States drug system. In general, the U.S. drug system is considered to be "closed," meaning that it is not readily open to foreign drug products. As previously discussed, all drugs entering the American marketplace must be FDA approved, whether made at home or abroad. But the job of the FDA has been complicated by the many FDA–approved drugs sold in the United States today being made in foreign countries. As a result of this new reality, combined with rising concern about counterfeit drugs, the FDA saw the need for further legislation clarifying exactly under what conditions drugs could be imported. Under the Prescription Drug Marketing Act of 1987, only the original drug manufacturer could reimport a drug made in the United States. Thus manufacturers of drugs in other countries must meet FDA standards and allow FDA inspection of their facilities in order to sell their products in the United States. These precautions guarantee that all drugs sold in the United States meet the same high standards of both safety and efficacy.

Amid all of this reasonably effective drug legislations, the rising costs of drugs has created more problems for regulatory authorities. As more and more Americans turn to Internet pharmacies for their medications, the FDA loses control over drug safety, prompting great concern. Although it is generally illegal to import drugs into the United States as an individual, loopholes in the law are exploited that allow sales of this type. The issue of personal importation was first addressed in 1954, when the FDA realized that some patients with serious medical conditions needed medicines that were still awaiting approval in the United States but were already approved elsewhere. This concern was raised again in 1988 when certain AIDS medications were not yet available in the United States. As a result, the FDA allows the personal importation of drugs under this type of specific circumstance. Enforcement of this policy, however, is quite difficult, and as a result Americans personally important thousands of drugs each year.

In the most recent bout of legislation concerning drug importation, the Medicare Prescription Drug, Improvement, and Modernization Act (MMA) of 2003 allows pharmacists and drug wholesalers to purchase drugs from Canadian manufacturers that meet U.S. guidelines for safety and efficacy. The act also allows for personal importation of a ninety-day supply of a drug, with a valid doctor's prescription, from a legitimate Canadian source. But section 1121 of the MMA includes a clause that the Secretary of the U.S. Department of Health and Human Services must activate the regulations regarding drug importation if he or she feels that such a policy will cause no risk to public safety. As of today, concerns regarding the real or perceived safety of drugs from Canada continue to thwart importation policies such as these.

SCOPE OF THE PROBLEM

Although limited information is available to measure the scope of drug importation in the United States today, holistic figures remain unknown. Officials and researchers have several problems when trying to gage the level of importation currently taking place. For one, many products are purchased in person at pharmacies across the border in Canada and Mexico, and thus enter the United States without any record. In addition, the sheer number of packages entering the country via various postal services makes estimates of drug importation difficult. Still, some studies have been conducted to give policymakers some scope of the problem.

According to the U.S. Customs and Border Protection (CBP), currently 355 "points of entry" exist for unapproved pharmaceuticals entering the United States.[3] Of these 355 entry points, 312 are ports, 29 are express consignments facilities, and 14 are international mail branches. (See Figure 16.1.) Based on relatively small pilot studies, the FDA believes that as many as 10 million packages of prescription drugs enter the United States annually, a figure that is also rapidly increasing from year to year.[4] The monetary

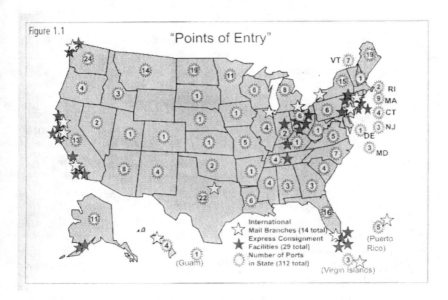

FIGURE 16.1. Points of entry. *Source:* Task Force on Importation (2004). Report on prescription drug importation. December. Washington, DC: U.S. Department of Health and Human Services, p. 11.

value of these packages is quite astounding. According to IMS Health, drugs crossing the Canadian-American border in 2003 alone were worth $695 million dollars ($408 million from Internet pharmacies and $287 million from physical border crossing sales).[5] Furthermore, HHS estimates that in 2003, 4.8 million packages of prescription drugs entered the United States via Canada. Based on the FDA's figure of 10 million packages entering annually, it can be estimated that yearly sales of imported drugs are worth more than $1.4 billion. At present, the monetary savings garnered by the purchasers of these 10 million packages of drugs are unknown, just as the relative safety and efficacy of those drugs remains a mystery.

WHAT DRUGS ARE IMPORTED
AND WHERE DO THEY COME FROM?

Similar to the figures quantifying the level of importation, both in the number of products and their monetary value, the types of drugs that are imported also remain elusive. Generally, it is believed that the majority of imported drugs are those that treat chronic conditions, such as hypertension and diabetes. It is also believed that imported drugs are more often sought by elderly patients, who may not be able to afford their medications otherwise. According to HHS, which recently acquired information on the subject from both the FDA and CBP, the following are some of the typical types/problems associated with imported drugs:

- *Improperly labeled drugs*—imported drugs sometimes have instructions in languages other than English.
- *Improperly packaged drugs*—drugs may be delivered in bags or envelopes rather than legitimate containers.
- *Controlled substances*—many imported drugs are classified as narcotics because of their abuse potential, and would normally be subject to regulation by the Drug Enforcement Administration (DEA).
- *Drugs withdrawn from the U.S. market for safety*—HHS cites Buscapina, or Dipyrone, which was taken off the market in 1977, as an example.
- *Foreign versions of FDA–approved Drugs*—the concern here is that foreign versions do not necessarily meet up with the safety and efficacy standards of the FDA.
- *Drugs that require titration*—many imported drugs, for example those that are related to thyroid conditions, that need to be carefully titrated for individual patients can be acquired without a prescription and thus with no legitimate monitoring.

- *Drugs with significant adverse drug-drug interactions*—HHS cites Zocor, Viagra, and Tramadol as examples.
- *Investigational products*—among imported drugs, some are not yet approved in the United States but are approved abroad. This occurs as a result of the varying prescription drug-approval practices of different nations.[6]

Recently, the U.S. government, which has become increasingly embroiled in the prescription importation debate, has attempted to pinpoint where the imported drugs are coming from. In doing this, it was found to be impossible to estimate the number or percent of FDA–approved drugs manufactured in foreign countries. Importantly, many of the drugs produced by American pharmaceutical companies are actually manufactured outside of the United States. Those facilities must be inspected by the FDA for quality control and must comply with all U.S. legislation regarding prescription drugs. For drug-manufacturing companies based in other countries that do not have FDA approval, as of today no system is in place for determining whether those drugs would comply with FDA standards. As a result, authorities do not know what percentage of imported drugs are actually in compliance with U.S. standards.

Because only FDA–approved drugs are considered to be safe and effective in the United States, even drugs manufactured in countries such as Canada, with comparable drug-approval processes and equally high safety and efficacy standards, are still considered unapproved drugs. That said, the vast majority of imported drugs are considered to be unapproved drugs. In its most recent studies, the FDA has concluded that Canada is responsible for the lion's share of all imported drugs, followed by Japan, India, the Netherlands, Taiwan, Thailand, Belize, Malaysia, Philippines, Nicaragua, Romania, Cambodia, Uganda, and the UK. Although considerable "foot traffic" is responsible for significant drug importation between Mexico and the United States, the Internet remains the primary mechanism for obtaining drugs from other countries. In 2001, it was estimated that somewhere between 300 to 400 Internet pharmacies specialized in the sale of imported drugs.[7] Today, it is believed that this figure is much greater.

In addition to Internet sales and foot traffic, additional avenues designed to facilitate the transfer of these drug to American consumers have recently appeared. Since 2000, the number of organized bus and train trips to Canada with the purpose of buying prescription drugs have steadily increased. In addition, some local and state governments have initiated their own imported prescription drug programs with cost savings in mind. As of today, only officials in Springfield, Massachusetts, and Montgomery, Alabama, have actually implemented such systems. In these cities, a Web site is set up specifically for city employees and others who can then buy drugs safely from Canadian pharmacies. In Montgomery, officials estimated that the city saved more than $500,000 by allowing its 4,100 employees and other retirees to buy drugs from Canada. More recently, Illinois Governor Rod Blagojevich requested permission from the HHS to import drugs from Canada to the entire state. The governor estimated that implementing such a plan could save the state as much as $56.6 million in prescription costs in addition to another $34.2 million in saving from out-of-pocket spending.[8] As a result of the increasing popularity of personal importation and more organized importation schemes, new businesses have emerged to streamline the process. Recently, a new type of pseudopharmacy began to appear called the "storefront pharmacy." These pharmacies, located in the United States, allow walk-in customers to buy drugs directly from Canada. When a patient walks into the storefront with a prescription, the pharmacy sends that prescription to a partnered pharmacy in Canada, that then mails the drug directly to the patient. Not surprisingly, this new type of pharmacy has been legally attacked by individual states, successfully in many cases, and deemed illegal. Nevertheless, operations such as these continue to surface.

REASON FOR CONCERN/POTENTIAL PROBLEMS

Although current knowledge about the extent and implications of drug importation is still lacking, its occurrence is no doubt widespread and increasing. The primary concern among policymakers who debate the issue is safety. In short, government officials, especially at the FDA, are concerned about imported drugs because of potential quality-assurance problems, the possibility of adulterated medicines and counterfeit drugs, labeling and language issues, and the use of medications in an unsupervised environment.

The principal concern of authorities regarding drug importation is that such drugs may not be equivalent to their American counterparts. One worry is that drugs may be subpotent, containing less active ingredient than the FDA–approved versions. In addition, though less common, a drug may be superpotent, containing too much of the active ingredient. In either of these cases the drug may not work as expected, cause additional or heightened side effects, or even do serious damage. Perhaps most frightening, patients taking subpotent drugs may not even realize the drug's deficiency until it is too late, the cumulative effect being an overall loss in therapeutic effect. Furthermore, even if the drug contains the same amount of active ingredient, it may have a number of additional ingredients that are different or exist in different proportions than expected. Experts recognize that even two pills that appear to be identical may be chemically different. Sub- and superpotency pose an especially acute threat to patients taking medicines with narrow therapeutic indications. These patients require specific titrated doses and continual close monitoring from a physician.

Clearly, legitimate risks are associated with imported medicines, but researchers have also indicated risks associated with reimported drugs. In most cases, reimported drugs, which are FDA–approved by definition, pose no danger to patients. Some concerns have been raised, however, regarding the containment and shipment methods as well as the labeling of these drugs. Researchers have pointed out that reimported drugs may be stored inappropriately (at inappropriate temperatures, lengths of time, etc.), and thus may lose therapeutic value. In addition, cases of mislabeled reimported drugs have occurred. In this scenario, foreign entities may purchase old or almost expired drugs, relabel them as new, and put them back on the market. The new labels may also contain false or inaccurate administration information or even be in another language. Concerns about labels and holding methods apply equally to both approved and unapproved drugs.

Internet Pharmacies

For a number of reasons, the bourgeoning Internet pharmacy business has also invited criticism and skepticism, especially regarding importation. Although the Internet is a useful tool for obtaining health information, it is also accompanied by the reality of fraudulent claims. The unsuspecting patient in search of affordable prescription drugs is left unassured that the online pharmacy is actually operating from the location it claims. Because it is incredibly easy for Internet pharmacies to misrepresent their location, the source of their products, whether their products were produced for consumption in their own country or for export only, and whether or not their drugs are FDA–approved, they create a buyer-beware scenario with little or no protection for regulatory bodies. Furthermore, many online pharmacies require the consumer to sign a disclaimer waiving their right to sue should an adverse reaction occur. Though this is true of most Internet pharmacies, one system, called the Verified Internet Pharmacy Practice Site (VIPPS), operated by the National Association of Boards of Pharmacy, evaluates online pharmacies for authenticity and provides a special logo to verified sites for consumers. Besides the possibility of fraudulent drugs, many Internet pharmacies do not require a prescription, which means drugs can be obtained without physician knowledge. As a result, the patient may take the drug improperly or remain unaware of potential drug-drug interactions.[9]

In all of the cases described, the full extent of their occurrence is unknown. However, cited examples of each exist and thus all of the scenarios must be taken seriously. For example, the FDA and HHS conducted their own research and found several fraudulent Internet pharmacies, which claim to operate out of Canada but actually reside in China or the Bahamas.[10] In addition, a study released by the General Accounting Office (GAO) found that of sixty-eight drugs purchased, each from a different Web site, forty-five were received without a prescription.[11] The full extent of actual health damage attributed to imported drugs will likely remain unknown. As of now, no national system for monitoring adverse events associated with imported drugs exists. Although the FDA maintains a system called MedWatch, which collects information on adverse drug events, it is not currently capable of distinguishing between approved and unapproved drugs. In addition, it is likely that many of the health repercussions of adulterated or otherwise fraudulent drugs will never be discovered, as they occur incrementally and over long periods of time. Although considerable risk is associated with importation as it stands today, the greatest dangers are associated with counterfeiting. (See Exhibit 16.1.)

COUNTERFEITING

What Are Counterfeit Pharmaceuticals?

Different types of counterfeit drugs exist, making it very difficult to agree on a single definition. The various types of counterfeit drugs include "rejects" that have been rejected by the manufacturer or regulatory authorities for quality reasons; "look-alikes," which contain little or no active ingredient; and relabeled medications that have expired but have been relabeled with a much later expiration date. According to the World Health Organization (WHO), a counterfeit pharmaceutical product is one that "is deliberately and fraudulently mislabeled with respect to identity and/or source. Counterfeiting can apply to both branded and generic products and counterfeit products may include products with the correct ingredients or with the wrong ingredients, without active ingredients, with insufficient active ingredient or with fake packaging."[12]

Where Is the Problem?

The magnitude of the counterfeiting problem, similar to the umbrella category of imported/reimported drugs, is very difficult to gauge. The prevalence of counterfeit drugs is generally known only when the perpetrators

EXHIBIT 16.1. Ordering prescription drugs from Canada over the Internet: How it works

1. For each medication requested, the patient must have a valid prescription issued by a physician licensed to practice medicine in the United States.

2. The patient completes and submits (online) or signs (hard copy) a health questionnaire and "customer agreement." The health questionnaire asks in varying degrees of detail about the patient's past medical history, family medical history, current medications, and drug allergies. The customer agreement is essentially a legal waiver.

3. The prescriptions (and completed forms, if hard copies are used) are sent to the company via fax or mail. Prescriptions for controlled substances and for medications that are not available in the United States are not honored.

4. The patient submits payment online using a credit card. (Most sites will not accept personal checks or money orders.)

5. A Canadian physician reviews the health questionnaire and submitted prescriptions and rewrites the prescriptions.

6. The medications are dispensed by a Canadian pharmacy. No more than a three-month supply is dispensed at one time, purportedly in accordance with what the FDA allows. Some sites state that they dispense medications only in the manufacturer's original container, so the amount dispensed may be more or less than the amount called for on the prescription (for example, a prescription may call for 90 tablets or 110 tablets, but the manufacturer's bottle of 100 tablets will be dispensed).

7. The medications are shipped to the patient. Usual delivery time is two to three weeks.

8. Refills may be initiated by the patient, by the online company (for example, the online company contacts the patient approximately three to four weeks before a refill is due to determine whether the patient wants the prescription refilled and whether there have been any changes in therapy), or shipped automatically.

Source: American Pharmacists Association. *Topics in Patient Care: Understanding Prescription Drug Importation.* 2003.

are caught, giving false impressions of the scale of the problem. WHO estimates that 10 percent of global pharmaceutical commerce involves counterfeit drugs, and annual earnings garnered from the sale of counterfeit pharmaceutical products are cited at $32 billion.[13]

To date, the majority of drug counterfeit rings have been traced to East Asian countries where the trade has developed enough to perfectly copy the packaging of the original drug. Experience has shown that substandard or counterfeit drugs are not manufactured for consumption in the country of origin, but are manufactured for export, one of the primary concerns of importation opponents.

Although counterfeiting is certainly not a new phenomenon, it has been the recipient of greater concern precisely as a result of its widespread and more frequent occurrence in recent years. In a WHO study on the reported cases of counterfeit drugs throughout the world, it was reported that developing countries of the Western Pacific (which include China, the Philippines, and Vietnam) made up the region with the most reported cases (48.7 percent), followed by developing areas of AFRO (Regional Office for Africa) with 19.7 percent. The industrialized areas of the Regional Office for Europe are third with 13.6 percent of all cases. (See Figure 16.2.) More recently, as pharmaceutical prices further increase and new markets for cheaper foreign drugs are developing, industrialized countries are increasingly becoming prime targets for counterfeiters.

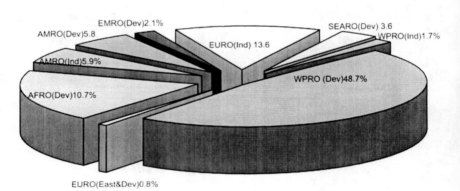

FIGURE 16.2. Geographical origin of cases (1982-1999) Total cases: 771. Countries are classified according to their WHO Regional Offices: AFRO— Regional Office for Africa; AMRO—Regional Office for the Americas; EMRO—Regional Office for the Eastern Mediterranean (includes most Middle East Countries and Pakistan); EURO—Regional Office for Europe; SEARO—Regional Office for South East Asia (includes India); WPRO—Regional Office for the Western Pacific (includes Australia, China, Philippines, and Vietnam). *Source:* Compiled from World Health Organization (1999). Summary of Counterfeit Drug Database as of April 1999. Unpublished report. Geneva: WHO Division of Drug Management and Policies.

Counterfeit Drugs Origins

With as much as 35 percent of the world's production of counterfeit pharmaceuticals originating within its borders, India is the leading country in counterfeit drug production.[14] Nigeria is second, responsible for 23.1 percent of counterfeit drugs, followed by Pakistan with a 13.3 percent share. Additional Asian countries excluding India and Pakistan account for 14.6 percent of the counterfeit drug production. (See Figure 16.3.) Though it is startling to see that the production of counterfeit drugs is so concentrated and yet its reach is so wide, more recent trends are even more disconcerting, indicating that occurrences of counterfeiting are increasing and the Western industrialized nations are more often targets for counterfeiters.

Dangers to Consumers

The specific dangers that counterfeit drugs pose to consumers depends to a great extent on the type of counterfeit, whether too little or no active ingredient exists, whether agents are substituted, or even whether harmful chemicals have been added. Drugs with a lack of active ingredient or a sub-therapeutic dose are harmful because they fail to deliver the expected, or in many cases, the essential treatment.[15] Drugs with substituted chemicals pose great and typically unknown dangers. Examples of the deleterious effects of counterfeiting are acute and worldwide in scope.

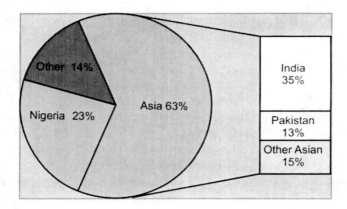

FIGURE 16.3. Origin of counterfeit drugs. *Source:* Compiled from World Health Organization (1997). Counterfeit Drugs: Report on Returned Questionnaires from Countries. Unpublished report. Geneva, Switzerland: WHO Division of Drug Management and Policies.

As the most problematic subset of the larger importation debate, counterfeiting is of great importance to drug regulators in the United States. From the current data available, which suggest that 10 percent of all pharmaceutical trade is counterfeit, it may be reasonable to extrapolate that, equally, 10 percent of imported drugs are counterfeit, though no such hard data exist.[16] Nevertheless, if health officials and policymakers are to implement safe importation programs, they will no doubt face serious challenges in confronting the ever-burgeoning counterfeit industry.

THE DRUG IMPORTATION DEBATE: PROFITS, SAFETY, AND INNOVATION

The drug importation debate is multifactorial, with at least three interest groups and concerned parties. U.S. government agencies, such as the FDA, are engaged in a balancing act between bolstering U.S. business enterprises with product safety and affordability for all Americans; some pharmaceutical companies themselves require large profits to reinvest in innovation; and, finally, the patients' primary concern is the acquisition of affordable prescriptions. For each stakeholder a trade-off exists, supporting business versus supporting the public for the government, earning profits versus supplying needed medications for pharmaceutical companies, and for many patients, affordable medications versus questions concerning drug safety and efficacy. For certain, most consumers would heartily welcome cheaper drugs, but how many would do so with even a small risk of obtaining substandard or harmful drugs?

The debate is also one that raises many questions: Why are drug prices so high in the United States, and conversely, why are they cheaper in most other countries? If high drug prices guarantee continued drug innovation, who is responsible for paying the bill—governments in developed nations, the citizens of those nations, the United States? Should the pharmaceutical companies accept more of the cost burden as well? How can the government create legislation that ensures the continued robustness of the American pharmaceutical industry while simultaneously ensuring the health of Americans? Which Americans are most effected by high drug prices and why? Finally, does drug importation/reimportation provide an answer capable of satisfying all vested interests? Clearly, each of these queries deserves an answer, since each comes ripe with its own complexities.

WHY ARE DRUGS SO EXPENSIVE?

As a result of high drug prices in the United States, many Americans are turning to other countries, especially to Canada, for their drugs. But why Canada? Americans who can't afford their drugs buy them from Canada because of its geographic proximity and equivalently high drug-safety standard.[17] Most important, however, drugs are cheaper in Canada—much cheaper. Prescription drugs in Canada range anywhere between 30 percent to 90 percent less expensive than their equivalent drugs in the United States.[18-20] This price differential is dependent on the type of drug in question, whether under U.S. patent, generic, or made in another country. The reduced prices also depend heavily on individual agreements worked out between pharmaceutical companies and the Canadian government. Unlike the United States, Canada, as with many other countries where drugs are cheaper, the government controls the price of drugs. They do this through a combination of controls on reimbursement, limits on rate of return of capital, and limits on overall spending.[21] The essential difference between nations such as Canada and the United States, when it comes to drug prices, is that in Canada a single arbiter of drug control exists. In other words, because health care is nationalized in Canada, as it is in many other nations around the world, a single government body is responsible for regulating national drug formularies and maintaining price caps for individual products. In Canada for example, the Patent Medicine Prices Review Board establishes the price manufacturers may charge for their products. In short, any drug manufacturer that wants to sell its products in Canada must negotiate and accept the price established by the Review Board if it wishes to sell its products in Canada at all. Conversely, the United States has no equivalent body, no single entity responsible for setting drug prices. Instead, *drug manufacturers* decide the price of a new drug and subsequently discount it to various managed-care organizations. Often, this means that the company, similar to any other company, whether manufacturing tires or refrigerators, charge what the demand will bear, the amount that people are willing to pay. As a result, drugs launched in the United States are often considerably more expensive than the same drugs in other countries. (See Figure 16.4.)

THE U.S. DRUG MARKET: WHO'S PAYING THE PRICE?

The U.S. market for prescription drugs is massive by anyone's standards. In 2003, prescription drug sales in the U.S. totaled more than $216.4 billion, representing almost half of all prescription drug sales worldwide. But this does not mean that Americans consumed half of all prescription drug prod-

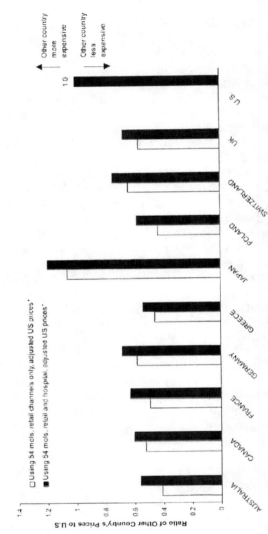

Price indices of innovator and licensed products in nine countries relative to the United States in 2003

All comparable 54 top-selling 2002 U.S. products, manufacturer prices for retail outlets (US$/kilo or IU), Weighted by U.S. consumption (kilos or IU)

FIGURE 16.4. Price indices of innovator and licensed product in nine countries relative to the United States in 2003.

ucts produced that year. It does mean that Americans paid more for their medicines, significantly more.

For the majority of Americans, those who are employed and receive health benefits, the cost of drugs remains a nonissue. For this group, the real price of drugs is masked by copays, which hide the real costs paid through employers to insurance providers, which in turn pay for prescription medications. But for the more than 45 million uninsured Americans, the cost of drugs, which must be paid for out of pocket, presents a more immediate and acute concern. The disproportionate level of coverage among Americans has led many researchers to conclude that the people most adversely affected by high drug prices in the United States are those among the lowest socioeconomic group, with no health insurance and no income to pay for high-priced medications. It is primarily the members of this group then that are forced to put their own health and often the health of their families in jeopardy by seeking out cheaper drugs from other countries. As one researcher states, "it is unfair that the burden of stimulating pharmaceutical company research is borne to the greatest extent by the most economically vulnerable Americans."[22] With so many people left unable to afford prescription medicines in the United States, one might ask, Why don't pharmaceutical manufacturers simply lower their prices? Again, a simple question with a complex answer.

PROFITS AND INNOVATION: FACT OR FICTION?

The pharmaceutical industry in the United States is without a doubt one of the greatest examples of American industry. Its development over the past century is nothing less than a brilliant success. The industry is responsible for the creation of thousands of medicines, many that are life saving or that significantly improve a person's quality of life. The particular success of the American pharmaceutical industry is the result of a complex system that protects and supports innovation through the granting of temporary monopolies (patents) while also bolstering a highly competitive, free-market atmosphere. Over the past century, this approach has fueled the fire of innovation, which continues to burn today. As proof, between 2000 and 2003, the United States was responsible for bringing to market 47 percent of all new active medical substances worldwide, a significant rise from the previous years.[23] As a result, the U.S. pharmaceutical industry earns billions of dollars in profit each year, employs hundreds of thousands of workers, and enjoys a spot as one the top industries in America. Seen in this light, it becomes clearer why government officials are not entirely enthusiastic about implementing measures that would hurt the industry.

For their part, individual U.S. pharmaceutical companies could reduce prices if they wanted too. They sell the same products in other countries sometimes for a price that is as much as 60 percent less. The debate here concerns a trade-off between profits and progress in the form of pharmaceutical innovation. The pharmaceutical industry argues that the price differentials between countries, and particularly the profits earned from the American market, the largest in the world, are reinvested to fund new research that in turn leads to new medicines. These industry experts purport that importation and reimportation, by limiting profits, also limit innovation, which negatively affects everyone. Interestingly, the pharmaceutical industry, unlike the FDA and HHS, does not raise concerns regarding the safety of imported drugs, as this argument, especially in the case of reimportation, might ultimately reflect poorly on the industry's own products. But evidence supports the industry's claims linking profits to innovation. For one, a commonly cited, though often contested figure for the cost of bringing a new drug to market, including the costs of conducting vast and expensive clinical trials, is $800 million.[24] In addition, it is known that for every drug that actually makes it through the rigorous FDA process and is released on the market, perhaps thousands of products never leave the lab. It is precisely the high costs of drug development, for the pharmaceutical industry, that justify high prices for those products that are on the market.

Although evidence supports the connection between large profits and R & D, it remains unknown at what point reducing profits will adversely impact innovation. However, there is no shortage of arguments supporting the idea that reducing some profit would not significantly impact R & D. For one, opponents argue that pharmaceutical manufacturers make considerable profits from products that utilize new formulations or delivery methods, drugs for which little new research is necessary. It is also argued by some that even with price reductions, innovation would continue with the massive yearly investment of the National Institutes of Health (NIH). According to one source, NIH funding was responsible for the majority of the most clinically significant drugs from 1965 to 1992.[25] Thus the argument goes that the American taxpayer is the real investor in pharmaceutical innovation. Finally, the pharmaceutical industry has been attacked for spending huge capital sums on marketing rather than on R & D. According to many reports, typical industry allocation of profits on advertising hovers around 18 percent, whereas investment in R & D remains around 12.5 percent. Thus, opponents argue that should price restrictions be put in place, manufacturers would reduce spending on marketing first, since R & D remains the lifeblood of the industry. Although the debate over the effect of importation on industry profits and ultimately on innovation will likely continue, the European model of parallel imports provides a research model for American policymakers and health researchers to consider.

LEARNING FROM THE EUROPEAN UNION AND THE SYSTEM OF PARALLEL IMPORTS

Although the debate over drug importation rages in the United States today, Europe has had experience with government-regulated importation for the past three decades. More specifically, twenty-five years ago, the original fifteen members of the European Union (EU) agreed on a system of commercial parallel trade for pharmaceuticals, more commonly called parallel importation (PI). Essentially, the enactment of PI within the European Union allows countries with relatively high drug prices, such as Germany, to import the same drugs, under certain conditions, from countries where the drugs are cheaper, such as Greece or Spain. The EU defines parallel importing as "legal importation of specific branded drugs, by licensed distributors, from one country's market into another." Within the EU, a licensed pharmaceutical distributor, within any member state, is legally allowed to purchase drugs from any other member state as long as the drug product has the same active ingredient and was manufactured by the same manufacturer. These distributors can then sell imported drugs to consumers in their own nations at lower prices. Although it is a relatively open system, important limitations are in place.

For one, member states are not allowed to import drugs from countries outside of the EU. Second, member states have the authority to restrict an import if it poses any threat to public health. Third, manufacturers can manage or limit their distribution to control the level of import/export. Fourth, individual drug manufacturers are permitted to block an import if it is found to be tampered with or relabeled in any way other than what is necessary to sell it in the receiving country. And most important, as already mentioned, only licensed distributors can sell imported drugs, thus personal importation is not permitted.

The EU system of parallel importation is relevant to the current U.S. debate on the subject primarily because the vast majority of research conducted regarding the PI system indicates that issues concerning product safety and efficacy are almost nonexistent. Furthermore, studies indicate that Europeans are not concerned about receiving fraudulent drugs from other EU member states. This indicates that such a policy, were it to be adopted in the United States might also prove critics concerned with safety, wrong. In addition, the EU experience has shown that importation does not necessarily negatively impact pharmaceutical innovation or create supply problems within individual nations.

But PI is also relevant because it illuminates certain peculiarities of the U.S. system, which are of concern. According to a recent study on PI in the EU, it was found that four conditions were necessary in order for consumers to benefit from this kind of importation:

- Consumers must have an incentive to seek out imported drugs, usually this being because they cost less. Because most EU governments have strict pharmaceutical price regulation systems in place, imported drugs are often no cheaper than those already sold from within the country.
- Consumers need to be aware that such a system exists and actively seek out venues that distribute imported drugs.
- A continual supply of imported drugs must be available for consumers to notice a long-term economic value.
- Consumers must not perceive imported drugs as to be any less safe and effective than locally sourced products. [26]

These conditions are interesting because they exemplify what is different about the U.S. system. First of all, because the government does not regulate drug prices (making them more costly than elsewhere), PI, if it were implemented in the United States, would likely take place on a much larger scale than in the EU, since the incentive is much greater. Assuming that this policy were implemented and parallel imports drastically increased, it is likely that pharmaceutical companies, which would most certainly be more affected in the United States since pharmaceuticals is the number-one market, would resort to drug limitations, curtailing the entire system. Thus, although the PI system in the EU shows that such a policy can be implemented without causing significant public health concerns, it does not suggest that an equivalent policy in the United States would lead to overall cheaper drug prices.

IS IMPORTATION/REIMPORTATION A VIABLE SOLUTION?

It remains clear that as long as Americans can obtain cheaper drugs from other nations with equivalent drug evaluation standards, the practice of importation/reimportation will continue. The extent to which economic benefits can accrue to consumers through the expansion of such a system, however, remains unclear. U.S. consumers seeking cheaper drugs have clear incentives to buy elsewhere. But forces beyond the consumer's control exist that will most certainly limit the benefits of importing drugs.

For one, the U.S. drug market is simply too large to implement drug importation on a grand scale. To take the Canadian example, Canada makes up 2 percent of the worldwide pharmaceutical market, whereas the United States makes up more than 50 percent.[27] As a result, the Canadian pharmaceutical supply is simply not large enough to meet U.S. demands, were they to grow drastically. Because any legislation in the United States permitting importation would most certainly place restrictions on where imports may come from, not enough imports would be available, and the exporting countries would stop exporting drug to the United States in order to sustain adequate drug supplies for themselves.

This situation is easily exacerbated by pharmaceutical manufacturers, who can place limits on product distribution to countries that export cheap drugs to other nations. In the case of Canada, this has already happened. Under pressure from the pharmaceutical industry, the Canadian government has increasingly been forced to enact legislation curbing the export of its drugs.[28,29] As pharmaceutical companies protect their interests by limiting distribution, drug shortages will increase prices in exporting countries, reducing the overall incentive for importation. Thus although drug importation may offer short-term savings, it does not provide a sound long-term viable solution to high drug prices.

THE FUTURE OF DRUG IMPORTATION/REIMPORTATION

As long as prescription drugs can be obtained at lower prices from various venues around the world, and as more people turn to the Internet to buy drugs, drug importation/reimportation will surely continue for the foreseeable future. On the other hand, the pharmaceutical industry will do everything in its power to maintain control over drug prices worldwide. As a result, distribution restrictions for various markets are likely to occur, which inevitably leads to tougher laws concerning the exportation of drugs and overall higher prices abroad. As this occurs, one future scenario could develop in which as prices increase abroad through product limitations and regulatory action, they decrease in the United States, evening out drug markets around the world. It is also likely that as importation continues to dig into industry profits, new measures such as creating different dosage forms, color-coding schemes, or packaging differences will be utilized. These measures would handicap importation laws that require imported drugs to be equivalent dosage forms, sizes, colors, and packaging.

In addition to these counterimportation measures, technological advances that support importation are also likely to play a more important role in the future. Particularly, the utilization of pedigree records (electronic or paper based) will be employed to track drugs along the distribution chain, thus increasing the culpability of drug handlers along the way. In addition, radio frequency identification (RFID) chips will be embedded within drug containers, making their location transparent at all times. Improvements in the ability to track drugs as they move from the manufacturer to the consumer will no doubt serve as partial deterrents to would-be counterfeiters. Furthermore, increased globalization will require improvements in communications capability between governments and thus, between drug regulatory authorities. As communication channels open up and as drug-evaluation systems of various nations become more transparent, the perceptibility of safety of drugs from abroad may increase. But the countervailing forces presented here will continue to collide in the future, with various interest groups putting pressure on government officials to both support and restrict importation, slowing any new legislative action.

CONCLUSION

With huge price differentials between the United States and other nations around the world, the proliferation of drug importation/reimportation is an understandable phenomenon. Increasingly, Americans are seeking cheaper prescription drugs and obtaining those drugs via Internet pharmacies or by physically carrying drugs across the border. Simultaneously, growing concerns exist that this phenomenon poses a significant safety threat to Americans since the importation phenomenon lies wholly outside of FDA oversight, making counterfeiting a growing reality. Whether grounded or baseless, these concerns, coupled with quarrels over resources for innovation and maintaining adequate drug supplies, define and shape the issue. Although the future of importation remains unknown, it can be expected to continue to provoke both support and controversy in the foreseeable future.

NOTES

1. Task Force on Drug Importation (2004). *Report on Prescription Drug Importation*. December. Washington, DC: U.S. Department of Health and Human Services.
2. U.S. Food and Drug Administration (2005). History of the FDA: The 1938 Food, Drug, and Cosmetic Act. Available at: http://www.fda.gov/oc/historyoffda/section2.html. Accessed on July 7/12, 2005.

3. Task Force on Drug Importation (2004), p. 11.

4. Task Force on Drug Importation (2004), p. 11.

5. IMS Health (2005). Canadian Cross-Border Pharmaceutical Sales: Q1/2002-Q12004. Fairfield, CT: IMS Management Consulting.

6. Task Force on Drug Importation (2004), pp. 13-14.

7. U.S. Food and Drug Administration (2003). Statement of John M. Taylor, Associate Commissioner for Regulatory Affairs before the U.S. House of Representative Committee on Energy and Commerce, Subcommittee on Oversight and Investigations. March 10.

8. Wilson, J.F. (2004). Cheaper Drugs in Foreign Markets Increase the Focus on Domestic Drug Prices. Annals of Internal Medicine 140(8): 677-680.

9. General Accounting Office (2004). Internet Pharmacies: Some Pose Safety Risks for Consumers. Report to the Chairman, Permanent Subcommittee on Investigations, Committee on Governmental Affairs, U.S. Senate. June.

10. U.S. Food and Drug Administration (2004). FDA News: FDA Test Results of Prescription Drugs from Bogus Canadian Website Show All Products are Fake and Substandard. July 13. Available at: http:www.fda.gov/bbs/topics/news/2004/NEW 01087.html.

11. General Accounting Office (2004).

12. World Health Organization (1999). *Guidelines for the development of measures to combat counterfeit drugs.* Geneva, Switzerland: WHO Department of Essential Drugs and Other Medicines. WHO/EDM/QSM/99.1.

13. General Accounting Office (2004).

14. World Health Organization (1997). Counterfeit Drugs: Report on Returned Questionnaires from Countries. Unpublished report. Geneva, Switzerland: WHO Division of Drug Management and Policies.

15. International Federation of Pharmaceutical Manufacturers and Associations (1997). Issue Paper: Counterfeiting of Medicinal Products. February. Geneva, Switzerland: IFPMA.

16. World Health Organization (1999).

17. Choudhry, N.K. and Detsky, A.S. (2005). A Perspective on US Drug Reimportation. *Journal of the American Medical Association* 293(3): 358-362.

18. Ibid 8.

19. Young, D. (2004). HHS Task Force Hears Concerns About Importation, Drug Prices. *American Journal of Health-System Pharmacy* 61(9): 868-869.

20. Young, D. (2004). Experts Debate Drug Importation. *American Journal of Health-System Pharmacy* 61(9): 874.

21. HHS Importation Task Force (2004). Presentation of Patricia M. Danzon, Listening Session #4, April 27.

22. Choudhry, N.K. and Detsky, A.S. (2005), p. 360.

23. Sources: *Scrip Magazine,* Scrip Review Issue, Script Yearbook, Scrip 1987 NCE Review, Scrip NCE Review, Scrip World Pharmaceutical.

24. Dimasi J.A., Hansen R.W., and Grabowski H.G. (2003). The Price of Innovation: New Estimates of Drug Development Costs. *J Health Econ* 22: 151-158.

25. National Institutes of Health (2000). *NIH Contributions to Pharmaceutical Development.* Bethesda, MD: NIH.

26. Gross, D. and Taylor, D. (2005). *Parallel Trading in Medicines: Europe's Experience and Its Implications for Commercial Drug Importation in the United States.* AARP Public Policy Institute.

27. War, C. (2004). Economic and Policy Implications of Reimportation: a Canadian Perspective. *Managed Care* 13: 17-20.

28. Canada May Ban U.S. Drug Sales When Supply Falls (2005). *Wall Street Journal.* June 30. Reuters News Service.

29. The Green Sheet (2005). Canada to Block U.S. Drug Imports With Legislation, Regulatory Action. July 11.

Chapter 17

Structure and Dynamics
of the Pharmaceutical Industry

Earlene Lipowski
Patrick McKercher

An examination of the structure and dynamics of the pharmaceutical manufacturing community illustrates how the industry adapts to economic, political, and technological change to preserve its functionality. Prior to WWII, pharmaceutical manufacturers in the United States operated as a segment of the chemicals industry. Unlike most industries in which growth is spurred by innovation in the methods of production, the pharmaceutical industry evolved as a distinct industrial entity based on discoveries in basic chemistry and innovations in chemical engineering.

The discovery of Tagamet (cimetidine) in the early 1970s marked an important turning point in the evolution of the industry, which was made possible by advances in science and technology. Tagamet was created using targeted drug design whereby new chemical entities are built to zone in on specific biological targets. The success of targeted drug design introduced an era of pharmaceutical innovation characterized by ever greater intensity in research and development (R & D) and higher returns on those investments. The products that resulted included novel treatments for herpes, AIDS, ovarian cancer, migraine, schizophrenia, depression, hypertension, and high cholesterol.[1]

At the start of the twenty-first century another conspicuous change was underway as the research emphasis shifted from chemistry to biotechnology (see also Chapter 18). Interdisciplinary research in biochemistry, cell biology, immunology, genetics, and molecular biology coupled with advances in information and imaging technologies drove these changes. A biotechnology sector emerged within the pharmaceutical industry during the 1990s, and within a decade the Pharmaceutical Research and Manufacturers of America was referring to all of its members as biopharmaceutical firms.[2] Independent of PhRMA, the Biotechnology Industry Organization, better known as BIO was formed in 1993 with the merger of two small associations: The Industrial Biotechnology Association (IBA), representing larger, established companies, and the Association of Biotechnology Companies (ABC), which tended to represent emerging companies and universities working specifically in biotechnology.

Developments in science and technology at the end of the twentieth century did not occur in isolation but were accompanied by significant social trends and economic developments. Even though science and technology provided unprecedented opportunities for investors, the 1990s was a time of rapidly rising health care expenditures, which forced examination of health policy and attempts to restructure health care delivery. Expanding government sponsored health programs, investor-driven health care organizations and managed care confronted the status quo in the pharmaceutical industry.

Public policy directed at the U.S. pharmaceutical industry provides some of the best examples of how government incentives foster innovations that have significant human and social value. However, these policies are not without controversy and criticism. The pharmaceutical industry faces myriad stakeholders including researchers, regulators, patients, payers, health care providers, and stockholders. The aims of the stakeholders for a substantial return on investment and the desire of consumers for readily accessible and affordable pharmaceuticals sometimes conflict. Although observable changes are taking place within the pharmaceutical industry, the pace of change and the ultimate outcome is difficult to forecast. Adaptation of the industry to societal pressures may be inevitable, but must take into account three traits that have been constants in the U.S. pharmaceutical industry: strong protection of intellectual property, demand for continuous innovation, and staunch defense of free market pricing.

INTELLECTUAL PROPERTY PROTECTION (IPP)

The pharmaceutical industry depends on patent protection to achieve a return on the sizeable investment of time and money required for new drug development. Current estimates are that an innovator firm can expect to spend fourteen years and nearly $900 million in research, testing, and regulatory approval before receiving the first dollar of revenue for a new drug product.[3] Profitability is closely tied to sales of patented drugs that are not threatened by generics or close therapeutic substitutes.

Patent laws were designed to give firms the ability to collect monopoly rents on innovations, and the pharmaceutical industry is a prime example of the benefits the law intended. The innovator firm either commercializes the product directly or licenses the rights to another firm while blocking rivals from introducing a competing duplicate product.

However, initial patents to protect expensive new products are not the only form of intellectual property protection (IPP) critical to the success of the pharmaceutical industry. A succession of statutes (see also Chapter 3) augment the patent system by (1) extending the term of the original patent, (2) shortening the period of time consumed by clinical testing and regulatory review, and (3) granting market exclusivity. At times laws and regulations produced by Congress and government agencies have resulted in multiple and additive protections for prescription drugs.

Table 17.1 summarizes the major legislative initiatives that have extended IPP for the pharmaceutical industry. Arguably the "single most important piece of legislation to affect the modern pharmaceutical industry" is the Hatch-Waxman Act of 1984. The act restored nearly all of the patent life that had been lost to FDA requirements for clinical trials and evidence review.[4]

Other measures passed in the 1990s considerably reduced the time required for clinical studies and FDA approval. The Prescription Drug User Fee Act (PDUFA) 1992 authorized the collection of user fees from pharmaceutical manufacturers to provide additional resources for the FDA to expedite the market-approval process. Pharmaceutical manufacturers accepted the fees, which were marginal in relation to the revenue that could be earned through faster approval and longer effective patent life. The Food and Drug Administration Modernization Act (FDAMA) of 1997 renewed the user fees and added fast-track authority that allowed the FDA to move more quickly on priority drugs. FDAMA also conferred six months market exclusivity to the end of an existing patent term for manufacturers that submit clinical studies specific to pediatric patients. Each of these acts has proven to be a powerful motivator to the industry. Altogether pharmaceutical industry experienced an increase of 2.1 years of patent protection from 1993-1999.[5]

Thus complex government requirements for market approval complement patent protection to enhance the competitive position of a drug product. Compared to pharmaceuticals, multifaceted electronic devices or machinery can involve the application of hundreds of patented components. In the industries in which products are complex and each component has multiple patents, factors such as secrecy, marketing savvy, and lead time work in conjunction with patent law to assure that patents and market exclusivity produce profits. Pharmaceuticals have relatively few patents per product.

Through its regulations the FDA protects innovator firms by creating de facto barriers to prospective competitors.[6] It is difficult for other firms, especially small new companies, to enter particular therapeutic markets when

TABLE 17.1. Laws that affect the patent life of prescription drugs.

Law	Description	Duration
1983 Orphan Drug Act	Exclusivity granted to drugs for indications with less than 200,000 U.S. patients. Protection from generic and other branded versions of the same drug for the same indication.	7 years from date of approval
1984 Hatch-Waxman Act	Exclusivity granted to new chemical entities to compensate for delays in regulatory approval process.	Up to 5 years from date of approval
	Exclusivity granted to modified versions of existing drugs with new clinical data, e.g., new dosage form or new clinical indication.	3 years from date of approval
	Automatic stay of approval of generic granted when holder sues for patent infringement.	Up to 30 months, or litigation concluded
	Exclusivity granted to first generic applicant prior to expiration patents for brand drug. Protection from approval of other generic versions during term of exclusivity.	Up to 180 days or until court declares patent invalid or not infringed
1992 Prescription Drug User Fee Act	Faster FDA review processes funded by establishment fees, new drug application fees and product fees paid by manufacturers.	FDA review reduced 2.1 yrs
1994 Uruguay Round Agreements Act	Set patent life to international standard for patents covering composition of matter, method of use, formulation, product by process.	20 years from date of filing
1997 FDA Modernization Act	Codified accelerated approval regulations and policies & procedures for fast-track approval.	FDA review reduced 2.1 yrs
	Granted in exchange for pediatric clinical trials requested by the FDA.	6 months added to life of patent or exclusivity

compliance with regulations represents substantial capital and time investment, demands a high level of technical expertise, and gives competing firms time to develop defensive marketing strategies. Although government policies on IPP and regulatory approval of new drug products surely have direct social benefits, they also have strategic implications for the industry.

R & D INTENSITY

The necessity for continuous innovation is a significant economic reality in the pharmaceutical industry. This is illustrated by the typical life cycle of a drug product (see Figure 17.1). The sales of the average new drug typically rise in a logarithmic pattern, achieving a peak roughly nine years after

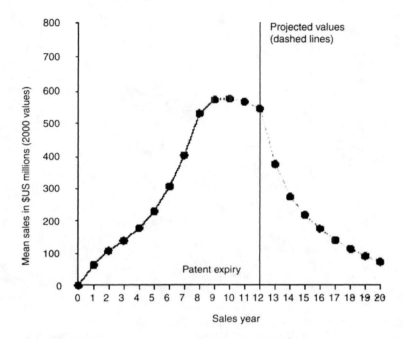

FIGURE 17.1. Actual and projected worldwide sales values for a representative sample product. *Source:* Grabowski H, Vernon J, DiMasi JA (2002). Returns on research and development for 1990s new drug introductions. *Pharmacoeconomics* 20(Suppl 3): 11-29. Reprinted with permission from Wolters Kluwer Health.

approval, after which sales tend to remain relatively stable until year twelve, at which point the patent expires and sales decline sharply due to competition from generically equivalent products.[7]

The life cycle pattern of products with the highest sales revenues is even more dramatic than the average drug (see Figure 17.2). Drugs in the top decile of sales include products that achieve blockbuster status by generating $1 billion or more in sales revenue per year. The top drugs tend to represent therapeutic breakthroughs and have a longer patent life than average, about fourteen years. However, they are prime targets for cost containment measures of health care payers and sales revenue drops dramatically after the patents expire.

Pharmaceutical benefits managers (PBMs) (see also Chapter 13) have become aggressive and adept at promoting the use of generic products in

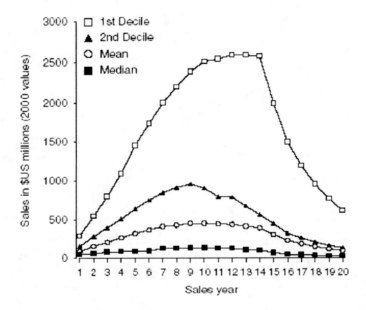

FIGURE 17.2. Worldwide sales profiles of 1990 to 1994 new drug introductions. *Source:* Grabowski H, Vernon J, DiMasi JA (2002). Returns on research and development for 1990s new drug introductions. *Pharmacoeconomics* 20(Suppl 3): 11-29. Reprinted with permission from Wolters Kluwer Health.

place of the brand-name innovator and at direct prescribing and dispensing toward less expensive alternatives within a therapeutic class. When Prozac (fluoxetine) lost its patent in 2001, Express Scripts reported that the market share of the generic version grew from zero to more than 20 percent of the market in eight months while the market share of the brand product fell from more than 25 percent to less than 5 percent. When Glucophage (metformin) lost its patent less than one year later, Express Scripts was able to produce a market shift of the same magnitude in the span of a single month.[8] More recently, PBMs have been able to extend the effect of generic availability to the entire therapeutic class. When a generic drug is the first in its therapeutic class, the sales of all brands in the entire class have dropped.[9]

Therefore life cycle management strategy for manufacturers with top-selling drugs relies more than ever on a vigorous defense of IPP and extensions that lengthen the effective patent life. For example, the original patent holders introduced a single isomeric form of Claritin as Clarinex and a single of isomer of Prilosec as Nexium when their respective patents expired.

The strategy added several years of effective product life. Despite efforts to defend intellectual property, however, the only true solutions for sustaining gross revenues is to continuously replace older products with completely new ones and introducing new medical entities addressing previously unmet medical needs.

U.S. public policy generally backs programs that provide economic incentives for pharmaceutical R & D, although the wisdom of some of these policies has come under attack. For example, when the Orphan Drug Act was passed in 1983 it was generally viewed as a model piece of legislation for stimulating R & D by rewarding new treatments for rare diseases with IPP. The incentive, seven years market exclusivity, resulted in the approval of 217 drugs designated as orphans by 2001.[10]

The majority of orphan drug products provide efficacious treatment, but the products presumably have limited sales potential to a small patient population. However, notable cases exist in which the innovator manufacturer realized expanded sales and profited handsomely. For example, the manufacturer of the first antiretrovirals for the treatment of HIV/AIDs benefited as the number of people infected grew well beyond the 200,000 that define an orphan condition. Manufacturers also profit when products for conditions with few treatment options are able to command high prices, or if the innovation proves effective for treating other, more prevalent diseases. Critics have questioned whether the Orphan Drug Act represents a net benefit to society whenever patient candidates for orphan drug therapies are grossly underestimated, resulting in significant sales and profits.

The development of drugs to treat endemic diseases in developing countries is another circumstance in which the economic incentive is not strong enough to stimulate pharmaceutical R & D. Although large in number, the populations with the greatest need for drugs to treat malaria or dengue fever cannot afford to pay the prices that prevail in the developed world. This situation leads to demands to override IPP and provide early or selective approval of generic formulations when useful but high-priced drugs exist.

Superior public policy would seek to preserve market exclusivity as a reward for firms willing to accept the inherent risk in finding innovative products while reducing the likelihood of what might be perceived as excessive profit. One suggestion has been to guarantee minimal sales at a preset price as an incentive for R & D efforts. Proponents of this approach also argue that it is likely to be efficient because a pharmaceutical manufacturer is in the best position to recognize promising research avenues and to deploy resources commensurate with the known sales potential.[11]

The U.S. government also provides support of pharmaceutical R & D through cooperative agreements between federal agencies and the industry.[12] The specific provisions are in the Bayh-Dole Act of 1980, Stevenson-

Wydler Act of 1980, and Federal Technology Transfer Act of 1986. Taken together, these acts supply the following directives and mechanisms for public-private collaboration.

1. *Active promotion of technology transfer.* Government-sponsored researchers are required to promote their discoveries to commercial firms. Each agency has a technology-transfer office whose role is to facilitate industry use and commercialization of publicly funded research.
2. *Cooperative Research and Development Agreements (CRADAs).* The National Institutes of Health (NIH) and government-funded university researchers are permitted to enter formal agreements with private entities for sharing personnel, services, equipment, resources, and knowledge on a specific project. The private sector partner is then able to secure exclusive rights to the products produced under the arrangement.
3. *Patent rights to government research.* Government agencies assist industry partners in obtaining patent protection on publicly funded research results if the firms agree to invest in additional R & D to commercialize their discoveries.
4. *Technology licensing.* NIH and other government agencies can grant licenses to private companies that use government-funded research findings in proprietary research or to develop the ideas into commercial products. Under technology licensing the government recovers some of its research investment through licensing fees.

When the products of public-private collaboration are successful, critics argue about whether it is appropriate for private business to profit without returning a share of the profit to government. The prevailing position, however, is that a public investment that is not commercialized is an even greater loss to society. Others maintain that government commercialization of discoveries is an unacceptable alternative in a free market system.

Evidence suggests that the introduction of innovative pharmaceutical products has slowed over the past decade despite increasing R & D expenditures and favorable public policy.[13] R & D expenditures roughly doubled in real terms from 1982 to 1992 as measured in capitalized and uncapitalized dollars. By 2001 R & D spending tripled the expenditures in 1992. R & D as a percentage of sales grew from 10 percent in 1980 to a peak of 17 percent in 1994 and then stabilized at 16 to 17 percent of sales to the present.[14] In 2005 R & D investment by the pharmaceutical industry totaled $38.8 billion.[15]

No published research demonstrates a correlation between the level of industry R & D spending and measurable advances in therapeutics.[16] Some speculation even exists that modern industry practices have contributed to the apparent decline in R & D productivity. That is, firms operating under continuous pressure for novel and distinctive products but unsure that they can satisfy stockholders' demands have come to depend more on the return on investment gained by aggressive marketing rather than from pioneering research on drugs. Whereas the ten largest pharmaceutical companies invest an average of 13.7 percent of revenue in R & D, the annual spending for marketing and promotion is 34.4 percent of sales.[17] Although information on the precise amount of the expenditures for research or promotion is difficult to access and allocate, it appears that spending on promotion relative to sales has remained relatively constant over the last decade.[18]

However, the focus of the industry R & D on blockbuster drugs is a strategy that is consistent with a greater marketing orientation. The industry concentrates resources on compounds likely to become blockbusters while deferring work on products not likely to generate a billion dollars or more in annual sales. Manufacturers launch new products with powerful marketing plans designed to overwhelm competitors and with strategies for rapid expansion to global markets.[19] Promotional allocations equal to sales in the first year decrease to 50 percent of sales in the second year, and drop to 25 percent of sales by the third year. Companies have been known to allocate five to ten percent of the first-year sales projections for promotions that take place up to two years before the product introduction.[20] What is not known is whether these strategic changes are just a temporary response to a shortfall of innovative new products or a more enduring change in the culture of the industry.

The fact remains that the traditional brand-oriented pharmaceutical industry is strongly influenced by competitive and economic factors. Research over the past four decades is consistent and clear: financial success is directly linked to the intensity of R & D and the contribution margins of innovative products it produces.[21,22,23]

PRICING AND PROFITABILITY

The pharmaceutical industry experienced a sharp rise in profitability during the 1970s and 1980s. From 1993 to 2002 it held first place in the Fortune 500 industry rankings in terms of net profit as a percent of revenues, and at or near the top in terms of returns as a percentage of either stockholders' equity or total assets. Net profit during this period ranged from lows of 14.4 and 14.3 percent in 1995 and 2003, respectively, to a peak of 18.9 percent in 1999 and remained above 18 percent through 2001. Commercial banks eclipsed the pharmaceutical industry in profitability in 2004, and the mining and crude oil industries surpassed both with spectacular gains in 2005. Despite falling to third in the 2005 rankings, the profitability of the pharmaceutical industry over the past three decades has been persistent and impressive, attractive to investors, and a target of criticism and scrutiny.

Fortune 500 rankings, however, reflect the median performance for the largest firms in the industry. Although profits are high in the aggregate, performance varies greatly across firms and across products within firms.[24] Profitability is highly skewed toward large returns for a small minority of products. The top decile of sales revenue accounts for 52 percent of total present value for the industry, an increase from 46 percent in the 1980s. Only one-third of products have present value in excess of the average R & D cost.[25] The profitability of the leading brand-oriented firms is increasingly driven by innovative products and best-in-class drugs. Profits are the industry's primary source of funding for its ongoing R&D.[26]

The mean return on investment (ROI) for the industry is 11.5 percent, which is slightly above the industry cost of capital of 11 percent as calculated by capital asset pricing model. Returns are described as modestly above cost of capital in the industry,[27] what Scherer describes in economic terms as a "virtuous rent seeking model."[28] That is, when profits are high the industry will increase R & D investments until profit margins fall in a self-regulating cycle.

What economists might describe as virtuous behavior vexes consumers and taxpayers. Prescription drug expenditures have been rising at double-digit rates, although several studies suggest that the increased spending is attributable to more than price hikes. The precise percentage varies across several studies, but increases in the prices of existing drugs explain only about 25 percent of the growth. More than 40 percent of the rise in expenditures is attributed to the increasing reliance on treatment with prescription drugs. The annual number of prescriptions rose from 7.8 per person in 1993 to 11.8 in 2003. Preference for newer, higher-priced drugs in place of older, less-expensive drugs accounts for the approximately one-third of the increase.[29] Thus, spending increases are the result of a combination of price, utilization, and adoption of innovation.

Irrespective of the reasons, increasing expenditures for consumers coupled with industry profitability has generated public controversy about the pricing policies of pharmaceutical firms. Concern about the value received in return for the mounting expense exists. Any defense of pharmaceutical pricing is complicated by the inherent nature of the product. The manufacturers incur high costs for development, but generally the cost of production is quite low. When most drugs can be produced for just "pennies per pill," it is difficult to explain why a price greatly exceeds the cost of production to customers who do not view these as discretionary purchases.

More than one study of drug pricing suggests that products have higher introductory prices for compounds when they represent a gain over existing treatment modalities or are intended for short-term use.[30,31,32] Conversely, introductory prices are lower than the prices of existing drugs when the products are close substitutes. This pattern is consistent with the position that prices for new drugs bear some relation to their clinical value and are responsive to price sensitivity. Apart from new drug introductions, average drug prices generally have followed price inflation trends in the overall economy.

Individual corporate pricing decisions are determined by considerations that are difficult to quantify. Industry experts suggest that the factors that determine drug prices take account of the company's market position and revenue targets, interest in the product, their current and future product portfolio, reimbursement trends among public and private insurers, switching costs in addition to production cost, clinical value, and patients' access to competing products. The impact of international price comparisons and price controls is becoming an increasingly important consideration for setting prices.[33,34]

INDUSTRY EVOLUTION AND CURRENT STRUCTURE

The pharmaceutical industry has been characterized so far as being highly dependent on intellectual property protection, under constant pressure for innovation, and dissected for its pricing practices. The firms that make up the Pharmaceutical Research and Manufacturers of America (PhRMA) fit this profile. Not all firms classified as pharmaceutical manufacturers fit the prototype of PhRMA members. The 2002 U.S. Commercial Census recorded 723 entities as pharmaceutical manufacturers, and only 263 employ more than 100 persons. PhRMA members include approximately 40 of the largest firms whose core activities involve basic and applied research followed by product development, clinical trials, FDA approval, and post-marketing surveillance.[35] At least two additional types of firms of all sizes exist with a significant presence in the pharmaceutical industry: firms focused on biotechnology and the generic, nonresearch based companies.

Nearly all the PhRMA members emerged from significant consolidation in the industry that has occurred since 1980. From 1960 to 1980 the trend had been for companies in the industry to divest themselves of consumer-market products, including over-the-counter (OTC) medicines, toiletries, and cosmetics, in order to concentrate fully on the growth and profits available in the prescription drug market. After 1980 the PhRMA companies went through a process of consolidation that created greater uniformity among the remaining firms in terms of size and product portfolios.[36,37] Thirty-two companies, all in business in 1980, were consolidated to form five of the companies that are now among the top ten manufacturers in the world: Pfizer, GlaxoSmithKline, Sanofi-Aventis, Novartis, and Bristol-Myers Squibb.[38]

The rising cost of research and development was often cited as the reason for the big mergers. However, mergers have not produced the efficiencies and increased R & D output that were sought. Industry observers speculate that company cultures were not always compatible and morale problems stifled creativity within the research enterprise.[39,40] The more cynical interpretation suggests that mergers and acquisitions please shareholders under the guise of strengthening the company's R & D irrespective of current products. Mergers effectively obfuscate the stock market and add short-term (five to ten years) value to the company. The maneuver thereby gives the company the time and resources it needs to carry out the long-term strategies and produce successful products.[41]

Drug products produced through biotechnology (see also Chapter 18) are distinct from drugs produced by the chemical processes that defined the traditional firms. Biotechnology draws its discoveries from biology and requires new science and different processes for R & D, manufacturing, and sales.[42] Products of biotechnology are predominantly specialty and injectable pharmaceutical products for which reimbursement obstacles and schemes differ from traditional oral chemical pharmaceuticals. Most biotechnology firms are smaller in size, more loosely structured, and more risk-tolerant than the established firms. These are characteristics that allow for greater innovation and rapid decision making. The primary activities of the biopharmaceutical firms include basic and applied research and product development, but they engage in clinical trials and new drug approvals to a lesser extent than PhRMA members.

Thousands of biotechnology ventures were launched in the 1990s, and several hundred have succeeded to the point that they form an important new sector in the industry. The big PhRMA firms have approached biotechnology somewhat cautiously. Their tendency is to invest in the biotechnology sector, postponing acquisitions and mergers until a promising drug prospect materializes. At that point an established parent company can get involved and provide the regulatory and marketing experience needed to introduce the drug to the global market.[43] The 2005 PhRMA *Industry Profile* reported separate statistics for the biotechnology sector but refers to all of its members as biopharmaceutical firms. Biotechnology accounted for $10.5 billion in research in 2004.[44]

Generic drug companies (see also Chapter 20) make up the largest sector of the pharmaceutical industry in terms of number of firms. Although most generic drugs are made by these companies, some are divisions of major companies that also produce brand name drugs. The Hatch-Waxman Act stimulated the development of the generic drug industry by introducing the Abbreviated New Drug Application (ANDA), which streamlined the approval process for products whose clinical efficacy was established. Hatch-Waxman provisions also gave generic manufacturers the authorization to begin product development and to file an ANDA prior to the expiration of the patent of a brand-name drug. The firm that receives the first approval is granted 180 days of market exclusivity as a reward for their initiative. The exclusivity provision also gives generic firms the incentive to challenge brand-name patents in order to be first to market among the competitors. On the strength of these incentives the proportion of prescriptions dispensed as generics rose from 18 percent in 1980 to more than 50 percent in 2003. [45]

The initial growth of the generic drug industry came about as firms perfected their skills in labeling and distributing their products. Producers of generic drugs relied on supply-chain management and manufacturing cost leadership to be successful in this niche.[46] More recently leading generic firms have begun to rely on their manufacturing capacity to achieve economies of scale.[47] This strategy reduces reliance on the producers of raw materials in addition to creating growth opportunities. Biogenerics are another attractive growth target as the first generation of biotechnology products loses patent protection in 2006. A critical development for the generic sector is pending the outcome of debates in Congress and at the FDA about whether generic biologics should be allowed and what the approval process will entail.[48,49]

Sales revenue for generic firms is disproportionately low relative to their numbers and share of the prescription market. Even though more than 50 percent of prescriptions are dispensed as generics, less than 10 percent of prescription expenditures come from the sale of generics. These figures have been stable in recent years. Any promotion of generic drugs by third party plans has largely been offset by the sales revenues of the newer, more expensive brand-name products.[50] However, experts are predicting that global generic sales will increase by 22 percent annually as new generic alternatives enter the market in the near future, whereas the sales of branded products will increase by less than 10 percent.[51]

The cost structure of the three industry sectors shown in Figure 17.3 effectively conveys their distinct character. Generic manufacturers survive on high volume sales with narrow profit margins and spend minimal amounts

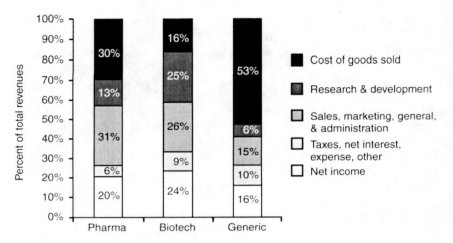

FIGURE 17.3. Comparison of expenses and net income, industry averages, 2001. *Source:* Centers for Medicare and Medicaid Services (2003). Health care industry market update: Pharmaceuticals. January 10. Office of Research Development and Information. Baltimore, MD: CMS. Available at: http://www.coms .hhs.gov/CapMarketUpdates/Downloads/hcimu11003.pdf.

on both R & D and marketing. Biotech firms spend heavily on research, producing relatively few products for sale. PhRMA members spend less on research than the biopharmaceutical firms and produce the bulk of the profitable products, spending heavily on sales and marketing.

TURNING POINT OR TIPPING POINT?

Societal pressures on the pharmaceutical industry are not new. Since the 1960s, important constituencies have been making paradoxical demands. Medical professionals and consumers want safe products and the rapid introduction of new discoveries to the market; stockholders and prescription buyers (often the same individuals) want low prices and lucrative investment opportunities.[52]

The publication of several books critical of the industry against the backdrop of product withdrawals and whistleblower claims created an exceptional year for media criticism of the industry in 2004. Not that there have not been similar exposés in the past, but 2004 was remarkable, for at least four books written by prominent physicians, including Drs. Marcia Angell[53] and Jerome Kassirer,[54] both former editors of the *New England*

Journal of Medicine, and Drs. John Abramson[55] and Jerry Avorn,[56] both Harvard Medical School faculty. At least three core issues are common to most critiques, and the outcry will be hard to ignore. They are (1) price levels per se and price differentials, (2) the cost and productivity of R & D, and (3) the nature of the market and promotional practices. Leading proposals for resolving these problems offered by the critics are (1) negotiated agreements on global pricing and price controls, (2) more sophisticated and targeted R & D, and (3) voluntary and mandatory restrictions on promotions and contracting arrangements. The magnitude and nature of the response from individual firms will determine if this is the onset of an historic transition within the industry.

Price Levels and Price Differentials

Prescription drugs are the most visible component of the health care market because prescription drugs represent the greatest out-of-pocket health expenditure for most consumers. Older persons use more prescription medicines and, if retired, likely face both a fixed income and diminishing prescription coverage. Managed care schemes increase prescription price awareness directly through patient cost sharing such as deductions and copayments, and indirectly by the increasing insurance premiums paid by employers and employees. Government programs pay for an increasingly larger proportion of the industry's products at prices that incense taxpayers.

Not only are high prices a concern but price differentials are potentially more infuriating. Cash customers pay prices nearly 15 percent more on average than customers with prescription insurance.[57] Consumers are abruptly confronted with the price differential between the brand and generic since regulatory changes and cost-containment measures promote generic replacements for the higher priced drugs as soon as the patents expire. Price differences between the U.S. and neighboring countries are not only inexplicably large and offensive to the public but viewed by consumers as sustained only by an FDA prohibition on parallel trade.[58,59,60]

Current public awareness of the prices and price differentials is unprecedented. Pharmaceutical manufacturers are in an increasingly untenable position. Any action perceived as limiting access to life-saving drugs for vulnerable populations intensifies the emotional response and contributes to price sensitivity of the public. Employer coalitions and politicians are apt to blame pharmaceuticals for driving the rise in health care expenditures that strains resources.[61] Public Citizen reported in 2004 that the pharmaceutical lobby spent more than $108 million dollars in lobbying the Medicare Prescription Drug, Improvement, and Modernization Act and came away with no provision for negotiation over prices to be paid for covered drugs. Every case of fraud or predatory pricing is front page news that generates more calls for price and reimbursement controls.[62]

Also, pressure on prices comes from awareness of competing products and the role that public policy may play in providing advantages to single-source suppliers.[63] In addition, direct-to-consumer (see also Chapter 19) advertising increases awareness of newer, more expensive drugs and allegedly creates unrealistic expectations for consumers. Questions are raised more frequently about whether the newer, higher cost prescription drugs represent a good value.[64]

Product R & D

Some firms have tried to spark innovation and productivity by reorganizing the R & D enterprise to emulate the small and more nimble biotechnology companies. Others have opted to promote their unique competencies such as knowledge management, team work, and relationships with key leaders in science or practice. A number have confined their pursuits to clinical areas with large patient populations with unmet needs. Alternatively they have focused on lifestyle drugs for which demand is driven by consumers with readily identified conditions who are willing and able to seek out the product whether it is covered by insurance or not.[65]

The cost of R & D continues to climb in large part due to the expense of clinical trials.[66] Drugs that are used for long periods to treat chronic diseases are the most attractive targets of research programs, but drugs for chronic disease require longer trials to demonstrate safety for their intended use. Studies that compare alternative treatments are increasingly needed to gain formulary access and assure product reimbursement. More complex studies are inherently more expensive, tend to require more subjects and increase the cost of patient recruitment. Firms have restructured to a more lean and flexible R & D operation, some outsourcing all but core activities.

Expertise in clinical trials and experience with the drug approval process effectively presents a barrier to new firms entering the industry. However, substantially new technology emerging from biotechnology and other advances such as nanotechnology can create a new experience curve that would nullify the historical advantage held by the current industry leaders. Industry leaders need to find a way to make the same technological leaps in order to compete with the new entrants.[67]

Wall Street seems to have taken note of these concerns. Investors fret that problems such as reduced discovery, safety worries, pricing pressure, and government regulation may be chronic rather than acute conditions. Stocks have not been bouncing back as quickly as they once did.[68] Market analysts are holding manufacturers more accountable for R & D expenditures.

Theories of industrial organization suggest that two ways exist to man-age risk in an industry heavily dependent on R & D. The first is to get larger. Increased size allows the firm to initiate and sustain more research projects, thereby increasing the chances that one project will pay off.[69,70] To date, however, the mega-mergers in the pharmaceutical industry have not gener-ated an increase in innovative new products. The alternative strategy is to develop networks for the discovery and development of drugs. Networks re-duce the risk posed to each firm and provide greater flexibility and adapt-ability. Evidence that suggests that the industry is moving toward a more networked structure includes the formation of strategic alliances between large firms and biotechnology companies, out-sourcing of R & D activities such as clinical trials, coordination between firms with products that com-plement drug products such as medical devices, and geographically locat-ing new R & D facilities near major universities or research centers.[71,72]

PROSPECTS FOR THE DOMESTIC PHARMACEUTICAL MARKET

A cursory overview of the market for pharmaceuticals gives a very posi-tive outlook. The aging of the population and long term treatment of chronic diseases present a promising future for the industry. Baby boomers are expected to exert their clout and demand better access to pharma-ceuticals. The implementation of drug coverage under the Medicare Mod-ernization Act of 2003 seems certain to increase demand.

A more thoughtful appraisal suggests that the future potential is apt to re-quire some strategic, and perhaps structural, changes in the pharmaceutical industry. The implementation of a Medicare prescription benefit poses some uncertainty for future profitability. Although the short-term impact is likely to bring increased sales, price discounts and cost-containment strate-gies are sure to follow. The market could shift, reducing the diverse set of customers who act as users, payers, and decision makers to a smaller num-ber of better-coordinated purchasing systems. Power shifts from sellers to buyers when revenues are concentrated in large volume sales to a small pool of purchasers: expenditures become more significant, buyers acquire more information and expertise, and the public sector maintains pressure to keep costs low.

A significant change in the character of the market for pharmaceuticals calls for reappraisal of the industry's promotional strategies. The open mar-ket taught drug manufacturers that the more sales representatives they employ, the higher their sales. From 1995 to 2002 the industry found itself in a virtual arms race as they tripled number of sales representatives to about 90,000. As the number of representatives in the field gathered negative reaction to sales tactics and showed signs of declining efficiency no one company seemed willing to be first to cut its sales force for fear of loosing ground to the competition.[73] Both AMA and the FDA saw fit to issue guidance designed to curb gift giving and other inappropriate sales practices. The prospects of market restructuring make reevaluation of promotional practices a more prudent course than additional regulation.

THE WORLD MARKET

Although scientific and technological advances pose new challenges, economic trends and political developments are creating a global marketplace. Globalization is not a newly emergent issue for the pharmaceutical industry, and is not an entirely negative prospect. Most major pharmaceutical companies have extensive operations and sales in foreign markets. However, the U.S. market is the largest and most profitable. The United States and Canada make up 70 percent of revenue for PhRMA members; sales to Europe and Asia account for an additional 23 percent.[74]

The negotiation of trade agreements that would open the world market for the U.S. pharmaceutical industry triggered a contentious debate over intellectual property rights. International enforcement of IPP is a matter that goes to the core of the entire PhRMA business model. PhRMA takes any threat to pharmaceutical patents seriously. The World Trade Organization (WTO) generated an agreement over trade-related aspects of intellectual property rights (TRIPS) that requires the least-developed countries to join other WTO member countries in providing twenty years of patent protection for pharmaceuticals by 2006.[75] However, the HIV/AIDs crisis in developing countries is a particularly sensitive issue where access to affordable drugs is concerned. Endorsement and implementation of the TRIPS agreement proved a lengthy ordeal. PhRMA may have won some battles in this arena, but whether their cause will prevail in the court of world opinion remains to be determined.

Business analysts suggest that ongoing disputes over the protection of IPP have begun to change the dynamics of the global pharmaceutical market. The global generic industry is strengthening and generating stronger competition. International generic manufacturers operate where margins are lower due to price controls. They are driving prices down ever further and accentuating the price disparity with brand-name drugs. On the other hand, these generic firms face limited sales potential in developing countries. To increase growth they are forced to turn to the large and lucrative market in the United States. Some firms have found it most advantageous to acquire or merge with U.S. companies that have an established sales and distribution infrastructure.[76]

In contrast with many observers, Kremer (2002) reasons that market and government failures in developing countries actually have greater implications for globalization of the pharmaceutical industry than U.S. government policy.[77] Multinational corporations operating in developing countries face small markets, different disease environments by reason of geography and poverty, weak health care systems, and widespread misuse of drugs. A lack of government regulation and enforcement stifle needed reforms.

Harmonization is another facet of globalization that confronts the industry, presenting both opportunity and risk. The European Agency for the Evaluation of Medicinal Products (EMEA) has adopted a centralized procedure for regulatory approval in all member states. The International Conference on Harmonization (ICH) aims to extend drug approval standards around the globe. Although the harmonization of requirements promises to simplify access to new markets for the industry, common standards would preclude the need for prohibitions on parallel importation. The outcome, expressed in economic terms, would be the removal of regulatory barriers that give innovator firms the structure that enables discriminatory pricing and supports monopoly rents. It also raises the prospect of collective decision making wherein firms routinely face an all-or-none decision for marketing approval and price.[78]

LOOKING TO THE FUTURE

To this point the response of the pharmaceutical industry to key issues has been reactive and defensive rather than proactive and innovative. A preferred strategy might be a series of mutually reinforcing initiatives to improve public relations. PhRMA took a step in that direction by naming former Congressman W.J. "Billy" Tauzin as its chief executive in spring of 2005. Mr. Tauzin's professed mission is "to rescue and restore the reputation" of the industry and rebuild trust.[79] He acknowledged that it will be at least two to three years to yield results.[80] To date, the industry has tried several approaches to improve their image, including restraint in direct-to-consumer advertising, more disclosure of clinical trials data and increasing access to drugs for the uninsured.[81] A broad mix of long range initiatives integrated with individual corporate strategies seems to be underway for shaping public perception and policy over the long term.[82]

A passive, wait-and-see strategy is not likely to be a viable option to the challenges facing the industry. At least two issues loom, one arising from scientific and technological developments and one that is political and economic in nature. First, scientific studies that mapped the genome and technological progress in bioinformatics are making an impact on the drug discovery process. The most recent drug treatments emerging from research in genetics foreshadow an era in which medicines can be tailored for individual patients. As the industry transitions to a new R & D paradigm based on these advances, the nature of these innovative treatments will require rethinking clinical trial designs and the revamping of manufacturing facilities and methods.[83]

The legal and economic challenges that accompany the introduction of personalized medicine could be as challenging as the scientific and technical hurdles.[84] Marketing efforts will confront differences in public opinion and controversial politics. It is not yet clear how quickly these new technologies will generate new products and how they will influence industry returns. Personalized medicine holds the promise of more efficient therapies, but at a price that will precipitate reimbursement dilemmas for payers. Industry executives predict that ten to twenty years may pass before personalized therapies can be incorporated into the mainstream of medical practice.[85,86]

CONCLUSION

In summary, the pharmaceutical industry continues to be highly profitable but likely to incur higher cost structure in the short term. Successful organizations must be able to navigate obstacles while maintaining motivation in the organization over the short term. At the same time, long-term success demands balancing the operation of two business models simultaneously, a chemical-based blockbuster model and the biotech individualized therapy model. Parts of the balancing act require being responsive to price sensitivity and the demand for increased transparency while maintaining the profit needed to fuel innovation; taking advantage of large size without loosing the agility that is characteristic of small, innovative firms; and thinking creatively about strategic alliances while capitalizing on unique competencies.

Government policy nurturing strong intellectual property protection and a relatively free market environment have been as instrumental as medical and pharmaceutical sciences to the viability of pharmaceutical industry. Negative sentiment evolved with drug recalls, pricing increases, conspicuous lobbying, and aggressive marketing. Negative sentiment invites legislation and regulations detrimental to the industry as currently configured.

The old system may give way to a heterogeneous mix of sectors. The current skill set of PhRMA members puts them in the best position to take on the development and worldwide marketing of widely used drugs that represent first-line therapy while the generic orientated firms focus on production and distribution efficiencies. The ultimate configuration of the pharmaceutical industry and the role of biopharmaceuticals will be shaped by the strategy, skill, resources, and luck that firms bring in response to change. A strategy of watchful waiting appears untenable.

NOTES

1. Grabowski H (2004). Are the economics of pharmaceutical research and development changing? *Pharmacoeconomics* 22 (Suppl 2):15-24.

2. Pharmaceutical Research and Manufacturers of America (2005). *Pharmaceutical Industry Profile 2005*. March. Washington, DC: PhRMA.

3. DiMasi JA, Hansen RW, Grabowski HG (2004). Assessing claims about the cost of new drug development: A critique of the Public Citizen and TB Alliance Reports. November 1. Boston, MA: Tufts Center for the Study of Drug Development, Tufts University.

4. Centers for Medicare and Medicaid Services (2003). Health care industry market update: Pharmaceuticals. January 10. Office of Research Development and Information. Baltimore, MD: CMS, p. 16

5. National Institute for Health Care Management Research and Educational Foundation (2002). A primer: Generic drugs, patents and the pharmaceutical marketplace. June. Washington, DC: NIHCM.

6. Eisenberg RS (2001). The shifting functional balance of patents and drug regulation. *Health Affairs* 20(5): 119-135.

7. Grabowski H, Vernon J, DiMasi JA (2002). Returns on research and development for 1990s new drug introductions. *Pharmacoeconomics* 20(Suppl 3): 11-29.

8. Frear RS (2002). The future of generics. Available at: http://www.express-scripts.com/ourcompany/news/outcomesconference/2002/slides/frear.ppt. Accessed January 2, 2006.

9. Saftlas H (2005). Healthcare: Pharmaceuticals. *Standard & Poor's Industry Surveys* December: 173 (28).

10. Barton JH, Emanuel EJ (2005). The patents-based pharmaceutical development process: Rationale, problems and potential reforms. *JAMA* 294: 2075-2083.

11. Kennedy CR, Harris FH, Lord M (2004). Integrating public policy and public affairs in a pharmaceutical marketing program: The AIDS pandemic. *Journal of Public Policy & Marketing* 23(2): 128-139.

12. Pharmaceutical Research and Manufacturers of America (2005).

13. Grabowski H (2004).

14. Grabowski H, Vernon J, DiMasi JA (2002).

15. Pharmaceutical Research and Manufacturers of America (2005).

16. Kennedy CR, Harris FH, Lord M (2004).

17. Barton JH, Emanuel EJ (2005).

18. Rosenthal MB, Berndt ER, Donohue JM, Frank RG, Epstein AM (2002). Promotion of prescription drugs to consumers. *NEJM* 346: 498-505.

19. Drews J (2003). Strategic trends in the drug industry. *Drug Discovery Today* 2003; 8: 411-420.

20. Grabowski H, Vernon J, DiMasi JA (2002).

21. Achilladelis B, Antonakis N (2001). The dynamics of technological innovation: The case of the pharmaceutical industry. *Research Policy* 30: 535-588.

22. Scherer FM (2001). The link between gross profitability and pharmaceutical R&D spending. *Health Affairs* 20(5): 216-220.

23. Grabowski H, Vernon J, DiMasi JA (2002).

24. Reinhardt UE (2001). Perspectives on the pharmaceutical industry. *Health Affairs* 20(5): 136-149.

25. Grabowski H, Vernon J, DiMasi JA (2002).

26. Scherer FM (2001).

27. Grabowski H (2004).

28. Scherer FM (2001).

29. Kaiser Family Foundation (2005). Prescription drug trends. November. Available at: http://www.kff.org/insurance/upload/3057-04.pdf. Accessed December 27, 2005.

30. Scherer FM (2001).

31. DiMasi JA (2000). Price Trends for Prescription Pharmaceuticals: 1995-1999. A Background Report Prepared for the Department of Health and Human Services Conference on Pharmaceutical Pricing, Practices, Utilization and Costs, August 8-9, 2000, Leavey Conference Center, Georgetown University, Washington DC. Available at: http://aspe.hhs.gov/health/reports/Drug-papers/dimasi-final.htm.

32. Keyhani S, Diener-West M, Powe N (2005). Do drug prices reflect development time and government investment? *Medical Care* 43: 753-762.

33. Freeman RA (2000). Pharmaceutical pricing: Practices and issues. U.S. Department of Health and Human Services Conference on Pharmaceutical Pricing Practices, Utilization and Costs, August 8-9, Washington, DC.

34. Kolassa EM (1997). *Elements of Pharmaceutical Pricing.* Binghamton, NY: The Haworth Press, Inc.

35. Pharmaceutical Research and Manufacturers of America (2005).

36. Achilladelis B, Antonakis N (2001).

37. Drews J (2003).

38. Projan SJ, Shlaes DM (2004). Antibacterial drug discovery: Is it all downhill from here? *Clin Microbiol Infect* 10(Suppl. 4): 18-22.

39. Cockburn IM (2004). The changing structure of the pharmaceutical industry. *Health Affairs* 23: 10-22.

40. Mervis J (2005). The hunt for a new drug: Five views from the inside. *Science* 309: 722-728.

41. Drews J (2003).

42. Cortada JW, Fraser HE (2005). Mapping the future in science-intensive industries: Lessons from the pharmaceutical industry. *IBM Systems Journal* 44: 163-183.

43. Anderson SJ (2003). *A New Structure for the Pharmaceutical Industry*. Unpublished M.A. thesis, Georgetown University, Washington DC, 2003.

44. Pharmaceutical Research and Manufacturers of America (2005).

45. Scherer FM (2001).

46. Batiz-Lazo B, Holland S The global pharmaceutical industry, 2004. General economics and teaching 0405002, EconWPA. Available at: http://129.3.20.41/eps/get/papers/0405/0405002.pdf.

47. Business Insight (2004). The pharmaceutical parallel trade outlook: Challenges to pharmaceutical companies across Europe and the US. London, UK: Business Insights.

48. Barrett A, Carey J, Capell K (2005). Biotech drugs: Where are the generics. *Business Week.* May 9, pp. 98-99.

49. Devine JW, Cline RR, Farley JF (2006). Follow-on biologics in the biopharmaceutical marketplace. *Journal of the American Pharmacists Association* 46(2): 193-204.

50. Kirking DM, Ascione FJ, Gaither CA, Welage LS (2001). Economics and structure of the generic pharmaceutical industry. *Journal of the American Pharmaceutical Association* 41(4): 578-584.

51. Whalen J (2005). Novartis expands generics range for $8.4 billion: Acquisition of two firms aims at growing demand for broader drug portfolio. *Wall Street Journal.* February 22, p. A1.

52. Schweitzer SO, Comanor WS (1999). The role of pharmaceuticals in the health care system. In Williams SJ, Torrens PR (Eds), *Introduction to Health Services*, Fifth Edition. Clifton Park, NY: Delmar Publications.

53. Angell M (2004). *The Truth About the Drug Companies: How They Deceive Us and What to Do About It*. New York: Random House.

54. Kassirer J (2004). *On the Take: How Medicine's Complicity with Big Business Can Endanger Your Health*. New York: Oxford University Press.

55. Abramsom J (2004). *Overdosed America: The Broken Promise of American Medicine*. New York: HarperCollins.

56. Avorn J (2004). *Powerful Medicines: The Benefits, Risks and Costs of Prescription Drugs*. New York: Knopf.

57. Centers for Medicare and Medicaid Services (2003).

58. Eisenberg RS (2001).

59. Kremer M (2002). Pharmaceuticals and the developing world. *Journal of Economic Perspectives* 16(4): 67-90.

60. Wagner JL, McCarthy E (2004). International differences in drug prices. *Annual Review of Public Health* 25: 475-495.

61. Kennedy CR, Harris FH, Lord M (2004).

62. Public Citizen (2004). The Medicare Drug War. Available at: http://www.citizen.org/documents/Medicare_Drug_War.pdf. Accessed December 30, 2005.

63. DiMasi JA, Paquette C. (2004). The economics of follow-on drug research and development: Trends in entry rates and the timing of development. *Pharmacoeconomics* 22(Suppl 2): 1-14.

64. Hensley S (2004). Scaled up. Biggest drug firm faces generics but has an edge: Its very bigness. *Wall Street Journal*. August 23, pp. A1, A6.

65. Batiz-Lazo B, Holland S (2004).

66. Grabowski H (2004).

67. Porter ME (1980). *Competitive Strategy: Techniques for Analyzing Industries and Competitors*. New York: Free Press.

68. Zuckerman G, Hensley S (2004). Drug-stock ills are hard to cure. *Wall Street Journal*. December 21, pp. C1, C4.

69. Anderson SJ (2003). *A New Structure for the Pharmaceutical Industry*. Unpublished master's thesis. Georgetown University, Washington, DC.

70. Cockburn IM (2004).

71. Anderson SJ (2003).

72. Cockburn IM (2004).

73. Batiz-Lazo B, Holland S (2004).

74. Pharmaceutical Research and Manufacturers of America (2005).

75. Kennedy CR, Harris FH, Lord M (2004).

76. Centers for Medicare and Medicaid Services (2003).

77. Kremer M (2002).

78. Batiz-Lazo B, Holland S (2004).

79. Clinton P, Wechsler J (2005). PhARMA's new face. *Pharmaceutical Executive* May 1. Available at: http://www.pharmexec.com/pharmexec/article/articleDetail.jsp?id=153 005&pageID=1&sk=&date. Accessed August 10, 2005.

80. Cusack B, Young J (2005). Tauzin promises 'pretty big changes' at PhRMA. May 4. Available at: http://www.hillnews.com/thehill/export/TheHill/News?Frontpage/050405/ tauzin.html. Accessed August 10, 2005.

81. Abboud L (2005). Stung by public distrust, drug makers seek to heal image. *Wall Street Journal*. August 25, pp. B1, B5.

82. Kennedy CR, Harris FH, Lord M (2004).

83. Cortada JW, Fraser HE (2005).

84. Grabowski H, Vernon J, DiMasi JA (2002).

85. Bonduelle Y, Pisani J (2003). *The Future of PhRMA: Back to Basics*. London: PriceWaterhouseCoopers.

86. Cortada JW, Fraser HE (2005).

Chapter 18

Health Policy and Economic Issues in Biotechnology and Pharmacogenetics

Louis P. Garrison, Jr.

INTRODUCTION

Henry Aaron, a leading American health policy analyst at the Brookings Institution, has characterized American's ongoing tension between cost containment and technical advance in graphic terms:

> The drama of rising health care costs should be seen as a saga of rapid and even reckless advance in technology, fueled increasingly by an entrepreneurial sense of adventure.[1]

Over the past 40 years, the U.S. health care system has been the most supportive of innovation and technology in the world. Many would argue that this is what lies behind the share (now 16 percent) of our GDP devoted to health care being significantly larger than in any other country.

But as Aaron suggests, Americans welcome innovation despite growing discomfort with total health care costs and the overall functioning of the system. For example, in a Research!America poll in 2005, 60 percent of polled persons said the United States does not have the best health care system, but citizen support for medical science is still strong.[2] In their recent (2006) national telephone poll, Americans said the following:

- 58 percent would increase societal spending for medical and health research.
- 51 percent would increase government funding for research.
- 67 percent would like to see three cents of every health dollar spent on prevention and public health research rather than only one cent.

- 57 percent would be willing to pay a dollar more for each prescription drug if the money would be used for additional research.
- 60 percent perceive clinical research as having great value.
- 63 percent would be willing to participate in clinical research. [3]

Yet, in terms of priorities, in the same poll, more Americans think it is *very important* to control the cost of health care (78 percent) and the cost of prescription drugs (75 percent) than think it *very important* to accelerate medical and health research (58 percent). Interestingly, the most cited (61 percent) barrier to research is "too many regulatory hurdles." Only 36 percent think that there are not enough researchers.

Americans generally view medical innovation favorably and see biotechnology and pharmacogenetics fields in this light. Yet, increasing cost-containment pressures are placing advances in these fields under the same scrutiny as traditional pharmaceuticals.

Since the cloning of the sheep Dolly in 1997, the completion of the sequencing of human genome in 2001, through to the ongoing hot debate about stem-cell research, genetics and biotechnology have captured the imagination of Americans. These fields are seen as the cutting edge of medical innovation. The purpose of this chapter is to (1) define and describe biotechnology and pharmacogenetics, (2) discuss what makes them unique from economic and policy perspectives, and (3) identify and discuss the key policy issues in a U.S. context.

WHAT ARE BIOTECHNOLOGY AND PHARMACOGENETICS?

Ho and Gibaldi (2003) define biotechnology as "An integrated application of scientific and technical understanding of a biologic process or molecule to develop a useful product."[4] One can distinguish between traditional small molecule pharmaceuticals (Rx) and large (or "macromolecule") biopharmaceuticals (bioRx). Biopharmaceuticals, also called biologics, have some advantages and disadvantages versus small molecule products: by being similar to naturally occurring substances in the body, they may have better bioavailability and have less toxicity. Yet, they are generally more complex to develop and especially to manufacture, and generally require intravenous administration.

Genomics and genetics are important to biotechnology as part of the production process, but we are using *pharmacogenetics*[5] here in a narrower sense to mean how drug response in humans is influenced by genetic variation.

Simply put, individuals (except identical twins) vary in the DNA sequence of their genome. The genome is the complete set of genetic material found in the nucleus of cells inherited from their parents with half coming from the mother and half from the father. DNA is a long, linear molecule made of bases of adenine, guanine, cytosine, and thymine. Particular stretches of base pairs can be identified as *genes,* and the actual nucleotide sequences in these stretches can vary among individuals, sometimes providing "information" that is predictive of observable differences among humans, i.e., genotype can be a predictor of phenotype—the physical appearance or a specific manifestation of a trait. For our purposes here, it is very important to understand that, for most common, complex diseases, the predictive power of genotype alone is often limited, and that environment (both at the cellular level and the level of individual lifestyle) is a significant contributor to phenotype. The occurrence of single genes predicting disease with very high likelihood is rare, e.g., Huntington's disease, cystic fibrosis, and Tay-Sachs disease. Nonetheless, these "monogenic" examples seem to dominate the public's perceptions and unduly influence their thinking about the potential impact of pharmacogenetics.

THE BIOTECHNOLOGY INDUSTRY AND ITS PRODUCTS

According to the Biotechnology Industry Organization (BIO),[6] at the end of 2003, nearly 1,500 biotechnology companies existed in the United States, of which slightly more than 300 were publicly held. The total market capitalization of the publicly traded companies was about $310 billion in April of 2005. Industry revenues grew from $8 billion in 1992 to $39 billion in 2003, and employment stood at nearly 200,000 at the end of 2003. Amgen, the largest biotechnology company, had sales of $12 billion in 2005, spent $2.3 billion (19.1 percent) on R & D, and 16,500 employees.[7] Pfizer, the largest pharmaceutical manufacturer, had sales of $51.3 billion, spent $7.4 billion on R & D (14.4 percent), and had 106,000 employees. For Amgen, the revenue per employee is about $727,000 and for Pfizer it is about $484,000. Given the apparently smaller relative R & D workforce, Pfizer is likely devoting more staff to sales and marketing. To some degree, this reflects the need to market small molecules for common conditions to a broad audience of physicians and patients. Table 18.1 lists U.S. sales of the top-selling small molecules and biopharmaceuticals in 2004.

The top selling small molecules are for the common chronic diseases of high cholesterol and gastrointestinal reflux, neither of which is life threatening in an acute sense. Interestingly, the top-selling biologics are

TABLE 18.1. Selected Top-Selling Pharmaceutical and Biologic Products in 2004[8]

Rank	Rx or BioRX	Product® (Company)	Indication	Sales ($billions)
1	Rx	Lipitor (Pfizer)	Hypercholesterolemia	$7.1
2	Rx	Zocor (Merck)	Hypercholesterolemia	$5.5
3	Rx	Prevacid (Tap)	Gastoint. Reflux	$4.0
4	Rx	Nexium (AstraZenica)	Gastoint. Reflux	$3.6
5	BioRx	Procrit (J&J)	Cancer anemia	$3.3
6	Rx	Zoloft (Pfizer)	Antidepressant	$3.0
12	BioRx	Epogen (Amgen)	Dialysis anemia	$2.5
17	BioRx	Aranesp (Amgen)	Anemia	$2.1
22	BioRx	Remicade (J&J)	Rheumatoid Arthritis	$1.8
24	BioRx	Neulasta (Amgen)	Low white cell count	$1.8
106	BioRx	Herceptin (Genentech)	Breast cancer	$0.47

Source: Adapted from NDC Health (2005). *The Top 200 Selling Drugs in 2004 by U.S. Sales.* Atlanta, GA: NDCHealth. Available at: http://www.drugs.com/top200_2004.html.

erythropoietins (EPOs) for anemia, with total sales of nearly $8 billion. Clearly, blockbusters play a major role in both the pharmaceutical and biotech industries.

AN ECONOMIC PERSPECTIVE ON BIOTECHNOLOGY AND PHARMACOGENETICS

In seeking to understand the economic impact and policy implications of biotech and pharmacogenetics it is useful to identify any distinguishing characteristics of them from an economic perspective.

Unique Economic Characteristics of Biotech Products

How do biologics products differ from traditional small molecule pharmaceuticals? The following characteristics stand out:

- Higher marginal costs of production
- Different safety profile

- Smaller markets
- Different regulatory pathway
- Less market competition

Of course, none of these characteristics—with the exception of the regulatory pathway—in and of themselves hold for all biotech products or fail to apply to some small molecules. Still, they can account for some of the unique structural features of the industry and related policy challenges.

Typically, biotech products are large molecules, such as monoclonal antibodies (MABs) or specific receptor proteins, which are complex and costly to manufacture. This implies that at the margin (per each dose) the cost is much more significant than for small molecules. Of course, marginal cost to the health care system also includes the costs of marketing and distribution. These can be high for both normal and biotech products, though the latter may be lower due to the generally smaller targeted audience. According to standard economic theory, a manufacturer with a patented product will behave as a profit-maximizing monopolist, setting price at the point at which marginal revenue equals marginal cost. Thus, marginal cost has some influence on the price level. However, the demand curve for these biotech products may be relatively more inelastic (i.e., less sensitive to price), so the margin between price and cost is often much higher than for small molecules. However, little direct evidence on this exists, as marginal costs of production and distribution are not readily observable.

Second, because biotech products often aim to copy or imitate naturally occurring proteins, they may be more likely to show efficacy and less likely to evoke certain types of adverse drug reactions (ADRs) in patients— though they can also carry risks of unwanted immune responses. Recently, a prominent example in Europe showed how changing the manufacturing process for one the top-selling erythropoetins (EPOs) resulted in a severe ADR in some patients (which also is a major factor in explaining why policies about "generic" entry differ for biologics).

At least for conditions such as anemia or neutropenia (white blood cell deficiency), it is reasonable to speculate that the proportion of patients responding and degree of response are greater and more pervasive and measurable in the target population than for many common small-molecule products. The populations for the best selling biologics tend to be smaller than for top selling drugs that focus on highly prevalent conditions such as high cholesterol or gastrointestinal reflux. By implication, the prices of the biologics per year tend to be higher per year or course of treatment.

In the United States, review and approval of new drugs and therapeutic biologics is conducted by the Center for Drug Evaluation and Research

(CDER), and the Center for Biologics Evaluation and Research (CBER) regulates other biologics, such as vaccine, blood products, certain devices, and cell- and tissue-based therapies. Review of therapeutic biologics was transferred from CBER to CDER in 2003 to ensure that the regulatory pathways for the product approval are the same. However, one major difference exists with important economic implications: no regulatory path is currently in place for "follow-on" biologics, analogous to the generic follow-ons that enter pharmaceutical markets after patents expire. The Hatch-Waxman Act (1984) facilitated generic entry (based on bioequivalence of the small molecule) by better defining and refining the processes around generic approvals. Generic compounds are not required to conduct a full-scale replication of the complete clinical trial program—Phase I to III. Generic companies can use the trial data from the patent-expired product to substantiate efficacy and safety. As yet, no such process for follow-ons to biologics exists in the United States. In contrast, the EU has a more defined process, calling these "biosimilars."

Another FDA special program—for so-called "orphan drugs" for rare diseases—is also important to biopharmaceuticals. In the twenty-four years since the passage of the Orphan Drug Act, 282 drugs and biologic products have received approval.[9] Major biopharmaceuticals have obtained approval for specific conditions under the Orphan Drug Act, which provides R & D tax credits and awards "data exclusivity" for the first product in class for a period of seven years if the target population is under 200,000. The aim is to promote innovations for rare conditions by limiting subsequent competition, by not allowing same-in-class competitors during the exclusivity period. Both branded, in-class, and generic follow-ons are excluded for this period. Approval under the Orphan Drug Act has limited competition for several major biological products.

Unique Economic Characteristics of Pharmacogenetics Products

How do pharmacogenetics-based products differ from traditional small molecule pharmaceuticals? The following characteristics stand out:

- A greater role for the diagnostic industry
- Potential impact throughout the product developmental life cycle—discovery, development, and marketing
- The paucity of current examples of products
- That pharmacogenetics-based diagnostics do not fundamentally different (from an economic perspective) from other diagnostics

Currently, fewer pharmacogenetics applications exist than do biologics. Indeed, the Royal Society in the UK recently concluded, "Pharmacogenetics is unlikely to revolutionize or personalize medical practice in the immediate future."[10] Garrison and Austin (2006) argue this is true for several reasons, though the impact of various factors—scientific challenges versus. economic barriers—is really an empirical question that remains open at the moment.[11] Before turning identifying those factors, let's first consider the state of the art.

CURRENT PHARMACOGENETIC APPLICATIONS

To this point only a limited number of pharmacogenetics applications exist. As shown in Exhibit 18.1, the major applications in drug labels were recently highlighted in a presentation by Dr. Felix Frueh, FDA genomics staff.[12]

The limited number of prominent pharmacogenetics applications is further illustrated in the review by Phillips and Van Bebber, providing an up-to-date and useful "systematic review of the cost-effectiveness analyses of

EXHIBIT 18.1. Known valid biomarkers

Genetic marker (drugs)

Safety Issue:

- TMPT (6-MP, azathioprine)
- UGT1A1 (irinotecan)
- CYP2C9/VKORC1 (warfarin)
- CYP2C6 (Strattera)

Efficacy issue:

- EGFR status (Erbitux, Tarceva)
- HER2/neu status (Herceptin)
- Philadelphia chromosome ~Bcr-abl (Gleevec)

Source: Adapted from Frueh, F. (2006). Qualification of genomic biomarkers for regulatory decision making. Presentation at the Annual DIA EuroMeeting, March 7, Paris, France. Available at: http://www.fda.gov/cder/genomics/presentations.htm. Accessed March 31, 2006.

pharmacogenomic interventions."[13] They find a paucity of studies—only eleven. The most commonly studied condition was deep vein thrombosis—four studies; three examined cancer, three examined viral infections, and one examined oral contraception. Factor V Leiden was the most frequently analyzed mutation, addressed in five of the studies. Seven of the studies addressed inherited mutations, three addressed acquired viral infections, and one a tumor mutation. Seven of the studies reported a clearly favorable cost-effectiveness ratio. The small number of studies and their limited breadth is indicative of the limited development and diffusion of pharmacogenetics-based technologies into common use, especially those based on inherited mutations.

The most commonly cited and recognized pharmacogenetics application is Herceptin (trastuzumab) for the 20-25 percent of women with breast cancer whose tumors have a specific genetic change that leads to over-expression of the cell receptor HER2; this also happens to lead to a more aggressive from of the cancer. Their tumors can be tested for overexpression of this gene, qualifying them to receive a chemotherapy regimen that includes this targeted product. Recent findings indicate a survival advantage for use of Herceptin in early stage breast cancer for women whose tumors overexpress HER2 in addition to the initial benefit demonstrated in metastatic breast cancer. It is also noteworthy in this case that the mutation is in tumor cells, and is not due to a mutation in the individual's inherited genome: it is a "somatic" rather "germline" mutation.

The recently approved Roche AmpliChip for testing for differences in drug metabolism among individuals is probably the next most prominent example of a potential application based on genetic variants among individuals. In principle, the AmpliChip could be applied to many drugs, such as warfarin, but its use is very limited at this point. Since other personal characteristics also apply in individual response, in many instances finding the optimal dose for a given patient will still be a matter of trial and error. How much knowing metabolism will help in more quickly finding the dose is an empirical matter.

ECONOMIC IMPACT ON DRUG DEVELOPMENT

The recent broad overview by Webster et al. provides a thorough, balanced perspective on the state of the field.[14] Economics was not their primary focus, but most of the issues they raise have an economic dimension. They introduce their piece by saying:

Pharmacogenetics is on the threshold of making a major impact in commercial labs and in the clinic. But, despite its promise and the heavy investment made in the technology, many companies still question whether there is a coherent business, health policy, or regulatory model emerging to shape the future development of pharmacogenetics.

Their search for a coherent model is aided by their useful taxonomy of areas of potential application of pharmacogenetics/pharmacogenetics, as shown in Exhibit 18.2. They conclude that most large pharmaceutical companies focus their investments on improving the efficiency of drug development: "These companies have little commercial interest in the applications of pharmacogenetics that are aimed at already licensed medicines, except where value can be added by extending product licenses. . . ." Although they see greater interest in preprescription genotyping among providers of health care and specialist diagnostic firms, they suggest that this is likely to take place mostly after linked drug-test combinations have been tested in clinical trials, and that this linkage will be made primarily in situations in which the linkage is required to make the drug viable for regulatory and commercial reasons.

They see it as unlikely that pharmacogenetic testing will be a regulatory requirement for all drugs:

> A drug that is highly efficacious across most of the population has a wide therapeutic index and that shows little inter-individual variability in kinetics and dynamics should not necessarily require pharmacogenetic testing. It would not be cost-effective to do so.

Nonetheless, they expect that most applications will at least address the question of pharmacogenetic variability in the CYP450 enzymes.

COST-EFFECTIVENESS OF PHARMACOGENETICS PRODUCTS

One way to consider the potential impact of personalized medicine is to ask: What are the characteristics of technologies and diseases that are most likely to be cost-effective? The cost-effectiveness of any given pharmacogenetics-based technology (such as a drug-test combination) will depend on the specific characteristics of that situation, and several factors will play a major role.

A brief review of relevant articles will illustrate the progression and refinement of this argument.

EXHIBIT 18.2. Taxonomy of pharmacogenetics impacts

Option 1: Using pharmacogenetics to discover better drugs

1a. Discovering drugs for specific genomic sub-groups (allelic variants of drug target).

1b. Discovering drugs that work in all sub-groups (ensuring leads work in all allelic variants).

Option 2: Pharmacogenetics to improve the safety of new drugs in development

2a. Early stage trial design and/or monitoring (for example, ensuring balanced trial population of cytochrome P450 variants).

2b. 'Rescue' of drugs that fail clinical trials owing to safety problems.

Option 3: Pharmacogenetics to improve the efficacy of new drugs in development

3a. Targeting late stage trials as "good responders" (prospective).

3b. 'Rescue' of drugs that fail clinical trials owing to lack of efficacy (retrospective).

Option 4: Improving the safety of licensed drugs

4a. Pre-prescription patient testing for risk of adverse drug reactions (ADRs) for example, thiopurine methyltransferase).

4b. Label and market extensions of drugs that have been restricted by ADRs (for example, abacavir).

4c. Improved post-marketing surveillance.

Option 5: Improving the efficacy of licensed drugs

5a. Pre-prescription patient testing to identify good responders.

5b. The use of efficacy data in drug marketing.

Source: Webster A, Martin P, Lewis G, and Smart A (2004). Integrating pharmacogenetics into society: In search of a model. *Nature Reviews Genetics* 5: 663-668. Reprinted with permission from Macmillan Publishers Ltd: *Nature Reviews Genetics,* copyright 2004.

Veenstra, Higashi, and Phillips (2000) applied a standard cost-effectiveness, decision-analysis framework to case of a linked pharmacogenetics-test and therapeutic intervention.[15] They conclude that ". . . pharmacogenetics likely will be cost-effective only for certain combinations of disease, drug, gene, and test characteristics, and that the cost-effectiveness of pharmacogenetic-based therapies needs to be evaluated on a case-by-case basis." They also identify several examples of drug-disease areas in which pharmacogenetics may be cost-effective, such as Herceptin for breast cancer, interferon/ribavirin for hepatitis C, and Tacrine for Alzheimer's disease.

Phillips, Veenstra, Oren, et al. (2001) conducted parallel literature reviews of drugs associated with adverse drug reactions (ADRs) and of drug-metabolizing enzymes associated with poor metabolism.[16] They identified twenty-seven drugs with ADR problems and were able to link sixteen of these to at least one enzyme with a variant allele (any of several forms of a gene usually arising through mutation) that causes abnormal metabolism. They recognize that this association is not necessarily causal and that it does not necessarily follow that a commercially viable pharmacogenetics test can be developed. More recently, Flowers and Veenstra[17] have refined the earlier Veenstra, Higashi, and Phillips analysis. They summarize the factors affecting cost-effectiveness in Table 18.2.

Variant allele refers to a specific version or variant of the gene that affects the response to the drug: the more common it is, the more aggregate health impact exists from identifying responders and also avoiding the effects of adverse effects in nonresponders. *Gene penetrance* refers to how often genotype leads to a particular phenotypic response. In the end, although identifying the useful questions to evaluate any given pharmacogenetics-based intervention, this analysis is still left with the conclusion that "it depends." Furthermore, the model takes the price of the therapeutic and the diagnostic as given. To understand better the incentives of pharmaceutical and diagnostic manufacturers to identify and pursue these opportunities, it is important to recognize that the prices charged for the drug and test are *endogenous*—chosen in the health care system by a combination of market forces, regulatory procedures, and price controls.

Rather than focusing on specific pharmacogenetics tests, one major study from Canada (Miller et al., 2002) examined their likely impact in the aggregate.[18] They distinguished among three types of tests:

1. Tests for fully penetrant genes: high predictive power; mutation causes disease in all.
2. Predisposition tests: highly, but not fully predictive; strong genetic component.
3. Risk factor tests: lower predictive power; cost of testing whole population amortized over responders.

They pointed out that, "predictive genetic tests cannot be meaningfully analyzed as one monolithic health technology." And Miller et al. concluded that full penetrance tests (given the limited number of monogenic diseases)

TABLE 18.2. Factors affecting cost-effectiveness of pharmacogenetics-based therapy-test combinations.

Factors and their features that favor cost-effectiveness of pharmacogenomic strategies		
	Factor to assess	**Features that favor cost-effectiveness**
Gene	Prevalence	Variant allele is relatively common
	Penetrance	Gene penetrance is high
Test	Sensitivity, specificity, and cost	High specificity and sensitivity
		A rapid and relatively inexpensive assay is available
Disease	Prevalence	High disease prevalence in the population
	Outcomes and economic impacts	High untreated mortality
		Significant impact on quality of life (QoL)
		High costs of disease management using conventional methods
Treatment	Outcomes and economic impacts	Reduction in adverse effects that significantly impact QoL or survival
		Significant improvements in QoL or survival due to differential treatment effects
		Monitoring of drug response is currently not practiced or difficult
		No, or limited, incremental cost of treatment with pharmacogenomic strategy

Source: Flowers CR, Veenstra D (2004). The role of cost-effectiveness analysis in the era of pharmacogenomics. *Pharmacoeconomics* 22(8): 481-493. Reprinted with permission from Wolters Kluwer Health.

are likely to have the lowest aggregate cost impact, whereas the aggregate costs of risk-factor tests are much less predictable. They argue that coverage decisions will have to be made on a case-by-case basis.

Two recent articles highlight another variant on the notion of personalized medicine based on economic differences rather than biological ones. Economists and other outcomes researchers have long argued that therapy choices should vary among individuals depending on their preferences regarding risk and benefit. For example, Califf says:

> The anticipated effect of personalized medicine also fits with the increasing belief that people should be responsible for their own decision making to the greatest extent possible; if they are given informa-

tion about the benefits and risks tailored to their biology and preferences ... they would make more rational health care choices.[19]

And Bala and Zarkin[20] make a similar point, arguing that cost-effectiveness should be done at the individual level. Califf also argues that our current clinical trial system is ill suited to support a move to personalized medicine. He calls for more large pragmatic trials, coordination of regulatory
and payment systems to support the needed studies, and provider education
in probabilistic thinking. He recommends a two-track system whereby provisional approvals would be followed by required larger, longer term
economic and outcomes studies.

The Economics of Pharmacogenetic Interventions

Only one published article—Danzon and Towse—that explicitly addresses the issue of incentives to develop pharmacogenetics-based linked
diagnostic therapeutics.[21] It is worthwhile to explain the framework they
use.

The economic incentives for a drug manufacturer related to introducing
a pharmacogenetics test are intuitive and fairly obvious. If a drug is already
on the market, the manufacturer has limited incentive to introduce a test that
would restrict the market size. The main reasons for doing so would be:
(1) if a higher price could be obtained for this smaller subset and/or (2) if it
is clear that some diagnostic test will be introduced during the life of the
product.

> Danzon and Towse formally analyze the economics of pharmaco-
> genetics using a standard microeconomic framework. Using a simple
> framework, they are able to delineate the basic economic impacts of a
> new pharmacogenetic test. In a theoretical model in which a test can
> identify the responders, the "social value" of testing depends on
> (1) the expected health benefit per responder, (2) the averted costs of
> treating non-responders, and (3) the cost of testing the entire popula-
> tion. They emphasize the viability of the testing will depend crucially
> on the ability of the firm to capture the extra health benefit provided
> through the targeted therapy. Also, they highlight the importance of
> price flexibility, saying "if the final drug price is unchanged, the inno-
> vative firm has no incentive to invest in pharmacogenetic testing in
> development that will result in a narrower indication."

In a recent paper, Garrison and Austin (2007) have extended this model
in two ways: (1) to recognize the value to the patient of reducing the uncer-

tainty and (2) allow the value to be captured by either the drug or diagnostic firm.[22] Their results are discussed in the following sections under pricing and reimbursement challenges.

Health Policy and Economic Issues in Biotechnology

The major health policy issues facing biotechnology today are the following:

* Regulation and generic competition
* Orphan drug status and investment incentives
* Pricing and reimbursement challenges

Regulation and Generic Competition

The erythropoietin products for treating anemia have been the biggest commercial success in biotechnology over the past decade. As indicated previously, current sales for the three top-selling products in the United States totaled more than $9.2 billion in 2004. But the patents are set to expire in the near future. As indicated, the FDA has no defined path for follow-on products to enter as "biogenerics" or "biosimilars." Prices for generic pharmaceuticals are, as would be expected, typically far below the comparable branded products, as competitive pressures push price toward short-run marginal cost (including a competitive rate of return).

The lack of a defined pathway does not in itself totally rule out competition within a drug class; for example, several branded anti–tumor necrosis factor biologics for rheumatoid arthritis are on market and in competition. On the other hand, the pressures to push price down substantially will only come through generic competition.

From a health policy perspective, it is important to keep in mind the role of the patents, as part of our intellectual property (IP) system. The need to encourage innovation through awarding intellectual property rights has its origins in the US Constitution. Article I, section 8 says Congress shall have power "To promote the progress of science and useful arts, by securing for limited times to authors and inventors the exclusive right to their respective writings and discoveries." Economists attribute this provision to the recognition by the founding fathers that information is a public good—one person's use of it does not make it unavailable to others. In addition, it's difficult to control and prohibit use of it. In the absence of property rights, a free market will tend to undersupply a public good. Patents, in effect, grant temporary monopoly rights to inventors. Economic theory predicts that monopolists will set price higher than is socially optimal in the short run, so that the quantity transacted will be smaller than is optimal as well. This results in a "welfare loss" in the short run that must be weighed against the social gain from having a higher rate of innovation in the long run.

On the pharmaceutical side, the Hatch-Waxman Act aimed to strike balance between protecting patents to encourage innovation and allowing generic entry to lower prices and improve access. Since the development of drugs typically takes eight to twelve years of the twenty-year patent life, and follow-on branded drugs in the same class are common, effective patent life and monopoly power can be very limited.

As the current biologics reach the end of their patent lives, it is unknown how common follow-on entry will be, and how the FDA will regulate it.

Orphan Drug Status and Investment Incentives

The "success" of the Orphan Drug Act in, aimed at rare and neglected disease, in stimulating drug development has probably far exceeded in the initial hopes of its supporters. Indeed, a recent article in the *Wall Street Journal* reports that nearly half of pipeline drugs in biotech companies are for orphan indications.[23] Prices can run into the hundreds of thousands of dollars for some patients for the rest of their lives. The article said that Genzyme Corporation had sales of $840 million on its drug for Gaucher's disease, which affects fewer than 10,000 people globally. Rep. Henry Waxman was reported to have commented, "We did not expect to see the high cost of orphan drugs." And he went on to say the price of drugs "is unfair across the board, and Americans everywhere are getting fed up."

Pricing and Reimbursement Challenges

With recent increases in drug and medical care prices, cost containment pressures are increasing and drug prices are under the microscope. The high or "premium" prices for biologics are increasingly in the spotlight. Given the widespread support among the general public for medical innovation, biologics—perceived as among the most innovative products—have been somewhat immune from scrutiny, and arguably have been able to attain some of the highest prices paid (reflected in high cost-effectiveness ratio, meaning fewer health gains for the money spent). This is not necessarily inequitable or inefficient: it depends on many other factors. But it does mean that these companies are receiving greater rewards for their innovations.

HEALTH POLICY AND ECONOMIC ISSUES
IN PHARMACOGENETICS

The major health policy/economics issues related to pharmacogenetics today are the following:

- Pricing and reimbursement challenges
- Genetic discrimination
- Patents
- FDA regulation

The focus here will be on the pricing and reimbursement. A brief comment is offered on each of the other three. First, however, it is necessary to review two concepts that color much of debate around health policy issues related to genetics.

Background: Genetic Determinism and Exceptionalism

In thinking about health policy and economic issues in pharmacogenetics, it is important to keep two prevalent views in mind—genetic determinism and genetic exceptionalism. Held in varying degrees by members of the public, they tend to influence their policy interests and prescriptions. We define these two views as follows:

- Genetic determinism: the belief that genes determine all aspects of physical or behavioral outcomes (i.e., phenotype).
- Genetic exceptionalism: the view that genetic information is fundamentally different from other kinds of medical information and, as a result, deserves special protection or regulation.

Generally speaking, "genetic determinism" is an erroneous position rooted in a monogenic (mis)perception of the impact of genetics. For most diseases and aspects of human behavior, genes alone have a very limited predictive power. Environment is at least—if not more—influential. Genetic exceptionalism is probably tied to genetic determinism in many people's minds: if genes are more highly predictive of disease or behavior, then they deserve special treatment. In fact, nongenetic factors, such as cholesterol levels, can be just as predictive of disease. Others argue genes are special because they provide information about family members, but so does nongenetic information such as infection with communicable diseases.

These misperceptions are not surprising given that most genetic tests currently used are for rare cases of single-gene disorders (for which gene and health outcome are tightly linked) or for paternity and forensic DNA testing. This has probably biased the public's perception too much in the direction genetic determinism and exceptionalism. But when it comes specifically to pharmacogenetics (e.g., testing to predict drug response), the public has very little experience since very few such tests exist. At the very least, in thinking about and formulating public policies we should at least question whether special provisions are needed for genetic or pharmacogenetic tests.

Pricing and Reimbursement Challenges

Like Danzon and Towse, Garrison and Austin (2007) argue that for products already on the market, given the limited ability to adjust market prices, drug companies have a very limited incentive to identify subgroups in which the risk-benefit ratio is better. Furthermore, diagnostic companies face an even more inflexible pricing and reimbursement system: reimbursement for diagnostics is more or less what economists would call an "administered pricing system" in which amounts reimbursed are based on some approximate projection of perceived costs and bear little relation to added value. This inflexible, administered pricing system can be a barrier to rewarding the innovation that is needed to sustain technological momentum in these fields.

Considering a number of scenarios, Garrison and Austin (2007) argue that incentives to develop a linked pharmacogenetics-based diagnostic therapeutic will depend on several factors: (1) whether the drug is already on the market (and priced) before the test is developed, (2) the extent to which drug and diagnostic prices are flexible and are value-based versus cost-based, (3) the competitiveness of the insurance market, and (4) the strength of the patent protection on the diagnostic versus the therapeutic.

Other Issues and Challenges

Briefly, it is worth mentioning three other policy issue areas in relation to economics and pharmacogenetics from an economic perspective. First, the issue of genetic discrimination raises both ethical and economic questions. Should life and health insurers be able to charge customers different rates based on their genetic markers? If insurers require tests for coverage, then potential customers may either avoid a test (even if it has some clinical value) or try to hide the results of the test (at the risk of subsequent denial of benefits if discovered). Allowing customers to obtain but not reveal tests could lead to "adverse selection" in the insurance market as those with positive tests (i.e., more likely to experience disease or death) seek more extensive insurance. Adverse selection can undermine insurance markets. Ossa and Towse analyze the trade-off between adverse selection versus discouragement of testing.[24] They argue that societal policy should take these into account, and that the results could differ depending on the specifics of a given test.

A second issue is: what should the FDA do to regulate and encourage the development of linked pharmacogenetic tests and pharmaceuticals? To the point, the FDA has not taken a strong proactive role in this. Their guidance on this covers "voluntary" genomic data submissions: companies are encouraged to collect genetic sample and to submit data based on these. Generally, the results from analyzing such samples are going to be only suggestive at best; clinical trials are powered to measure the primary endpoint on an efficient sample, and not in a subgroup of patients. In the case of Tarceva for non-small-cell cancer, the FDA required the company to analyze subgroups based on a biomarker test of the presence of epidermal growth factor receptors. The results were included in the label, though the test is not required for prescription as its predictive power is still under debate.

A final issue concerns patents. Although "gene patents" are allowed if they met the standard patent criteria (unique, nonobvious, useful, full disclosure, etc.), some controversy remains about whether they should be. Nonetheless, it is also becoming clearer that pharmacogenetic response to drugs is a complex phenomenon that could be affected by many genes. If multiple patent holders on the panel of genes best predict some outcome, how will the licensing and royalty issues be resolved, and will this be a major barrier to developing such complex tests? Should patent reform or organized patent pools be encouraged to address these potential problems?

CONCLUSION

The health and economic policy challenges facing these two innovative, related fields of biotechnology and pharmacogenetics have some commonalities, but also some major differences. First, the incentives to innovate in both could be greatly affected by regulatory and reimbursement policies. How the regulatory issues regarding follow-on biologics are handled could have profound implications for that industry. Potential pharmacogenetics applications would be affected should the FDA move behind the current voluntary guidance to requiring more biomarker testing throughout product development. Both biologics and linked diagnostic-therapeutic products would be affected by major changes in the reimbursement environment, e.g., required cost-effectiveness evaluation to obtain coverage and reimbursement (as occurs in the UK). Indeed, a good argument can be made that to promote the optimal level of innovation, some policy changes are needed to provide a supportive regulatory, legal, and payment environment.

This chapter only scratches the surface of the myriad fascinating economic and policy issues facing the dynamic fields of biotechnology and pharmacogenetics. In his seminal 1978 book *Who Shall Live?* Victor Fuchs identified the "technological imperative" as one the major factors influencing how medical care is provided in the United States: physicians desire to use whatever technologies are at their disposal regardless of the benefit-cost ratio.[25] This imperative continues to this day, but is increasingly coming up against the pressures to contain costs. How this trade-off is handled in the policy realm will have much to say about whether these fields remain on the cutting edge of science and medical practice.

NOTES

1. Aaron HJ (2003). Should public policy seek to control the growth of health care spending? *Health Affairs* January: W3/28-36.

2. Research!America (2005). *American Speaks: Poll Data Summary,* Volume 6. Alexandria, VA: United Health Foundation.

3. Research!America (2006). *National Survey, 2006.* United Health Foundation Alexandria, VA: United Health Foundation. Available at: http://www.research america.org/ polldata/index.html. Accessed March 31, 2006.

4. Ho RYJ and Gibaldi M (2003). *Biotechnology and Biopharmaceuticals: Transforming Proteins and Genes into Drugs.* Wilmington, DE: Wiley-Liss.

5. We do not distinguish here between pharmacogenetics and pharmacogenomics, though some use these terms to mean different things.

6. Biotechnology Industry Organization (2006). Biotechnology industry facts. Available at: http://www.bio.org/speeches/pubs/er/statistices.asp. Accessed March 31, 2006.

7. Hoovers (2006). Amgen Inc. Available at: http://www.hoovers.com/amgen-inc./—ID__12623—/free-co-factsheet.xhtml. Accessed March 30, 2006.

8. NDC Health (2004). The top 200 selling drugs in 2004 by U.S. sales. Atlanta, GA: NDC Health. Available at: http://www.drugs.com/top200_2004.html.

9. Haffner ME (2006). Adopting orphan drugs: Two dozen years of treating rare diseases. *NEJM* 354(5): 445-447.

10. The Royal Society (2005). *Personalised Medicine: Hopes and Realities.* September. London: The Royal Society.

11. Garrison LG and Austin MJF (2006) Linking pharmacogenetics-based diagnostics and drugs for personalized medicine. Health Affairs, 25(5): 1281-1290.

12. Frueh, F (2006). Qualification of genomic biomarkers for regulatory decision making. Presentation at the Annual DIA EuroMeeting, March 7, Paris, France. Available at: http://www.fda.gov/cder/genomics/presentations.htm. Accessed March 31, 2006.

13. Phillips KA, Van Bebber SL (2004). A systematic review of cost-effectiveness analyses of pharmacogenomic interventions. *Pharmacogenomics* 5(8): 1-11.

14. Webster A, Martin P, Lewis G, and Smart A (2004). Integrating pharmacogenetics into society: In search of a model. *Nature Reviews Genetics* 5: 663-668.

15. Veenstra DL, Higashi MK, Phillips KA (2000). Assessing the cost-effectiveness of pharmacogenomics. *AAPS PharmSci* 2(3): E29.

16. Phillips KA, Veenstra DL, Oren E, et al. (2001). Potential role of pharmacogenomics in reducing adverse drug reactions: A systematic review. *JAMA* 286(18): 2270-2279.

17. Flowers CR, Veenstra D (2004). The role of cost-effectiveness analysis in the era of pharmacogenomics. *Pharmacoeconomics* 22(8): 481-493.

18. Miller F, Hurley J, Morgan S, et al. (2002). Predictive Genetic Tests and Health Care Costs. January 10. Toronto: Ontario Ministry of Health and Long-Term Care.

19. Califf RM (2004). Defining the balance of risk and benefit in the era of genomics and protenomics. *Health Affairs* 23(1): 77-87.

20. Bala MV, Zarkin GA (2004). Pharmacogenomics and the evolution of heathcare: Is it time for cost-effectiveness analysis at the individual level? *Pharmacoeconomics* 22(8): 495-498.

21. Danzon P, Towse A (2002). The economics of gene therapy and of pharmacogenetics. *Value in Health* 5(1): 5-13.

22. Garrison LG and Austin MJF (2007). The economics of personalized medicine: Incentives for value creation and capture. Forthcoming *Drug Information Journal.*

23. Anand G (2005). How drugs for rare diseases became lifeline for companies. *Wall Street Journal,* November 15, p. A1.

24. Ossa DF and Towse A (2004). Genetic screening, health care and the insurance industry. Should genetic information be made available to insurers? *Eur J Health Economics* 5: 116-121.

25. Fuchs, VF (1978). *Who Shall Live?* New York: Basic Books.

Chapter 19

Promoting Pharmaceutical Products

Alan Lyles

INTRODUCTION

Pharmaceutical products have a long history of promotion. Such promotion by the pharmaceutical industry has been directed at medical professionals and more recently it has been directed at the general public. These efforts include activities as diverse as having a pharmaceutical company's pharmaceutical sales representative (PSR, previously called a *detail person*) meet with physicians, scheduling presentations for physicians' continuing education, arranging lunches and lectures for medical students and residents, advertising in scientific journals, and promotional activities targeting potential consumers. Promotional spending in the pharmaceutical industry has grown substantially, from $9.3 billion in 1996 to $25.3 billion in 2003—a 272 percent increase in unadjusted dollars (see Table 19.1). Although these are distinct activities, the goal is a consistent, reinforced message across the communications.

Consolidations in the pharmaceutical industry through mergers and acquisitions has generally impeded rather than facilitated bringing new products to market. For an industry whose members' shares are publicly traded, the consequence of slowing revenue generation can be swift and brutal—particularly when the past record of earnings has been stellar. Consequently, expanding the use of existing products will be even more crucial over the next five years. The challenge of innovation as the path to revenue growth is captured in a twelve-year analysis of New Drug Applications (NDAs) to the U.S. Food and Drug Administration (FDA). The National Institute for Health Care Management examined NDAs covering 1989 to 2000: priority-review new molecular entities (NMEs) represented 15 percent of approvals for new drugs during this period (153 of 1,035), while 65

TABLE 19.1. Total U.S. pharmaceutical product promotional spending, by type, 2003 (in millions U.S. dollars).

Promotional spending	2003	2002	2001	2000	1999	1998	1997	1996
DTCA	3,235	2,638	2,679	2,467	1,848	1,317	1,069	791
Office	4,455	5,327	4,789	4,038	3,607	3,386	2,785	2,458
Hospital	819	873	702	765	713	671	579	552
Medical journal advertising	448	437	425	484	470	498	510	459
Sub-total	8,957	9,275	8,595	7,754	6,368	4,943	4,916	4,260
Free product samples	16,373	11,909	10,464	7,954	7,230	6,602	6,047	4,904
Total	25,330	21,184	19,059	15,708	13,598	11,545	10,963	9,164

Percent share by type of promotional spending								
Office	18	25	25	26	27	29	25	27
DTC	12.8	12.5	14.1	15.7	13.6	11.4	9.8	8.6
Samples as	64.6	56.2	54.9	50.6	53.2	57.2	55.2	53.5
Medical journal advertising	1.8	2.1	2.2	3.1	3.5	4.3	4.7	5.0

Source: IMS Health (2006). Total U.S. Promotional Spend by Type, 2003. Available at: http://www.imshealth.com/ims/portal/front/articleC/0,2777,6599_44304 752_44889690,00.html. Accessed on: April 5, 2006.

percent contained already marketed active ingredients.[1] The importance of marketing and advertising as an integrated strategy with research and development is obvious.

LEGISLATION, REGULATION, AND OVERSIGHT

The American Medical Association (AMA)'s Council on Pharmacy and Chemistry, established in 1905, had a large impact on medical journal advertising policies and on physician prescribing decisions. Although the council was established to fight patent medicines and their advertising, it also affected consumer access to drug information. "The council ... would not approve any drug that was directly advertised to the public, or whose 'label, package or circular' listed the diseases for which the drug was to be used."[2] To place an advertisement in a medical journal, a manufacturer had first to comply with the AMA's requirement for disclosure of the product's content and its testing through the Bureau of Chemistry established by the Federal Food and Drugs Act of 1906.[3] As Paul Starr observed, the consequence of these actions changed the direction of the Federal Food and Drugs Act of 1906.[2] Instead of consumers having more accurate label information, they now had to rely on physicians as the source for drug information.

The Bureau of Chemistry was divided into two units in 1927 and in 1930 was renamed the Food and Drug Administration (FDA). The 1938 Food, Drug, and Cosmetic Act replaced the 1906 law. It mainly concerned requirements for proof of safety prior to marketing new drugs, and the Wheeler-Lee Amendment (1938) placed all drug advertising under the Federal Trade Commission (FTC), not the FDA.[4] FTC jurisdiction meant that the criteria for requirements and constraints were those of commercial communications. It was not until the Kefauver-Harris Amendment (1962) that oversight of prescription drug advertising became an FDA authority,[5] and regulation began to reflect the difference between drugs and consumer goods. Regulatory oversight of prescription drug promotions now resides in the Division of Drug Marketing, Advertising, and Communications (DDMAC).

Advertising and promotion of pharmaceutical products are restricted to approved uses, although physicians may legally prescribe marketed drugs for other, or off-label, uses. When off-label uses are promoted by manufacturers, or suspected of being promoted, possible actions include investigations ranging from communication reviews by the DDMAC to inquiries and possible Justice Department litigation.

The determination of a drug's status as prescription-only versus over-the-counter (OTC) was inconsistent until the Durham-Humphrey Amendment of 1951.[6] Prior to this law, each pharmaceutical company could decide whether a drug was a prescription-only product or not, and manufacturers might come to a different decision regarding the same drug. The FDA could, of course, contest these decisions through the courts. Following the Durham-Humphrey Amendment, prescription-only products, known as legend drugs, carried the legend "CAUTION: Federal law prohibits dispensing without a prescription."

Rapidly unfolding basic science discoveries and subsequent medical applications rested, in part, on a patent system that protected the intellectual property of the firm awarded the patent for the product or process. Legislation encouraged researchers and universities to work with drug companies to file patents and bring the benefits of their discoveries to the public. As more of the products dispensed in pharmacies were manufactured by large drug companies rather than being compounded by pharmacists, drug manufacturers became a more potent stakeholder in setting the prices for prescription products. Patent protection providing a period of potential monopoly on drugs, coupled with the costs of expanding manufacturing, research, and development infrastructure, led manufacturers to increase their revenues through more active product promotion. Initially these activities targeted physicians through detailing and medical journal advertisements.

From the 1950s through the 1980s, drug product promotions were mainly advertising in medical journals, sponsoring continuing medical education, and detailing physicians. Detail persons, or pharmaceutical sales representatives, are salespeople responsible for meeting with physicians, presenting information regarding their employer's products, answering doctors' questions, and, in the end, persuading physicians to write more prescriptions for the product(s) they are "detailing." Drug manufacturers' direct access to prescribing physicians has been the foundation of pharmaceutical product promotion for decades. This model is seen as Path A in Figure 19.1.

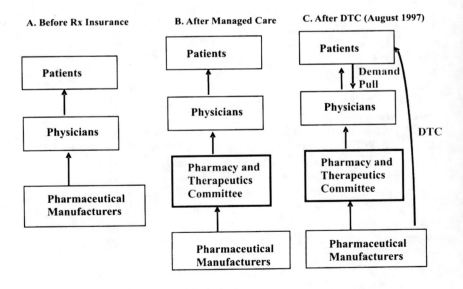

FIGURE 19.1. Evolution of pharmaceutical product communications.

Prescription Drug Costs

Beginning in the early 1980s, cost containment efforts were relatively successful for hospital and physician expenditures. However, annual drug cost increases throughout the 1990s outpaced the rates of increase in hospital and in physician costs. As more employers looked for opportunities to reduce their operating costs, pressure existed to lower or at least restrain the growth in health insurance premium costs. Drug cost trends generally defied these pressures and required cross-subsidization through savings achieved in other sectors, such as hospital and physician payments (see Table 19.2).

Promoting Pharmaceutical Products

Virtually everyone in the United States has been exposed to prescription drug advertisements intended for consumers—these advertisements are on

TABLE 19.2. Annual change per capita in health care spending and gross domestic product (GDP), 1994-2004.

	Change in Spending on Type of Health Care Service						
Year	All services	Hospital inpatient	Hospital outpatient	Physician	Rx drugs	Other	GDP
1994	3.5%	−2.3%	8.0%	2.1%	5.1%	12.3%	4.9%
1995	4.2	−3.7	7.0	2.6	10.7	8.6	3.4
1996	4.2	−4.6	7.0	2.2	10.8	12.0	4.4
1997	5.6	−5.4	8.9	4.1	11.4	11.8	5.0
1998	7.1	0.0	7.7	5.6	13.6	7.6	4.1
1999	9.9	2.6	11.6	6.7	18.1	5.5	4.8
2000	9.3	4.0	9.8	7.7	14.2	4.4	4.8
2001	11.3	8.6	14.5	7.8	13.5	9.1	2.1
2002	10.7	8.2	13.0	7.9	13.1	6.2	2.5
2003	8.4	6.1	11.1	6.4	8.9	5.8	3.9
2004	8.2	6.2	11.3	6.4	7.2	6.0	5.6

Notes: GDP is in nominal dollars. Estimates differ from past reports due to data revisions by Milliman and the Bureau of Economic Analysis. Health care spending data are the Milliman Health Cost Index ($0 deductible). Gross domestic product is from the U.S. Department of Commerce, Bureau of Economic Analysis. *Source:* Strunk BC, Ginsburg PB, and Cookson JP (2005). Tracking Health Care Costs: Spending Growth Stabilizes at High Rate in 2004. Center for Studying Health System Change. Data Bulletin # 29. June. Available at: http://www.hschange.org/CONTENTS/745/.

television, in newspapers and magazines, on the radio, and available on the Internet. However, the target of these promotions, consumers, cannot directly purchase the marketed product. In addition, the same communication about the product should contain a balance of the most important evidence about both its therapeutic benefit and risks. These advertisements should reflect the intended audience's medical sophistication. Drugs differ from other consumer products in that although caveat emptor may guide commerce, it is not applicable in medicine. Instead, behavioral models such as the physician being the agent for the patient, the *learned intermediary,* and ethical codes emphasizing *beneficence* provide guidance and preferred standards in health care.

Direct-to-consumer (DTC) communications were, however, just 12.8 percent of pharmaceutical marketing and advertising expenditures in 2003 (see Table 19.1).[7] Marketing pharmaceutical products directly to consumers, although pervasive, is just the most visible aspect of pharmaceutical product promotion. Samples of free products in 2003 represented 64.6 percent, physician office promotions were 17.6 percent, and medical journal advertising was just 1.8 percent of total U.S. pharmaceutical product promotional spending.

The trends and relative types of promotional spending have changed since the FDA issued a draft guidance on direct-to-consumer broadcast advertisements in 1997.[8] Although overall promotional spending grew 272 percent (in absolute dollars) from 1996 to 2003, the share for DTC increased from 8.6 to 12.8 percent, and for free drug samples from 53.5 percent to 64.6 percent. The promotional strategy shift is starkly reflected in the declining share for medical journal advertising—from 5 percent in 1996 to 1.8 percent in 2003. Whether this represents waning support for peer-reviewed publications or a reallocation based on return-on-investment calculations, it has challenged nonpromotional, peer-reviewed journals to seek other revenue sources.

Pressure to Reduce Pharmaceutical Expenditures

Private health insurance paid just 1.3 percent of prescription drug expenditures in 1960, public programs paid only 2.7 percent, and the remainder (96 percent) was paid directly by individuals.[9] During this period of predominantly out-of-pocket payments by patients for their prescription drugs, patients' independent access to prescription drug information was further limited by the American Pharmacists Association's Code of Ethics for Pharmacists then in force: "the pharmacist does not discuss the therapeutic effects or composition of a prescription with a patient. When such questions are asked, he [or she] suggests that *the qualified practitioner* is the proper person with whom such matters should be discussed" [emphasis added].[10]

In recent years, third parties have had risk and financial responsibility for larger portions of pharmaceutical costs. Insurance products that offered a prescription drug benefit, including managed care health insurance, have grown in popularity; by 1996, individual payments for prescription drug expenditures in the United States declined to just one-third of total expenditures. Managed care enrollment increased substantially during the last two decades of the twentieth century; from 1980, with enrollments of nine million, 81 million people were members of managed care plans by 1999.[11] This represented a major shift in the pharmaceutical products market: instead of having millions of individuals paying for prescription drugs that had been selected by individual physicians, large organizations were financially responsible for much of the cost of products covered under the insured person's policy. This model is seen in as Path B in Figure 19.1.

Distinct trends began to converge. As professionalism grew in medicine and pharmacy and purchasers became more powerful, control of pharmaceutical expenditures became a priority; these forces collectively form a foundation for the demand for DTC. The rise of DTC spending followed a period of rapid expansion of managed care plan enrollments in the 1980s and 1990s. These insurance products provided the financial means for more people to obtain prescription drugs, yet for pharmaceutical manufacturers, managed care plans' benefit designs began to present a barrier to their direct communications with physicians (see Figure 19.1). Managed care plans began with open access to FDA–approved pharmaceutical products, initially subject to nominal cost sharing by the insured—typically a fixed copayment amount per prescription dispensed. During periods of expanding health plan enrollments, the rate of increase in prescription drug costs outpaced costs for other benefits (see Table 19.2).[15] This trend prodded insurers and health plans to become more active in the oversight and management of pharmaceutical product use by those they insured.

As a form of oversight, the pharmacy and therapeutics committee (P & T committee) evolved to become a vital organizational resource for assessing the adequacy or strength of evidence to support the use of alternative drugs and making recommendations regarding them to health plans, providers, employers, and insurance companies. To maintain a clinical and safety rather than primarily a financial focus, a centralized decision-making body of drug therapy experts, the pharmacy and therapeutics committee, was interposed between the pharmaceutical company, its pharmaceutical sales representative(s), and the prescribing physician. It is this committee that assesses the strength of the evidence for candidate products and where each product's use fits the clinical needs of the covered population. P & T committees increasingly requested evidence to support benefit coverage and the extent of coverage of specific drug products, producing a rapid increase in the number of economic studies of pharmaceuticals[12] and the birth of the discipline of pharmacoeconomics. Initially the absence of practice guideline standards led Drummond (1992) to question whether pharmacoeconomics, as then practiced, was actually science or another form of marketing.[13,14]

Health plans, insurance companies, and managed care plans had turned to the use of drug lists, known as formularies, to influence prescription drug utilization and costs.[16] These formularies were, at first, *open*—meaning that the list was for information and posed no restriction or financial barrier to access for marketed drugs. Subsequent insurance benefit designs used *partially closed* and *closed* formularies, under which only selected products were covered by the individual's insurance policy. The formulary has been used to implement the prescription drug benefit by linking the insured's cost sharing to different tiers or levels of product support within the formulary: two tiers consisting of generic and brand products; three tiers consisting of generic, brand, and nonpreferred brands; and four tiers consisting of generic, brand, nonpreferred brand, and lifestyle or other designated products. The extent of the insured's cost sharing increases at each tier, clearly intending to influence the prescriber to use and the patient to request a product from a lower tier if possible.

These changes created competition among pharmaceutical products for favorable formulary placement. The insertion of the P & T committee as a decision-making body and its influence on medication use within an insurance or health plan substantially altered the relative effectiveness of marketing activities. For example, physician detailing by pharmaceutical sales representatives as a marketing strategy based solely, or primarily, on physician communications and their autonomous prescription decision authority had to change.

Although fourth-tier products may require 100 percent payment by the insured, including those products on the formulary may permit their costs to be applied toward a patient's deductible. These approaches to drug product selection influence the extent and specific use of pharmaceutical products. They were, over time, augmented by utilization management techniques such as physician prescription profiling, requiring prior authorization for certain drugs and limiting the prescribing of some classes or drugs to specific physicians or specialties.[17]

Although physicians still have the professional prerogative to prescribe any marketed product they determine to be appropriate, as a practical matter insurance coverage or the extent of coverage of specific products for their patients pressure them to prescribe products endorsed by the pharmacy and therapeutics committee.

Although the FDA mandated the inclusion of information on benefits and risks of oral contraceptives in a patient package insert (PPI) in 1970, this was an isolated accomplishment for more accessible consumer information on approved drugs—a pilot PPI program was cancelled in 1982. Instead, the FDA elected to rely on voluntary, private sector actions to provide patients with product-specific information on risks and benefits.

During the period of definitively classifying drugs as prescription-only or OTC and evolution of regulatory authority over advertising them, advertisements and promotional activity by pharmaceutical companies generally excluded the public. From the Durham-Humphrey Amendment (1951) to the early 1980s, marketing emphasized physicians and, to a lesser extent, physicians-in-training. Starting with a public advertisement of the price for a branded version of ibuprofen,[18] a pneumococcal vaccine advertisement and then an advertisement for acyclovir, the move to promote prescription products directly to consumers had begun.[19] The shift from general, or help-seeking promotions to one based on a specific product was influenced by the campaign for Oraflex (benoxaprofen). Side effects and deaths attributed to this product lead to its removal from the market—voluntarily, by the manufacturer—and then to the commissioner of the FDA's request in 1983 for a moratorium on DTC advertising. During the moratorium, the regulatory implications of communications that balanced safety with risk were assessed.

In ending the moratorium, the commissioner decided that consumers would receive sufficient protection if the guidelines for physicians remained in place but were applied to communications for all audiences.[20] These standards required *product-claim* advertisements to include a *brief summary* and to provide *fair balance* between the health benefits and risks posed by use of the product. In addition, a drug advertisement could not be false, misleading, or lacking in material facts.[21] These requirements, however, presented a dilemma for advertising claims for a specific product to a lay audience since the brief summary was an extensive compilation of a prescription drug's *adverse event profile, contraindications, warnings, and precautions*. The prospect of including all of this information in a broadcast communication, such as a television or radio advertisement, was impractical since the available time was too short to include it all. It was also unappealing to manufacturers since the comprehensive discussion of all, even rare, side effects might defeat their purpose.

Besides a product-claim advertisement, the FDA also recognizes two other types: *help-seeking* (ads that only include information on medical conditions) and *reminder* advertisements (ads that mention the pharmaceutical product but make no claim regarding its uses).[22] These alternatives are not, in a strict sense, advertisements since they do not actively promote a particular product (unless it is the only treatment for the condition mentioned in the help-seeking advertisement or the general public already knows the use(s) of the product in the reminder advertisement). Other than benefiting from a possible class effect, pharmaceutical companies would gain little from these types of promotional expenditures; consequently, they were a small component of the overall industry's promotional strategy.

The requirements and restrictions on broadcast drug advertisements intended for consumers were revised, and the FDA issued a draft guidance in 1997, with a provision for review after two years (the resulting final guidance was not materially different from the draft). The draft guidance for industry on DTC broadcast advertisements permitted such advertisements subject to several requirements: broadcast advertisements must contain a *major statement* of the most important risks and *adequate provision* by which consumers could obtain the full package label information. The adequate-provision requirement would be met by having four alternative sources for complete information identified in each advertisement, varied to accommodate different information seeking preferences and abilities: (1) a telephone number (toll free) from which the complete information can be read to the caller, (2) a print advertisement in a widely available publication, (3) a suggestion to ask a physician or pharmacist, and (4) an Internet page.

Marketing pharmaceutical products presents some of the most sophisticated examples of lessons learned from applied social science, yet pharmaceutical promotions to consumers, began in earnest in 1997, pose unique challenges to a marketing industry built on hyperbole.

CURRENT PRACTICE

Direct-to-Consumer Advertising

Arguments used by the proponents and opponents of DTC advertising have remained essentially the same since the draft guidance in 1999. Those who favor DTC advertising argue that it raises awareness of new therapies among consumers, motivates people to see a physician, and reinforces medication adherence for those taking prescription drugs. Some of the arguments raised by opponents to DTC are that: it does not give sufficient attention to nonpharmacologic options, does not promote the use of generic medications when feasible, requires physician time to dissuade patients who make inappropriate medication requests, understates the risk of pharmacotherapy, and makes some consumers believe that they have all of the information needed to decide about their own pharmacotherapy.[23] This model of communication is seen as Path C in Figure 19.1.

From DTC's start under the FDA's 1997 guidance on broadcast communications, *Prevention* magazine has annually surveyed consumer awareness, understanding, and reactions to DTC advertising. Its telephone survey of a nationally representative adult sample in 2003-2004 had a ± 3 percent margin of sampling error.[24]

Consumer awareness of specific advertised products has increased markedly: from 3 of 13 drugs in the 1999 survey to 8 of 11 in the 2003-2004 survey. This overall change is even more dramatic for heavily promoted products: respondents identifying the condition that a drug is used to treat increased from 44 percent to 76 percent for Drug A, from 64 percent to 75 percent for Drug B, 63 percent to 72 percent for Drug C, and 41 percent to 61 percent for Drug D.

The effectiveness of product-specific DTC advertising as determined by recall varies by product, gender, age, health status, and other attributes of those reporting exposure to DTC advertising. Overall, 21 percent believe that "almost everyone" will experience the advertised benefits, and only 5 percent reported believing that "hardly anyone" will. The corresponding views on side effects were that 7 percent believed "almost everyone" would experience them and 15 percent believed that "most people" would, while 25 percent believed "hardly anyone" would.[25] According to the president of the Pharmaceutical Research and Manufacturers of America (PhRMA), "we have not done a good job about educating the patients of America that all drugs come with significant side effects."[26] Twenty-five percent reported the "benefit" information in drug advertisements to be "very clear," but 15 percent felt it was "not too clear"; the corresponding perceptions for risk information were 18 percent and 25 percent—suggesting a potential imbalance in perceived risk/benefit messages.[27] One example of the adverse consequences of a patient's belief concerning risks and benefits comes from a September 2005 consumer survey. It reported that 31 percent of adults polled reported that they had not filled "a prescription that your doctor gave you because you felt it was unnecessary."[28]

The current dampening of confidence in the FDA's regulating drug safety is coupled with DTC advertising since the products being withdrawn were some of the most heavily promoted and now actively litigated. For example, rofecoxib (Vioxx) promotional expenditures were $159.5 million in 2000, the year following marketing approval. Another COX-2, celecoxib (Celebrex), had $80.1 million in promotional expenditures during the same period.[29] The subsequent discovery of the potential exposure to cardiac risks in the millions of persons who had used rofecoxib has reinforced concerns about the safety of marketed drugs and how much is or is not known when they are approved by the FDA. In a July 21, 2005, survey by Harris Interactive, 52 percent of respondents agreed that it is a good idea to forbid direct-to-consumer advertising for some period of time after the FDA has approved a new drug so that doctors have time to become familiar with the drug; 36 percent favored a mandatory ban, and 16 percent preferred a voluntary ban. For respondents aged 65 and older, the percent agreeing with some type of restriction increased to 55 percent.[30]

To provide more time to gain understanding and data about possible actions and side effects in a broader population, several drug manufacturing companies have announced that they would voluntarily forego DTC advertising in the initial period following a new product's marketing approval. For example, Bristol-Myers Squibb decided to withhold DTC advertising for the first year following a new drug's marketing approval, and Pfizer pledged a six month moratorium.[31]

Educational level is strongly associated with a consumer's overall determination that "DTC advertising provides enough information to decide if benefit of using advertised drugs outweigh risk" —a surprising 32 percent of consumers believed that the advertisements do provide enough information. This response is highest for those with the lowest educational attainment and lowest for those with the highest educational attainment: 43 percent for those with "less than high school" education believed this, whereas just 36 percent of "high school graduates," 28 percent of respondents with "some college" and 23 percent of "college graduates" agreed with this statement.[32]

Prevention's survey indicates that the additional sources that FDA requires DTC advertising to include for consumers to obtain more complete information are infrequently sought. Recall and follow-up to obtain additional information from the adequate-provision sources that advertisements provide are consistently dismal. Only 26 percent remembered that a print advertisement was mentioned, and one-third did not recall the mention either of a Web site or of a toll-free telephone number as additional information sources.[33] Reported actual use of these sources is equally bleak: 4 percent sought print advertisements, 17 percent used a Web site, and 8 percent used the toll-free telephone number mentioned in the advertisement. Although 23 percent of respondents overall used at least one of the sources, many of these people were caregivers and were not seeking information for themselves.[34] Use of additional information sources varied by age: "Boomers" (ages 40 to 59) were highest and "Matures" (ages 60 and over) were lowest, despite greater use of prescription drugs an average by the "Matures" group.

Consumers Union is an independent, nonprofit testing and information organization serving only consumers, and serve as a comprehensive source for unbiased advice about products and services, personal finance, health and nutrition, and other consumer concerns.[35] The Consumers Union position is that more transparency and more complete safety information are needed for prescription drugs. To that end, it has three advocacy offices and a Consumer Policy Institute to advance its "Prescription for Change" campaign whose goal is to give all consumers access to safe, effective, and affordable prescription drugs.[36]

Advertising legend drugs to consumers may deemphasize nonpharmacologic treatments or actions to take prior to using pharmaceutical products. However, some consumers who have been exposed to DTC advertising do report making lifestyle changes as a result of such advertisements (21 percent) and seeking information about the condition mentioned in the drug advertisement (20 percent).[37]

DTC advertising is effective. It does provide information, but its role in marketing communications is to influence; the main function of DTC advertising is to enhance sales of advertised products. Over the first seven years of the *Prevention* survey, the percent of respondents who reported asking their doctor for an advertised drug spans the narrow range from 26 percent to 30 percent.[38] The survey results suggest that a patient's assessment of the adequacy of the benefit and risk information in advertisements influences whether they are more or less likely to speak with their doctors about the advertised drug. Forty-two percent of those who believed that they have enough information to balance risk and benefit spoke with their doctor, but just 27 percent of those who did *not* believe they had enough information spoke with a physician [39] These results are similar for men and women, but differ by generation. Overall 26 percent asked their doctor for an advertised drug, but this was lower for those over 40 years old and higher for those under 40: for 18 to 25 years it was 32 percent, for 26 to 39 years it was 31 percent, for 40 to 59 years it was 25 percent, and for those aged 60 and over it was just 15 percent.[40]

The bottom line, as it is said, is the bottom line. How do physicians respond to patient requests for an advertised prescription drug? The trend, based on annual consumer reports of their physician's prescribing the requested product, has been steadily increasing since 2000: 71 percent in 2000, 77 percent in 2001, 79 percent in 2002, and 84 percent in 2003.[41] In 2003, physicians prescribed a different drug to 7 percent of the requestors, and a declining percentage of those requesting a specific product left the doctor's office with no prescription: 19 percent in 2000, 13 percent in 2001, 11 percent in 2002, and 8 percent in 2003.

The apparently positive financial return on investment for DTC advertising may represent an appropriate expenditure by society in meeting its citizen's needs for previously untreated diseases—if rational pharmacotherapy is being practiced. Addressing this question requires moving beyond the conventional research methodology used in DTC advertising: much of the data regarding DTC advertising rely on surveys, opinions, and recall. A recent randomized trial provides empiric evidence on the prescribing consequences of DTC advertising as it is currently practiced and regulated.

Kravitz, et al.(2005) reported a randomized trial of DTC–related prescription drug requests to family physicians and internal medicine physicians.[42] Standardized patients (SPs) were calibrated with scripts that supported either a diagnosis of major depression or of adjustment disorder (that is, without major depression). Each standardized patient made one of three different prescription drug requests to a primary care physician who had been randomly selected from a panel of such physicians: (1) for an advertised, brand-name product; (2) for a drug to treat depression, but not specifying a particular product; or (3) no drug request. As might be expected, standardized patients with major depression frequently received antidepressant medication: 53 percent of those making brand-specific requests received an antidepressant, 76 percent of those making general drug requests received an antidepressant, but just 31 percent of those who made no drug request received an antidepressant. When a brand name drug was requested by a standardized patient with major depression, 27 percent received the requested brand, 26 percent received a different antidepressant, and 47 percent received no pharmacotherapy.

However, 34 percent of those *without* major depression also received antidepressant drugs: 55 percent of those who had made a brand-specific request, 39 percent of those who made a general drug request, and 10 percent of those who had not requested a drug. Unexpectedly, 67 percent of persons without major depression who had requested a brand-name drug for depression received a prescription for that product. These data question both differential diagnosis and treatment of major depression in primary care practice. The impact of DTC advertising on usual primary care practice appears both to encourage appropriate pharmacotherapy and to stimulate inappropriate drug demands and prescribing.

Promoting prescription drugs to consumers has some elements in common with selling various brands of detergent—including free trial offers, rebates, and utilization incentives such as offering a free refill after a certain number of filled prescriptions for that product. These promotions blur the distinctions between formulary tiers and lower the consumer/insured person's out-of-pocket costs for some branded products. Such promotions potentially lead to greater utilization of these products than of multisource or generic drugs in the same therapeutic class. Although pharmaceutical companies assert that these actions can raise consumer awareness of legitimate alternatives, opponents to such practices note the temporary savings relative to the longer term costs once the patient begins to refill his or her prescriptions. Currently, only Massachusetts prohibits the use of coupons for prescription drugs.[43]

OTHER FORMS OF PROMOTION AND REACTIONS TO THEM

Medical School Faculty: A Reaction to DTC

Commercial Alert, a nonprofit advocacy group whose mission is "to keep the commercial culture within its proper sphere, and to prevent it from exploiting children and subverting the higher values of family, community, environmental integrity and democracy,"[44] presented a petition for FDA's November 1-2, 2005, public hearings in which it requested that DTC advertising be prohibited. According to Thomaselli (2005), the petition was endorsed by more than 200 faculty from medical schools.[45] From testimony given by Gary Ruskin, Executive Director of Commercial Alert, at that November 2005 FDA hearing:

> Prescription drug advertising pressures health professionals to prescribe particular medications . . . This intrudes in the relationship between medical professionals and patients, and disrupts the therapeutic process . . . Prescription drug advertising is not educational. It is inherently misleading because it features imagery and omits crucial information about drugs and their proper use, as well as about side effects and contraindications that can be found on the full FDA-approved label . . . [DTC advertising] should not exist unless accompanied by the full FDA-approved label. Nor should drug ads be allowed to display imagery that is primarily emotive and not educational. Drug ads on TV and radio should be prohibited because they cannot meet this standard for truthfulness.[46]

Promotion to Physicians: Detailing

Promoting pharmaceutical products to consumers may create demand, but ultimately it is the physician who writes the prescription. Consequently, promotions to physicians and a search for the most effective ways to promote products to physicians have been a high priority of pharmaceutical manufacturers.

Data from Lehman Brothers, reported in Merx (2005), estimate the average sales per pharmaceutical sales representative at $1.9 million—a substantial amount individually and an impressive total when multiplied over the approximately 100,000 sales representatives (according to Verispan as cited by Merx).[47] These 100,000 salespeople worked with the approximately 782,200 physicians in the United States in 2000, or about one sales person per 7.8 physicians.[48]

Some health plans and providers restrict the frequency and content of sales representatives' contacts with physicians, residents, and others. The University of Michigan Health System prohibits unscheduled visits, all gifts, and drug samples. Kaiser Permanente (California) requires sales representatives to have scheduled appointments with doctors and it prohibits the use of drug samples. The Johns Hopkins Hospital's Pharmaceutical Sales Representative (PSR) Policy (October 2004)[49] requires a PSR to register with the Department of Pharmacy and to have scheduled the mandatory appointment at least three days in advance. PSRs "may not be the speaker for the [educational] program [or in-service] and may not attend any conference, program or meeting at which patient-specific information or quality assurance activities are discussed." In addition, Johns Hopkins' policy requires that "all promotional or information material provided by a PSR must be explicitly requested by JHH faculty or staff. Unsolicited distribution of materials is not permitted." (Johns Hopkins Hospital, 2004) The Henry Ford Hospital has had a similar policy for more than a decade.

Among other professional functions, a pharmaceutical sales representative provides free drug samples to physicians. The use of free drug samples of brand-name products might be supported as making a medication available to poor patients who otherwise may not be able to obtain the drug. However, noting that no free samples of generic drugs exist, Dr. Jack Billi of the University of Michigan Medical School explained that the use of brand-name drug samples actually, complicate initiation and continued medication use by indigent patients since they will confront the branded product's price when a refill is needed.

A risk exists that some promotions to physicians may violate federal fraud, abuse, and antikickback statutes. The Office of Inspector General (OIG) of the U.S. Department of Health and Human Services developed compliance program guidance for federal health care programs participants to "encourage the use of internal controls to efficiently monitor adherence to applicable statutes, regulations and program requirements."[50] OIG's guidance provides both a structure and process of internal controls that would mitigate the risk of violations. The OIG's compliance program guidance for pharmaceutical manufacturers, issued in 2003, cautions manufacturers regarding the practice of paying physicians to meet with pharmaceutical sales representatives, to visit Internet sites, or similar activities as "highly susceptible to fraud and abuse" and strongly discouraged these practices.

The OIG guidance also expressed concerns about arrangements in which something of value might be given to physicians, such as "entertainment, recreation, travel, meals, or other benefits in association with information or marketing presentations; and, gifts, gratuities, and other business courtesies" since they "potentially implicate the anti-kickback statute."

Increasing reliance on physicians as invited lecturers, members of a speaker bureau, or consultants requires clear adherence to this guidance. According to Verispan data cited in Hensley and Martinez (2005), the number of pharmaceutical-company-sponsored presentations in 1998 employing company sales representatives was about equal to those using physicians as presenters (60,000), whereas those using physicians increased to 237,000 in 2004 but those using company sales representatives had only increased to 134,000.[51]

Gifts to Physicians

The American Medical Association's Council on Ethical and Judicial Affairs provides guidance on gifts to physicians from industry in Opinion 8.061.[52] Opinion 8.061 was reviewed by an AMA Working Group and it stands as the profession's position. Under AMA's ethics guidelines, a gift is only acceptable if it benefits a patient or is "of modest value." One of the AMA's goals for these guidelines is to provide the basis for industry to train its sales representatives regarding physician expectations. A second goal is to avoid even the appearance of conflict of interest, as well as to prevent actual conflicts from arising.

Promotion to Physicians: E-Detailing

The Internet is a growing adjunct to in-person physician detailing. A 2002 survey of senior pharmaceutical company executives reported an anticipated decline in the importance of conventional marketing (advertising promotion, sales force, print media, conference events, and seminars) but an increase in the importance of general Web sites, company Web sites, call centers, and e-detailing. Of those activities expected to grow in importance, the largest gain by 2007 is expected to be in e-detailing.[53] Internet physician detailing, or e-detailing, reached 206,280 physicians in 2003. Physicians cited the following as the main reasons for participating in e-detailing (listed from high to low):

Do it on their own time, honoraria for learning about products, less disruptive than a representative, complements representative's information, control over a representative's information, curious about technology, learn what other MDs think, prefer over representative visits, preferred Pharma information source, replace representative visits.[54]

The Internet can be a means to promote products to physicians, but it also provides patients with condition- and product-specific information. Only 17 percent of consumers acted on a DTC advertising offer of a Web site for more complete product information on benefits and side effects of an advertised drug, but 35 percent of Americans over 15 years old using the Internet are seeking health information.[55] The difficulty of regulating the accuracy of Internet communications led the FDA to develop consumer guidelines for "Health Information On-Line" as early as 1996.[56]

More recently, stealth marketing using the Internet has grown beyond just spam. Although word-of-mouth marketing is not currently linked to the promotion of pharmaceutical products, within the advertising industry word-of-mouth, or "buzz marketing" is achieving prominence. The Word of Mouth Marketing Association (WOMMA) foresees increasing use of buzz marketing and, in its code of ethics, addresses the public concern about duplicity and misrepresentation of individuals with marketing firms in the initiation and maintenance of word-of-mouth campaigns. From the WOMMA Code (2): The Honesty ROI: Honesty of Relationship, Opinion, and Identity: "We practice openness about the relationship between consumers, advocates and marketers. We encourage word of mouth advocates to disclose their relationship with marketers in their communications with other consumers. We don't tell them to be open and honest about any relationship with a marketer and about any products or incentives that they may have received."[57]

Medical Students: A Response to Promotions to Physicians

Medical students, through the American Medical Student Association (AMSA), organized a national Counterdetailing Initiative in which first- and second-year medical students provide "the latest sources of unbiased, evidence-based, and clinically-applicable information on pharmaceuticals" to physicians in their offices, while third- and fourth-year students on clinical rotations distribute cards containing this information.

The mission of AMSA's Counterdetailing Initiative is to educate medical students about evidence-based medicine, specifically evidence-based prescription practices, to empower students through activism to teach themselves, fellow students, and physicians about existing clinical guidelines, "to introduce sources of unbiased and expert-reviewed information on pharmaceuticals to resident physicians, attending physicians, and practicing physicians in the community; and to educated medical students and physicians about the effect of pharmaceutical promotions on prescription habits."[58]

Pharmaceutical Manufacturers

Writing that the "APA [American Psychiatric Association], AMA [the American Medical Association]and public policy officials, among others" are concerned about DTC advertising, Moran (2005) reported on the Pharmaceutical Research and Manufacturers of America's (PhRMA's) fifteen voluntary guiding principles covering DTC advertising.[59] These voluntary guiding principles[61] come at a time of heightened concern about the safety of marketed prescription drugs, the information provided to and the relationships between physicians and industry, and the clarity and completeness of DTC advertising risk communications.

These guiding principles discourage reminder advertisements (guiding principles # 3 and # 4), urge companies to time consumer promotions so that they are not distributed until after new drugs are detailed to physicians (guiding principle # 6), and propose the use of advertisements that discuss general health issues rather than individual pharmaceutical products (guiding principle # 14). TNS Media Intelligence data cited in Hensley identified name brand advertising expenditures at $4.08 billion versus $362 million for advertisements not linked to a branded drug. Under the PhRMA guidelines, this mix would be expected to change. As yet, no independent study evaluating compliance with these voluntary guidelines exists.[60]

CONCLUSION

Pharmaceutical product promotions will continue to be a "full court press" with specific communications for consumers, physicians, health plans, and pharmacy benefit management firms. As manufacturers face the risky prospect of relying on innovation for future growth, the path of earnings through marketing appears more certain.

All participants in the selection and use of prescription drugs will continue to receive promotions for pharmaceutical products. These promotions will increase in amount and sophistication as the opposing forces for cost control meet the demands for revenue growth by publicly traded companies.

DTC advertising of prescription drugs will not be prohibited for two main reasons: (1) First Amendment protections on commercial communications will likely supersede the FDA's claim to regulatory oversight, and (2) some evidence that the public desires the information that is, perhaps imperfectly, communicated in these advertisements. The public's demand for more information and more credible information about prescription drugs will increase as baby boomers age and consumer-directed health plans with high deductibles push more prescription drug costs to patients' out-of-pocket expenses.[62]

Consequently, advertising and promoting pharmaceutical products will increase, innovate, and cover a broader spectrum. Recent initiatives such as e-detailing and word-of-mouth marketing are just two examples of promotions that creatively employ technology. The ascendancy of advocacy and interest group politics assures that FDA and OIG guidelines will continue to be contested. The content of promotional activities will continue to be assessed for balance and absence of bias in communicating gains and risks from pharmaceutical products. As with existing laws governing drug efficacy, safety, and communications, those governing promotional activities will likely lag actual practice. The limits of regulations will be tested, and the interactions among FDA and OIG guidance, consumer demand, and the marketplace will persist in producing novel, durable, and dynamic challenges.

NOTES

1. National Institute for Health Care Management (2006). Changing Patterns of Pharmaceutical Innovation. May 2002. Available at: http://www.nihcm.org/final web/innovations.pdf. Accessed April 5, 2006.

2. Starr P (1982). *The Social Transformation of American Medicine*. New York: Basic Books, Inc.

3. Federal Food and Drugs Act of 1906 (The "Wiley Act"). Pub. L. No. 59-384, 34 Stat. 768 (1906).

4. Federal Food, Drug, and Cosmetics Act. Pub. L. No. 75-717, 52 Stat. 1040 (1938), codified as amended 21 U.S.C. §§ 301 et seq. "Federal Food, Drug, and Cosmetics Act," June 25, 1938.

5. Food, Drug, and Cosmetic Act 1962. Kefauver-Harris Amendment, 21 U.S.C. Section 355.

6. Durham-Humphrey Prescription Drug Amendment of 1951. 1997. 21 U.S.C.§ § 353,355.

7. IMS Health (2004). Total U.S. Promotional Spend by Type, 2003. Available at: http://www.imshealth.com/ims/portal/front/articleC/0,277,6599_44304752_4488 9690,00.html. Accessed April 5, 2006.

8. Food and Drug Administration (1999). Guidance for Industry: Consumer-Directed Broadcast Advertisements. August. Available at: http://www.fda.gov/cder/ guidance/804fnl.htm. Accessed April 15, 2006.

9. Centers for Medicare and Medicaid Services (2004). National Health Source Expenditures, Selected Calendar Years: 1980-2003. Available at: http://www.cms .nhs.gov/statistics/??/historical/tables.pdt. Accessed May 25, 2004.

10. American Pharmaceutical Association (1952). Code of Ethics of the American Pharmaceutical Association. *Journal of the American Pharmaceutical Association* 41(2:2): 20-21.

11. Centers for Disease Control and Prevention (2004). Health, United States, 2003. Table 132: Health Maintenance Organizations (HMOs) and Their Enrollment According to Model Type, Geographic Region, and Federal Program: United States, Selected Years 1976-2002. Available at: www.cdc.gov/nchs/data/hus/hus03.pdf. Accessed October 20, 2004.

12. Elixhauser A, Halpern M, Schmier J, and Luce BR (1998). Health Care CBA and CEA from 1991 to 1996: An Updated Bibliography. *Medical Care* 36(5 Suppl): MS1-9, MS18-147.

13. Drummond MF (1992). Economic Analysis of Pharmaceutical: Science or Marketing? *Pharmacoeconomics* 1(1): 8-13.

14. Drummond MF (1998). A Reappraisal of Economic Valuation of Pharmaceuticals: Science or Marketing? *Pharmacoeconomics* 14(1): 1-9.

15. Strunk BC, Ginsburg PB, and Cookson JP (2005). Tracking Health Care Costs: Spending Growth Stabilizes at High Rate in 2004. Center for Studying Health System Change. Data Bulletin #29. June. Available at: http://www.hschange .org/CONTENT/745/.

16. Lyles A and Palumbo FB (1999). The Effect of Managed Care on Prescription Drug Costs and Benefits. *Pharmacoeconomics* 15(2): 129-140.

17. Lyles A (2006). Formulary Decision-Maker Perspectives: Responding to Changing Environments. In Pizzi JT and Lofland JT, *Economic Evaluation in U.S. Health Care: Principles and Applications* (pp. 113-142). Sudbury, MA: Jones and Bartlett Publishers.

18. Pines WL (1999). A History and Perspective on Direct-to-Consumer Promotion. *Food and Drug Law Journal* 54: 489-518.

19. Basara LR (1992). Direct-to-Consumer Advertising: Today's Issues and Tomorrow's Outlook. *Journal of Drug Issues* 22(2): 317-330.

20. Federal Register (1985). Direct-to-Consumer Advertising of Prescription Drugs; Withdrawal of Moratorium. September 9. *Federal Register* 50(174): 36677-36678.

21. Food and Drug Administration (1999). Prescription Drug Advertising. 21 Code of Federal Regulations Pt. 202.1(e).

22. Federal Register (1995). Direct-to-Consumer Promotion: Public Hearing. August 16. *Federal Register* 60(158): 42581-42584.

23. Lyles A (2002). Direct Marketing of Pharmaceuticals to Consumers. *Annual Review of Public Health* 23: 73-91.

24. *Prevention* Magazine (2005). *Consumer Reaction to DTC Advertising of Prescription Medicines.* Seventh Annual Survey, 2003-2004. Emmaus, PA: Rodale Press.

25. *Prevention* Magazine (2003-2004). See Tables 15, 16, 20, and 21.

26. Berenson A (2005). Big Drug Makers See Sales Decline With Their Image. *New York Times.* November 14.

27. *Prevention* Magazine (2003-2004). See Table 24.

28. Prescription Drug Compliance a Significant Challenge for Many Patients, According to New National Survey. Available at: http://www.harisinteractive.com/news/allnewsbydate.asp?NewsID=904. Accessed on: April 16, 2006.

29. IMS Health (2001). Leading 10 Products by U.S. DTC Spend, 2000. Available at: http://www.imshealth.com/ims/prtal/front/articleC/C,2777,6599_40054629_1004776,00.html. Accessed April 24, 2006.

30. Harris Interactive (2005). Majority of U.S. Adults Think it is a Good Idea to Forbid Direct-to-Consumer Advertising for New Prescription Drugs when They First Come to Market. *Wall Street Journal* Online/Harris Interactive Health-Care Poll 4(14): 1-5. Available at: http://www.harrisinteractive.com/news/newsletters/wsjhealthnews/WSJOnline_HI_Health-CarePoll2005vol4_iss14.pdf.   Accessed April 9, 2006.

31. Hensley S (2005). Drug Makers Seek to Transform Advertising. *Wall Street Journal* Online. August 29. Available at: http://online.wsj.com/artcle-print/JB1125 2681442925007.html. Accessed October 14, 2005.

32. *Prevention* Magazine (2003-2004). See Table 22.

33. *Prevention* Magazine (2003-2004). See Table 25.

34. *Prevention* Magazine (2003-2004). See Table 27.

35. Consumers Union (2006). About Consumers Union. Available at: http://www.consumersunion.org/aboutcu/about.html. Accessed April 16, 2006.

36. Consumers Union (2006). About the Prescription for Change campaign. Available at: http://www.consumersunion.org/campaigns/prescription/about.html. Accessed April 16, 2006.

37. *Prevention* Magazine (2003-2004). See Table 60.

38. *Prevention* Magazine (2003-2004). See Table 54.

39. *Prevention* Magazine (2003-2004). See Chart 12.

40. *Prevention* Magazine (2003-2004). See Table 55.

41. *Prevention* Magazine (2003-2004). See Table 58.

42. Kravitz RL, Epstein RM, Feldman MD, Franz CF, Azari R, Wilkes MS, Hinton L, and Franks P (2005). Influence of Patients' Requests for Direct-to-Consumer Advertised Antidepressants: A Randomized Controlled Trial. *Journal of the American Medical Association* 293(16): 1995-2002.

43. Krasner J (2006). Drug Coupons May Be No Bargain: Legislators Fear They Could Push Health Costs Up. *Boston Globe.* April 6. Available at: http://www.boston.com/business/healthcare/articles/2006/04/06/drug_coupons_may_be_no_bargain/.

44. CommercialAlert (2006). Our Mission. Available at: http://www.commercialalert.org. Accessed April 16, 2006.

45. Thomaselli R (2005). 200 Medical School Professors Condemn DTC Advertising. Available at: http://adage.com/news.cms?newsId=46542. Accessed October 28, 2005.

46. CommercialAlert (2005). Testimony of Gary Ruskin, Executive Director of Commercial Alert Before the U.S. Food and Drug Administration Hearings on Direct-to-Consumer Prescription Drug Advertising. November. Available at: http://www.commercialalert.org/dtctestimony.pdf. Accessed April 15, 2006.

47. Merx K (2005). Drug Marketing: Freebies For Doctors Curbed. *Detroit Free Press.* July 12. Available at: http://www.freep.com/money/business/pharmrep123_20050712.htm.

48. Bureau of Health Professions (2001). National Center for Health Workforce Analysis: U.S. Health Workforce Personnel Factbook. Table 101. Estimated Supply Of Selected Health Personnel And Practitioner-To-Population Ratios, Selected Years: 1970-2000. Health Resources and Services Administration, U.S. Department of Health and Human Services. Available at: http://bhpr.hrsa.gov/healthworkforce/reports/factbook.htm. Accessed April 15, 2006.

49. Johns Hopkins Hospital (2004). *Johns Hopkins Hospital Pharmaceutical Sales Representatives Policy.* October 1. Baltimore, MD: Johns Hopkins.

50. Federal Register (2003). OIG Compliance Program Guidance for Pharmaceutical Manufacturers. May 5. *Federal Register* 68(86): 23731-23743.

51. Hensley S and Martinez B (2005). To Sell Their Drugs, Companies Increasingly Rely on Doctors. *New York Times.* July 15, p. A1.

52. American Medical Association Council on Ethical and Judicial Affairs (2005). Gifts to Physicians: Ethical Opinions and Guidelines. Opinion 8.061. Available at: http://www.ama-assn.org/ama/pub/category/4001.html. Accessed April 15, 2006.

53. IMS Health (2004). How Relevant is e-Detailing? August 9. Available at: http://www.imslhealth.com/imsp/portal/front/articleC/0,277,6599_54702271_5470351,00.html. Accessed April 5, 2006.

54. Boehm, El (2003). Forrester Research, CBI's eDetailing Conference Proceedings, September 2003. Cited in What Are Doctors Saying About e-Detailing? Available at: http://www.imshealth.com/ims/portal/front/articleC/0,2777,6599_ 54 70 2273_54703544,00.html. Accessed April 5, 2006.

55. National Telecommunications and Information Administration (2006). A Nation Online: How Americans Are Expanding Their Use of the Internet. Available at: http://www.ntia.doc.gov/ntiahome/dn/html/toc.htm Accessed April 18, 2006.

56. Food and Drug Administration (1996). Health Information On-Line. *FDA Consumer Magazine* 30(5). Available at: http://www.fda.gov/fdac/features/596_info.html.

57. Word of Month Marketing Association (2006). Word of Mouth Marketing Code of Ethics. Available at: http://www.womma.org/ethicscode.htm. Accessed April 15, 2006.

58. American Medical Student Association (2006). American Medical Student Association's Counterdetailing Initiative. Available at: http://www.amsa.org/prof nextlevel.cfm. Accessed April 6, 2006.

59. Moran M (2005). Complaints Lead Drug Firms To Modify Ad Guidelines. American Psychiatric Association. *Psychiatric News* 40(17): 1. Available at: http://pn.psychiatryonline.org/cgi/content/short/40/17/1-b Accessed April 18, 2006.

60. Moran M (2005).

61. Pharmaceutical Research and Manufacturers of America (2005). PhRMA Guiding Principles Direct to Consumer Advertisements About Prescription Medicines. Available at: http://www.phrma.org/files/2005-11-29.1194.pdf. Accessed April 16, 2006.

62. Berndt ER (2005). To Inform or Persuade? Direct-to-Consumer Advertising of Prescription Drugs. *New England Journal of Medicine* 352: 325-328.

Chapter 20

Competition: Brand-Name versus Generic Drugs

Jeff J. Guo
Christina M.L. Kelton

To encourage new drug development, the government grants pharmaceutical companies patents for their discoveries that allow them to obtain monopoly profits and charge monopoly prices for a period of time. Because bringing a new drug to market costs, on average, more than $800 million,[1] drug companies would not undertake the risks associated with developing new drugs without the opportunity to be rewarded for their efforts. When the innovator company's patent expires, generic companies begin to enter the market, and eventually the market starts to resemble a competitive market. The speed at which the transformation occurs depends on how quickly generic (multiple-source) drugs are substituted for branded (single-source) medications, and public policy can influence this speed.[2] When the market becomes competitive, efficiency of resource allocation is restored as price approaches marginal cost. This chapter is devoted to understanding competition in pharmaceutical markets and to understanding public policies that serve either to limit competition or enhance competition in those markets.

Patents are key to the length of time that a firm captures monopoly profits. On the one hand, the government rewards innovation with patents that are "long enough." The Hatch-Waxman Act of 1984 (which added Section 156 to the U.S. Patent Act) permits patent term extension for up to five years for human drug products. The act restores a portion of the patent term during which the patentee must wait for the Food and Drug Administration's (FDA's) review of its drug. The Uruguay Round Agreements Act of 1994 (which amended Section 154 of the U.S. Patent Act) extended the patent length for all U.S. patents (including those on pharmaceuticals) from seventeen to twenty years. The FDA's Modernization Act of 1997 helps to accelerate the drug review process by reducing or simplifying many of the regulatory obligations imposed on drug manufacturers. The Patent Term Guarantee Act of 1999 requires the federal Patent and Trademark Office to compensate firms for delays of more than three years in processing patents. The Best Pharmaceuticals for Children Act of 2002 gives drug companies a six-month patent extension if they test the safety of their drugs in children.

On the other hand, upon patent expiration, the government wants to encourage the entry of generic manufacturers in order to create a competitive market as soon as possible. The Hatch-Waxman Act of 1984 gives the FDA the authority to accept Abbreviated New Drug Applications (ANDAs) for generic entry. Generic manufacturers must demonstrate only bioequivalence to the patented drug in order to be approved by the FDA through the ANDA process. The time period between patent expiration and generic drug entry was shortened from three to four years before 1984 to one to three months in the 1990s.[3] The first approved ANDA, in 1984, was for generic disopyramide, marketed as Norpace and used in the treatment of cardiac arrhythmia. Since that time, 8,019 ANDAs have been submitted to the FDA through December 31, 2000.[4]

U.S. pharmaceutical companies have been innovative. They have nearly doubled their research and development (R & D) investment every five years since 1980, from $2 billion in 1980 to $8.4 billion in 1990, and to $31 billion in 2002.[5] Over the past decade, R & D costs have risen annually at the rate of 7.4 percent above inflation.[6] Between 1990 and 2004, the Food and Drug Administration approved a total of 1284 new drug applications.[7] Indeed, as it turns out, the newer, more expensive patented medications are currently replacing the older medications faster than generic entry reduces the costs of older medications going off patent, and this trend is the basis for the current pharmaceutical cost increases. Schondelmeyer reported that the proportion of generic drug utilization in Medicaid programs actually declined from 54 percent in 1995 to 51 percent in 1998.[8]

Double-digit annual increases in pharmaceutical costs for more than a decade have put the current system under tremendous pressure and have caused academics and policymakers to revisit the trade off between innovation encouraged by the patent system and social welfare enhanced by competition. According to a 2002 report prepared by the National Institute for Health Care Management,[9] the explanations for the rising trend in drug expenditures include declining buyer price sensitivity due to better insurance coverage for drugs; an increase in the number of prescription medicines available, especially for chronic conditions; an increase in the diagnosis of diseases in an aging population; and more aggressive marketing of prescription drugs to doctors and patients. These four factors underlie both an increase in the number of prescriptions written (an increase in drug utilization) and an increase in the average price per prescription. Lichtenberg[10] showed that the replacement of older drugs by newer, more expensive drugs (as previously discussed) was the single most important reason for the increase in the average level of pharmaceutical prices.

The private sector is responding to the rising costs of pharmaceuticals through the use of drug formularies, the emergence of pharmaceutical benefits management companies, and the expansion of mail-order pharmacies. In the public sector, state Medicaid programs are adopting preferred drug lists, prior authorization programs for more expensive drugs, and either require or encourage substitution of generic drugs in an attempt to slow their soaring expenditures. Drug acquisition costs for Medicaid are reduced further by rebates given by the pharmaceutical manufacturers. The Omnibus Budget Reconciliation Act of 1990 requires drug manufacturers to rebate a portion of a drug's price back to states and to the federal government. The rebate is approximately 15 percent of average wholesale price (AWP) for brand-name drugs and 11 percent of AWP for generics.[11] The Medicare program will likely face the same cost pressures with its new prescription drug benefit and be required to adopt cost-containment strategies as well.

PRESCRIPTION DRUG MARKETS IN THEORY

One could easily make the argument that each specific generic compound is its own market, hence each patented, single-source medication gives its manufacturer a monopoly in that market. Due to the unique characteristics of each medication, no single-source medication is a perfect substitute for any other. Some patients benefit more from some drugs whereas others benefit more from other drugs. In addition, physicians tend to have their preferred medications. Upon expiration of a branded drug's patents, the monopoly disappears. Companies marketing the same generic entity provide direct competition to the branded drug company, bringing competition to the market, though, as we will describe, not necessarily via a lower price for the branded drug. For older drugs in large markets, fifty or more companies may be competing for sales of a given generic entity. For these markets, the perfectly competitive economic model may be most appropriate as generic firms compete by driving price down to marginal cost. Much of the literature in economics journals in the 1990s focused on drug price trends and how they related to patent expiry and generic entry. The 1984 Hatch-Waxman Act facilitated the entry of generic drug products, and research examined the results of the act, emphasizing the determinants of entry, the speed of entry, and the resulting change in price and market share for the branded and generic drugs in the market.[12,13-21]

The pharmaceutical sector has also been described as a group of differentiated oligopolies (markets with a few sellers, each offering a product similar to the others).[22] Although a firm may hold a patent for a specific drug, it must often compete in a market consisting of several different drug entities (single- and multiple-source) that treat the same or similar indications. The Bertrand-Nash model of differentiated oligopoly assumes price competition by branded pharmaceutical companies marketing different chemical entities usable for the same therapeutic purpose. With product differentiation, quantity demanded of a drug depends not only on its own price (inversely) but also directly on the prices of substitute products. A substitutability parameter α determines how closely the drugs substitute for each other. In a duopoly equilibrium presented in Elzinga and Mills,[23] the equilibrium price $= 1 / (2 + \alpha)$, showing that drug prices are high when substitutability is low, and vice versa. Oligopolist direct-to-consumer advertising is an attempt to lower α as well as to increase overall demand.

Missing from oligopoly characterizations are purchasers who possess monopsony (single, large buyer) buying power, giving them the ability to negotiate lower drug prices. Pharmaceutical benefits managers and health maintenance organizations (HMOs) maintain formularies and encourage the use of generic drugs or older, less expensive branded drugs. Significant buyer power comes specifically from the ability to take advantage of any between-brand competition in a market.[24-26] Elzinga and Mills[27] argue that hospital buyers and HMOs are able to increase the substitutability parameter α, bringing down prices for those buyer groups. As we discuss, we found that one large hospital buyer was able to obtain 65 percent discounts on some of the older anti-infective medications that it purchased.

Finally, even if using an economic model, we could mimic well the market structure of a pharmaceutical market at a particular point in time; often these markets are quite dynamic. New drugs constantly replace older, less effective medicines. New categories of medicines develop around "blockbusters." For example, the market for antiulcer gastric medications, which did not exist prior to 1977 when Tagamet was introduced by SmithKline, is now on its third generation of drugs capable of fighting ulcers. All three generations (histamine H_2-receptor antagonists or H_2RAs, coating agents, and proton pump inhibitors or PPIs) are now available simultaneously, with the different generations competing, at least loosely, with one another in some markets.

PRESCRIPTION DRUG COMPETITION
IN PHARMACEUTICAL MARKETS

Without a single theoretical model of market structure that fits the entire pharmaceutical sector (with oligopoly, monopoly, monopsony, and perfect competition all applicable for certain aspects of firm behavior), we turn to empirical observations to see how different types of competition affect drug prices and utilization of both branded and generic drugs. In our empirical analysis, we distinguish between innovator, single-source pharmaceutical companies selling brand-name products, and generic manufacturers of bioequivalent drugs. We distinguish as well among three different market definitions —wide, narrow, and single generic compound—since drugs can be loose, close, or perfect substitutes for one another, respectively, depending on how the market is defined. With these distinctions, various types of competition occur between the two types of firms and in the different sized markets. We discuss separately some empirical results for each of the following four types of competition:

- *Intermarket* ("wide market") competition, which occurs between drugs in different "narrow markets" within the same therapeutic class, for example between the PPIs and the H_2RAs
- *Interbrand* ("narrow market") competition, which occurs between drugs in the same narrow market, for example, competition between two different PPIs (e.g., Protonix and Nexium) or between two different H_2RAs (e.g., Tagamet and Zantac)
- *Brand-generic* competition, which occurs between a brand-name drug and generic manufacturers of the same generic compound
- *Generic* competition, which occurs between generic manufacturers, again of the same generic compound

We have studied these four types of competition for two different buyer groups (the Medicaid market and the nonprofit hospital market) and for a number of different therapeutic classes: antidepressants, antipsychotics, oral chemotherapy medicines, anti-infectives, and antiulcer gastric medications. In this chapter, we discuss our antiulcer results for the Medicaid market (Ohio Medicaid only)[28] and our anti-infective results for a system of nonprofit hospitals in southwestern Ohio.[29]

Intermarket Competition

Three types of antiulcer gastric medications exist: histamine H2-receptor antagonists (H2RAs), coating agents, and proton pump inhibitors

(PPIs). Both H2RAs and PPIs reduce the production of acid in the stomach, though they are chemically and pharmacologically unrelated drug classes. The currently marketed H2RA drugs are cimetidine (Tagamet), famotidine (Pepcid), nizatidine (Axid), and ranitidine (Zantac). The available PPI agents are esomeprazole (Nexium), omeprazole (Prilosec), pantoprazole (Protonix), lansoprazole (Prevacid), and rabeprazole (Aciphex). Carafate is a gastric mucosa protectant or coating agent. Instead of inhibiting acid secretion, sucralfate (Carafate) acts by forming a protective coating over the ulcer, which in turn promotes healing. These ten drugs are listed in Table 20.1, along with their manufacturers and dates of market introduction. Following mergers between Astra and Zeneca as well as between Glaxo and SmithKline, these ten drugs are currently produced by eight different manufacturers.

A systematic replacement of older, less expensive H_2RAs by the newer, more expensive PPIs has occurred in the Ohio Medicaid market. The number of PPI prescriptions increased from 57,600 in the first quarter 1997 to 235,500 in the third quarter 2002. The number of prescriptions for H_2RAs and coating agents combined decreased from 148,300 to 91,588 over the same time period. Average reimbursement per prescription ("price") for PPIs increased from $105 in 1997 to $129 in 2002. Meanwhile, over the same time period, the average price for H_2RAs decreased from $72 to $20. The average price for coating agents decreased as well. Of course, with both utilization and price moving in the same direction, the cost (utilization times average price) to Medicaid of the proton pump inhibitors clearly increased over this time period, whereas the cost of the other antiulcer medications fell. The overall cost to Ohio Medicaid of antiulcer gastric medica-

TABLE 20.1. Anti-ulcer gastric medications

Generic name	Label	Market	Company	Date introduced
cimetidine	Tagamet	H2RA	SmithKline	1977
ranitidine	Zantac	H2RA	Glaxo	1983
famotidine	Pepcid	H2RA	Merck	1986
nizatidine	Axid	H2RA	Lilly	1988
sucralfate	Carafate	Coating agent	Aventis	1981
omeprazole	Prilosec	PPI	Astra	1989
lansoprazole	Prevacid	PPI	TAP	1995
rabeprazole	Aciphex	PPI	Janssen & Eisai	1999
pantoprazole	Protonix	PPI	Wyeth-Ayerst	2000
esomeprazole	Nexium	PPI	AstraZeneca	2001

tions rose from $17 million in 1997 to $32.4 million in 2002. Direct competition between the two classes is limited since physicians and patients are essentially free to select a drug from either group. Some cost savings are achieved when clinical practitioners adopt a step-down therapy by switching from a more potent PPI therapy to a less expensive H_2RA medication once patient symptoms are alleviated.

Interbrand Competition

As far as narrow-market competition is concerned (between branded drugs in the H_2RA class or between two branded PPIs), several specific outcomes can be expected. Accounting for other factors that affect average reimbursement per prescription or drug utilization, we should observe a decline in both prices and market shares of branded drugs when entry of a new branded drug into the market occurs. Neither competitive effect, however, is observed in the Ohio Medicaid market, at least in part because the market overall was growing so rapidly over these five years. In fact, Guo, Kelton, et al.[30] found no statistically significant effect of new brand entry on either price or utilization of other branded drugs.

Figure 20.1 shows the trends in brand-name prescriptions for all ten of the antiulcer gastric medications studied. The only PPI with decreasing utilization during this time period is Prilosec. The utilization of Prevacid steadily increased throughout the 1997 to 2002 period. Prescriptions for Protonix, Aciphex, and Nexium have also risen. Since a single drug manufacturer, Astrazeneca, supplies both Prilosec and Nexium, the declining share for Prilosec may be due to a strategic move by a single company rather than to competition. Meanwhile, utilization of Axid, Carafate, Pepcid, and Zantac (the H_2RAs) fell (in Zantac's case, precipitously) during the study period. Tagamet, already on the market for twenty years, had a small number of prescriptions from 1997 to 2002. No new H_2RAs were introduced, however, so the declining shares are not due to new branded entry in the H_2RA market, but rather to the increasing use of PPIs and generic versions of the H_2RAs.

Figure 20.2 shows the trend in reimbursement per prescription for the branded medications. The entry of the three new PPIs, Aciphex, Protonix, and Nexium, had no effect on the prices for Prilosec or Prevacid, the two PPIs sold throughout the period. Nexium and Aciphex were introduced at similarly high prices, and those prices continued to rise. Protonix was introduced at a lower price; its price increased over time as well. The prices for the H_2RAs were variable, and several show declines over time. However, the timing of the price drops does not coincide with the introduction of the

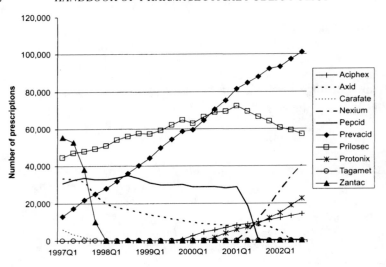

FIGURE 20.1. Quarterly prescriptions for branded antiulcer gastric medications: 1997-2002. *Source:* Guo JJ, Kelton CML, et al.(2004). Price and Market-Share Competition of Anti-Ulcer Gastric Medications in the Ohio Medicaid Market. *Int J Pharmaceutical Medicine* 18(5): 271-282. Reprinted with permission from Wolters Kluwer Adis.

new PPIs, implying that other factors (such as the entry of generic competitors) were responsible for the price movements.

Generic Competition to the Branded Drug

For antiulcer medications reimbursed by Ohio Medicaid, compelling evidence for competition between generic manufacturers and the brand-name manufacturer for the same compound was found, primarily with respect to market share of the branded medication. As Figure 20.3 shows, the number of Zantac prescriptions decreased sharply from 58,000 in 1997 to nearly zero in 1998 after its generic counterpart ranitidine entered the market. Prescriptions for ranitidine increased from 13,159 in the third quarter 1997 to 49,575 in the third quarter 2002. (Zantac 75 was introduced in the over-the-counter [OTC] market in April 1996, before the beginning of our study period, and following Pepcid AC and Tagamet HB in 1995. Hence, the large drop in prescriptions of Zantac throughout 1997 is due more to the substitution of ranitidine than to the OTC version of the medication.) As shown in Figure 20.4, the cost per Zantac prescription to Medicaid decreased sharply

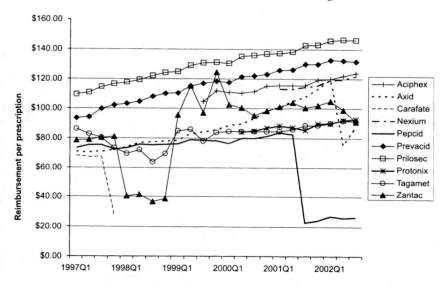

FIGURE 20.2. Quarterly average reimbursement per prescription for branded antiulcer gastric medications: 1997-2002. Guo JJ, Kelton CML, et al. (2004). Price and Market-Share Competition of Anti-Ulcer Gastric Medications in the Ohio Medicaid Market. *Int J Pharmaceutical Medicine* 18(5): 271-282. Reprinted with permission from Wolters Kluwer Adis.

in 1998 after the entry of ranitidine, then increased in 1999 and remained at the relatively higher reimbursement rate through the third quarter 2002.

The conclusions from Figures 20.3 and 20.4 are reinforced by statistical results in Guo, Kelton, et al.,[31] in which we found a statistically significant (*p* value = 0.000) negative effect of the number of generic companies on the market share of the relevant branded drug (in our case, Tagamet, Zantac, Pepcid, and Carafate) that experienced generic entry during this time period. No statistically significant long-term effects of generic entry on branded-drug price were found.

Generic Competition

For Ohio Medicaid, it is only the fourth type of competition that leads to significantly lower prices for drug payers. Depending on the size of the market, the number of generic manufacturers can rise to fifty or more. At the end of our time period, nineteen different companies sold the generic

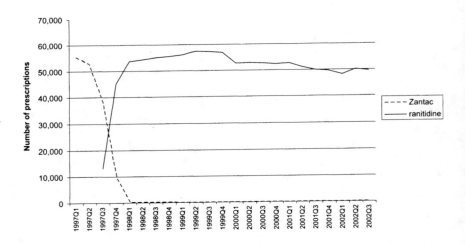

FIGURE 20.3. Quarterly Prescriptions for Zantac versus ranitidine: 1997-2002.

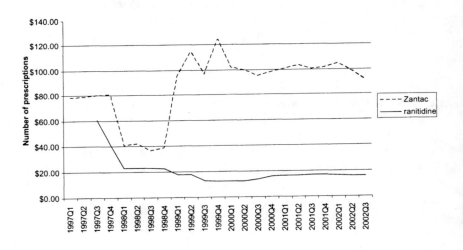

FIGURE 20.4. Reimbursment per prescription for Zantac versus ranitidine: 1997-2002.

ranitidine to purchasers reimbursed by Medicaid. Eventually, with enough entry, the price is driven down to the marginal production cost. However, the decline takes awhile. Notice in Figure 20.4 the abrupt, then slower, decline in the price of ranitidine as entry of more manufacturers occurs. Figure 20.5 looks specifically at the relationship between average reimbursement per prescription and the number of generic manufacturers. The average price per prescription, as seen in Figure 20.5, fell from $60.82, when ranitidine was first marketed, to $16.02 in 2002. In Guo, Kelton, et al.,[32] we found a statistically significant effect (p value = 0.047) of number of generic competitors on the reimbursement per prescription for generic drugs (ranitidine, cimetidine, famotidine, and sucralfate).

Buyer Power

Pharmaceutical companies face different types of purchasers, such as hospitals, clinics, and retail pharmacies. Companies are able to price discriminate across the various purchasers depending on buyers' relative market power, that is, their relative ability to take advantage of the latent competition between pharmaceutical companies. In this section, some of the results of a study that examined specifically the purchasing behavior of a

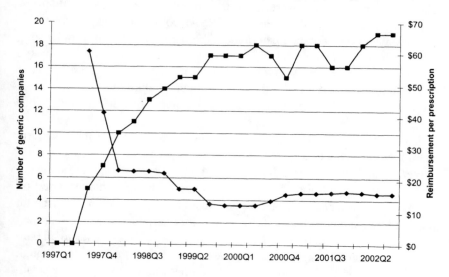

FIGURE 20.5. The relationship between reimbursement per prescription and number of generic competitors for ranitidine: 1997-2002.

buyer with significant power in negotiation are summarized.[33] The buyer is a nonprofit, six-hospital system that serves a substantial community base in southwestern Ohio and provides medical services to a large number of uninsured and underinsured individuals. The objective of this buyer is to keep costs to a minimum by negotiating vigorously with its medical vendors. Whereas Ohio Medicaid had no formulary during our study period, the hospital buyer we studied has a strict formulary that is updated on a monthly basis. The buyer, along with other health care providers, has seen its drug costs rise dramatically over the past decade, although at a rate of 11 percent between 2000 and 2001 compared to the national average of 18 percent and Ohio Medicaid's increase of 23 percent (from $996 million in 2000 to $1.23 billion in 2001).[34]

We studied price discounts (percentage discount of the buyer's transaction price from AWP) across twenty-three narrow anti-infective markets, in which the buyer had from weak to strong bargaining power depending on the number of competitive options that it had available, and also depending on a number of other factors, such as the amount of overall business conducted with each manufacturer. Out of the twenty-three markets, twenty were defined based on their six-digit American Hospital Formulary Service classification, and three were markets defined by indication (methicillin-resistant staphylococcus aureus or MRSA, community-acquired or CA pneumonia, or nosocomial pneumonia). Table 20.2, excerpted from Dusing, Guo, Kelton, and Pasquale,[35] shows the average discounts received by the buyer in each of the markets. On average, the buyer received a 46 percent discount relative to AWP. For the hospital buyer, unlike for Ohio Medicaid, we were able to find statistical evidence of competitive effects for all four types of competition discussed previously.

This empirical study suggested that the addition of one more generic manufacturer leads to a 2.44 percentage point increase in the discount received by the buyer on its brand-name or generic purchases of the same generic drug. The addition of one more branded drug to a market based on therapeutic class leads to an 0.55 percentage point increase in the discount received by the buyer. The addition of one more branded drug to an indication market (which cuts across several therapeutic classes) leads to an 0.56 percentage point increase in the discount received by the buyer. Although evidence of intermarket and interbrand competition exists, again the strongest competitive effects occur only when generic manufacturers enter the market.

TABLE 20.2. Market Expenditure and Weighted Average Discount Received by Buyer in 23 Anti-Infective Markets

Market*	Average annual expenditure	Weighted average discount
Amebicides	$487.58	22.27
Aminoglycosides	$108,660.63	47.82
Anthelmintics	$318.88	29.16
Antifungals	$1,045,944.46	41.79
Antimalarials	$1,352.50	24.95
Antiretrovirals	$267,556.37	56.45
Antituberculosis agents	$35,690.99	29.86
Antivirals	$221,333.61	38.77
Carbapenems	$310,636.06	45.56
Cephalosporins	$1,160,516.60	59.57
Chloramphenicol	$792.77	26.07
Macrolides	$245,247.85	42.33
Penicillins	$1,113,029.74	46.87
Quinolones	$1,192,407.83	37.97
Sulfonamides	$825.08	65.81
Tetracyclines	$21,547.91	65.09
Urinary anti-infectives	$5,179.09	27.52
Miscellaneous antibiotics	$100,470.89	27.19
Miscellaneous anti-infectives	$79,290.08	35.18
Miscellaneous beta-lactam antibiotics	$126,889.23	60.42
Overall average	**$6,038,178.15**	**46.31**
C.A. pneumonia	$1,914,163.41	39.92
MRSA	$474,852.60	47.02
Nosocomial pneumonia	$1,496,232.13	37.27
Average for indication submarkets	**$3,885,248.14**	**39.77**

*Dollar amounts for indication submarkets are counted as well in AHFS submarkets.

Source: Dusing, ML, Guo JJ, Kelton CML, Pasquale MK. (2005). Competition and Price Discounts for a Hospital Buyer in the Anti-Infective Pharmaceutical Market. *Journal of Pharmaceutical Finance, Economics and Policy* 14(2): 59-85. Reprinted with permission from The Haworth Press, Inc.

GENERIC DRUG ENTRY AND PATENT SETTLEMENTS
IN PHARMACEUTICAL MARKETS

The Hatch-Waxman Act of 1984 allows generic entry within one to three months of patent expiration. It grants the first successful generic applicant a 180-day marketing exclusivity, after which other generic manufacturers are allowed to enter the market as well. With substantial monopoly profits at stake, however, it is not surprising that brand-name pharmaceutical companies try to maintain their monopolies as long as possible, by patent extension litigation or by agreement with potential generic manufacturers to delay competition.

Since the passing of the 1984 act, drug companies have raised patent infringement issues, through lawsuits involving more than 130 different brand-name drugs.[36-38] A lawsuit brought against a potential generic competitor triggers an automatic thirty-month stay on that company's generic drug approval, potentially delaying significantly the marketing of generic alternatives. Extending patent life by patenting molecular modifications of the original drug is another common strategy. For example, Bristol-Myers Squibb's (BMS's) BuSpar (buspirone) was patented in 1980 and approved by the FDA in September 1986 to treat anxiety. U.S. sales of the drug were $709 million in 2000, making BuSpar the fifth highest selling drug for the company in that year. Six years prior to patent expiration, which was to occur in late 2000, BMS settled its patent litigation with Schein Pharmaceuticals, which had challenged BMS's patent, for $72.4 million. Then, one day prior to the patent's expiration in November 2000, BMS received a new patent on extended-release BuSpar and requested a delay of any generic buspirone entry; Mylan Laboratories was about to deliver the first truckload of generic buspirone when it was forced to stop delivery. In late November 2000, Mylan and Watson Pharmaceuticals (which had been approved to market a different dosage form of buspirone) jointly filed a lawsuit to contest the validity of the new BuSpar patent. In March 2001, the generic companies won the lawsuit and were allowed to sell generic buspirone; they captured two-thirds of buspirone sales by June 2001. In October 2001, BMS appealed this decision, which triggered the automatic delay under the Hatch-Waxman Act. Only in February 2002 was the case finally settled without further BuSpar patent extension. BMS had successfully delayed full generic entry for fifteen months in the U.S. market.[39]

In summer 2002, the U.S. Federal Trade Commission (FTC) issued a report on generic entry, after reviewing twenty complex legal cases between brand-name drug companies and first generic drug applicants.[40] Final settlements in these cases included seven patent license agreements (in which the generic applicant obtained a license to use the brand-name company's patents on the patented drug in question prior to patent expiration), two supply agreements (in which the generic company is allowed to market the brand-name company's product), and nine agreements with brand payments (from the brand-name company to the generic applicant). The FTC found that the thirty-month stay provision was susceptible to manipulation and was being used to create entry barriers for generic companies. Moreover, no limit was placed on the number of thirty-month stays that could be requested. GlaxoSmithKline was able to obtain five thirty-month stays for Paxil. The FTC made a number of recommendations, including limiting the number of thirty-month stays to one per ANDA.

An alternative to bringing legal action surrounding patent infringement is collusion with the first FDA-approved generic drug company in order to delay generic entry.[41] For example, Hoechst (now Aventis) and Andrx entered into an agreement in which Andrx was paid millions of dollars to keep the generic alternative (diltiazem hydrochloride) to Hoechst's Cardizem CD (a calcium channel blocker for the treatment of hypertension) off the market. Because this collusion violated U.S. antitrust law, thirty states filed a class-action lawsuit in 2002 against Aventis and Andrx. The final settlement required the two companies to give compensation of $80 million to consumers (state Medicaid programs and insurance companies) for their overpayment for Cardizem CD from 1998 to 2003.[42]

Similarly, Abbott entered into an agreement with Geneva in order to deter Geneva from entering the market with a generic version of Abbott's Hytrin (an alpha-adrenergic blocking agent for treatment of hypertension and prostate cancer). Abbott paid Geneva $4.5 million per month to delay generic drug entry.[43] When the FTC and the FDA intervened, Geneva was required to waive its right to a 180-day exclusivity period for its generic drug.

POLICIES TO INCREASE GENERIC DRUG UTILIZATION

Once therapeutically equivalent, generic alternatives to a brand-name pharmaceutical are available, eventually at a significantly lower price than their branded counterpart, most purchasers will select the lower-priced generic substitutes. However, because the savings are so substantial in doing so, public policies are developed to reinforce these natural competitive market forces. Most states in the United States have passed drug-product substitution laws that allow pharmacists to dispense a generic drug even when a prescription calls for a brand-name drug. According to the National Association of Boards of Pharmacy,[44] forty-one states as of November 2001 permitted pharmacists to substitute a generic drug unless the doctor indicated in writing "no substitution" or unless the brand was "medically necessary" (a designation that could appear either in a specific area of the prescription as an option to be "checked" or somewhere on the prescription in the doctor's handwriting, depending on the state). Of those states, twelve of them mandated pharmacists to substitute a generic drug unless specifically overridden by a doctor's orders. In addition, forty-one states required that the patient/consumer give consent or be informed of generic substitution. Fifteen states required that pharmacists use the FDA's "therapeutic equivalency list" when making judgments about generic substitutions.

Furthermore, many managed care organizations have increased the cost-sharing burden placed on consumers with higher and tiered copayments for pharmaceuticals. In the spring of 2000, 80 percent of health plans with prescription benefits were offering three-tier copay options.[45] The tiered structures commonly assign generic drugs the lowest copay, formulary brand-name drugs a somewhat higher copay, and nonformulary brand-name drugs a higher copay still. This copayment structure provides an incentive for the patient/consumer to choose generic drugs. The tiered copayment structures have been shown to reduce by 15 to 22 percent utilization of brand-name drugs.[46,47] Interestingly, no significant differences in physician office visits, inpatient, or emergency room use rates were found with the introduction of tiered copyament structures.[48]

Together, the Medicaid and Medicare programs pay for approximately one quarter of all prescription drugs purchased in the U.S. market.[49] Medicaid spending for prescription drugs has increased, on average, 18 percent per year since 1997, and reached $27.5 billion in 2003, accounting for 12 percent of the Medicaid budget. According to the Kaiser Commission on Medicaid and the Uninsured, Medicaid policies designed specifically to increase the use of generics include higher dispensing fees for pharmacists for generics, lower copays for generics, generics on the state preferred drug list, and physician education.[50] Medicaid's cost of generic drugs is kept down through two programs: the federal upper limit program and the state maximum allowable cost (MAC) programs, with the latter usually broader and more aggressive than the former. States with established MAC programs have reported annual savings of up to 4 percent.[51]

However, as discussed earlier in this chapter, as some patents expire, other new branded medications enter the market, and even whole new classes of medications come into existence—at patented monopoly prices. It appears that, as these new drugs are requested by patients and prescribed by their physicians, the share of generics generally decreases. Generic drugs account for only between 15 and 20 percent of total Medicaid drug spending.[52] In other words, the innovative new drugs that the patent system encourages are having a more powerful effect on the overall cost of medication than is the creation of competitive markets, through generic entry, for older drugs. For example, selective serotonin reuptake inhibitors (SSRIs) in the U.S. Medicaid program increased their market share among antidepressants from 13 percent in 1991 to 57 percent in 2004, while the traditional, primarily generic tricyclic antidepressant (TCA) market share decreased from 74 percent in 1991 to 12 percent in 2004 (see Figure 20.6).[53] Overall, the market share for single-source antidepressants increased from 38 percent in 1991 to 72 percent in 2001 due to the increasing use of SSRIs. After the patent on Prozac expired in 2001, the share started to decrease and fell to 53 percent by 2004 (see Figure 20.7).[54] The proportion of branded atypical antipsychotics used for patients with bipolar disorder in a U.S. managed care Medicaid population increased from 8 percent in 1998 to 20 percent in 2002, while the share of the traditional generic lithium mood stabilizer decreased from 10 percent in 1998 to 6 percent in 2002 (see Figure 20.8).[55] Total expenditure on antipsychotics in the U.S. Medicaid program increased sharply from $135 million per quarter in 1991 to $1.25 billion per quarter in 2004 specifically because of the increased use of branded atypical antipsychotics and the decreased use of generic typical antipsychotics.[56] Yet another example involves oral cancer drugs. Over the period 2002 to 2004 the conventional breast cancer drug therapy (tamoxifen) was replaced by newer, and considerably more expensive, branded medications such as Femara, Arimidex, and Taxotere.[57]

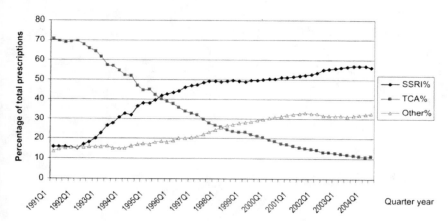

FIGURE 20.6. Market-share percentages among three antidepressant therapeutics (SSRIs, TCAs, others) in the U.S. Medicaid program: 1991-2004. *Source:* Guo JJ, Kelton CML, et al. (2005). Market-Share Competition of Antidepressants in the US Medicaid Programs. [unpublished] ISPOR Annual Conference. May. Washington, DC.

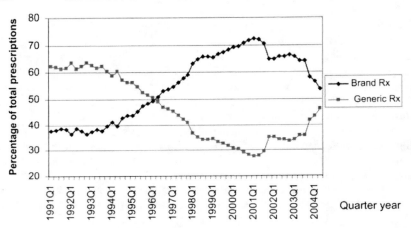

FIGURE 20.7. Percentages of brand-name and generic antidepressant prescriptions in the U.S. Medicaid program: 1991-2004. *Source:* Guo JJ, Kelton CML, et al. (2005). Market-Share Competition of Antidepressants in the US Medicaid Programs. [unpublished] ISPOR Annual Conference. May. Washington, DC.

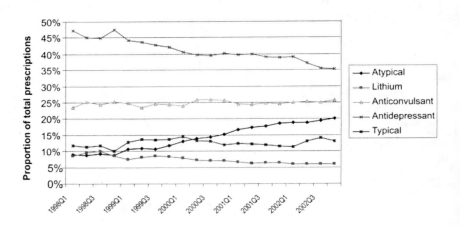

FIGURE 20.8. Prescription percentages for Medicaid patients with bipolar disorder: 13,471 patients from 1998 to 2002. *Source:* Excerpted from Guo JJ, Keck PE, et al. (2004). Price, Utilizaiton, and Market-Share Competition of Anti-Psychotics in the US Medicaid Programs. [Unpublished] American College of Clinical Pharmacy Annual Meeting. October. Dallas, TX.

CONCLUSIONS

In its efforts both to encourage new drug innovation and to keep medicines affordable for pharmaceutical payers, the U.S. government has compromised, for new brand-name medications, with a monopoly market structure for a period of time followed by intense generic competition. The transition from the monopoly to the competitive structure can be rough because of the substantial monopoly profits lost after competition. The legal system handles cases of alleged patent infringement by generic drug companies, which may delay entry of generic alternatives.

Once generic drugs are available, public and private payers encourage the use of generic substitutes through copay systems, preferred drug list, or physician and patient education. Although brand-generic and generic competition serve to reduce drug costs after patent expiration, it is much more difficult to harness the power of intermarket and interbrand competition. Only a purchaser with significant buying power, that a formulary allows, for example, can force loose branded substitutes to compete for a spot on that formulary. Only such a purchaser, moreover, can counteract the rise in drug costs caused by the introduction of new, high-priced medicines by requiring the use of older, less expensive medications to keep costs down, assuming of course that no significant difference in safety and efficacy exists between the lower-cost and the higher-cost alternatives.

NOTES

1. Berndt ER (2002). Pharmaceuticals in U.S. Health Care: Determinants of Quantity and Price. *The Journal of Economic Perspectives* 16: 45-66.

2. Although we appreciate that generic companies may brand their products as well, we use the term "branded" in this chapter to refer to the innovator company's brand.

3. Cook A (1998). How Increased Competition from Generic Drugs Has Affected Prices and Returns in the Pharmaceutical Industry. Congressional Budget Office Report. Washington, DC: CBO.

4. Federal Trade Commission (2002). *Generic Drug Entry Prior to Patent Expiration: An FTC Study.* July. Washington, DC: FTC.

5. Pharmaceutical Research and Manufacturers of America (2004). Research and Development Report. Washington, DC: PhRMA.

6. DiMasi JA, Hansen RW, Grabowski HG (2003). The Price of Innovation: New Estimates of Drug Development Costs. *Journal of Health Economics* 22: 151-185.

7. Center for Drug Evaluation and Research (2005). *NDAs Approved in Calendar Years 1990-2004 by Therapeutic Potential and Chemical Type.* March. Rockville, MD: U.S. Food and Drug Administration.

8. Scholdelmeyer S (2000). Patents, Intellectual Property, Innovation and Prescription Drugs: Do the Rules Benefit Consumer? Presentation made at a congressional briefing. September 25.

9. National Institute for Health Care Management (2002). *Prescription Drug Expenditure 2001: Another Year of Escalating Costs.* May. Washington, DC: NIHCM.

10. Lichtenberg FR (2000). *The Benefits and Costs of Newer Drugs: Evidence from the 1996 Medical Expenditure Panel Survey.* Working Paper No. 404. Center for Economic Studies. Munich, Germany: Institute for Economic Research.

11. Crowley JS, Ashner D, Elam L (2003). *Medicaid Outpatient Prescription Drug Benefits: Findings from a National Survey, 2003.* December. Kaiser Commission on Medicaid and the Uninsured. Washington, DC: The Henry J. Kaiser Family Foundation.

12. Cook A (1998).

13. Bae JP (1997). Drug Patent Expirations and Speed of Generic Entry. *Health Services Research* 32: 87-101.

14. Caves RE, Whinston MD, Hurwitz MA (1991). Patent Expiration, Entry, and Competition in the U.S. Pharmaceutical Industry. *Brookings Papers Microeconomics,* pp. 1-66.

15. Frank RG, Salkever DS (1992). Pricing, Patent Loss and the Market for Pharmaceuticals. *Southern Economic Journal* 59: 165-179.

16. Frank RG, Salkever DS (1997). Generic Entry and the Pricing of Pharmaceuticals. *Journal of Economics and Management Strategy* 6: 75-90.

17. Grabowski HG, Vernon JM (1992). Brand Loyalty, Entry, and Price Competition in Pharmaceuticals After the 1984 Drug Act. *Journal of Law and Economics* 21: 331-349.

18. Griliches Z, Cockburn I (1994). Generics and New Goods in Pharmaceutical Price Indexes. *American Economic Review* 84: 1213-1232.

19. Hudson J (1992). Pricing Dynamics in the Pharmaceutical Industry. *Applied Economics* 24: 103-112.

20. Hurwitz MA, Caves RE (1998). Persuasion or Information? Promotion and the Shares of Brand Name and Generic Pharmaceuticals. *Journal of Law and Economics* 31: 299-320.

21. Scott Morton FM (1999). Entry Decisions in the Generic Pharmaceutical Industry. *RAND Journal of Economics* 30: 421-440.

22. Elzinga KG, Mills DE (1997). The Distribution and Pricing of Prescription Drugs. *International Journal of the Economics of Business* 4: 287-299.

23. Elzinga KG, Mills DE (1997).

24. Snyder CM (1996). A Dynamic Theory of Countervailing Power. *RAND Journal of Economics* 27: 747-769.

25. Snyder CM (1998). Why Do Larger Buyers Pay Lower Prices? Intense Supplier Competition. *Economic Letters* 58: 205-209.

26. Ellison SF, Snyder CM (2001). *Countervailing Power in Wholesale Pharmaceuticals.* MIT Department of Economics Working Paper No. 01-27. Available at: http://econ-www.mit.edu/faculty/download_pdf.php?id=222.

27. Elzinga KG, Mills DE (1997).

28. Guo JJ, Kelton CML, Pasquale MK, Zimmerman J, Patel A, Heaton PC, Cluxton RJ (2004). Price and Market-Share Competition of Anti-Ulcer Gastric Medications in the Ohio Medicaid Market. *International Journal of Pharmaceutical Medicine* 18: 271-82.

29. Dusing ML, Guo JJ, Kelton CML, Pasquale MK (2005). Competition and Price Discounts for a Hospital Buyer in the Anti-Infective Pharmaceutical Market. *Journal of Pharmaceutical Finance, Economics, and Policy* 14(2): 59-85.

30. Guo JJ et al. (2004).

31. Guo JJ et al. (2004).

32. Guo JJ et al. (2004).

33. Dusing ML et al (2005).

34. Ohio Department of Job and Family Services (2005). *Ohio Medicaid Expenditure Annual Report 2000, 2001, 2002.* Medicaid Department. Columbus, OH: ODJFS.

35. Dusing ML et al. (2005).

36. From 1992 to 2002, patent infringement cases involved many well-known drugs such as BuSpar, Capoten, Cardizem CD, Cipro, Claritin, Lupron, Neurontin, Paxil, Pepcid, Pravachol, Prilosec, Procardia XL, Prozac, Vasotec, Xanax, Zantac, Zocor, Zoloft, and Zyprexa.

37. Federal Trade Comission (2002).

38. National Institute for Health Care Management Research and Education Foundation (2002). *A Primer: Generic Drugs, Patents and the Pharmaceutical Marketplace.* June. Washington, DC: NIHCM Foundation.

39. NIHCM Foundation (2002).

40. Federal Trade Commission (2002).

41. Federal Trade Commission (2000). *Antitrust Actions in Pharmaceutical Services and Products.* May. Washington, DC: FTC.

42. Office of the Attorney General (2003). Attorney General Announces Cardizem CD Settlement. January. Virginia. Richmond, VA: Office of the Attorney General.

43. Federal Trade Commission (2002).

44. National Association of Boards of Pharmacy (2005). *Survey of Pharmacy Law.* May. Mount Prospect, IL: NABP.

45. Motheral BR, Fairman K (2001). Effect of a Three-Tier Prescription Copay on Pharmaceutical and Other Medical Utilization. *Medical Care* 39: 1293-1304.

46. Motheral BR, Fairman K (2001).

47. Motheral BR, Henderson R (1999). The Effect of a Copay Increase on Pharmaceutical Utilization, Expenditures, and Treatment Continuation. *American Journal of Managed Care* 5: 1383-1394.

48. Motheral BR, Fairman K (2001).

49. Dusing ML et al. (2005).

50. Crowley JS, Ashner D, Elam L (2003).

51. Abramson RG, Harrington CA, Missmar R, Li SP, Mendelson, DN (2004). Generic Drug Cost Containment in Medicaid: Lessons from Five State MAC Programs. *Health Care Financing Review* 25: 25-34.

52. Abramson RG et al. (2004).

53. Guo JJ, Chen Y, Jing YH, Kelton CML, Patel NC (2005). Drug Utilization and Market-Share Competition Among Antidepressant Medications in US Medicaid Programs. International Society of Pharmacoeconomics & Outcomes Research Annual Conference, May 15-18, Arlington, Virginia.

54. Guo JJ et al. (2005).

55. Guo JJ, Keck PE, Li H, Jang R, Carson W (2004). Evolution of Mood Stabilizer Utilization Among Patients with Bipolar Disorder in a Managed Care Medicaid Population. American College of Clinical Pharmacists Annual Meeting, October 24-26, Dallas, Texas.

56. Guo JJ, Jing YH, Kelton CML, Chen Y, Louder A, Patel NC (2005). Drug Price, Utilization, and Market-Share Competition Among Antipsychotic Medications. Ohio Pharmacists Association Annual Conference, April 15, Columbus, Ohio.

57. Malott SA, Chen Y, Pruemer J, Guo JJ (2005). Price Trends and Utilization Patterns of Breast Cancer Drug Therapy in the US Medicaid Systems. Ohio Pharmacists Association Annual Conference, April 15, Columbus, Ohio.

Chapter 21

Drug Insurance Design

Earle "Buddy" Lingle

INTRODUCTION

Who pays for pharmaceuticals has greatly evolved over the past forty years. When Congress passed Medicare and Medicaid in 1965, only about 7 percent of expenditures for pharmaceuticals were paid by insurers and public programs, that is, third-party payers.[1] However, by 2004 the percentage of payments for prescription drugs had climbed to 75 percent.[2] This substantial increase has provided third parties with influence over the prescribing, dispensing, and use of prescription drugs. This change has contributed to an ongoing struggle involving employers/payers and the pharmaceutical industry over controlling costs.

Controlling the cost of a drug benefit is important to increasing the profits of employers (by limiting their employee benefit costs) and third parties (who act on behalf of employers) as well as restraining the expenditures of publicly funded programs. In this chapter, references to "third parties" will be directed to organizations that are responsible for benefit management and/or the payment of services in lieu of the patient. These may include private insurance companies, managed care organizations, pharmaceutical benefits managers, and government programs such as Medicaid.

The purpose of this chapter is to provide the reader with information regarding the different policies and programs third parties utilize to help control costs. These may be mechanisms that directly control reimbursements or others that are intended to assure the appropriate use of therapies. For our purposes these policies and programs will be divided into the following categories:

- Prescribing restrictions
- Patient cost sharing
- Utilization controls

- Product cost controls
- Pharmacist reimbursement

PRESCRIBING RESTRICTIONS

Prescribing restrictions are controls put in place by payers that limit the choice of pharmaceutical products available to be prescribed. They may vary from rigid lists of drug products that may not be prescribed to lists of suggested products. Most allow some appeal process by which a patient may receive a restricted product. The following are the typical programs used to restrict prescribing in drug benefit programs.

A *formulary* may be defined as a preferred list of drug products that are deemed essential for the rational treatment of patients. Formularies were first developed for use in the hospital setting. They were formed to decrease inventory costs and promote prescribing of appropriate therapy. As third party drug benefit programs increased in number and size, formularies became more accepted for use in outpatient care settings.

Generally, formularies vary by the amount of information they provide and their restrictiveness. Formularies may be lists that provide guidance as to which drug products will be reimbursed by a third party and/or they may be designed to provide a prescriber with therapeutic information about a drug product. With the advent of personal digital assistant (PDA) and other electronic systems, formularies may also provide cost comparisons of various products within a therapeutic category.

One method used to characterize the restrictiveness of formularies is through the use of the terms *open formulary* and *closed formulary*. An open formulary is one that is perceived to by fairly unrestrictive and/or its use is voluntary. It is usually little more than a list of most prescribed products and serves as a guide to prescribing and payment. A closed formulary is more restrictive regarding the number of medications included and it is usually mandatory. The drug products that are allowed are usually organized by therapeutic category.

Decisions regarding the inclusion and exclusion of drugs from a formulary are usually made by a pharmacy and therapeutics committee (also known as a P & T committee). This committee usually consists of members who are knowledgeable about pharmacotherapeutics and includes practicing physicians and clinical pharmacists. Managed care groups and pharmaceutical benefits managers (PBMs) many times also include medically trained professionals with an expertise in pharmacoeconomics. A P & T committee will usually make formulary decisions based on the primary criteria of safety and efficacy and effectiveness (see also Chapter 23, which discusses health technology assessment). If various drug products have similar safety and efficacy profiles then product cost will also be a factor in decision making. Most formulary policies usually include an appeals process by which a physician or patient can appeal the exclusion of a drug product from a formulary. Approval of this appeal is usually based on the medical necessity of the patient receiving the excluded drug.

Formularies have been criticized for various reasons. Physicians have maintained that they hinder their ability to prescribe the most appropriate medicine for a patient and, therefore, they negatively impact patient care. Prescribers and the pharmaceutical industry may also express a concern that some therapeutically effective pharmaceuticals are omitted because of their cost. Some opponents, including the pharmaceutical industry, maintain that restriction of access to pharmaceuticals may not have the desired impact on expenditures because other medications or services are substituted if the preferred drug cannot be prescribed.[3]

Prior approval programs (also known as prior authorization, PA) have been used by some third parties instead of or in conjunction with a formulary. Most PA programs consist of access restrictions for drug products within certain therapeutic categories. As with formularies, if a specific drug is not included as a covered drug then the physician or pharmacist must justify its need. Some third parties also have PA programs related to restrictions on products or dosage forms prescribed, length of therapy, diagnoses, and patient's age.

State Medicaid programs have used PA programs because they are not allowed by law to employ a formulary. With the passage of the Omnibus Budget Reconciliation Act of 1990 (OBRA-90) state Medicaid programs were limited in restricting Medicaid recipients' access to most prescription drugs. The act provided that state Medicaid programs must cover drug products if they are marketed by companies with federal drug rebate agreements. (Several drug classes were allowed to be restricted, including agents for weight gain or anorexia, agents to promote fertility, agents for cosmetic purposes or hair growth, agents for symptomatic relief of cough and colds, agents for smoking cessation, prescription vitamins and mineral products [except prenatal vitamins and fluoride products], nonprescription drugs, outpatient drugs requiring purchase of tests or monitoring services from the same manufacturer, Drug Efficacy Study Implementation [DESI] drugs, barbiturates, and benzodiazepines.) States were required to cover all new drug products approved by the FDA for at least six months after approval. Beyond the six months, prior approval (PA) programs were popular methods by which states attempted to control utilization. The subsequent passage of OBRA '93 repealed the requirement that new drugs be covered without restriction. It allowed states to exclude, restrict, or place on PA recently approved drugs. OBRA '93 did establish various criteria a state must meet when establishing a formulary, including the requirement that drugs excluded from a formulary (except from the categories previously listed) must be made available by way of a prior approval program. In many ways, prior approval programs have become de facto formularies. The requirements of OBRA '93 make formularies and PA programs essentially the same in functionality. In some instances, the process of making a PA request may be more restrictive than overriding a formulary exclusion.

A *preferred drug list* (PDL) is another method used to restrict prescribing. A PDL (see also Chapter 22) is essentially a group of prior-approval programs. Each therapeutic category will have "preferred" drugs that will not require prior approval before being dispensed. A *step-therapy* program (also called step protocol) is often used in conjunction with a formulary or prior approval program. Its purpose is to begin therapy with a drug product that is deemed to be the most cost-effective. Patients would begin their therapy with a "first-line" drug product. If therapeutic failure occurred, the prior approval process would allow the dispensing of a "second-line" drug product.

Step therapy has become a particularly popular program as new generic products enter the market and as prescription-only products become available over the counter (OTC). For example, as proton pump inhibitors (PPIs) became available over the counter and at a lower cost, many third parties made them a first-line therapy.

Aside from the prescribing restrictions mentioned previously, most third-party programs make decisions that will not allow coverage of certain drug products or drug categories. Most of these decisions are based on concerns about the safety of a drug product or because its use is not considered medically necessary. For example, many plans no longer cover barbiturates or benzodiazepines because alternative therapies are considered more effective and safer. Certain therapeutic categories of drug products that are thought of as "lifestyle" drugs may also be excluded from coverage. These include drug products used for cosmetic purposes as well as those used to treat erectile dysfunction.

The *coverage of OTC products* is another decision that third parties must make. Traditionally, third parties have been hesitant to cover OTCs because of difficulty controlling the reimbursement process, the potential for fraud by patients, the large number of products, and difficulty in knowing their ingredients, as well as the inability to provide the information to health care professionals for inclusion in their patient profiles.

Because of the potential cost differential between OTC products and prescription-only drug products, third parties have begun to increase their coverage. The switch to OTC status for an allergy medication was actually initiated by WellPoint Health Networks, a managed care organization, which petitioned the FDA for switching the drug product from prescription status to OTC. As the number of these switches has increased, the coverage of OTCs by third parties has also risen. Some third parties believe that the coverage of OTCs is such a cost-effective strategy that they require a prescription be written for the OTC and a dispensing fee is paid to the pharmacy. Other third parties reduce or waive patient cost sharing if the patient utilizes an OTC instead of the prescription-only product.

PATIENT COST SHARING

Almost all drug insurance plans require the patient to share in the cost of their prescriptions. By doing so, third parties believe that excessive and/or unnecessary utilization will decrease. The basis for this is that when a good or service is fully covered (i.e., price equals zero), the patient will demand the quantity of goods or services corresponding to a price of zero. Co-payments are used to make a patient evaluate the financial cost for using a drug compared to the need or potential benefit to the patient. Hopefully, this will deter excess utilization. However, if the cost-sharing amount is too high, the concern that arises is that both necessary and unnecessary utilization will be decreased. If this occurs, a patient's health may worsen and more expensive medical care services may be ordered.

Several different types of patient cost sharing exist that a third party may implement. A common type is a *deductible*. This is the amount of eligible expense that a patient must pay from his or her own pocket before benefits begin. For example, if a patient has a $250 deductible then he or she must pay the first $250 of "eligible" expenses before the drug benefit begins.

Although not a method of cost sharing, the concept of *eligible expenses* is important to the understanding of cost sharing and various other aspects of third-party drug benefit programs. Examples of noneligible expenses include payments for a drug that is not on the third party's formulary. Therefore, if a prescribed drug is not on the formulary then the amount the patient pays for that prescription would not be included toward the deductible the patient must meet.

A second type of patient cost sharing is *coinsurance*. This represents a portion of prescription costs that a patient must pay, and is usually implemented as a fixed percentage of the costs. When combined with a deductible, coinsurance will be paid by the patient once the deductible has been met. For example, a 20 percent coinsurance policy will result in a $20 payment for a $100 prescription once a deductible is met.

Another type of cost sharing is the *copayment* (or copay). A copayment is a specific, fixed amount a patient must pay per prescription. It is usually due to the pharmacy when services are rendered. For example, if a patient has a drug benefit plan that includes a $10 copayment, then the patient would be expected to pay $30 if he or she has three prescriptions dispensed. A complication with copayments is that the actual cost of generic prescriptions may be less than the copayment. Many third parties have established policy that the copayment is the lower cost; the patient will pay the prescription's actual cost (product cost plus pharmacist's fee for dispensing) if is lower than the copayment.

Recently, most private third-party drug benefit plans and Medicare Part D plans have implemented the use of *tiered copayments*. The purpose of a tiered copayment system is to steer patients away from using the more expensive medications and toward using lower-cost drugs. Only a small minority of drug benefit plans do not use tiered copayments.

Tiered systems may include two-tier, three-tier, or four-tier plans. A two-tier plan will have two categories of drugs, usually preferred drugs (generics) and nonpreferred (brand-name drugs). The nonpreferred tier will have a higher copayment than the preferred tier. A three-tier plan may have a preferred (generics), preferred brands (brand-name drugs without generic substitutes), and nonpreferred brands (brand-name drugs with generic substitutes) tiers, with three different copayments. The intent is to drive utilization away from the more expensive, nonpreferred brand drugs. In 2004, the average copayments for a three-tier plan were $10 for generics, $21 for preferred brands, and $33 for nonpreferred brands.[4] A four-tier plan may include the three tiers described as well as a fourth tier that includes lifestyle drugs, cosmetic drugs, and/or injectable drugs. Frequently, a patient will be responsible for the full cost of prescriptions for medications in the fourth tier.

UTILIZATION CONTROLS

Although many cost-containment tools used by third parties attempt to indirectly control utilization, some directly limit utilization. Some of these methods include limits on the number of prescriptions a patient may receive, the quantity of doses that may be dispensed, or a patient's annual prescription drug expenditures. These utilization controls limit access or make the patient share in the costs. Other methods limit utilization after a review and evaluation of a patient's therapy regimen. These mechanisms control utilization by requiring the use of a therapeutically equivalent but lower-cost option.

Limiting the number of prescriptions a patient may receive over some time period (most frequently per month) are found in public programs such as Medicaid more often than in private programs. Limits on days supply or quantity of doses per prescription can be either minimum or maximum limits. A maximum quantity limit (e.g., thirty-day supply or one hundred doses) is used to help prevent wastage in the event a medication order is stopped because of ineffectiveness or adverse drug events. A common reason why a minimum limit might be implemented is to supply greater quantities of chronic medications. For example, a third party may require a ninety-day supply of medication to treat hypertension in lieu of a thirty-day supply. This would be implemented to decrease the number of dispensing fees paid to pharmacies and/or decrease the handling and shipping charges for mail-order prescriptions.

Some drug benefit programs have placed dollar reimbursement limits that may be implemented on a monthly, quarterly, semiannual, or annual basis. The standard drug insurance plan for the Medicare Part D drug benefit has a deductible and then coverage with coinsurance; however, when a recipient reaches a monetary limit of $2,250 he or she has no coverage until another $2,850 in prescription drug expenditures occurs. Therefore, the standard Medicare drug benefit uses a unique structure with an expenditure limit that serves as a coverage gap until an additional benefit begins when total expenditures reach $5,100.

Although these direct controls on utilization should decrease a third-party's prescription drug costs, the principal concern with their use is what happens once patients meet their limits.[5] When this occurs the concern is that a patient will not get the medication he or she needs and that the utilization of other medical care services will be substituted, resulting in greater costs. This is the main reason these controls are not frequently used.

Drug utilization review (DUR) (see also Chapter 27) is another method by which utilization may be controlled. With the passage of the Omnibus Budget Reconciliation Act of 1990 (OBRA-90), all state Medicaid programs were mandated to have DUR programs for their outpatient drug programs. The use of DUR programs by private third parties also has greatly expanded. DUR may take various forms but, in general, it includes any system that is used for monitoring and managing drug utilization. DUR serves two general purposes: to (1) facilitate appropriate drug use and (2) manage costs by reducing inappropriate drug use. Although DUR has frequently focused on assuring appropriate physician prescribing, it also includes pharmacist dispensing as well as patient's adherence to drug therapy regimens.

PRODUCT COST CONTROLS

Two components to prescription drug costs exist: the cost of the drug product and reimbursement to the pharmacy for services rendered. Pharmacy reimbursement for services will be considered in the next section. Because a significant cost of the pharmacy benefit is the drug product cost, payers give significant attention to determining the proper method by which they should reimburse for drug products.

Third parties attempt to reimburse pharmacies at their actual cost to purchase. This is also known as the *actual acquisition cost* (AAC). Reimbursing product costs at the pharmacy's AAC is difficult to achieve because of the various discounts, rebates, and deals that pharmacies receive. In addition, these factors will vary depending on if the drug product is purchased from a wholesaler or direct from the manufacturer, and on the volume of product ordered. The most accurate method for determining AAC is to perform audits of pharmacies' invoices; however, this method is cost prohibitive because of the large number of pharmacies that would need to be audited and because prices keep changing. Therefore, third parties have developed different product cost estimates in an attempt to reimburse pharmacies at their approximate purchase price. The following are various methods that have been used.

Third parties have used the average wholesale price of a drug product to assist in calculating a product reimbursement. *Average wholesale price* (AWP) is a suggested wholesale price of a drug. In other words, it is the manufacturer's published price recommended for wholesalers to sell a drug product to a pharmacy. However, because of the discounts that wholesalers provide pharmacies, it is a higher price than what the pharmacy usually pays. Because of this reason, it is rarely used alone as the method for determining drug-product reimbursement.

Because AWP is not an accurate estimate of product cost and AAC is too expensive and too difficult to determine, third parties have employed a calculation using AWP to determine the *estimated acquisition cost* (EAC). EAC uses an estimate of the discounts a pharmacy receives expressed as a percentage and deducts that from the AWP. For example, a third party may reimburse pharmacies for drug products at AWP–15 percent. Even though this estimate only approximates pharmacies' actual costs, it is simple and inexpensive to implement.

In state Medicaid programs the EAC formulae vary from AWP–16 percent in New Hampshire to AWP–5 percent in Alaska.[6] Some states have different EAC calculations for brand name versus generic drugs. For example, Connecticut's Medicaid program calculates product reimbursement at AWP–12 percent for brand-name drug products and AWP–40 percent for generics. Some states also vary their EAC formulae by the type of pharmacy submitting prescription drug claims. Michigan reimburses independent pharmacies (one to four stores under the same ownership) at AWP–13.5 percent, whereas it reimburses chain pharmacies (five or more pharmacies under the same ownership) at AWP–15.1 percent.

EAC has also been calculated using the wholesaler acquisition cost (WAC). It also is a published price, but it is defined by law as a manufacturer's price to a wholesaler or direct purchasers.[7] It does not include discounts, rebates, or other reductions in price. Third parties reimburse pharmacies based on the WAC plus a specified percentage that represents the markup that a wholesaler would add to their cost before selling the drug product to a pharmacy. For example, the Ohio Medicaid program reimburses pharmacies at the lower of WAC+9 percent or AWP–12.8 percent.[8]

The use of maximum allowable cost payments was first introduced in the Medicaid program in the 1970s. It was an attempt to take advantage of variation in prices of multiple source products. *Maximum allowable cost* (MAC) limits are payment limits for multisource drug products that have different market prices. MACs take advantage of the difference in prices of brand-name drugs and generic drugs and limit the product cost reimbursement to the lowest price at which the product is available. MAC limits undergo periodic review and may either be increased, decreased, or discontinued depending on the availability and prices of generic drug products. Pharmacies may dispense a more expensive brand-name drug, but they will be reimbursed only at the MAC limit.

Most third parties use a "lowest of" provision in their contracts with pharmacies to assure that they are paying the pharmacy's best price. The third party will reimburse the pharmacy the lowest prescription price based on (1) the EAC plus a dispensing fee (dispensing fees will be discussed in the next section), (2) the MAC limit (if available) plus a dispensing fee, or (3) the pharmacy's usual and customary charge. The *usual and customary* charge is the pharmacy's price to a cash-paying customer.

The use of a third party's selected method of product reimbursement is not readily apparent to a patient. However, it may be an important issue regarding the patient's access to pharmacy services. If a third party reimburses a pharmacy at a lower price than the pharmacy's actual cost or reimburses an inadequate dispensing fee, the pharmacy may decide to not participate in that drug benefit plan. This decision would also be affected by the third party's reimbursement for pharmacy services.

Related to drug product costs but not a pharmacy reimbursement method, manufacturer *rebates* have become an important tool for third parties to recoup product costs they have paid. Rebates are payments from a manufacturer to a third party based on the utilization of the manufacturer's drug products over a period of time. This results in a discount back to the third party.

Third parties will often require rebates in order for a manufacturer to have its drug products available to the benefit plan's insured patients. Usually access to a drug product is related to including the product on a restrictive formulary or to granting the product "preferred" status on a preferred drug list (PDL). Rebates are negotiated between the third party and the manufacturer and may be based on a specific drug or on a bundle of drugs. Manufacturers prefer to negotiate based on a bundle and will use their newer, innovative drugs as leverage to get their other drugs covered by the plan.[9] Third parties prefer to negotiate by the specific drug.

Rebates were mandated for the Medicaid program through the OBRA-90 legislation in an attempt to ensure that Medicaid would receive the "best price" that manufacturers offer public or private third parties. Some states recognized the potential to produce additional savings for drug product costs and implemented "supplemental" rebates. States persuaded manufacturers to provide these additional rebates by excluding them from their prior authorization programs if supplemental rebates were provided to the state.

The use of *mail order* may be included in several different sections of this chapter. It may be discussed under "Prescribing Restrictions" since formularies and prior approval programs are used extensively in mail-order programs. It could be discussed in the "Utilization Controls" section since mail order often uses quantity limits. It might even be discussed under "Patient Cost Sharing" since mail order offers lower copayments to entice patients to receive their prescription drugs in such a manner. However, it is included under this section, "Product Cost Controls," because a major reason for mail order's professed cost savings is due to lower product costs. Because of the large volume of prescriptions that mail-order facilities dispense, they are able to purchase medications in bulk, resulting in larger product discounts. In addition, the economies of scale for such facilities provide lower operating costs and enable them to accept lower reimbursement for their dispensing functions.

PHARMACY REIMBURSEMENT

In addition to reimbursing pharmacies for the drug product, third parties also pay pharmacies for their services. Although most of the payments are to pay for dispensing of the medication, pharmacies are also being reimbursed for other services they provide. The most common form of pharmacy reimbursement is the *dispensing fee*. The advantages for third parties paying for pharmacy services through a dispensing fee include the simplicity to administer, good predictability of dispensing costs, it provides no incentives to the pharmacy to dispense a more expensive drug product, and it is viewed by pharmacy as being "professional." The dispensing fee offered to a pharmacy should cover the pharmacy's cost to process and dispense the prescription, including personnel and building expenses, and should also provide some profit. Some pharmacies may not be concerned about a low dispensing fee if they are able to purchase the drug product at a price below what they are reimbursed.

Dispensing fees in state Medicaid programs range from $1.75 in New Hampshire to $5.77 in Louisiana.[10] To encourage the dispensing of generic drug products, some states provide higher dispensing fees for generics than for brand-name products. States may also differentiate their dispensing fees based on whether the dispensing pharmacy is a retail pharmacy, institutional pharmacy, or long-term care pharmacy. Utah also provides higher dispensing fees for rural pharmacies compared to pharmacies in urban areas.

Some third parties may also pay pharmacies for nondispensing services. These services have been called various names, including cognitive services and pharmaceutical care. (See also Chapter 27.) The challenge for a third party is to differentiate between services provided by pharmacists when dispensing a prescription medication and those services that are not related to this function. When third parties have reimbursed for nondispensing services they have usually based payments on the resources used and the time spent in providing the services. Chapter 27 covers this topic in more depth.

A less popular form of pharmacy reimbursement is *capitation*. Capitation is a payment for services to be rendered over a specific period of time, and is based on the number of patients who will receive services at that pharmacy. Capitation reimbursement holds several advantages for pharmacies. With capitation a pharmacy is paid for services before services are provided, thereby alleviating potential cash-flow problems resulting from the filing of prescription claims. Also, the pharmacy is paid whether or not a patient receives any services during the specified time period. Advantages also exist for third parties in that administrative costs are decreased since claims are not processed and the third party will have a more predictable expenditure for pharmacy services. In addition, the third party expects that the pharmacy would have an economic incentive to eliminate unnecessary utilization and decrease costs since it is only being paid one capitation fee per patient.

Even though advantages exist for pharmacies and third parties, capitation has failed to become a popular reimbursement mechanism. The main reason for its lack of use is because the proper amount of reimbursement is difficult to estimate. With the high price of prescription drug products, a change or addition of one prescription for a patient could produce a significant loss for a pharmacy. Because pharmacists do not have final authority to change a physician's prescription, their ability to influence utilization and expenditures is limited. Therefore, an unnecessary burden of risk would be placed on pharmacies unless third parties would allow capitation payments to vary with utilization. However, this would negate the advantages of the capitation reimbursement method.

Pharmacy reimbursement is still evolving as third parties attempt to implement product reimbursement that most closely approximates actual product acquisition cost. However, pharmacies have long relied on product reimbursements to be greater than acquisition costs in order to offset inadequate dispensing fee reimbursements. This difference is being lessened lower as third parties refine their product reimbursement methods. Pharmacists also continue to promote reimbursement for their nondispensing services. The new Medicare drug benefit and its medication therapy management program may facilitate the recognition of pharmacy services and their reimbursement.

SUMMARY

The evolution of drug benefit programs continues as the share of prescriptions paid by third parties increases. Since prescription drug spending is expected to increase at a greater rate than inflation, third parties will continue to work to decrease their expenditures. The influence of third parties and their use of methods to control prescribing, utilization, product costs, and reimbursement will shape the future of drug benefits. However, it is imperative that third parties and health care providers remember that a drug benefit will directly affect the utilization and expenditures for other medical care. In some instances, a more expensive drug benefit will result in a complete benefit package that will provide higher quality care at a reduced total cost.

NOTES

1. Centers for Medicare and Medicaid Services (2006). National health expenditure data: Overview. Available at: http://www.cms.hhs.gov/NationalHealthExpend Data/.

2. Smith C, et al. (2006). National health spending in 2004: Recent slowdown led by prescription drug spending. *Health Affairs* 25:186-196.

3. Murawski MM and Abdelgawad T (2005). Exploration of the impact of preferred drug lists on hospital and physician visits and the costs to Medicaid. *American Journal of Managed Care* 11: SP35-SP42.

4. Kaiser Family Foundation/Health Research and Educational Trust (2004). *Employer Health Benefits: 2004 Annual Survey*. September. Washington, DC: Kaiser Family Foundation. Available at: http://www.kff.org/insurance/7148/upload/2004-Employer-Health-Benefits-Survey-Full-Report.pdf.

5. Soumerai SB et al. (1991). Effects of Medicaid drug-payment limits on admission to hospitals and nursing homes. *New England Journal of Medicine* 325: 1072-1077.

6. Centers for Medicare and Medicaid Services (2005). Medicaid prescription reimbursement information by state: Quarter ending March 2005. Available at: http://www.cms.hhs.gov/MedicaidDrugRebateProgram/08_MdPresReimInfo.asp

7. Office of Inspector General (2005). *Medicaid Drug Price Comparisons: Average Manufacturer Price to Published Prices*. June. U.S. Department of Health and Human Services. OEI-05-05-00240. Washington, DC: Government Printing Office.

8. Centers for Medicare and Medicaid Services (2005).

9. Hoadley J (2005). *Cost Containment Strategies for Prescription Drugs: Assessing the Evidence in the Literature*. March. Washington, DC: Kaiser Family Foundation.

10. Centers for Medicare and Medicaid Services (2005).

Chapter 22

Evidence-Based Preferred Drug Lists

John Santa

Prescription drugs are now at the center of multiple health policy debates. Outpatient prescription drugs under Medicaid increased from $6.9 billion to $26.6 billion between 1993 and 2003. The rate of increase in cost also remains substantial due to increased utilization, increased prices, and substitution of less expensive drugs with more expensive drugs. Substantial resources have been shifted to drugs from other sectors including basic eligibility. Fewer individuals are covered under Medicaid because of these increases in costs.

The sophisticated information policies used in the marketing and sales of prescription drugs significantly influence Medicaid expenditures. The business model that has evolved emphasizes competition among a few large pharmaceutical companies who dominate consumer and prescriber information rather than multiple smaller companies competing on the basis of price for similar drugs. Although "breakthrough" drugs are encouraged and desired, the bulk of dollars spent purchasing prescription drugs go to "me too" drugs marketed as "blockbuster" drugs. The marginal benefits of many of these drugs are difficult to determine in the overwhelming barrage of information unleashed on consumers and prescribers.

The purchasing process for prescription drugs has become complex because of this business model. Price competition can occur only if sellers (in this case pharmaceutical companies) believe that buyer's information will be sufficiently credible with patients served by the buyer (most of whom are third parties such as Medicaid) to establish that some products are similar to others despite overwhelming seller information to the contrary. Not surprisingly, pharmaceutical companies also know that unless buyers (since they are third parties) are also actually willing to do what it takes to enforce their decision, the consequences of failing to compete on price will be minimal.

The purchasing process is also made more difficult by the multiple steps that occur behind closed doors. Although rationale exists for some price negotiation to be private, virtually all purchasing steps in the prescription drug purchasing process are concealed. Little information is shared with physicians, enrollees, or patients that explains how and why a drug is chosen for a formulary. Concealing such information helps the seller to avoid price competition.

In the case of public purchasers, the purchasing process is no less complex and suffers many of the same challenges. The pharmaceutical industry has been able to obscure the purchasing process by convincing the federal government to agree to a national discounting system in which state Medicaid programs are provided rebates (discounts after the fact based on volume) but must keep information about the rebate secret. Other federal government programs are not precluded from more effectively using their buying power. For example, the VA (U.S. Department of Veterans Affairs) has received substantially lower prices than state Medicaid programs through their use of formularies.

Preferred drug lists (PDLs) are one policy approach to correcting the current imbalance in market forces. PDLs use evidence and pricing information to arrive at a list of drugs deemed to be of better value for the Medicaid program and its recipients. In contrast to more restrictive formularies, PDLs allow easier access to nonpreferred drugs through a variety of authorization mechanisms. Both PDLs and formularies use information, pricing, and implementation strategies to develop and deliver program approaches. The different approach PDLs create allows public policymakers to encourage market approaches, including price competition. Each of these strategies is crucial in establishing credibility, motivating price competition, and implementing effectively to maximize outcomes.

Two-thirds of state Medicaid programs now have (PDLs). PDLs have become an important part of efforts to bring better value to Medicaid patients and taxpayers as they shift purchasing to less expensive but equally effective alternatives at a lower price or a larger rebate.

This chapter will focus on PDLs as designed and implemented by Medicaid pharmacy programs, especially those explicitly using evidence to make decisions. Federal regulation allows state Medicaid programs to implement PDLs. PDLs offer more flexibility for both Medicaid programs and their patients. State Medicaid programs are in the midst of implementing PDLs that take different approaches to the three steps of information, pricing, and implementation. Key differences have begun to emerge. State Medicaid PDLs offer an interesting policy contrast to private formularies. Most PDLs pursue a more classic, market-oriented approach to purchasing than do private formularies. They offer a unique opportunity to evaluate the contrast between state and federal policy, and between price competition policy approaches and information competition strategies.

Pharmacists are playing lead roles in the formulation, implementation, and evaluation of PDL approaches. All the stakeholders involved rely on pharmacists to provide both quantitative and qualitative information about options available. Pharmacists are influencing and leading major health policy and health economic initiatives as a result.

PREFERRED DRUG LISTS (PDLS)

Preferred drug lists are authorized under a series of federal statutes and regulations.[1] Medicaid regulations with regard to PDLs have been challenged in several court cases. For the most part, pharmaceutical companies have argued that state governments cannot pursue PDLs because of existing Medicaid statutes, such as the federal Medicaid rebate agreement, or because of concern over price fixing. Although states have prevailed in most of these cases, they have shaped the approaches states take to designing and implementing PDLs.

States move through information, pricing, and implementation steps in the development of a PDL. The challenge for pharmacists involved in these efforts is to anticipate and adjust to the local conditions that make every PDL effort unique. Substantial variation in prescribing practices exists. Variation is caused, among other things, by significant variability in implementing evidence and subjective regional preferences promulgated by experts in that region. A variety of factors may influence prescribers—evidence is only one. A decision in one region may be greeted with acclamation while in another region decried. Most prescribers have poor information systems that provide little or no cumulative information about their prescribing practices. The marketing approach used by the pharmaceutical industry reinforces this variation and makes it difficult to appreciate because of the disorganization of information at the provider and purchaser level. A policy change as significant as a PDL should be done carefully if it is to be successful over the long term. Several steps are needed to succeed.

Making the Case

Public programs operate in very different environments than private programs. The information step for public programs always begins by "making the case" for a change in policy. Given that public resources are in play and the lives of less-fortunate citizens could be affected, the public deserves to understand and support the case for change. The "public" includes pharmaceutical companies who can be expected to make their case effectively in both private and public forums. Making the case for any initiative involving prescription drugs requires program administrators to describe all the factors potentially at play. These include the following:

- The legal framework of public programs related to health is shaped by federal law, state law, and waivers (explicit exceptions) from federal law that a state has been granted by the federal government. Waivers are provided for a variety of reasons—innovation, differences and preferences in states, and a desire to modernize an approach without federal legislation. Medicaid law remains fundamentally the same as in the 1960s when the original legislation was passed. Coverage of prescription drugs, for example, is not required under federal Medicaid law—it is an optional benefit that requires approval of a waiver. No state's legal framework is identical. From the outset, a program designer must understand the legal framework their effort would fall under, the weaknesses and strengths of that framework and the political process the framework operates under.
- The patient population of any public program, especially Medicaid, is very different from the population usually covered in a private program. Large numbers of vulnerable populations are covered in public programs—patients with chronic diseases, especially mental health conditions, non-English speaking populations, poor frail elderly, and disabled individuals. Eligibility for public benefits plays a key role in any program approach. Who is eligible and for how long? Medicaid programs are known for significant turnover in eligibility, especially when income levels are considered.
- Medicaid financing can vary significantly from state to state. Financing is always a combination of federal and state dollars, but the portion of each (expressed as the "match rate") can vary significantly depending on the economy of a state and the type of program being funded. State financing of Medicaid can come from various sources, many of which may provide a variable stream of dollars—tobacco taxes or provider taxes for example. Every funding source has unique characteristics influencing timing, predictability, and commitment. Savings are also important resources—if savings accrue, for what purpose will they be used and how will they be reported?
- Executive and legislative branch leadership changes frequently in response to elections and national/state/local politics. As a result, leadership of agencies and key legislative committees change. Governors and legislators of states have to balance budgets. Governors have to execute programs consistent with legal frameworks.

- The practitioner community is key to any proposal. Practicing physicians and pharmacists are effective in swaying decision makers. A proposal that fails to capture the support of those "in the trenches" is unlikely to go far. The astute policymaker frequently asks: Are genuine health outcomes for citizens being improved here or are financial health outcomes for providers and manufacturers actually the focus? It is not uncommon for health strategies to be justified solely or in large part not on the basis of improvement in health outcomes but on the basis of improvement in reimbursement rates.
- The administrative capabilities of public programs, especially those related to Medicaid, are particularly scrutinized. Proposals need to take into account the past successes or failures agencies have had administering programs. Since most PDLs involve preauthorization in the implementation phase, this aspect is especially important (discussed in further detail later in the chapter).
- Key information is needed to make the case for any change. This information needs to effectively blend local information with information from outside the jurisdiction involved. Local information is needed for credibility and relevance in order to get local buy in. Outside information helps decision makers to see that unusual circumstances are not in play (mismanagement, unusually sick patient population) and that potential solutions do exist. If a policymaker is not able to provide key information defining the policy change and why it is needed, the effort is likely lost—information will be provided by special interests who will modify the policy to their liking or defeat it when the time comes.
- Transparency of information should be considered when any policy concerning prescription drugs is considered, simply because no sector in the health care industry makes decisions related to prescription drugs transparently. The public's trust of pharmaceutical companies is in decline. Explicit decision making and a transparent conflict of interest process go a long way in establishing a different kind of "case" for whatever policy process is proposed.

These factors need to be organized into an efficient policy proposal that can be read, presented, and understood by policymakers. The case for a policy should attract and bind multiple stakeholders committed to its success. The proposal needs to set the stage with data that define the clinical and financial problems and the consequences of action and inaction. The essentials of a PDL policy should be described with clear-cut goals and accountabilities articulated. The administrative costs and projected savings should be emphasized. Any potential adverse clinical outcomes should be addressed directly and hopefully minimized through proactive measures. Local decision making should be emphasized.

Politics

Politics is everywhere in most health care organizations, and public organizations are no exception. Any industry that is responsible for 15 percent of the gross domestic product has acquired significant political influence throughout the political process. Change will not occur easily, quickly, or without a political debate.

Pharmacists experienced in the political process are a valuable resource as they are able to understand both political and operational issues and find the most effective ways to influence the policy debate. Staff with little experience can be overwhelmed quickly by all of the issues common in a political debate. The executive branch has to make government work. The governor and agency heads are ultimately responsible for implementing the budget and delivering value for taxpayer dollars. Key executive decision makers must act in concert with the governor and other executive agencies to communicate effectively and honestly to the legislature. They must defend their agency's performance and budget to the governor, the legislature, and other agencies. The executive branch has to make day-to-day decisions and explain those decisions to the public.

In Oregon in 2001, then Governor Kitzhaber was faced with a dilemma. Prescription drug spending was on track to exceed hospital costs, minimizing the expansion of Medicaid he had hoped to achieve related to the Oregon Health Plan. Every dollar saved went to reducing the number of uninsured people, assuring that equity and value would be preserved. On the other hand, the pharmaceutical industry lobby had succeeded in defeating every attempt to reform prescription drug purchasing by Medicaid through a dominant information strategy emphasizing the possible risks to the vulnerable and the administrative hassles likely to affect prescribers.

Legislatures are the major decision makers when it comes to budget resources, but they convene intermittently and rarely have the resources to be involved in the day-to-day challenges of specific programs. Legislatures formalize group decision making processes. Success in the legislature occurs when individuals successfully employ group decision making processes. Legislative leaders need to understand a proposal if they are going to prioritize and support it. They are able to focus on specific problems, especially programs that are perceived by a significant stakeholder as threatening or unsuccessful. The consequences of legislative action in such circumstances can be unpredictable. A poorly administered prior authorization program for example can plague an agency at the legislature for many years after, even if the program has been improved or abolished. An ineffective information system can endanger an agency's credibility. A compromised purchasing process can result in significant restructuring and replacement of key staff.

In Oregon in 2001 legislators were divided regarding prescription drug issues. Some were concerned about the dominance of the industry's business approach, others were concerned about the state's budget, which was vulnerable to recession and limited by the voters reluctant to approve any new taxes. Legislatures are usually about priorities and compromise. Ultimately Governor Kitzhaber made prescription drug reform his first priority. Legislators made other issues theirs. The legislation creating Oregon's evidence-based prescription drug program passed in the early morning hours of the last day of the legislative session. During the subsequent 2003 session however the legislature approved a law prohibiting preauthorization by Medicaid related to its PDL, significantly impairing its implementation. An experienced lobbyists commented, "It's the next vote that is the most important."

The judicial branch of government provides both proactive (through consultation) and reactive (through litigation) advice and resources to other branches of government. Legal advice and counsel is available to agency staff to explain the boundaries created by statute or the implications of proposed rules or legislation. Agencies are usually well served to take advantage of these resources early on. The judicial branch is also available to respond to legal challenges. Such challenges should be considered part of the process. In fact, when it comes to pharmaceutical issues, some observers feel that a legal challenge is an indicator of success. Multiple legal challenges have been mounted to state PDL efforts. States have prevailed in all of the challenges mounted so far.

States can use enforcement of current law to counter misuse and abuse within an industry. The judicial branch of government also has significant enforcement powers and can initiate action if industry fails to follow the law. Multiple lawsuits have been initiated by states' attorneys general with several resulting in awards or settlements in the many millions of dollars.[2]

Oregon's prescription drug reform was challenged early on based on language in the Oregon statute related to evidence. Oregon prevailed in the suit and continues to administer the program. Oregon's attorney general has played a lead role in several successful suits alleging inappropriate marketing of pharmaceutical products.

THE INFORMATION PROCESS

The key to successful PDLs in the public sector, especially in a Medicaid program, is getting off to a credible, positive start that establishes a long-term commitment to accept resource constraints, help the sick, protect the worst off, respect autonomy, sustain trust, and promote inclusive decision making.[3] The first way to do this is to commit to a drug information process that rises above any available in the private sector and sets a standard for public purchasing that can be defended from the most vigorous critics. These critics will surely be present since control of information is a major strategy for success in the current business model favored by industry. An information process that sets a high standard will be hard for even the most vocal critic to oppose and will provide high ground to enable a PDL process to begin.

Several states' Medicaid programs and private nonprofits have decided to pursue the most rigorous and transparent information process for influencing drug purchasing decisions. Oregon began this process in 2001 when it began its PDL effort by committing to making decision related to comparative effectiveness and safety of drugs in a therapeutic class based on a public, evidence-based, transparent process.[4] Oregon's experience using an evidence-based practice center (EPC) to provide evidence-based comparisons of the effectiveness of various medications used for the same therapeutic purpose through the use of systematic reviews and synthesis of pertinent research findings has generated information that is comprehensive, credible, and timely. EPCs are centers designated by the Agency for Healthcare Research and Quality[5] that have expertise and experience in doing systematic reviews of important topics decision makers need clarity on, whether for future research, purchasing, or medical direction to patients and practitioners.[6] EPCs usually do so through systematic reviews, comprehensive analysis of all of the relevant research on a topic done by a researcher neutral to any specific objective, or finding in the research field.

Oregon's initial success became the foundation for the collaborative Drug Effectiveness Review Project (DERP). DERP now involves fifteen state Medicaid programs and two private nonprofit organizations. DERP contracts with three evidence-based practice centers to conduct systematic reviews comparing drugs in the largest classes. Twenty-six drug classes are scheduled to be reviewed. Exhibit 22.1 lists the drug classes reviewed. At the time of the preparation of this chapter, twenty-five have been completed. The reports on these reviews are available to the public.[7]

The systematic review process contrasts with the expert review process most of us are familiar with. Although expert processes are valuable, they have been shown to potentially have significant biases related to the re-

EXHIBIT 22.1. DERP drug classes

1. Proton pump inhibitors
2. Long-acting opiods
3. Statins
4. Nonsteroidal anti-inflammatory drugs
5. Estrogens
6. Triptans
7. Skeletal muscle relaxants
8. Oral hypoglycemics
9. Overactive bladder, drugs to treat
10. ACE inhibitors
11. Beta-blockers
12. Calcium channel blockers
13. Angiotensin II
14. Second generation antidepressants
15. Antiepileptic drugs in bipolar mood disorder and neuropathic pain
16. Second generation antihistamines
17. Atypical antipsychotics
18. Inhaled corticosteroids
19. ADHD and ADD, drugs to treat
20. Alzheimers, drugs to treat
21. Antiplatelet drugs
22. Thiazolidinedione
23. Newer antemetics
24. Sedative hypnotics
25. targeted Immune Modulators
26. Inhaled beta antagonists

search interests or experience of the expert. Expert reviews also may not include all relevant research and may not fully disclose conflicts of interest that users may find important. The following are the key elements of the systematic review process used by evidence-based practice centers in DERP:

- Formulation of key questions
- Finding evidence
- Selecting and evaluating evidence
- Synthesizing and presenting evidence
- Conducting peer review
- Revising draft documents into final systematic reviews
- Maintaining and updating reviews

Each step is important in providing local decision makers with relevant, reliable information as they address purchasing, coverage, and quality of care issues related to pharmaceutical products.[8]

Formulating Key Questions

The most important and sometimes most difficult step in starting the systematic review process is to establish the questions that the review of research literature is to answer. Even top quality research that answers an irrelevant question is useless to decision makers and wasteful of personnel and other resources.

It is important to spend the time needed to engage fully in the process of identifying key questions. This step cannot be left to one party. Decision makers need advice on exactly how to phrase questions clearly, and in ways suitable for an evidence-based process, so that they can obtain the information they need for decision formulation. Researchers need this dialogue to ensure that the work they are doing is relevant to the decisions being considered. Reviews of prescription drug classes must specify which drugs, for which outcomes, using which indicators of those outcomes, in what type of studies. Outcomes and indicators are particularly important. How important are process outcomes versus clinical outcomes? Should a good quality randomized, head to head trial carry more weight than twenty fair quality placebo controlled trials that allow indirect comparisons of the two drugs?

In the DERP, a dialogue is convened between the participating organization and the researchers assigned to the class of drugs under review. This dialogue carefully specifies the populations to be addressed (adults, children, specific disease states, etc.), the interventions (specific drugs included in the class) to be studied, the clinical (death, myocardial infarction, stroke) or process (serum cholesterol, blood pressure) outcomes.

Participating organizations have time to gather input about the key questions from parties that will be affected by the policies in question, including patients, pharmacists, pharmaceutical companies, and practitioners. This feedback helps ensure that the concerns of patients and practitioners are thoroughly considered. Specifying clear and appropriate key questions *in advance* helps ensure that evaluations of the evidence are not biased and that the evidence is interpreted without regard for preexisting opinions.

The DERP has taken the additional step of making draft key questions available to the public for comments and including those comments in final decisions regarding key questions. This commitment to a public process reinforces the importance of transparency and explicit decision making. It stands in contrast to the implicit and proprietary process prevalent in private sector industry efforts related to prescription drugs.

When the dialogue is completed, the key questions will do the following:

- Specify the clinical conditions (diagnoses, diseases) of interest for the particular review.
- Define the populations, interventions, and outcomes (expected benefits, potential risks or harms) of interest for the systematic review.
- Distinguish intermediate outcomes (e.g., laboratory test results or biometric measures) from true health outcomes (e.g., death, morbidity, functioning, quality of life) and focus the research on true health outcomes.
- Identify those types of studies felt sufficiently reliable and valid to contribute to a decision making process (randomized controlled trials, observational trials).
- Use terminology that makes it clear that the evidence-based review seeks to present a specific type of information—evidence regarding the issue—not to make decisions or recommendations for decision makers.

Finding Evidence

In an electronically connected world, finding all the information needed to make good decisions sounds easy. Although finding some information is easier than ever, the diversity of sources for information pertinent to the types of decisions under consideration requires knowledgeable and skilled personnel as well as access to a wide array of computer-based and hard copy sources of research literature. Such resources will help ensure that the greatest possible amount of relevant information is obtained and analyzed.

Search efforts are focused on major databases of the world's medical literature and other resources such as systematic reviews found in the Cochrane Library. The specifics of the search are provided in the systematic review. In addition, the EPCs can accept published or unpublished information from all reasonable sources if the party submitting the information allows the information to be made public so that it can be openly compared to other information acquired by more traditional methods. The DERP actively solicits submission of information from the public, including the pharmaceutical industry. Information related to indications not approved by the FDA but of interest to participants in DERP is included. The focus on clinical information is reinforced by exclusion of any information on price or cost. The solicitation follows the clinical information format of the Academy of Managed Care Pharmacy (AMCP) protocol, except that information submitted is not considered proprietary. The AMCP protocol provides a reasonable, standardized approach for pharmaceutical companies to follow.[9] Additional elements can be required if needed. The proprietary approach suggested by the AMCP contrasts with the DERP approach. This difference has catalyzed a healthy debate regarding the importance of transparency of clinical information.

DERP also does not include information regarding cost, including cost-effective analysis, since relevant cost information is usually proprietary and highly variable depending on volume and likelihood of market shift in response to price. DERP focuses on the first step—are drugs in the same class homogeneous? If homogeneity is present, cost-effectiveness is directly proportional to daily price or treatment course price. This focus on the first step has also prompted concern from proponents of cost-effectiveness analysis. Such analyses are of course dependent on heterogeneity being present and often contain economic models that are proprietary. This debate has also helped decision makers to understand the importance of each step in developing sound policy and the importance of keeping as much of the process as possible transparent.

Selecting Evidence

The body of evidence found may be overwhelming or minimal. Separating information expected to be useful from potentially irrelevant or misleading data is a special challenge, even when key questions have been well specified. Thus, an important step is to specify, in advance, the sources of "admissible" evidence related to the key questions. This is referred to as "stating the eligibility criteria" for material that will be included or excluded from consideration in the review process. The evidence-based process calls for EPCs to take the following factors into account in describing evidence to be selected and retained:

- Which databases or other sources and information to include
- What limits relating to language, year of publication, and similar details should be considered
- What types of publications to include and exclude
- What types of research studies to include and exclude

When considering the types of research that will be accepted, although randomized controlled trials (RCTs) involving head-to-head comparisons of drugs may be the optimal design for this process, they are not the only evidence that may be valuable to or necessary for decision makers. Figure

22.1 shows an often used "pyramid" of evidence helpful in identifying the general reliability and validity of study methodologies. RCTs with placebo controls, although not as reliable for comparison purposes, may be a source of important information when other comparative approaches are lacking. Moreover, large, well-designed studies other than RCTs are often critical sources of data on populations not typically included in RCTs, on longer-term outcomes, and on potential adverse events. The need for internal validity needs to be weighed with the importance of generalizability.

Once the eligibility criteria have been identified, the process of searching for relevant evidence begins by reviewing titles and abstracts of research studies, and then reviewing entire articles reporting on such investigations, against the eligibility criteria already stipulated, and deciding which items to use and which to set aside. One systematic reviewer usually takes the lead in reviewing all the relevant articles. A second reviewer independently reviews each article and all conclusions or summaries in the systematic review. If an article or study is excluded from consideration, the reason for doing so is recorded as part of the final documentation.

Once the acceptable sources of information have been identified, the information in them is abstracted into detailed "evidence tables" that provide crucial information on study purpose and design, populations, diagnoses or conditions, interventions, outcomes, and other data. Examples of evidence table elements for a systematic comparative drug review are provided in Exhibit 22.2. Evidence tables provide more information for the reader than a citation and better specific information on key methodology issues than abstracts. Average reviews however still may have evidence tables running hundreds of pages in length.

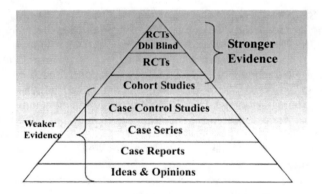

FIGURE 22.1. Types of study design.

EXHIBIT 22.2. Evidence table elements

Author	Method of randomization
Year	Allocation concealment
Setting	Number of adverse events
Purpose	Most common adverse events
Population characteristics	Withdrawals
Intervention	Intention to treat analysis
Control	Outcomes
Eligibility criteria	

Synthesizing and Presenting Evidence

Synthesis of evidence is the process of analyzing and combining all good information gleaned from the review of research studies and findings relevant to the key questions formulated at the outset. Analysts typically rely heavily on information from evidence tables for this task. This step, and the overall presentation of evidence, can be done in qualitative terms, through text discussion of the evidence, and in quantitative terms, through statistical combination of information in a technique known as meta-analysis.

A critical element of the evaluation of the evidence involves two related steps: grading the quality of individual studies and rating the strength of the overall body of evidence. These are formal steps for which well-recognized methods exist. For a systematic review to be defensible, it is imperative that both of these judgments be made in a clear and consistent manner.

Review of the quality of individual studies relies on study design *and* conduct. Study design alone is insufficient. The best-designed study can provide poor evidence if the conduct of the study does not rigorously follow good research practice. The quality of a study is often summarized as providing good, fair, or poor evidence, and reviewers must clearly state how the review uses each category of evidence. For example, does the review consider (but down-weigh) poorly designed or conducted studies or exclude them altogether? This may be particularly important when quantitative syntheses are performed. Another consideration is that study quality may not, by itself, be sufficient. A very good study that has only limited applicability to a key question may not be as helpful as a fair study that is directly related to the question at hand. Often, systematic reviews will focus particular attention on a limited number of high-quality, critical studies, from which key evidence can be highlighted in more detail.

Evidence tables are created to allow those decision makers who wish to do so the opportunity to examine the entirety of the evidence. For ease of presentation, summary tables derived from detailed evidence tables may also be desirable. Other approaches to presenting information about the magnitude of benefits and harms, such as "balance sheets" that provide results in terms of the number of patients who would benefit or be harmed by undergoing a particular intervention, can be used. Forest plots and other graphic approaches allow multiple studies to be presented for comparative purposes.

As all the evidence is organized into evidence tables, summary tables, and text, reviewers then need to make some assessment of the overall quality and applicability of the evidence. The questions at this stage involve the cumulative quality of the studies (are studies mostly of good quality, mostly of fair or only poor quality, or a mix), the quantity of the data (e.g., numbers of studies and aggregate sample sizes), and consistency (e.g., do the studies show consistent results or are some clearly negative and some positive). Again, the entire body of evidence is often characterized as good, fair, or poor, and typically the limitations of the literature are discussed.

In synthesizing all this information, reviewers may also address a variety of other questions of concern to policymakers. These include but are not limited to:

- What do the largest studies show compared to smaller ones?
- What populations have been studied and are those populations relevant to the question at hand? What critical populations have been excluded or ignored?
- Have "real life" outcomes of concern to patients been studied, or have outcomes been limited largely to biologic or physiologic measures?
- Have risks and harms been reported as thoroughly as benefits?

All these preceding steps will then be assembled into a draft systematic review, complete with background, methods, results, discussion, evidence tables, summary tables, and citations. This draft is then subjected to external peer review.

Conducting Peer Review and Revising the Draft into a Final Systematic Review

Peer review is the act of soliciting critiques from national and international experts and potential users of the systematic review. Peer reviewers are asked to comment on factual matters, presentation, interpretation, missing information, readability/usability, and similar matters. The aim is to identify omissions, unwarranted conclusions or inferences, unintentional bias, inadvertent over- or underemphasis, and unnecessarily tedious, obscure, or misleading writing. Peer review is an integral part of the standards required by the Agency for Healthcare Research and Quality for developing systematic reviews. Comments from reviewers are all given serious consideration.

Peer reviews can be solicited through distribution of hard copies of the draft review to previously identified outside reviewers. As long as any conflict of interest is made explicit, any qualified individual can constructively contribute to a systematic review. In the DERP the draft report is also posted on the project Web site enabling the public to make comments. Again the commitment to public input and transparency is reinforced.

Following peer review (or beginning while peer review is still ongoing), the authors of the systematic review begin necessary revisions. All legitimate points raised by the peer review and public comments are addressed in the final draft of the systematic review. For example, if reviewers note important missing data or studies, these are obtained and data from them are added to evidence tables and text, as appropriate.

Once the authors have completed the final evidence report, they will then make it available for dissemination as determined by the participating organizations. The authors of the report may also submit the report, or a shorter article summarizing it, for publication in a scientific journal. These journal publications further enhance the credibility and impact of the reports and of the evidence-based process within the scientific community. The DERP posts all final reports on the project Web site, making them available to the public on an ongoing basis. Participating organizations make the final reports and other documents public at their public venues.

Maintaining and Updating Reviews

Even the best information can become outdated, sometimes quickly (within months) and sometimes over a longer period (two to three years). The DERP updates reviews once every seven to twenty-four months. Each update consists of a new literature search that seeks additional data or analysis from studies published in the interim; of particular significance will be newly published systematic reviews on the same or a related topic and results from clinical trials or large observational studies.

A commitment to updates allows the information process to acknowledge errors and omissions, constantly improve, and continually reinforce the importance of starting the decision process correctly. Stability in the information process is also reinforced. Decision makers can return to a familiar format and more easily deal with new information added to a familiar synthesis.

Resources

The approach previously outlined can seem daunting at first. However, substantial resources are available to assist those interested in using the best information. Significant numbers of systematic evidence-based reviewers are interested in prescription drugs throughout the world. Many of these reviewers are pharmacists whose expertise and credibility is substantial.

Resources spent on original research are substantial. Resources currently devoted to systematic reviews represent a very small fraction of research resources. More attention and emphasis on such approaches would better enable policymakers to understand the body of research evidence, draw conclusions, and set priorities for future research from the perspective of the population they represent. Funding for systematic reviews needs to come from organizations not dominated by manufacturers or private purchasers since they have conflicts that would bias or create a perception of bias compromising the review. Public purchasers involved in Medicaid and Medicare have a unique opportunity to fund systematic reviews and turn over the conduct of such reviews to organizations such as EPCs that they have no control over.

Several existing organized systematic review efforts should be considered when prescription drug information is desired from a systematic review. These sources include:

- The Drug Effectiveness Review Project[10]
- The Cochrane Collaborative[11]
- The Agency for Healthcare Research and Quality Evidence-Based Practice Centers[12]
- The U.S. Preventive Services Task Force[13]
- National Institute for Clinical Excellence (NICE)[14]
- U.S. Department of Veterans Affairs[15]

THE PRICING PROCESS

Purchasing prescriptions drugs, as with many health services and products, requires knowledge of the principles of competition, specifics of a variety of regulations (what does the FDA actually regulate), and a determination to make each work in favor of the public purchaser. Prescription drug sellers will do everything possible to avoid or moderate any strategy that might promote price competition. Any seller, particularly those with billions of marketing and sales resources, would prefer to compete based on sales and marketing information rather than price. They will be very knowledgeable about regulations, and will use tools that provide any advantage to them to moderate price competition. Their strategy will often include the use of practitioner and patient advocacy groups to influence the public (and private) purchaser. These latter strategies can be countered more effectively if the information process has been conducted in public with multiple opportunities for advocacy groups to engage. Once an information base is established and decision makers have a sense of a product and its comparative performance, it is time to turn to the pricing process.

Much of the pricing process is proprietary. Competition may be enhanced if prices during the negotiation process are confidential. However, the stage for a favorable negotiation can be set if the buyer has credibly established that drugs in a class are homogeneous and that the source of information closest to being "perfect" supports that decision. Effective PDLs allow states to be much more successful in pricing negotiations if they are sufficiently confident in their information and prior authorization approaches such that they will not be the first to compromise on pricing. This means that the pharmacist team members must feel certain that alternatives to higher priced drugs are equally effective and available.

When differences in effectiveness or adverse events is supported by the evidence, a cost-effectiveness analysis (CEA) should be considered to provide some sense to decision makers of what differentials in price are justified. The methodology used in cost-effectiveness analysis is still evolving, leading to highly variable quality.[16] Pharmacists should be careful to analyze these studies to make certain that the evidence used to drive the analysis is consistent with the best quality synthesis of the evidence in the class. A CEA based on weak or unrepresentative evidence is of little use and can potentially confuse and deceive purchasers. Costs used in CEAs are also important to appreciate. They may or may not be the same costs that a purchaser will incur.

A variety of pricing strategies makes it possible for pharmaceutical companies to be competitive when they decide to do so. Pricing can vary depending on size of tablet, time to patent expiration, length of the PDL commitment, number of other similar drugs on the PDL, effectiveness of the prior authorization approach, current market share, market share in the total market, and influence of the PDL process on other public and private purchasers. Almost always purchasers will rely on pharmacists to sort through all of the possible pricing approaches to arrive at a comparable pricing methodology—cost of a daily dose, cost of a treatment course, etc.

Some consideration should be given to ways in which practitioners, patients, and taxpayers can be better informed of the pricing process without disclosing offered prices. The public is better informed if it can correlate the pricing strategy of a company with the evidence. For example, a product that has no evidence supporting superiority in its class that is priced ten to twenty times that of its least-expensive competitor obviously is counting on a strategy other than one based on evidence to succeed. Taxpayers have a right to understand how a jurisdiction can agree to pay such a price differential when no rationale exists to do so. Stockholders surely have a right to understand how the company they have invested in plans to justify such a price to buyers. An explicit discussion of that strategy informs practitioner and patient advocates regarding the real world in which pharmaceutical drugs are marketed and sold.

Rebates are a common mechanism used in Medicaid markets to reward companies for competitive pricing and purchasers for shift in market share. Rebates are additional discounts provided to states (and private purchasers) dependent on volume prescribed, proportion of market share, and in some cases shift in market share. Rebates provide a mechanism for price competition since Medicaid prices are fixed by federal statute. Rebates pose many difficult problems. Their calculation requires significant amounts of information that is available only some time after the point of sale. Rebates present budgeting challenges in terms of predicting when these additional "revenues" will arrive and how the rebates will be allocated when they do arrive. This mechanism often results in rebates being used for a variety of other purposes than those directly related to the prescription drug benefit. Although this may seem advantageous, in some circumstances it undermines the credibility of administrative and budget processes. Rebates are often linked to a variety of other pharmaceutical company objectives—other products, disease management programs, selection after patent expiration, etc. Rebates result in the purchasing process being more implicit than explicit, an approach that favors the seller in these circumstances. For now rebates are a "necessary evil" that has been created by a health care system that is increasingly dysfunctional. Acknowledging and understanding the perverse incentives that rebates can result in is important.

IMPLEMENTATION

The key process in implementation is the process chosen to interact with practitioners and patients, usually preauthorization (PA). Preauthorization can range from straightforward phone and online communication to complex data submission and evaluation. The most important factor in a PDL's credibility is the ease and efficiency of the prior authorization process (PA).

The information step allows a state to be a credible purchaser. The pricing step when coordinated well with the information step creates price competition. The PA process communicates the decision made by the state down to the practitioner-patient relationship. The prior authorization process becomes the "face" of the Medicaid program. It must be easily accessible, professional, evidence-based, constantly committed to evaluation, and open to change when evaluation suggests it do so. The designers of the PA approach need to consider key decisions, service issues, and strategies that can support PA.

The first step in assuring that a PA process is credible is to ensure that the program uses evidence for key implementation decisions. Key decisions include number of drugs on the PDL, "grandfathering" of current prescriptions, requirement for PA for refills, and acceptance of PA information from physician substitutes (nurses, medical assistants, disease managers, pharmaceutical companies).

Key decisions can often be better informed by a thorough knowledge of the drug, the disease, and the evidence regarding both. For example, evidence clearly establishes that second-generation antidepressants are effective 65 percent of the time. Ineffectiveness of one does not predict ineffectiveness of another. Selection of a single agent for a PDL means that prior authorization calls will frequently be made due to treatment failures 35 percent of the time. Two to three drugs should be considered for the PDL to avoid this. Allowing patients to remain on antidepressants that are working should be considered since requiring change when treatment is working would mean that a drug with 100 percent effectiveness for that patient would be discontinued and replaced by a drug that is likely effective 65 percent of the time.

Adequate service levels are key. Telephone, e-mail, and faxed requests should be answered within a reasonable time frame 90 percent or more of the time. Decisions should be made based on the initial request 90 percent or more of the time. When decisions cannot be made initially a substantial portion should be made within twenty-four to seventy-two hours. An emergency prescription of the requested medicine should be available in such circumstances. Any unsuccessful PA should be reviewed by a pharmacist or physician for correctness. Cumulative information should be available to managers to assess performance frequently—preferable on a daily basis. If possible, the prior authorization process should be done locally. Decisions made from a distance are always more likely to be questioned.

Several strategies can support and enhance the PA process. Providing efficient summaries of the evidence regarding the drugs in question can be useful, even if the authorization is approved for a drug not on the PDL. Working with care coordinators, disease managers, and others involved in the care of patients on multiple prescription drugs can result in significant movement toward the PDL. Dispensing pharmacists need to understand and support the PDL. They are capable of informing patients and practitioners of the evidence regarding prescription drug use. Formal efforts to do "academic detailing" of practitioners to explain the PDL and evidence supporting it can increase use of the list and reduce PAs.

Other approaches have been taken to encourage the use of PDLs in Medicaid programs, especially in states where the pharmaceutical industry has succeeded in limiting the use of PA or the state has experienced difficulties effectively operating PA. A variety of approaches can often be used to moderate the concerns of practitioners and patients regarding PA. These approaches vary in their success, depending on the degree they result in practitioners considering the evidence supporting their planned prescribing.

Voluntary PDLs can result in change in prescribing especially if they are accompanied by academic detailing. The resources need to do academic detailing however are substantial and reduce the cost saving of the PDL. When coordinated with private purchasers to inform practitioners and patients of the evidence, voluntary approaches can have a significant market effect. This may not however translate into savings for taxpayers that a Medicaid agency can identify.

PA approaches that simply require practitioners to communicate their need for an exception are significantly more effective than voluntary efforts because they result in practitioners evaluating the PDL options prior to using resources for a call. PA approaches that require that practitioners justify their need for an exception are more effective still, though they require a more sophisticated approach on the Medicaid program's part. PA programs that provide feedback to practitioners can improve the quality and cost-effectiveness of practitioners, especially those who have no organized information system. Pharmaceutical companies know how practitioners are prescribing. Ironically, most practitioners have no idea what their overall prescribing pattern is over a period of time.

Anecdotal evidence across state programs suggests that the effectiveness of implementation of a PDL varies based on how effective PA is. Voluntary efforts result in small market-share shifts, academic detailing in moderate shifts, and PA in large market-share shifts. If evidence is used wisely, the overall clinical and administrative outcomes will clearly favor the PDL approach.

Many practitioners acknowledge the evidence but are influenced to prescribe by a variety of other factors. They are often not aware of substantial differences in price or the persistence of brand loyalty. They may be in denial of the evidence demonstrating the effectiveness of marketing and sales strategies on practitioners and patients. An effective PA program can increase evidence-based practice and competition.

Implementing a PDL should start as the case is made for one. The same stakeholders crucial for making the case should be involved throughout the process as the effort moves along. It is particularly important that practitioners, pharmacists, and consumers be involved in the information step. The details of the prior authorization approach should come as no surprise to all the parties. The best position to be in for the pharmacy program is to commit to doing each step in a transparent way, collaborating with those whose approach is constructive.

Communication should use every medium—one on one for key stakeholders, public meetings, Web site, stakeholder newsletters, and any media outlet interested in the topic. The latter is particularly important. Government is often wary of the media, sometimes for good reasons. Information about prescription drugs however is so dominated by the industry and so opaque to practitioners and the public that an approach welcoming discussion of controversial topics and conducting as much of the process in public as possible provides needed communication to practitioners and patients. All communication with the industry should be made public. Every opportunity to communicate with the industry is also an opportunity to communicate to the public and to improve trust.

Communication to practitioners and pharmacists is especially important. They should be involved as decision makers in the information process through public processes. Conflict-of-interest issues, transparency, and explicit decision making should be highlighted in these processes and made explicit whenever possible. Practitioners and pharmacists are acutely aware of these issues and will welcome the opportunity to make decisions in environments free of pharmaceutical industry influence. Practitioners and pharmacists with conflicts should be included in the process as participants but not as decision makers. Their conflicts should be disclosed to the public if they desire to participate. Expectations regarding relationships between academic medical centers and pharmaceutical companies may be changing.[17] An implementation approach that sets a high standard regarding transparency and conflict of interest will set itself apart from the industry's usual approach.

State practitioner associations should be provided with information about the process as soon as it is available. Private purchasers should be informed of the information process and encouraged to engage in it in order to provide every opportunity to shift the information focus from a sales approach to an evidence approach. Every opportunity to share evidence regarding effectiveness and safety of drugs on the PDL should be pursued.

Reasonable time lines should be used for implementation with sufficient flexibility allowed to adjust to those issues that either evidence or further public discussion warrants. Credibility and trust is more important in the long run than quick market-share shifts. A period of voluntary compliance is often helpful since word of classes being added to the PDL, specific drugs on the PDL, and directions on how to pursue PAs can take time to sink in. Practitioners are used to formularies and PA but they are also frustrated with multiple formularies and PDLs each with different sets of procedures. High-volume prescribers of targeted drugs should be focused on in terms of both evidence and how the PA process works. High-utilization patients should also be focused on to minimize miscommunication and transitions that result in over or under utilization

The PDL/PA program should constantly be evaluated and improved, starting with the information process and moving through the entire sequence. Constant changes, adjustments, and improvements will be needed to maintain credibility. Acknowledgement of errors, changes in evidence, and other important changes reinforces trust and accountability. Feedback to practitioners and pharmacists should be included in this process. Those who disagree with the process should be given every opportunity to interact with the process, starting with the information process.

Evaluation

Several outcomes are important to measure and share with decision makers. These include financial outcomes, service levels, and clinical outcomes both direct and indirect.

Financial Outcomes

Financial outcomes can be measured in a variety of ways. Analysis of the costs for specific classes is particularly useful. Market-share graphs enable decision makers to see what approaches have resulted in significant market-share shifts. Cost trends by class put any PDL intervention in perspective. Overall savings can be projected for specific classes. Financial outcomes should include the administrative costs of the PDL/PA systems and any costs to the system overall generated by the PDL—increase in physician visits for example. Measuring the financial outcomes of clinical events is more of a challenge. If the evidence base is substantial and the populations studied similar to those of the Medicaid program, it is reasonable to make assumptions that the evidence from these more rigorous studies can be used to project effectiveness and adverse event rates. Financial outcomes should also include at least some estimate of the impact of any savings, i.e., if the savings were used to insure more people the positive impact of that coverage should be estimated.

Service Levels

Service levels can be measured in a variety of ways—waiting times, call duration, PAs generated on first call, appeal rates, average time for appeal decision, etc. These results should be constantly fed back to operations staff with agreed-upon goals for improvement and strategies to reach those goals. Complaints about the PA process should be sought after and shared with operations staff. Satisfaction of key stakeholders including the PA staff should be measured.

Clinical Outcomes

Clinical outcomes are particularly difficult to measure on an ongoing basis. Databases that would allow this type of analysis can, however, be established and made available to program analysts and researchers. CMS has recently announced that it will make databases of Medicare prescription drug use and other databases available to researchers. Process outcomes such as hospitalizations, visits, or duplicated prescriptions are easier to measure than are clinical outcomes. Access to laboratory databases may allow indirect measures of clinical success or failure such as cholesterol, hemoglobin A1c, etc. More robust clinical events, such as symptomatic events including death, are more difficult to measure and attribute. Integrated systems can more easily take on these challenging approaches.

Ultimately these issues can only be resolved with ongoing large practical clinical trials that monitor the effects of drugs.[18] This approach seems to be too complex until one acknowledges the billions of dollars being spent on prescription drugs. PDLs have brought attention to the medical and economic importance of measuring and acting on evidence related to comparative benefits of services and products. Hopefully we will all benefit locally as robust global efforts produce evidence on this important topic.

SUMMARY

PDLs represent a significant opportunity for pharmacists to engage in, implement, and lead the policy process. The states participating in the Drug Effectiveness Review Project have repeatedly been able to engage policymakers, practitioners, and patients in a rational decision-making process related to prescription drugs. Some DERP states (Oregon and Washington) were able to understand and weigh the evidence regarding cardiac effects of COX-2 inhibitors in 2002 and exclude higher risk agents from their PDLs years prior to the FDA's decision to limit the availability of COX-2s. Explicit discussion of the evidence regarding the effectiveness of PPIs, long-acting opioids, sedative hypnotics, and many other drug classes has led to increased price competition. The availability of systematic drug class reviews have led to more transparent discussions of mental health drugs—their benefits, risks, and costs—something the industry has tried to dominate despite the substantial impact on Medicaid, families and patients.

The policy issues confronting the field of pharmacy, as manifested in PDLs, are similar to those of health care as a whole. The success of the pharmaceutical industry business model has both direct and indirect effects on the health care industry. Pharmacists have an obligation to understand these policy issues and provide knowledgeable advice and counsel to those they serve regardless of whether they are involved with buyers, sellers, practitioners, or patients. Pharmacists will be especially important in translating evidence in the three steps of the purchasing process—information, pricing, and implementation.

NOTES

1. Centers for Medicare and Medicaid Service (2006). Medicaid Drug Rebate Program: Overview. Available at: http://www.cms.hhs.gov/MedicaidDrugRebate Program.

2. National Association of Attorneys General (2005). Consumer Protection. Available at: http://www.NAAG.org/issues/issue-consumer.php.

3. Burton, S.L. et al. (2006). The Ethics of Pharmaceutical Benefit Management. *Health Affairs*20(5): 150.

4. Oregon Health and Science University (2006). Drug Effectiveness Review Project. Available at: http://www.ohsu.edu/drugeffectiveness.

5. Agency for Healthcare Research and Quality (2006). Advancing Excellence in Health Care. Available at http://www.AHRQ.gov.

6. Agency for Healthcare Research and Quality (2006). Evidence-Based Practice Centers. Available at: http://www.AHRQ.gov/clinic/epc.

7. Oregon Health and Science University (2006).

8. The text that follows describing the systematic evidence-based review process is modified from a paper written for the Drug Effectiveness Review Project by Mark Gibson, Mark Helfand, Kathleen Lohr, and John Santa.

9. Academy of Managed Care Pharmacy (2006). What's New. Available at: http://www.AMCP.org.

10. Oregon Health and Science University (2006).

11. The Cochrane Collaboration (2006). The Reliable Source of Evidence in Health Care. Available at: http://www.cochrane.org/index.htm.

12. Agency for Healthcare Research and Quality (2006). Evidence-Based Practice Centers.

13. Agency for Healthcare Research and Quality (2006). U.S. Preventive Services Task Force (USPSTF). Available at: http://www.AHRQ.gov/clinic/uspstfix.htm.

14. National Institute for Health and Clinical Excellence (2006). Providing National Guidance on Promoting Good Health and Preventing and Treating Ill Health. Available at: http://www.NICE.org.uk.

15. U.S. Department of Veterans Affairs (2006). Pharmacy Benefits Management Strategic Healthcare Group. Available at: http://www.pbm.va.gov.

16. Bell, C.M. et al. (2006). Bias in Published Cost Effectiveness Studies: Systematic Review. *BMJ* 332(7543): 699-703.

17. Brennan, T.A. et al. (2006). Health Industry Practices That Create Conflict of Interest. *JAMA* 295: 429-433.

18. Tunis, S.R. et al. (2003). Practcial Clinical Trials: Increasing the Value of Clinical Research for Decision Making in Clinical and Health Policy. *JAMA* 290: 1624-1632.

Chapter 23

Recent Developments in the Health Technology Assessment Process

Paul C. Langley

THE ROLE AND EMERGENCE OF FORMULARY SUBMISSION GUIDELINES

Formulary submission guidelines are a set of informational and analytical standards that have been put in place by a health care system to support the assessment of health technologies. *Health technology assessment* refers to the evaluation of individual drug products, devices, and associated therapeutic interventions as well as more broadly based multiple product/device assessments as part of disease area and therapeutic class reviews. The latter can include support for clinical guidance recommendations within disease and therapeutic areas (see also Chapter 22).[1] Health technology assessment requirements are typically directed toward drug and device manufacturers. The request by a pharmacy and therapeutics committee or its equivalent for a technology assessment dossier, which in the United States is at the discretion of the committee, can support both an individual or one-time-only product or device evaluation as well as disease area or therapeutic class reviews. In the latter a request for a dossier is sent to all manufacturers with products (including devices) within the disease area or therapeutic class. Disease area and therapeutic class reviews are becoming more widespread. This reflects recognition of the importance of ongoing comparative product assessments, given the continually changing competitive landscapes, with new products entering the marketplace and increasing cost pressures on health care systems (with the need to justify therapy choices and premiums for benefit packages to employers). A process of ongoing health technology assessments can support not only formulary decisions and product positioning within a formulary but also the activities of specialty pharmacies in which patients are recruited into disease management programs to ensure the appropriate use and monitoring of high-cost therapies (e.g., biologics and home monitoring devices).

From an assessor's perspective, the standards set in a health technology assessment guideline detail (1) the information that should be supplied to the committee and (2) the analytical techniques that the committee believes are appropriate to evaluating the prospective impact of introducing a drug product (or device) into their treating environment. In asking manufacturers and others to subscribe to a particular format, guidelines establish minimum informational and analytical standards to support drug-impact assessments. Assessments focus on three areas of interest:

- The comparative clinical or therapeutic case for the product, with emphasis on claims for treatment effect and the product safety profile
- The cost-effectiveness case for the product in which the incremental therapeutic benefits from moving an "average" patient to the product are matched against incremental cost of treatment
- The system impact case for the product in which the forecast impact of moving patients to the product is assessed in terms of the impact on the annual budgets supporting patients in that disease or therapeutic area and the expected health benefits of the treating population

In establishing informational and analytical standards, assessors seek transparency in the case made for a product and a commitment by manufacturers to making meaningful product comparisons. This is seen in requests for pragmatic, randomized, active comparator trials as well as in health care systems developing framework for product assessments. This extends to recruiting academic groups to undertake independent review of products in a disease area together with an assessment of the case made by a manufacturer in the dossier submitted to the pharmacy and therapeutics committee. All too often, unfortunately, manufacturers are seen as putting forward a selective "best case" for their product and eschewing comparisons with competitor products. In focusing on placebo comparisons to support claims for superior treatment effects, manufacturer-sponsored claims for and product cost-effectiveness are often seen as problematic.

The submission of a dossier to support a technology assessment is only the first step. As will be emphasized here, health care systems are becoming increasingly reluctant to take product claims at face value. In part, this reluctance reflects concerns with the "independence" of authors submitting pivotal clinical papers, for which the research has been supported by a manufacturer and a potential conflict of interest exists.[2] The latest guideline to authors, published by the *Journal of the American Medical Association,* is a case in point. The guideline requests an independent audit of statistical analyses as part of the peer review process.[3] In more general terms, claims for products in terms of treatment effect, safety profile, cost-effectiveness, and system impacts should been seen as provisional —they are hypotheses as to anticipated product performance. Irrespective of the apparent face validity of a claim for product performance, health care systems are asking for such claims to be monitored and verified as part of ongoing disease area and therapeutic class reviews. As will be discussed here, requirements for product claims to be put in empirically evaluative terms and to be monitored and verified over the product life cycle represent a major innovation in health technology assessment requirements.

The Emergence of Guidelines

Australia was the first country to introduce (and mandate) formulary submission guidelines (in August 1992—they were last revised in 2002), followed shortly thereafter by the Province of Ontario, Canada.[4,5] The Australian guidelines have as their principal rationale the need to ensure efficiency in the delivery of health care from a national perspective. Manufacturers are required to submit a dossier to the Pharmaceutical Benefits Advisory Committee (PBAC) if they want their product to be considered for subsidy under the Pharmaceutical Benefits Scheme—the national Australian formulary for products available through community pharmacies. Standards required by the PBAC are highly prescriptive, asking the manufacturer to make a comparative clinical, cost-effective, and budgetary impact case for the product. If the PBAC considers that the manufacturer has made a justifiable case, the manufacturer then enters into contract negotiations with the authorities to agree unit price for the product and any restrictions on patient access. In putting together a cost-effective and budget impact case for their product two points are worth noting: first, the unit product price that the manufacturer utilizes in the cost-effective and budget impact case need not be the final price agreed with the authorities and, second, the guidelines include a mandatory resource item classification and unit costs for modeling cost-effectiveness claims.[6]

No doubt the Australian guidelines have set the standard for other countries that have introduced health technology guidelines as part of their product assessment process. Even so, it should be noted that in Australia it is left up to the manufacturer to make a submission for product subsidy. If a manufacturer, after marketing approval has been received, decides not to submit a dossier—or where a dossier has been rejected—then the patient pays the full price determined by the manufacturer for the product. In other countries (e.g., the United States) unsolicited dossiers are not accepted—a health care group has to request a dossier for formulary review. In other countries, a product can be listed and subsidized with the decision to review the product for clinical recommendation left to the discretion of the authorities (e.g., England and Wales). A number of other countries have issued guidelines, although only in a handful of cases are they required as part of the process of formulary assessment (Portugal, the Netherlands, Denmark, Norway, Sweden, Finland, and New Zealand). In other countries—France, Spain, Italy, Germany—guidelines are peripheral to product assessments and typically take a backseat to a clinical review, followed by an assessment of anticipated market share and product affordability for the health system.[7]

Since the publication of the Australian guidelines in 2002, technical standards in cost-effectiveness analyses have changed significantly. Although outside the scope of the present chapter, four developments are of particular importance. These are the following:

1. The requirement to integrate more closely pooled clinical claims for the product and its comparators (to include procedures) with the modeled claims for cost-effectiveness and system or budgetary impact
2. The need to deal comprehensively with uncertainty in evaluating claims for treatment effect, cost-effectiveness, and system impact through the application of techniques such as probabilistic sensitivity analyses
3. The requirement for claims to be expressed in cost-per–quality adjusted life year (QALY) terms, in which the default is health-related quality of life measured through the application of a generic instrument
4. The development of independent "gold standard" cost-effectiveness and system impact model frameworks in lieu of models developed individually by manufacturers to support cost-effectiveness and system impact claims

The adoption of new standards is seen particularly in the health technology assessment activities of the National Institute for Clinical Excellence (NICE) in the UK, the Scottish Medicines Consortium (SMC), and Pharmac in New Zealand.[8-10] In terms of influence, NICE is by far the most important of these agencies in setting technical standards, in requiring manufacturers to express claims in generic cost-per–QALY terms (the "reference case"), and in contracting academic and associated groups for independent assessments of products as part of disease area and therapeutic class reviews. This latter activity is noteworthy in that independent assessors in the UK have, in large part, rejected the claims and models put forward by manufacturers as selective and self-serving in favor of de nouveau model structures to support claims for products by place in therapy and as a key input to clinical guidance for product utilization within the National Health Service.[11]

From a global perspective, it is worth noting a key requirement of the SMC process. Once a product has received marketing approval for the UK, a health technology assessment—to include clinical, cost-effectiveness and system impact claims—has to be submitted to the SMC. The results of the assessment are published within three months. This means that, where a manufacturer is attempting to coordinate product launch in key European markets and the United States, the SMC acts as the global assessment watchdog. If the SMC is not prepared to endorse a product for use within the Scottish NHS, finding claims for cost-effectiveness unsupported, it will have a negative impact on submissions made to other health care systems—including the United States.

The United States has no national guidelines set for health technology assessment. Although the federal government, through the Agency for Healthcare Research and Quality (AHRQ), has supported a program of health technology assessment, the heterogeneous structure of health care delivery in the United States (as opposed to a single-payer system) has precluded agreement on the need for a national standard for health technology assessments. The notable exception here is the report of the U.S. Panel on Cost-Effectiveness in Health and Medicine and its recommendations for health technology assessments.[12] Unfortunately, this report, although widely reported, had little immediate impact on decision makers, although the authors of the report clearly played a major role in pointing to the need for health technology assessments and the establishment of the International Society for Pharmacoeconomics and Outcomes Research (ISPOR). Although ISPOR has played a key role in proposing analytical standards in outcomes research and in promoting health technology assessment activities, ISPOR has not developed guidelines for formulary submissions.

Even though federal agencies have stepped back from recommending health technology assessment standards, this may change with the commitment by the Centers for Medicare and Medicaid Services (CMS) to cost-effectiveness assessments under the Medicare Prescription Drug, Improvement, and Modernization Act 2003, the initiative for standards and processes in health technology assessment rests with individual health plans, pharmacy benefit management companies, and independent interest groups.

The emergence of formulary submission guidelines can be traced back to the publication in 1996 of guidelines for Foundation Health of California and two papers published in 1997 (Langley and Sullivan; Langley and Martin) which described, respectively, the rationale for guideline development together with an overview of the Foundation Health guidelines.[13-15] The next set of guidelines to be issued was released by Regence Blue Shield (now The Regence Group) in June 1997 (revised 1999).[16] These gained considerable recognition in the US and, in fact, were the initial template for the Academy of Managed Care Pharmacy Guidelines. These were followed by guidelines issued by Blue Cross and Blue Shield of Colorado and Nevada in October 1998.[17] In the fall of 2000, the Academy of Managed Care Pharmacy (AMCP) also issued guidelines.[18]

It is the AMCP guidelines that have received the most exposure and that many consider the de facto U.S. standard, although limited evidence exists as to how far the AMCP guidelines as a whole have been implemented by health care systems. The AMCP guidelines were revised and reissued in the fall of 2002, with a further revised version released in the spring of 2005.[19] Finally, in 2001 WellPoint Pharmacy Management issued its own guidelines, based on the initial AMCP format, followed by the release of completely redrafted guidelines in 2004, revised in February 2005, and with a further revision in the fall of 2005.

STANDARDS AND GUIDELINES

In terms of the development of formulary submission guidelines in the United States and the distinction between *standards* and *guidelines,* it is worth noting the contribution of an early paper by Langley and Sullivan. Although this paper was not the first to point to the need for guidelines and their development in U.S. health care, it is important because it presents an early template for the informational and analytical structure of guidelines in the U.S. market.

The Langley and Sullivan paper first draws a distinction between *standards* and *guidelines.* This is a crucial distinction: the term *guidelines* refers to evidentiary requirements mandated by drug purchasers, whereas the term *standards* refers to the analytical techniques that are designed to evaluate treatment effects and the modeling of cost-effectiveness claims. Ideally, it is argued, guidelines should allow considerable latitude in the range of analytical techniques that may be used by those making the submission. The paper cautions, however, that accepted analytical standards may not be appropriate if the purchaser is asking for a systems-impact or prevalence-impact perspective rather than a traditional cost-effectiveness approach in which the focus is on decision-model based incremental cost-outcome claims.

For Langley and Sullivan the issue of perspective is critical: the perspective proposed is that of the health care purchaser. The economic-impact assessment focuses on the direct costs of therapy interventions and the outcomes specific to the membership of the health system; community-wide claims take second place. As detailed in Langley and Sullivan, in the last resort, the perspective of formulary submission guidelines should be the impact, in systems terms, of the introduction of a new therapy on the total direct costs of treating patients in a therapy or disease area and the outcomes profile experienced by the patient group.

Langley and Sullivan suggest a formulary submission format. This comprises ten parts:

Part I: Product Description—A pharmacological profile of the product including name and chemical composition, approved indication, principal pharmacological action, course of treatment, concomitant drug therapies, contraindications and adverse effects.

Part II: Displace in Therapy—A description of principal treatment options, place of proposed product, and a profile of drugs used in that treatment area.

Part III: Comparator Products—The identification of drugs for which the new drug is expected to be substituted, including a pharmacological profile of the comparators, present distribution of these drugs, and anticipated patterns of substitution.

Part IV: Therapy Intervention Framework—The development of a framework for evaluating the impact of the new product, identifying the principal treatment options in the disease or therapy area, the processes of treatment, the drug and medical resources consumed, the cost profiles, and the principal outcomes of therapy.

Part V: Supporting Clinical Data—A summary of the principal supporting clinical trial data and the relevance of these data to the case being made in terms of the therapy intervention framework.

Part VI: Pharmacoeconomic Supporting Data—A review of relevant health technology assessment studies for the proposed product in the disease or therapy area, with particular attention to the relevance of the study to the treating population under consideration.

Part VII: System Impact Assessment—Costs—For the three years following product launch, an assessment of the cost impact, taking into account rate of product uptake, characteristics of the treating population, patterns of substitution for other products, and net impact on resources used to support therapy.

Part VIII: System Impact Assessment—Outcomes—Given the choice and justification of outcomes, the anticipated impact of introducing the product in net terms on the outcomes profile of the treating population, under proposed patient switching scenarios.

    Part IX: Costs and Outcomes—Overall Assessment—A concise description of the estimated cost and outcome impact for the proposed patient switching scenarios.

    Part X: Bibliography and Supporting Materials—A detailed bibliography, copies of key clinical references, and a spreadsheet model.

    The important point to note is the distinction drawn by Langley and Sullivan between the claims for a product in "cost-effectiveness terms" and the claims for a product in "system impact terms." The former is concerned with, typically, a modeled claim for cost-effectiveness based upon a decision framework representing therapy intervention points and the natural course of the disease. Modeled claims are expressed in net-benefit or incremental-net-benefit terms, with the advocates of a new drug therapy arguing a "value proposition" that health systems should be willing to pay for the claimed incremental clinical or quality-of-life benefit attributable to patients switching to a new therapy. The latter systems approach is concerned with the impact patient switching on the total costs of delivering health care and on the overall net clinical or quality-of-life benefits (including the distribution of benefits) to those patients who have switched. The systems approach requires forecasts of the characteristics of patients who are expected to move and the associated forecasts of the associated resource utilization impacts. Finally, whereas the cost-effectiveness claim is based upon a model that tracks the course of the disease, the systems approach requires claims to be made in budget period terms.

    Have guidelines proposed by Langley and Sullivan stood the test of time? In general terms, yes, although four points are worth making. First, in emphasizing the importance of a systems perspective, the Langley and Sullivan approach focused on a requirement that is still dominant (in, for example, the AMCP guidelines) in their emphasis on modeled claims for cost-effectiveness. This may seem paradoxical given that as far back as 1992 the Australian guidelines were asking for a detailed assessment of the impact of introducing a new drug on both the national community pharmacy and medical budgets. Second, the Langley and Sullivan proposals clearly did not put sufficient emphasis on the need to monitor and validate both cost-effectiveness and system-impact claims. Given that claims for product impact are (by definition) hypotheses, then claims should not only be put forward in empirically evaluative terms, but submissions should suggest how claims should be monitored and validated. Third, the Langley and Sullivan approach does not address the issue of resource allocation (implicit in a systems perspective) in which health systems have to decide which products to support. This is now receiving attention through the NICE reference case requirement for generic cost-per–QALY claims. It is worth noting that a reference case had been advocated by the U.S. Panel on Cost Effectiveness in Health and Medicine in 1996, with the New Zealand guidelines in 1999 mandating a reference case in 1999. Finally, the Langley and Sullivan paper is now dated in terms of the technical standards required in modeled cost-effectiveness claims. Specifically, a greater appreciation of the need to take adequate account of the treatment of modeled and, in particular, parameter uncertainty in product cost-effectiveness claims now exists. This is seen in the emphasis on probabilistic sensitivity analysis in the NICE guidelines and the somewhat uncompromising advocacy for this technique by leading health economists.[20]

THE WELLPOINT GUIDELINES: BACKGROUND

The WellPoint guidelines are important, first, because they represent a major innovation in the process of health technology assessment by a U.S. pharmacy benefit management group and, second, because they integrate the process of monitoring and validating claims with regular disease area and therapeutic class reviews. This latter point is worth emphasizing: WellPoint is committed, through its advocacy of an outcomes-based formulary, to claims monitoring and validation.[21] In establishing provisional claims, to support initial product listing, the focus is on clinical systematic reviews and pooled or meta-analysis of treatment effect—where the claims for treatment effect are appropriate to the characteristics of the target population within the WellPoint health system and the claims made are considered useful for health care decision making. An essential part of such advocacy is to base physician practice on the concept of "evidence-based medicine" in eliminating unproductive practice pattern variations in the delivery of health care, a position that is strongly endorsed by WellPoint senior management.[22]

Given this focus on relevant outcomes claims, WellPoint recognizes the importance of taking a life-cycle perspective in evaluating drug impacts. As the competitive landscape changes following the entry of new products, health systems need to be appraised continually of how the entry of new products, changing pricing structures (e.g., genericization), and changing clinical and safety evidence may lead to a reconsideration of prior formulary decisions—hence the importance in the WellPoint guidelines of the commitment to a process or ongoing disease area and therapeutic class reviews.

Manufacturers, in making submissions to WellPoint, are advised that claims must not only be presented in empirically evaluative terms but that manufacturers are under an obligation to monitor and validate claims. This represents a major step forward in health system management, where, all too often in the past, modeled claims (which include clinical claims based on pivotal, placebo-controlled trials) have been taken at face value. With the possible exception of requirements for pharmacovigilance studies, manufacturers have been under no obligation to demonstrate the face validity of modeled claims; indeed, many have been reluctant to even address the question.

The WellPoint guidelines are also groundbreaking given the role Well-Point plays as a pharmaceutical benefit management (PBM) group. As a PBM, WellPoint's influence extends beyond those lives managed directly by WellPoint to the services WellPoint provides through pharmacy management to other clients.

No single guidelines exist to document. Rather, WellPoint has a series of supporting documents. These are: (1) guidelines to support new products, indication, and formulation; (2) guidelines to support product reevaluations as part of disease area and therapeutic class reviews;[23,24] (3) two technical assessment frameworks to identify questions asked by assessors for the two sets of guidelines;[25,26] (4) a comprehensive overview of the evidentiary and analytical standards required in health-technology assessments;[27] and (5) a brief description of the process of health-technology assessment within WellPoint.[28]

THE WELLPOINT GUIDELINES: NEW PRODUCTS, INDICATIONS, AND FORMULATIONS

In introducing the new product (new indication and new formulation) guideline, WellPoint emphasizes that the principal reason for putting guidelines in place is to support WellPoint's commitment to an outcomes-based formulary. Following its commitment to evidence-based medicine, Well-Point is concerned that interventions (products and procedures) are evaluated in terms of outcomes achieved—outcomes that may, in the first instance, be modeled, but that have to be assessed empirically for their performance within the WellPoint treating population. This emphasis on treating initial claims as provisional hypotheses, although in a sense unsurprising, in fact represents a significant step forward in the charge placed upon manufacturers to demonstrate, as expeditiously as possible within the WellPoint population, that claims made can be substantiated.

The WellPoint new product guidelines comprise seven sections. These are:

The WellPoint Outcomes-Based Formulary

A brief overview of the WellPoint outcomes-based formulary concept, emphasizing the ongoing reevaluation of products over their life cycle, details of the evaluation process, and a statement of the standards expected in literature searches.

Product Description and Indication

In common with other guidelines. WellPoint asks for a comprehensive description of the new product (to include the product insert). A full description of current product utilization is requested (to include off-label use), together with details on future indications being sought.

Target Population, Treatment Patterns and Outcomes

This section requires manufacturers to provide a comprehensive epidemiological profile of the disease state; this sets the stage for evaluating the number at risk within the WellPoint system. Elements considered for the profile include (1) a classification of the disease state, (2) characteristics of the target patient population, (3) characteristics of potential subpopulations, (4) annual incidence/prevalence, (5) annual treatment incidence/prevalence, (6) underlying trends, and (7) identification of risk factors. WellPoint also requires a comprehensive assessment of treatment patterns within the disease state together with a statement of the place of the new product in therapy. Comparator therapies (defined as those that the new product is expected to substitute against) are to be identified together with the expected outcomes of therapy. In specifying the outcomes of therapy, WellPoint emphasizes that in assessing competing therapies, the focus is on effectiveness and safety. WellPoint has a well-defined hierarchy of clinical evidence, with naturalistic, active comparator trials that are appropriate to the target WellPoint treating population at the apex.

Clinical Assessment

The clinical assessment mandated by WellPoint is intended to produce an unbiased estimate of the clinical efficacy and effectiveness against comparator therapies. The first step in the clinical assessment is a systematic literature review (with search procedures detailed) for the product and comparators. The second step is to provide a summary of each clinical study identified as relevant (data elements are described). The third step is to generate, for each product, a meta-analysis for the product and comparators (including summaries of existing meta-analyses). In selecting studies for inclusion in meta-analyses, WellPoint requires a quality assessment to be undertaken and to include only those studies that meet appropriate score cutoff points. The third step is to provide an overall statement of the clinical advantage of the product. The fourth step asks manufacturers to point to any differential treatments effects and the possible existence of subgroups. Finally, manufacturers are asked to consider the generalizability of trial-based claims to the target WellPoint population.

Cost-Outcome Assessment and Product Claims

Where a modeled claim for product impact is being made, WellPoint will place the greatest weight on claims based on active comparator, pragmatic clinical trials. At the same time, WellPoint requires summaries to be provided of all relevant health economic studies in the disease area (data elements are described). Since modeled claims for cost-effectiveness are typically expressed in decision-model terms, manufacturers are expected to justify the model structure and the parameter assumptions (and to link these back to the clinical meta-analyses). The manufacturer must take due account of both modeled and parameter uncertainty. The decision framework must reflect the approved indication and the proposed place of the product in therapy within the WellPoint system. The perspective adopted for the modeling should be WellPoint's, with a focus on the direct costs of care incurred by the health care system. Outcomes should be expressed in effectiveness and intention-to-treat terms. WellPoint is also concerned with how scarce health care resources are allocated within the WellPoint system and, although not mandating a generic cost-per–QALY case, argues for manufacturers to present a reference case as part of their submission. In presenting summary results of cost-effectiveness claims, WellPoint's preference is for results to be expressed in probabilistic sensitivity analysis terms (to take account of parameter uncertainty). WellPoint requires any modeled claim to be submitted in electronic-spreadsheet terms.

Budget and System Impact Claims

Presenting a cost-outcome claim is only part of the case to be made for a product. WellPoint also requires a systems-impact claim to be presented—

and one that, once again, is empirically evaluative. Claims for system impact are typically driven by forecasts of the number and characteristics of patients who are expected to be moved to (or initiated to) a new therapy. Claims for system impact should include (1) claims for patient moving scenarios, (2) resource utilization impact claims, (3) budget impact claims, and (4) population outcome claims. Again, these claims should be expressed in terms that make them amenable to empirical assessment with a spreadsheet model provided. Budget impact claims should be presented for the first three years following product entry to the WellPoint system.

Monitoring and Validating Claims

From WellPoint's perspective, manufacturers are expected to monitor and validate claims made for their product. In their initial submission, manufacturers are expected not only to identify evaluative claims but to propose also how these claims are to be monitored and validated (e.g., proposed prospective study design). Manufacturers can opt for either experimental or nonexperimental designs. Claims could be assessed via naturalistic or pragmatic, active comparator prospective trials or through nonexperimental observational studies. The choice is at the discretion of the manufacturer.

THE WELLPOINT GUIDELINES: REEVALUATING PRODUCT CLAIMS

Unlike the AMCP and guidelines such as those in place in the UK (NICE) and Australia (PBAC), the WellPoint guidelines pay particular attention to the monitoring and validation of claims for product performance made by manufacturers. Although this might seem paradoxical, guidelines such as those proposed by the AMCP appear to take modeled or synthetic claims made for product performance at face value: no provision is made for monitoring and validating claims as part of ongoing disease area or therapeutic class reviews. This is clearly unacceptable; the changing competitive environment in virtually all disease areas means that the health systems must reassess initial decisions to invest in particular products. Indeed, even if new products do not enter the marketplace, that manufacturers typically follow a policy of annual (and even semiannual) price increases (typically in excess of inflation) means that initial claims for cost-effectiveness and systems impact should be revisited.

The WellPoint guidelines for product reevaluations falls under six heads.

The WellPoint Outcomes-Based Formulary

This introduction follows from the new product guideline, in presenting an overview of the WellPoint outcomes-based formulary concept, emphasizing the ongoing process of disease area and therapeutic class reviews supporting reevaluation of products over their life cycle, details of the evaluation process, and a statement of the standards expected in literature searches.

Update of Product Description and Indication

As part of the reevaluation of the product, manufacturers are asked as part of the disease area and therapeutic class review, to detail any changes in product description and indication since the previous evaluation. In addition, manufacturers are asked to detail the utilization of product (to include off-label utilization) since the last submission.

Review of Target Population, Treatment Patterns, and Outcomes

WellPoint asks that previous claims as to the epidemiological profile of the product, descriptions of treatment patterns, and the place of the product in therapy be reevaluated. The epidemiological profile should be updated, together with any evidence to support claims for changing treatment patterns and qualifications as to the place of the product in therapy. If the competitive landscape has changed, this needs to be detailed in terms of possible comparator change. Manufacturers are also asked to update the results of their trial programs, noting in particular any active comparator, pragmatic trial results.

Revised Clinical Assessment

The role of the clinical assessment is to provide an unbiased estimate of the clinical efficacy and effectiveness of the product and comparator products. In a reevaluation submission, manufacturers are expected to provide an update of the assessment provided in their previous dossier for both their own product and comparator products. New data should be identified via systematic reviews with appropriate clinical summaries and, if necessary, revised meta-analyses and a restatement of the product's clinical advantage.

Revised Cost-Outcome Assessment and Product Claims

WellPoint expects manufacturers to justify any claims for the continuing validity of an initial or previous cost-effectiveness claim. Prior modeled constructs should be revisited and, if necessary, reestimated (e.g., with revised treatment effect estimates). Literature summaries need to be revised, if necessary the reference case revisited with a revised summary of cost-outcomes claims. As far as validation of prior claims is concerned, manufacturers should restate the initial claims for cost-effectiveness, describe how these were proposed to be monitored and validated, detail how the monitoring was carried out, and present results as to the extent to which claims were met.

Evaluation of Budget and System Impact Claims

Given prior claims as to budget and system impacts, manufacturers are asked to detail previous claims, describe the monitoring and validation process, and present results as to the extent to which these claims were met. This should be in terms of (1) resource utilization claims, (2) pharmacy budget impact claims, (3) medical budget impact claims, (4) aggregate budget impact claims, and (5) outcome claims.

DISCUSSION

Although WellPoint takes the position that all claims for product impact—whether clinical, cost-effective, or systems focused—are provisional, this does not mean that the highest technical standards should not be applied in making the case for the product. This starts with a requirement for comprehensive and well-documented literature reviews to support epidemiological profiling, clinical evaluations (to include unpublished trial data), and health-technology assessments. Manufacturers are encouraged to support claims for the place of a product in therapy, resources used to support therapy pathways, and choice of comparator products and procedures through evaluations of both public and private data sets (e.g., Medicare 5 percent Standard Analytical Files, administrative claims data). Manufacturers also have to undertake critical reviews of the clinical literature, apply exclusion/exclusion criteria and quality checks to identify studies for meta-analyses, report meta-assessments of treatment effects, and link these to outcome assumptions for modeled claims for cost-effectiveness. In the hierarchy of clinical data, the greatest weight is attached to active comparator, naturalistic clinical trials.

Wellpoint also puts forward as the default outcome measure, quality of life. This is seen as a final-outcome measure, with concerns expressed that if claims are based on intermediate or surrogate measures, these need to be linked quantitatively to final outcomes. The manufacturer has the choice of measure, although the relevance of the underlying quality of life construct needs to be justified. WellPoint does not insist on a reference case being made to support a product. However, where a manufacturer has made prior submissions to other agencies involving a generic cost-per–QALY instrument (the EQ-5D is mentioned explicitly), then, if preference weights are available for the United States, WellPoint would expect the cost-per–QALY case to be presented.

The technical standards required to support cost-effectiveness claims are similar to those proposed by agencies such as NICE. Manufacturers are expected to present decision-theoretic claims that accommodate both modeled and parameter uncertainty. Manufacturers are expected to apply probabilistic sensitivity analyses and to present results in the form of cost-effectiveness acceptability curves against willingness-to-pay levels for incremental benefits. WellPoint, in judging the merits of a cost-effectiveness claim, require a clear justification of assumptions that support parameter estimates. These include linking treatment effect claims (in distributional terms) to meta-analyses, with claims for resources to support therapy justified by administrative claims data and even patient chart reviews. All resource utilization assumptions are expected to be detailed as the basis for predicting resource-utilization impacts. Resource units are to be identified by CPT (current procedural terminology) code. Each CPT code is to be accompanied by its resource-based relative value unit, with manufacturers assigning a relative value multiplier to give a unit-cost estimate. This allows WellPoint, when the model is being evaluated in spreadsheet form, to apply its own multiplier.

That WellPoint asks for manufacturers to supply an electronic version of their modeled claims for cost-effectiveness does not mean that such claims are taken at face value. As already noted, independent assessments of cost-effectiveness claims undertaken in the UK have typically put the model structures and choice of comparator therapy submitted by manufacturers to one side in favor of de nouveau modeling framework, which provides for a comprehensive (yet indirect) assessment of competing cost-effectiveness claims and the potential place of products in therapy. There is no reason why WellPoint, given resources committed to technology assessments, should not follow the same path. Indeed, WellPoint may be forced to follow in NICE's footsteps and even mandate a common model framework for submissions in selected disease and therapeutic areas. In this context it is worth noting that, at the time of writing, commercially available model structures exist that provide a common reference point (or reference case) for product assessments (e.g., diabetes).Where the Wellpoint guidelines differ from NICE (and the AMCP) is in requiring claims to be expressed in empirically evaluative terms. This means that claims for cost-effectiveness should be amenable to empirical assessment either through prospective experimental studies—a "direct" test of cost-per–QALY claims—or through observational studies. These might involve claims for resource sparing, which could be assessed retrospectively, or for clinical impacts that could evaluated through a sample of patient charts.

Exactly the same standards apply to claims for system impact. These claims are expected to be formulated in budget-year terms (for each of the first three years following formulary listing) and to detail (1) forecasts of the rate of uptake of the new therapy and (2) the characteristics of patients who move to the new therapy. These forecasts provide the basis for re-source-impact claims (which can be tracked from administrative claims data in CPT terms) and estimates of pharmacy and budget impact, utilizing relative value multipliers.

The results of claims monitoring and validation are expected to be pre-sented as part of a new dossier for disease area and therapeutic class re-views—which initiates a further series of claims and requirements for mon-itoring and validation. These are expected to continue through the life cycle of the product. WellPoint sees the duty of the manufacturer as one of engag-ing in an ongoing dialogue with WellPoint (and other health systems) to evaluate the extent to which claims can be justified—and to identify cir-cumstances under which claims may have to be modified. If a product fails to live up to initial claims or its position is weakened by the entry of new products, WellPoint recognizes the reality of possible product disinvest-ments or product repositioning decisions.

The process of reevaluation is a key input to the efficient delivery of health care services; to accept at face value modeled or synthetic claims for a product is absurd. Although modeled claims may be accepted as the basis for an initial formulary decision, manufacturers are expected to commit themselves to invest in studies (both experimental and nonexperimental) to monitor and validate claims. Moreover, the WellPoint time lines are rela-tively short: with two to three years between disease area and therapeutic class reviews, manufacturers are expected to be diligent and timely in demonstrating the case for their product.

In focusing on the monitoring and validation of empirical claims, Well-Point sees itself as being in the forefront of both effective and efficient for-mulary management. WellPoint seems to be under no illusions as to the magnitude of the task it has set and the resources it will have to commit to ensure the evaluation process is successful. The questions remain, however, as to how manufacturers see their role and the evidence they bring to the table. If the evidence presented to support initial and subsequent reviews is considered incomplete, how far will WellPoint go in requesting resubmissions, undertaking independent modeled cost-effectiveness and system impact assessments, and denying formulary access? Will WellPoint be able to demonstrate that the introduction of these guidelines and the evaluation process have led to greater efficiencies in health care delivery and, inevitably, cost savings?

Finally, no doubt we are at a critical point in the commitment to health technology assessments and the standards expected of manufacturers by health care systems in the United States and countries with a well-developed commitment to and expertise in health technology assessments, such as the UK. Perhaps the single most important challenge lies in the choice of modeled framework and associated techniques to underwrite cost-effectiveness and system-impact claims. From a health system perspective, the effective management of limited health care resources requires model frameworks that allow multiple product comparisons and assessments of the place of individual products in therapy sequences over meaningful treatment horizons—particularly for chronic therapies. In short, we are not far from a situation in which health care systems will recommend (or possibly mandate) a model structure to support disease area and therapeutic class reviews. Manufacturers will be expected to make their case in this context—or at least provide a compelling case for a competing model structure.

If "gold standard" model structures are proposed by health technology assessment groups, these will have a profound impact on the process of product development. Manufacturers will be faced with their claims for cost-effectiveness and system impact being judged against a published "reference case." The need to populate a "reference case" model structure will drive protocol designs and pooled assessments of treatment effect. The reference case will also be a key input to pricing decisions and the positioning of a product in target patient populations. Evidentiary and analytical standards will still be in place, but will be subsumed within a common model framework. In the United States, health systems such as WellPoint and federal agencies such as CMS—and even possibly the AMCP and ISPOR—will play a key role in setting disease and therapeutic area model standards. Although it is unlikely that agreement will be reached on a national model standard for disease and therapeutic areas, the emphasis on monitoring and validation of evaluative claims will very likely drive a new model construct and health technology assessment agenda.

NOTES

1. The term *health technology assessment* is used here as it is considered more comprehensive (in embracing the assessment of devices and treatment interventions as opposed to individual drug products) than terms such as *pharmacoeconomics* and *outcomes research.*

2. JE Bekelman, L Yan, CP Gross (2003). Scope and Impact of Financial Conflicts of Interest in Biomedical Research: A Systematic Review. *JAMA* 289: 454-465.

3. PB Fontanarosa, A Flanigan, CD DeAngelis (2005). Reporting Conflicts of Interest, Financial Aspects of Research, and Role of Sponsors in Funded Studies. *JAMA* 294(1): 110-111.

4. Department of Health and Ageing (2002). *Guidelines for the Pharmaceutical Industry on Preparation of Submissions to the Pharmaceutical Benefits Advisory Committee.* September. Canberra, Australia: Department of Health and Ageing.

5. Ministry of Health (1994). *Ontario Guidelines for Economic Analysis of Pharmaceutical Products.* Toronto, Ontario, Canada: Ontario Ministry of Health, Drug Programs Branch.

6. Department of Health and Ageing (2002). *Manual of Resource Items and their Associated Costs.* September. Canberra, Australia: Department of Health and Ageing.

7. A direct link exists to all guidelines documents from the International Society for Pharmacoeconomic Research Web site: http://www.ISPOR.org.

8. National Institute for Clinical Excellence (2004). *Guide to the Methods of Technology Appraisal.* April. London, UK: NICE.

9. Scottish Medicines Consortium (2002). *Guidance to Manufacturers: Notes for the Completion of the New Product Assessment Form.* Glasgow, Scotland: SMC.

10. Pharmaceutical Management Agency (1999). *A Prescription for Pharmacoeconomic Analysis,* Version 1. Auckland, New Zealand: PHARMAC.

11. Woolacott N, Hawkins N, Mason A, et al. (2005). *Efalixumab and Etanercept in the Treatment of Psoriasis.* February. York, UK: Centre for Reviews and Dissemination/Centre for Health Economics, University of York.

12. MR Gold, JE Siegel, LB Russell, et al. (1996). *Cost-Effectiveness in Health and Medicine.* New York: Oxford University Press.

13. PC Langley, RE Martin, E Burton (1966). *Guidelines for Formulary Submission.* October. Rancho Cordova, CA: Integrated Pharmaceutical Services and Foundation Health Corporation.

14. PC Langley and SD Sullivan (1996). Pharmacoeconomic Evaluation: Guidelines for Drug Purchasers. *Journal of Managed Care Pharmacy* 2(6): 671-677.

15. PC Langley and RE Martin (1997). Managed Care Guidelines for Economic Evaluation of Pharmaceuticals. *American Journal of Managed Care* 3(7): 1013-1021.

16. Regence BlueShield Pharmacy Services (1999). *Guidelines for the Submission of Clinical and Economic Data Supporting Formulary Consideration.* Seattle, WA: Regence BlueShield, University of Washington.

17. PC Langley (1999). Formulary Submission Guidelines for Blue Cross and Blue Shield of Colorado and Nevada. *Pharmacoeconomics* 16(3): 211-224.

18. Academy of Managed Care Pharmacy (2000). *Format for Formulary Submissions.* October. Alexandria, VA: AMCP.

19. Academy of Managed Care Pharmacy (2005). Format for Formulary Submissions, Version 2.1. *Journal of Managed Care Pharmacy* 11(5): Sb.

20. K Claxton, M Sculpher, C McCabe, et al. (2005). Probabilistic Sensitivity Analysis for NICE Technology Assessment: Not an Optional Extra. *Health Economics* 14(4): 339-348.

21. B Sweet, CG Tadlock, W Waugh, A Hess, A Nguyen (2005). The WellPoint Outcomes Based Formulary: Enhancing the Health Technology Assessment Process. *Journal of Medical Economics* 8: 13-25.

22. LD Schaeffer, DE McMurty (2004). When Excuses Run Dry: Transforming the US Health Care System. *Health Affairs (Milwood)* October 7 (Suppl. Web Exclusives): VAR117-120.

23. WellPoint Pharmacy Management (2005). *Drug Submission Guidelines for New Products: New Indications and New Formulations.* September. Health Technology Assessment Guidelines. West Hills, CA: WellPoint Pharmacy Management.

24. WellPoint Pharmacy Management (2005). *Drug Submission Guidelines for Re-evaluation of Products: Indications and Formulations.* October. Health Technology Assessment Guidelines. West Hills, CA: WellPoint Pharmacy Management.

25. WellPoint Pharmacy Management (2005). *Health Technology Assessment Guidelines: Assessment Report for New Products, New Indications and New Formulation Submissions by Manufacturers.* September. West Hills, CA: WellPoint Pharmacy Management.

26. WellPoint Pharmacy Management (2005). *Health Technology Assessment Guidelines: Assessment Report.*

27. WellPoint Pharmacy Management (2005). *Health Technology Assessment Guidelines: Evidentiary and Analytical Standards in Health Technology Assessments for the WellPoint Pharmacy Management System.* September. West Hills, CA: WellPoint Pharmacy Management.

28. WellPoint Pharmacy Management (2005). *Health Technology Assessment Guidelines: The Process of Health Technology Assessment for the WellPoint Outcomes Based Formulary.* September. West Hills, CA: WellPoint Pharmacy Management.

Chapter 24

Why Is Medication Use Less Than Appropriate?

David P. Nau
Duane Kirking

Medications are one of the key tools in the therapeutic management of disease. However, they are not always used in an ideal, or appropriate, manner.[1,2] When medications are not used appropriately, patients may experience adverse events or fail to achieve their therapeutic goals. In turn, this results in suboptimal quality of life and wasted resources for our society.

Less-than-appropriate medication use has been underappreciated and underevaluated. Programs to control rapidly escalating medication costs may not be consistent with efforts to use medications more effectively, especially if the result is increased medication use or cost. Fortunately, that narrow perspective is changing. Outcomes research has shown that appropriate medication use may reduce other health care costs. In addition, contemporary disease- and medication-based monitoring systems are better at detecting inappropriate use, especially underutilization, than traditional systems that examined only medication.

Hepler and Strand (1990) have used the term *drug-related morbidity* to describe the phenomenon of therapeutic malfunction—the failure of a therapeutic agent to produce the intended therapeutic outcome.[3] This concept encompasses both treatment failure and the production of new medical problems. Considering that drug-related morbidity accounts for at least 7 percent of hospital admissions and billions of dollars in unnecessary health care expenditures, drug-related morbidity is an important public health issue.[4-6]

Drug-related morbidity is often preceded by a drug-related problem (DRP).[7] A DRP is an event or circumstance involving drug treatment that actually or potentially interferes with the patient experiencing an optimum

477

outcome of medical care. Strand and colleagues delineated eight categories of drug-related problems:

1. *Untreated indications.* The patient is in need of a drug that was not prescribed.
2. *Improper drug selection.* The wrong drug is being used.
3. *Subtherapeutic dosage.* Too little of an appropriate drug is being used.
4. *Overdosage.* The patient receives too much of an appropriate drug.
5. *Failure to receive drug.* The patient does not obtain/use the drug that was prescribed.
6. *Adverse drug reaction.* An unintended and potentially harmful effect of a drug.
7. *Drug interactions.* Undesirable consequences of drug-drug or drug-food interactions.
8. *Drug use without indication.* The patient is taking a drug for which he or she has no medical need.[8]

Drug-related problems may arise due to inappropriate prescribing, inappropriate dispensing/administration of the drug, inappropriate behavior by the patient, inappropriate monitoring of the patient, or patient idiosyncrasy. Although idiosyncrasy is inherently unpreventable, most of the other causes of DRPs can be prevented. The following section of this chapter will provide a framework for examining the causes of inappropriate medication use.

A FRAMEWORK FOR EXAMINING INAPPROPRIATE MEDICATION USE

Hepler and Grainger-Rousseau's (1995) conceptualization of a pharmaceutical care system offers a good framework for examining the potential sources of drug-related problems (see Figure 24.1).[9] A pharmaceutical care system begins with a patient seeking care, and requires that someone (a health care professional and/or the patient) recognizes the patient's health problem and assesses the patient's need for medication therapy. Ideally, a therapeutic plan is then developed that may include the prescribing of a medication along with explicit goals and monitoring parameters. The medication is then dispensed to the patient along with advice on its proper use. The patient then receives the medication and participates in the monitoring of his or her progress toward the therapeutic goals. If the goals are not being met or an adverse drug-related event occurs, the therapeutic plan can be modified to resolve the problem. The monitoring and active management of

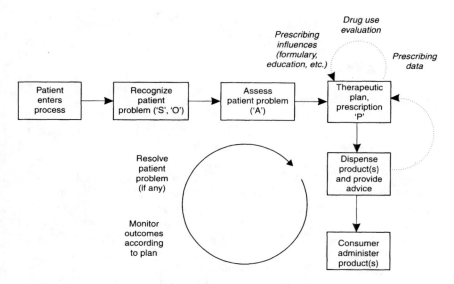

FIGURE 24.1. Monitoring outcomes changes the medications use process into a pharmaceutical care system. Abbreviations: A = assessment; O = objective evidence; P = plan; S = subjective evidence. *Source:* Hepler CD, Grainger-Roussea T-J (1995). Pharmaceutical care versus traditional drug treatment. Is there a difference? *Drugs* 49: 1-10, p. 6. Reprinted with permission from Wolters Kluwer Health.

the drug regimen should continue as long as the patient requires the medication.

Hepler's pharmaceutical care system is similar to the drug-use process described by Knapp and colleagues in the 1970s.[10] Hepler's model builds upon the Knapp model by adding the functions of drug monitoring and management to denote the importance of ongoing attention to the patient and drug regimen. Hepler and Grainger-Rousseau (1995) suggest that three key elements are necessary for proper functioning of a pharmaceutical care system: (1) initiating therapy, (2) monitoring therapy, and (3) managing (i.e., correcting) therapy. Appropriate initiation of therapy requires the recognition and assessment of the patient's signs and symptoms to generate an appropriate diagnosis and therapeutic plan. It also entails the prescribing of a drug that, based upon the knowledge of the prescriber and information available to the prescriber, would be the most appropriate product for the individual patient. Furthermore, the patient must obtain the prescribed medication (most often from a pharmacy that presumably has dispensed the appropriate medication along with appropriate advice to the patient) and must begin using it. Given the numerous steps and people involved in the initiation of drug therapy, it is easy to identify many potential reasons for failures in this process.

Problems with Initiation of Therapy

If patients do not recognize a potential health problem that could be treated with a medication, or do nothing about a recognized problem, then the initiation of drug therapy will not occur. Patients may not recognize a problem because the problem may be asymptomatic or because they lack an understanding of the significance or meaning of symptoms. They may also choose not to seek the advice of a health professional due to fears of what they may be told, or because of a distrust of providers. They may also lack access to health care due to an inability to pay for services or geographic barriers.

Once a patient accesses the health care system, an evaluation of his or her signs or symptoms should be conducted. However, if the patient is unable to communicate clearly with the provider, an accurate assessment of the problem becomes difficult. The provider may also lack the necessary skills or equipment to accurately diagnose the problem, or may not give adequate attention to the patient's problem. If the problem is not correctly diagnosed, it is unlikely that appropriate drug therapy will be prescribed.

Once the diagnosis is made, the clinician then needs to decide whether a drug is warranted for treating the patient. If so, the selection of the drug (along with an appropriate dose, route, duration, and instructions) can be challenging. Given the thousands of drug products that are available, and the characteristics of the patient (e.g., age, weight, renal function, cognitive function), the clinician is tasked with selecting the most appropriate therapy for the disease in the patient at that time. The task is made more complex for the physician by having to deal with multiple payers who may each specify in their formularies a different preferred drug for a given condition, as well as by advertisements that lead patients to request specific products, or by conflicting data from clinical trials. Most often, the clinician is working from his or her memory of the numerous products indicated for a particular disease, and uses simple decision rules to reduce the complexity and uncertainty inherent in product selection (e.g., "If the patient is a child with uncomplicated otitis media, and no other health problems, I prescribe amoxicillin"). Numerous studies have been conducted of how physicians select drug products. The detailed findings of these studies are beyond the scope of this chapter.[11-15]

Once the prescription for drug therapy is generated, the ambulatory patient generally obtains the medication from a pharmacy. The pharmacist is charged with confirming the appropriateness of the medication for the patient and then dispensing the product, along with instructions on proper use, to the patient or caregiver. Although the pharmacist should be able to detect problems with the prescription (e.g., an overdose of chloral hydrate for an infant), this does not always happen. An individual pharmacist may lack the knowledge of appropriate drug therapy, or may be too busy in the hurried environment of many community pharmacies to adequately review the prescription. Systems operating on the pharmacy computer have criteria to assist in identifying potential problems with prescriptions, however the alerts generated by these systems may not always provide clear guidance on the action to be taken by the pharmacist, and a high-volume of low-risk alerts may lead to high-risk alerts being overlooked.[16,17] Another challenge for the pharmacist is the lack of information regarding the patient's medical condition. However, the patient's diagnosis and other pertinent clinical information are not often immediately available to the pharmacist. This review process is sometimes called prospective drug utilization review (PDUR). Chapter 26, which discusses various types of drug utilization reviews, provides additional detail on the strengths and weaknesses of computerized systems supporting PDUR.

If the pharmacist has deemed the prescribed therapy to be appropriate, then the correct drug and information need to be provided to the patient or the patient's caregiver. Within hospitals, the product is usually provided by the pharmacy to a nurse who then administers the drug to the patient. However, hospitals may also have medications stocked within a nursing unit, and the pharmacist may be bypassed altogether. This limits the opportunity to double-check the order prior to the drug's administration. Regardless of setting, numerous steps are involved with the dispensing and/or administration of a drug product, and often several personnel are involved in processing the drug order before the product reaches the patient. This creates many opportunities for error.

Numerous factors are involved in dispensing-related medication errors. Errors often result from a combination of human factors and systems failures. Some of the most frequently cited factors include: (1) the lack of a consistent dispensing process or unclear roles within the process, (2) a workload that exceeds the capacity of the personnel and dispensing process, (3) excessive distractions in the dispensing process, (4) unclear handwritten prescriptions, (5) similar drug names that can easily be confused, (6) products or packaging that look identical, (7) lack of training for personnel, and (8) failure to communicate with patients.

Pharmacist-patient communication is important for at least three reasons. First, it provides the pharmacist with information to assess the appropriateness of the prescribed regimen. Second, talking to the patient about the prescribed medication can reveal potential medication errors before the patient receives the medication (e.g., the pharmacist had interpreted the handwritten prescription as being for a cardiovascular drug, but the patient says that she was prescribed the drug for breast cancer). Last, the pharmacist can provide the patient with information regarding the appropriate use of the medication and can confirm that the patient understands the information.

Unfortunately, verbal communication between pharmacist and patient does not always occur. Several reasons for this exist. Some pharmacists perceive that patients do not want to talk to them, and thus they do not attempt to initiate a dialogue. However, research has indicated that many patients want more information about their medications.[18] Even when pharmacists do attempt to communicate drug-related information, the patient or caregiver may have difficulty engaging in a productive dialogue if they feel ill or are distracted by a sick child. A financial disincentive discourages pharmacy personnel from spending time talking with patients since payment to the pharmacy is based on sale of the product regardless of whether the pharmacist and patient converse about the medications. Thus, spending time in conversation with patients detracts from dispensing more prescriptions and maximizing revenue. In addition, patients may expect to receive their medications within a few minutes of presenting the prescription and the pharmacist may feel compelled to minimize the processing time for prescriptions by not talking with patients. Finally, some pharmacists feel apprehensive about talking with patients and may avoid conversations altogether.[19]

Perhaps the most important participant in a pharmaceutical care system is the patient. The patient ultimately decides if, and how, he or she will take the medication. Patients may choose not to fill the prescription or may alter the regimen in ways that are not conducive to optimal outcomes. This may stem from concerns over side effects or addiction, a perceived lack of effectiveness of the drug, or may be due to an inability to pay for the medications. In addition, it may be difficult for some patients to manage a complex drug regimen that involves many medications or complicated directions. Thus, patients may unintentionally miss doses because of the burden involved. More detail on patients' use of medication is found in Chapter 28.

Problems in Monitoring and Managing Drug Therapy

The monitoring and management of drug therapy are crucial elements of the pharmaceutical care system since they facilitate the identification of problems with the initial therapeutic plan or problems with the patient's use of the medications. However, these are also the elements of pharmaceutical care that are most often neglected. The ongoing management of drug therapy may not happen if clinicians or patients fail to monitor the progress toward the therapeutic goals or if they fail to act despite the monitoring data clearly showing the need for change in the plan.

Philips and colleagues (2001) have used the term *clinical inertia* to describe the "failure of health care providers to initiate or intensify therapy when indicated."[20] Clinical inertia is due to at least three problems: overestimation of care provided, use of soft reasons to avoid intensification of therapy, and practice organization not being designed for achieving therapeutic goals. Several studies have noted that physicians overestimate their care provided for chronic illnesses, including overestimation of the extent to which they screened for, and monitored, diseases such as diabetes and coronary heart disease.[21,22]

Even when monitoring data indicates that the therapeutic goal is not being achieved, physicians may use "soft" reasons to justify their decisions not to intensify therapy. For example, if the physician perceives that control of the disease has improved, then he or she may be reluctant to intensify therapy despite the therapeutic target not being achieved.[23] Physicians may also choose not to intensify therapy if they perceive that the patient would not adhere to the intensified therapy.[24] These barriers may stem from concerns over side effects, a belief that the therapeutic targets proposed in clinical guidelines may not be appropriate for a specific patient, or a lack of physician training to "treat to goal."[25]

Many physicians were not trained to intensify drug therapy until therapeutic targets were achieved.[26] In addition, many practice sites are not organized to systematically identify patients who are not achieving the therapeutic goal and to prompt action for further monitoring or intensification of therapy. Many practices are organized to focus on the patient's current medical complaint without attention to the ongoing control of chronic disease. For example, a sixty-five-year-old woman with diabetes may present to the physician's practice to discuss menopausal symptoms. The physician may discuss menopause but then fail to identify that the patient has not had an assessment of glycemic control for the past two years. Although office-based quality improvement initiatives have been developed in recent years to counter this problem, the majority of physician practices are still not engaging in quality improvement efforts toward this aim.[27,28]

Many quality improvement efforts have recognized the important role that nonphysician providers can play in a pharmaceutical care system. Nurses and pharmacists can play a significant role in educating and monitoring patients with chronic illnesses, and with identifying those patients in need of therapy modification. Since pharmacists often encounter patients monthly for drug refills, they are in an excellent position to collect objective monitoring information (e.g., blood pressure, hemoglobin A1c) and solicit subjective feedback from patients regarding their experience with the drugs (e.g., side effects, symptom resolution) to identify those patients in need of further evaluation by a physician. Many health systems, particularly the Veterans Health Administration in the United States, have begun to have pharmacists play a significant role in adjusting drug therapy to promote achievement of the therapeutic targets. A recent multistate project demonstrated that community pharmacists who provided enhanced services to diabetes patients helped the patients achieve better health and reduced total health care expenditures.[29] Unfortunately, these innovative models of care are not widespread.

Problems with Information Flow

A crosscutting theme regarding the suboptimal use of medications is the poor flow of information throughout the pharmaceutical care system. In order for clinicians to make informed decisions regarding the initiation or modification of drug therapy, they need to have timely access to objective and subjective data regarding the patient. In order for pharmacists to evaluate the appropriateness of a prescribed drug, they need to have information such as the patient's diagnosis, weight, and other medications. The patient also needs to know the therapeutic goals, how to appropriately use the medication, how to self-monitor for side effects and therapeutic effectiveness, and how and when to contact various clinicians.

It is important to recognize that information flow, by itself, does not always lead to better decisions or greater achievement of therapeutic goals. Electronic prescribing systems have the potential to decrease several types of medication errors, however they may also create other types of errors.[30] Furthermore, providing pharmacists with more information about the patient does not necessarily lead to better care by pharmacists.[31] This is particularly true if the pharmacy's operations are not designed to facilitate interaction between patients and pharmacists.. Nonetheless, increasing the electronic connectivity between providers and with patients reduces barriers that impede the appropriate initiation, monitoring, and management of drug therapy.

HOW OFTEN DO PROBLEMS OCCUR
IN THE USE OF MEDICATIONS?

Hundreds of studies have been conducted over the past several decades that document myriad problems with the use of medications. We selected examples of studies from each of the eight categories of drug-related problems as defined by Strand and colleagues,[32] as well as from the literature on medication errors It is important to note that the evidence presented in the category of *adverse drug events* is not limited to reports of idiosyncratic drug reactions, and includes reports of both preventable and nonpreventable adverse drug events.

Adverse Drug Events (ADEs)

A recent study using the National Ambulatory Medical Care Survey estimated that there were 4.3 million ambulatory visits in the United States during 2001 for the treatment of an adverse drug event.[33] This equates to 15 visits per 1,000 population with nearly half of these visits being to a hospital emergency department. The authors of this national study also found that the elderly and women were most likely to receive care for an ADE.

In 1995, Bates and colleagues (1995) found that adverse drug events occurred in 6.5 percent of all adult, nonobstetrical, hospital admissions.[34] They estimated that 28 percent of the ADEs were preventable. A study of pediatric patients found that ADEs and potential ADEs occurred in 2.3 percent and 10 percent, respectively, of admitted patients.[35] Yet another study found that ADEs occurred in more than 12 percent of patients within three weeks of discharge from a hospital.[36] The majority of these ADEs were judged to be preventable or ameliorable. Other studies of ADEs have shown similar results.[37] Changes to the inpatient medication-use system such as computerized physician order entry, clinical decision-support programs (See also Chapter 29), and pharmacist involvement with the medical team have been shown to decrease the risk of medication errors and ADEs.[38-42]

Untreated Indications

The patient may have a need for drug therapy (a drug indication), but is not receiving a drug for that indication. It has been estimated that less than half of persons who qualify for lipid-modifying therapy are receiving it.[43] The treatment of hypertension is only slightly better, with 59 percent of persons with hypertension receiving drug therapy.[44] Although it is possible that some persons with dyslipidemia and hypertension could achieve control of their disease without a medication, only 20 percent of patients with coronary heart disease achieve their goal for LDL cholesterol, and 34 percent of hypertensive patients achieve their blood pressure goal.[45,46] However, the proportion of diabetic patients receiving drug therapy for dyslipidemia increased from 28 percent in the early 1990s to 56 percent by 2000.[47] Increases were also seen in the use of drug therapy for hypertension and glycemic control in the same population. Thus, an improvement in the treatment of chronic disease has occurred in recent years, although many people still do not receive drug therapy when needed.

Inappropriate Prescribing

Examples of inappropriate prescribing include: (1) selecting a drug that will not be effective for treating the patient's condition (i.e., wrong drug), (2) selecting a dose that is too low to be effective, (3) selecting a dose that is too high and potentially harmful, or (4) selecting a drug that is inappropriate based upon the patient's comorbidities or concurrent drug use (drug-disease or drug-drug interactions). Researchers of inappropriate prescribing often combine some of the aforementioned categories when reporting the results of their studies.

A recent trend is to examine the use of potentially inappropriate medication (PIM) in the elderly based on criteria developed by Beers and colleagues (1991).[48,49] The Beers criteria focus on drugs that may be inappropriate for use in the elderly due to their propensity to cause adverse drug events in this population. The elderly are an important population for medication-use studies since they may be more vulnerable to adverse drug-related events and often use many medications.

Lau and colleagues (2004) used the Beers criteria to identify potentially inappropriate medication use among elderly nursing home residents.[50] They found that more than 50 percent of residents experienced inappropriate prescribing of medications. Specifically, 40 percent of residents experienced inappropriate drug selection, 11 percent had excess dosage, and 13 percent had a drug-disease interaction. In a follow-up report, Lau et al. (2005) determined that residents who experienced inappropriate prescribing had greater odds of hospitalization in the month following exposure to PIM.[51]

Curtis and colleagues (2004) examined the frequency of PIM in noninstitutionalized elderly patients using prescription claims from 1999.[52] They found that 21 percent of older adults received at least one drug included on the revised Beers list, and 15 percent received at least two drugs of concern. Rigler et al. (2005) compared the frequency of PIM in three cohorts with the Kansas Medicaid program (nursing home residents, recipients of home and community-based services for the frail elderly, and ambulatory patients).[53] They found that PIM occurred in 38 percent, 48 percent, and 21 percent, respectively, of nursing home residents, frail elderly, and ambulatory patients.

One limitation of the numerous studies of PIM in the elderly is that they frequently assess the use of individual medications that are considered inappropriate regardless of the patient's diagnoses or concurrent use of other drugs. To overcome this limitation, Zhan and colleagues (2005) examined the frequency of six drug-drug combinations and fifty drug-disease combinations that place the elderly at risk for adverse drug events.[54] Using data from two national surveys regarding ambulatory visits, they estimated that 0.74 percent of visits involving two or more prescriptions had at least one inappropriate drug-drug combination, and 2.58 percent of visits involving at least one prescription had an inappropriate drug-disease combination. Thus, when more stringent criteria are used to assess PIM in the elderly, the rate of inappropriate prescribing appears much lower.

It is not just the elderly who may have inappropriate drugs prescribed. Some hospitalized patients receive antibiotics that are not appropriate for the identified or suspected pathogen.[55] Patients with mental health disorders may also receive drugs that are not appropriate for their diagnoses.[56] For example, some patients with depression receive only tranquilizers, perhaps because a physician failed to recognize that the patient's sleep disorder stemmed from depression.[57]

Even when appropriate drugs are selected, the prescribed dose may be insufficient to achieve the desired therapeutic benefit. A study of the California Medicaid population revealed that two-thirds of patients using antidepressants were receiving a subtherapeutic dose.[58] The majority of patients with diabetes receive drug therapy that is inadequate to achieve glycemic control.[59-61] Specialists are marginally better than primary care physicians at intensifying therapy in response to elevated blood glucose levels, but the majority of diabetes patients still do not receive intensification of drug therapy when warranted.[62] Pain control medications are also underdosed frequently, particularly in terminally ill patients.[63,64]

Doses that are too high may also be prescribed. One reason for excessive doses is the failure of the prescriber to account for a patient's renal impairment.[65] This is particularly important for drugs with a narrow therapeutic index that are excreted in the urine (e.g., aminoglycosides, digoxin). Many U.S. hospitals have developed pharmacokinetic dosing services to ensure that renally impaired patients receive appropriate doses of medications.[66] Small children, particularly infants, require weight-based dosing of many drugs to ensure that they do not receive overdoses. However, medication overdoses, particularly related to oncology medications, continue to occur in hospitalized children.[67] The drug class most commonly associated with overdoses in nonhospitalized children is analgesics, particularly acetaminophen.[68] Overall, approximately 7.5 percent of all overdoses treated in emergency centers in the United States are due to errors in prescribing, dispensing, or monitoring drug therapy.[69]

Failure to Receive Drug

Even if the patient is prescribed a drug when appropriate, and an appropriate medication and dose are selected, the patient may not receive the drug. A survey of Medicare beneficiaries in 2003 found that four in ten seniors did not take all of the medications prescribed for them in the past year.[70] The reasons most frequently given for not taking all of their medications were: (1) the costs were too high, (2) they didn't think the drugs were helping them, and (3) the drug made them feel worse. Approximately 26 percent of subjects did not fill a prescription or cut their dose of a drug because of cost concerns, and 25 percent stopped taking a drug because it made them feel worse or they perceived the drug was not helping. Subjects who had prescription drug benefits were less likely to go without medication due to the cost of medications.

The reasons for suboptimal adherence to medications may depend partly on the type of drug therapy regimen and may be multifactorial. A study of lipid-lowering therapy identified that only 26 percent of elderly patients maintained a high level of use of statin drugs over five years, with the greatest decline in adherence occurring in the first six months of therapy.[71] A similar study noted that only 31 percent of patients were adherent at three years after initiation of therapy, with the greatest decline happening in the first three months.[72] This study also noted that the short-term effectiveness of the drug therapy was associated with higher adherence in subsequent months. Thus, patients may be more likely to discontinue therapy with statin drugs when they see no improvement in their cholesterol levels and do not feel better. The perceived lack of effectiveness, when coupled with the high cost of statin drugs, may be leading to the high discontinuation rates of these drugs.

Side effects may also contribute to poor adherence with some drug regimens. In particular, antidepressants may produce undesirable side effects such as lethargy and sexual dysfunction, with about one-third of depressed patients discontinuing therapy prematurely.[73] Side effects are also noted frequently as a contributing factor in poor adherence to highly active antiretroviral therapy (HAART).[74] However, side effects alone do not explain much of the variance in medication nonadherence, and they are most likely weighed against the perceived benefits of the medication when patients decide whether to continue taking a medication.[75,76] Many patients taking antidepressant or antiretroviral drugs discontinue their regimens when their "concerns" about the medications exceed the perceived "necessity" of the medications.[77,78]

Drug Use Without Indication

In this category, the patient is taking a drug for which he or she has no medical need. According to the 2003 National Survey on Drug Use and Health, an estimated 6.3 million Americans are using prescription drugs for nonmedical purposes (See also Chapter 25).[79] This represents 2.7 percent of the U.S. population over the age of twelve. However, an estimated 4 percent of twelve- to seventeen-year-olds reported past-month prescription drug abuse. The rate of prescription drug abuse among American youth has increased considerably since 1990.[80]

Some "nonindicated" drug use stems from overprescribing of drugs by physicians. For example, the majority of patients with an upper-respiratory infection receive antibiotics despite the lack of effectiveness of antibiotics for these conditions.[81-82] It is estimated that 17 to 20 percent of the patients who receive antibiotics lack an indication for the drug.[83-84] The high rate of nonindicated antibiotic utilization may be partly driven by patients' misunderstandings about antibiotic effectiveness for viral infections, physician desires to satisfy patients' demands, and marketing campaigns for new antibiotics.[85]

Medication Dispensing/Administration Errors

Although many of the drug-related problems listed in the preceding sections could result from errors in diagnosis, prescribing, consumption, or monitoring of patients, it is also important to examine errors in the dispensing or administration of medications. Considerable variation in the rates of dispensing errors has occurred across numerous studies in ambulatory settings. However, a recent, well-conducted study provided a national benchmark rate of 17 errors out of every 1,000 prescriptions dispensed (1.7 percent).[86] Approximately 6.5 percent of the errors were judged as having the potential for clinically significant consequences for the patient. Given that 3 billion prescriptions are dispensed in the United States each year, an estimated 51 million dispensing errors occur annually.

Medication errors also occur within institutional settings. In 2002, a study of 36 hospitals and skilled-nursing facilities found that 19 percent of doses were in error, with 7 percent of errors being potentially harmful.[87] The most common types of errors involved giving the drug at the wrong time or omitting a scheduled dose. Given the frail health of many persons in hospitals and nursing homes, these medication administration errors can be particularly devastating.

Although the aforementioned studies derived their estimates of errors via observation of pharmacists or nurses, the public's perception of errors is also important. In 2002, the Commonwealth Fund conducted a nationwide survey regarding consumer perceptions of health care quality.[88] Some 22 percent of respondents reported that they or a family member had experienced a medical error, and 16 percent had (at some point in their lives) received the wrong medication or wrong dose of medication. A more recent survey of an insured population found that about 18 percent of respondents had experienced an error by an ambulatory pharmacy at some point in their lives, with 6.8 percent of subjects experiencing an error within the past year.[89] Despite the personal experiences of the public with medical error and media attention to this issue, only 6 percent of the public and 5 percent of physicians viewed medical errors as one of the nation's most important health issues.[90] Concerns about errors ranked far below concerns about the costs of medical care and prescription drugs.

CONCLUSION

Why is medication use less than appropriate? Upon reviewing the evidence from this chapter, we conclude that a short, simple answer to that question exists: complexity and uncertainty. If only the solutions were as simple.

The medication use system is amazingly complex. Although we may commonly equate medication use with consumption by the patient, the management of medication use involves physicians, pharmacists, nurses, and other health professionals as well as those involved in the organization and financing of health care. In addition, these persons work in a mélange of physical settings, adding to the complexity. To make such a complex system operate well, information and other elements of collaboration must be shared across providers who may be in separate physical locations.

The thousands of different medications that make up our armamentarium and the unique characteristics of individual patients make the selection of medication regimens complicated even in the best system of care. Coupled with this complexity is uncertainty as to how individual patients may respond to a drug and uncertainty generated by conflicting clinical trial results. While the complexity and uncertainty of health care create challenges in initiating and managing drug therapy for an individual patient, the same factors complicate our efforts to build a better medication-use system.

Uncertainty as to the frequency and nature of drug-related problems and uncertainty about the effectiveness of various system-level interventions complicate our efforts to modify an already complex medication-use system. The complexity of research on drug-related problems heightens this uncertainty. For example, definitive assessment of the preventability of adverse drug events is not always possible. Furthermore, the extent and nature of drug-related morbidity in the elderly have been obfuscated by the proliferation of studies that examine "potentially inappropriate medications" with varying criteria. Thus, it isn't clear how many elderly patients are experiencing actual drug-related morbidity versus "potential" drug-related problems.

Also contributing to the uncertainty is the difficulty in detecting and measuring some types of drug-related problems. For example, the untreated indication is harder to detect than a drug-drug interaction. More broadly, errors of omission (not doing what is needed) may be more difficult to identify than errors of commission (doing something wrong) since no sentinel event may occur and no easily-accessed data may exist in the case of omissions. Thus, the frequency of untreated indications is less well-known than the frequency of drug-drug interactions, and the prevention of untreated indications may be more challenging.

If complexity and uncertainty are the root causes of many drug-related problems, then quality improvement efforts for the medication use system should focus on methods to reduce complexity and uncertainty. Information systems (see also Chapter 29) that facilitate better decision making and improve both the nature and content of communication between all the participants in health care will go a long way toward reducing drug-related problems. Teamwork, systems-thinking, and continuous learning from successes and failures are also essential components to building a safe and effective medication-use system. At the same time, the importance of the individual must not be overlooked. The strong covenantal relationship between provider and patient can establish an environment that facilitates a truly helpful dialogue. Once we develop a better understanding of how to improve the quality of the medication-use system, we can design payment systems and health care policies that facilitate the appropriate use of medications.

Achieving these steps toward improved medication use will be a challenge, because they require not only considerable resources but also substantial changes in behavior. In addition, new programs may introduce problems of their own. The following suggestions do not represent a complete solution to inappropriate medication use but rather serve to stimulate discussion among policymakers on defining the best ways to achieve that end.

1. Continue to heighten awareness of the extent and severity of drug-related morbidity to consumers, health care providers, and government and other payers.
2. Support further development and use of systems designed to prevent medication errors, provide evidence-based guidance supporting optimal medication choice, and incorporate managed care formularies and other benefit design tools. These systems would include, for example, computerized physician order entry systems and other aspects of the electronic medical record and bedside barcode systems to match patients' with their therapies.
3. Enhance information systems such as prospective and retrospective drug utilization programs that use individualized criteria to identify patients in need of drug therapy modification. Such systems need to incorporate findings as they become available from the growing field of pharmacogenomics, which will allow closer matches of specific medications with the patients most likely to benefit from them.
4. Refine and expand use of systems by health professionals and patients to report medication adverse effects and errors. Examples of current programs include the FDA's MedWatch program and the USP's Medmarx program.
5. Create mechanisms that allow all involved health professionals to share medical and medication records with due regard for HIPAA and other confidentiality considerations.
6. Encourage multidisciplinary care teams that facilitate communication between health professionals and with patients.
7. Use those teams to increase patients' participation in the decision-making process, including care plan goals and therapy follow-up.
8. Hold providers and health systems accountable for inappropriate care and provide incentives for achieving appropriate care.
9. Support research to provide rigorous assessment of the aforementioned activities in terms of how well they function and how to make them perform better. Although many of the activities are conceptually sound and supported by limited empirical evidence, more research to assure their optimal use is needed.

Virtually all individuals and groups involved in health care need to be part of this medication optimization agenda. Key roles exist for certain organizations. National Committee for Quality Assurance (NCQA), Joint Commission On Accreditation of Healthcare Organizations (JCAHO), and other accrediting organizations can use their combined regulatory and health-practice orientation to emphasize the importance of quality in medication use. Health professional organizations can assure that decisions incorporate both the science and art of health care. Similarly, consumer organizations need to insist that the perspectives of their constituencies are appropriately represented. Employers, government, and other payers of care can use their financial influence to assure that changes incorporate principles of cost-effective care. Through a concerted effort by these and all interested parties, the elusive goal of optimal medication use can be achieved.

NOTES

1. Manasse HR (1989). Medication use in an imperfect world: Drug misadventuring as an issue of public policy, Part 1. *Am J Hosp Pharm* 46: 929-44.

2. Manasse HR (1989). Medication use in an imperfect world: Drug misadventuring as an issue of public policy, Part 2. *Am J Hosp Pharm* 46: 1141-52.

3. Hepler CD, Strand LM (1990). Opportunities and responsibilities in pharmaceutical care. *Am J Hosp Pharm* 47: 533-543.

4. Johnson JA, Bootman JL (1995). Drug-related morbidity and mortality: A cost-of-illness model. *Arch Intern Med* 155:1949-1956.

5. Bootman JL, Harrison DL, Cox E (1997). The health care cost of drug-related morbidity and mortality in nursing facilities. Arch Intern Med 157: 2089-2096.

6. Winterstein AG, Sauer BC, Hepler CD, Poole C (2002). Preventable drug-related hospital admissions. *Ann Pharmacother* 36: 1238-1248.

7. Strand LM, Morley PC, Cipolle RJ, Ramsey R, Lamsam GD (1990). Drug-related problems: Their structure and function. *DICP Ann Pharmacother* 24: 1093-1097.

8. Strand LM, Morley PC, Cipolle RJ, Ramsey R, Lamsam GD (1990).

9. Hepler CD, Grainger-Rousseau T-J (1995). Pharmaceutical care versus traditional drug treatment. Is there a difference? *Drugs* 49: 1-10.

10. Knapp DA, Knapp DE, Brandon BM, West S (1974). Development and application of criteria in drug use review programs. *Am J Hosp Pharm* 31: 648-658.

11. Denig P, Haaijer-Ruskamp FM, Zijsling DH (2002). How physicians choose drugs. *Soc Sci Med* 1988;27:1381-6.

12. Denig P. Scope and nature of prescribing decisions made by general practitioners (2002). *Quality & Safety in Health Care* 11: 137-143.

13. Groves KEM, Flanagan PS, MacKinnon NJ (2002). Why physicians start or stop prescribing a drug: Literature review and formulary implications. *Formulary* 37: 186-194.

14. Schwartz RK, Soumerai SB, Avorn J (1989). Physician motivations for nonscientific drug prescribing. *Soc Sci Med* 28: 577-582.

15. Segal R, Wang F (1999). Influencing physician prescribing. *Pharm Pract Manage Q* 19: 30-50.

16. Chrischilles EA, Fulda TR, Byrns PJ, et al. (2002). The role of pharmacy computer systems in preventing medication errors. *J Am Pharm Assoc* 42: 439-448.

17. U.S. Pharmacopeia Drug Utilization Review Advisory Panel (2000). Drug utilization review: Mechanisms to improve its effectiveness and broaden its scope. *J Am Pharm Assoc* 40: 538-545.

18. Kimberlin C, Brushwood D, Allen W, et al. (2004). Cancer patient and caregiver experiences: Communication and pain management issues. *J Pain Symptom Manage* 28: 566-578.

19. Anderson-Harper HM, Berger BA, Noel R (1992). Pharmacists' predisposition to communicate, desire to counsel and job satisfaction. *Am J Pharm Educ* 56: 252-258.

20. Phillips LS, Branch WT, Cook CB, et al. (2001). Clinical inertia. *Ann Intern Med* 135: 825-834.

21. McBride P, Schrott HG, Plane MB. et al. (1998). Primary care practice adherence to National Cholesterol Education Program guidelines for patients with coronary heart disease. *Arch Intern Med* 158: 1238-1244.

22. Drass J, Kell S, Osborn M, et al. (1998). Diabetes care for Medicare beneficiaries. Attitudes and behaviors of primary care physicians. *Diab Care* 21: 1282-1287.

23. El-Kebbi IM, Ziemer DC, Gallina DL, et al. (1999). Diabetes in urban African-Americans. XV. Identification of barriers to provider adherence to management protocols. *Diab Care* 22: 1617-1620.

24. El-Kebbi IM, Ziemer DC, Gallina DL, et al. (1999). Diabetes in urban African-Americans. XV. Identification of barriers to provider adherence to management protocols. *Diab Care.* 1999;22: 1617-1620.

25. Phillips LS, Branch WT, Cook CB, et al. (2001).

26. Phillips LS, Branch WT, Cook CB, et al. (2001).

27. Phillips LS, Branch WT, Cook CB, et al. (2001).

28. Institute of Medicine (2005). *Crossing the Quality Chasm.* Washington, DC: National Academy Press.

29. Garrett DG, Bluml BM (2005). Patient self-management program for diabetes: First-year clinical, humanistic, and economic outcomes. *J Am Pharm Assoc* 45: 130-137.

30. Institute for Safe Medication Practices (2005). It's time for standards to improve safety with electronic communication of medication orders. Available at: http://www.ismp.org/MSAarticles/improve.htm. Accessed August 29.

31. Weinberger M, Murray MD, Marrero DG, et al. (2002). Effectiveness of pharmacist care for patients with reactive airways disease. *JAMA* 288: 1594-1602.

32. Johnson JA, Bootman JL (1995).

33. Zhan C, Arispe I, Kelley E, et al. (2005). Ambulatory care visits for treating adverse drug effects in the United States, 1995-2001. *Joint Commission Journal on Quality and Patient Safety* 31: 372-378.

34. Bates DW, Cullen D, Laird N, et al. (1995). Incidence of adverse drug events and potential adverse drug events: implications for prevention. *JAMA* 274: 29-34.

35. Kaushal R, Bates DW, Landrigan C, et al. (2001). Medication errors and adverse drug events in pediatric inpatients *JAMA* 285: 2114-2120.

36. Forster AJ, Murff HJ, Peterson JF, Gandhi TK, Bates DW (2003). The incidence and severity of adverse events affecting patients after discharge from the hospital. *Ann Intern Med* 138: 161-167.

37. Lazarou J, Pomeranz BH, Corey PN (1998). Incidence of adverse drug reactions in hospitalized patients: A meta-analysis of prospective studies. *JAMA* 279: 1200-1205.

38. Leape LL, Bates DW, Cullen DJ, et al. (1998). Systems analysis of adverse drug events. *JAMA* 274: 35-43.

39. Bates DW, Leape LL, Cullen DJ, et al. (1998). Effect of computerized physician order entry and a team intervention on prevention of serious medication errors. *JAMA* 280: 1311-1316.

40. Evans RS, Pestotnik SL, Classen DC, et al. (1998). A computer-assisted management program for antibiotics and other antiinfective agents. *N Engl J Med* 338: 232-238.

41. Leape LL, Cullen DJ, Clapp MD, et al. (1999). Pharmacist participation on physician rounds and adverse drug events in the intensive care unit. *JAMA* 282: 267-270.

42. Kucukarslan SN, Peters M, Mlynarek M, et al. (2003). Pharmacists on rounding teams reduce preventable adverse drug events in hospital general medicine units. *Arch Intern Med* 163: 2014-2018.

43. National Cholesterol Education Program (2002). Third Report of the expert panel on detection, evaluation, and treatment of high blood cholesterol in adults. NIH Pub. No. 02-5215. Bethesda, MD: National Heart, Lung and Blood Institute.

44. Chobanian AV, Bakris GL, Black HR, et al. (2003). Seventh report of the joint national committee on prevention, detection, evaluation, and treatment of high blood pressure. *Hypertension* 42: 1206-1252.

45. National Cholesterol Education Program (2002).

46. Chobanian AV, Bakris GL, Black HR, et al. (2003).

47. Saydah SH, Fadkin J, Cowie CC (2004). Poor control of risk factors for vascular disease among adults with previously diagnosed diabetes. *JAMA* 291: 335-342.

48. Beers MH, Ouslander JG, Rollingher I, et al. (1991). Explicit criteria for determining inappropriate medication use in nursing home residents. *Arch Intern Med* 151: 1825-1832.

49. Fick DM, Cooper JW, Wade WE, et al. (2003). Updating the Beers criteria for potentially inappropriate medication use in older adults: results of a US consensus panel of experts. *Arch Intern Med* 163: 2716-2724.

50. Lau DT, Kasper JD, Potter DEB, Lyles A (2004). Potentially inappropriate medication prescriptions among elderly nursing home residents: their scope and associated resident and facility characteristics. *Health Serv Res* 39: 1257-1276.

51. Lau DT, Kasper JD, Potter DEB, Lyles A, Bennett RG (2005). Hospitalization and death associated with potentially inappropriate medication prescriptions among elderly nursing home residents. *Arch Intern Med* 165: 68-74.

52. Curtis LH, Ostbye T, Sendersky V, et al. (2004). Inappropriate prescribing for elderly Americans in a large outpatient population. *Arch Intern Med* 164: 1621-1625.

53. Rigler SK, Jachna CM, Perera S, Shireman TI, Eng ML (2005). Patterns of potentially inappropriate medication use across three cohorts of older Medicaid receipients. *Ann Pharmacother* 39: 1175-1181.

54. Zhan C, Correa-de-Araujo R, Bierman AS, et al. (2005). Suboptimal prescribing in elderly outpatients: Potentially harmful drug-drug and drug-disease combinations. *JAGS* 53: 262-267.

55. Hecker MT, Aron DC, Patel NP, et al. (2003). Unnecessary use of antimicrobials in hospitalized patients. *Arch Intern Med* 163: 972-978.

56. Edgell ET, Summers KH, Hylan TR, Ober J, Bootman JL (1999). A framework for drug utilization evaluation in depression: Insights from outcomes research. *Med Care* 37: AS67-AS76.

57. Wells KB, Katon W, Rogers WH (1994). Use of minor tranquilizers and antidepressant medications by depressed outpatients: Results from the Medical Outcomes Study. *Am J Psychiatry* 151: 694-700.

58. McCombs JS, Nichol MB, Stimmel GL (1990). The cost of antidepressant drug therapy failure: A study of antidepressant use patterns in a Medicaid population. *J Clin Psychiatry* 51: 60-69.

59. Grant RW, Cagliero E, Dubey AK, et al. (2004). Clinical inertia in the management of type 2 diabetes metabolic risk factors. *Diab Med* 21: 150-155.

60. Shah BR, Zinman B, Hux JE, van Walraven C, Laupacis A (2005). Clinical inertia in response to inadequate glycemic control: Do specialists differ from primary care physicians? *Diab Care* 28: 600-606.

61. Wetzler HP, Snyder JW (2000). Linking pharmacy and laboratory data to assess the appropriateness of care in patients with diabetes. *Diab Care* 23: 1637-1641.

62. Shah BR, Zinman B, Hux JE, van Walraven C, Laupacis A (2005).

63. Cleeland CS, Gonin R, Hatfield AK, et al. (1994). Pain and its treatment in outpatients with metastatic cancer. *N Engl J Med* 330: 592-596.

64. Larue F, Colleau SM, Brasseur L, Cleeland CS (1995). Multicentre study of cancer pain and its treatment in France. *BMJ* 310: 1034-1037.

65. Olyeai A, de Matos A, Bennet W (2000). Prescribing drugs in renal disease. In Brenner B. (Ed.), *The Kidney,* Sixth edition (pp. 2606-2653). Philadelphia, PA: WB Saunders Co.

66. Pedersen CA, Schneider PJ, Scheckelhoff DJ (2003). ASHP national survey of pharmacy practice in hospital settings: Monitoring and patient education—2003. *Am J Health-Syst Pharm* 61: 457-471.

67. Liem RI, Higman MA, Chen AR, Arceci FJ (2003). Misinterpretation of a Calvert-derived formula leading to carboplatin overdose in two children. *J Pediatr Hematol Oncol* 25: 818-821.

68. Litovitz TL, Klein-Schwartz W, Rogers GC Jr, et al. (2002). 2001 annual report of the American Association of Poison Control Centers Toxic Exposure Surveillance System. *Am J Emerg Med* 20: 391-452.

69. Litovitz TL, Klein-Schwartz W, Rogers GC Jr, et al. (2002).

70. Safran DG, Neuman P, Schoen C, et al. (2005). Prescription drug coverage and seniors: Findings from a 2003 national survey. *Health Affairs* W5: 152-166.

71. Benner JS, Glynn RJ, Mogun H, et al. (2002). Long-term persistence in use of statin therapy in elderly patients. *JAMA* 288: 455-461.

72. Benner JS, Pollack MF, Smith TW, et al. (2005). Association between short-term effectiveness of statins and long-term adherence to lipid-lowering therapy. *Am J Health-Syst Pharm* 62: 1468-1475.

73. Pampallona S, Bollini P (2002). Patient adherence in the treatment of depression. *Brit J Psychiatr* 180: 104-109.

74. Samet JH, Libman H, Steger KA, et al. (1992). Compliance with zidovudine monotherapy in patients infected with Human Immunodeficiency Virus, Type 1: A cross-sectional study in a municipal hospital clinic. *Am J Med* 92: 495-502.

75. Gao X, Nau DP, Rosenbluth A, et al. (2000). The relationship of disease severity, health beliefs and medication adherence among HIV patients. *AIDS Care* 12: 387-398.

76. Walsh JC, Horne R, Dalton M, et al. (2001). Reasons for non-adherence to antiretroviral therapy: patients' perspectives provide evidence of multiple causes. *AIDS Care* 13: 709-720.

77. Aikens JE, Nease DE, Nau DP, et al. (2005). Adherence to maintainence-phase antidepressant medication as a function of patient beliefs about medication. *Ann Fam Med* 3: 23-30.

78. Horne R, Buick D, Fisher M, et al. (2004). Doubts about necessity and concerns about adverse effects: identifying the types of beliefs that are associated with non-adherence to HAART. *Int J STD AIDS* 15: 38-44.

79. Office of Applied Studies (2003). 2003 National Survey on Drug Use and Health. Substance Abuse and Mental Health Services Administration. Rockville, MD:.U.S. Department of Health and Human Services. Available at: http://www.oas.samhsa.gov/nhsda.htm (last accessed on August 27, 2005).

80. Office of Applied Studies (2003).

81. Gonzales R, Steiner JF, Sande MA (1997). Antibiotic prescribing for adults with colds, upper respiratory tract infections and bronchitis by ambulatory care physicians. *JAMA* 278: 901-904.

82. Watson RL, Dowell SF, Jayaraman M, et al. (1999). Antimicrobial use for pediatric upper respiratory infections: reported practice, actual practice, and parent beliefs. *Pediatrics* 104: 1251-1257.

83. Akkerman AE, Kuyvenhoven MM, van der Wouden JC, Verheij TJM (2005). Analysis of under- and overprescribing of antibiotics in acute otitis media in general practice. *J Antimicrob Chemother* July 20:1-6.

84. Jelinski S, Parfrey P, Hutchinson J (2005). Antibiotic utilization in community practices: Guideline concurrence and prescription necessity. *Pharmaoepidemiol Drug Saf* 14: 319-326.

85. Avorn J, Solomon DH (2000). Cultural and economic factors that (mis)shape antibiotic use: The nonpharmacologic basis of therapeutics. *Ann Intern Med* 133: 128-135.

86. Flynn EA, Barker KN, Carnahan BJ (2003). National observational study of prescription dispensing accuracy and safety in 50 pharmacies. *J Am Pharm Assoc* 43: 191-200.

87. Barker KN, Flynn EA, Pepper GA, et al. (2002). Medication errors observed in 36 health care facilities. *Arch Intern Med* 162: 1897-1903.

88. Davis K, Schoenbaum SC, Collins KS, et al. (2002). *Room for Improvement: Patients' Report on the Quality of Their Health Care.* New York: The Commonwealth Fund.

89. Nau DP, Erickson SR (2005). Medication safety: Patients' experiences, beliefs and behaviors. *J Am Pharm Assoc* 45: 452-457.

90. Blendon RJ, DesRoches CM, Brodie M, et al. (2002). View of practicing physicians and the public on medical errors. *N Engl J Med* 347: 1933-1940.

Chapter 25

Diversion, Abuse, and Other Nonmedical Use of Prescription Drugs

Bonnie B. Wilford
Robert L. Dupont

INTRODUCTION

The use of controlled prescription drugs to treat a variety of disorders has been controversial for decades and remains so today. Such controversy notwithstanding, DuPont (2005) observes that two facts are beyond dispute:

1. The majority of patients who use prescription opioids, stimulants, or sedatives in a medical context do so with generally good results and with no evidence of abuse of the prescribed medication or any other substance.
2. Such medications are federally "controlled" precisely because their nonmedical use and abuse constitute a public health problem that deserves appropriate attention.[1]

He further notes that, in the course of the public debate about nonmedical use of prescription drugs, many individuals and groups focus on one of these facts to the exclusion of the other. For example, some in the addiction-treatment field and in law enforcement have focused solely on the abuse of opioids intended for the treatment of pain, while some medical practitioners and patient organizations have focused only on the benefits associated with such use. Yet reasonable discussion and sound public policy cannot be achieved by looking only at one of these facts and ignoring the other. Health care providers and policymakers must accurately identify and quantify the real problem of diversion and abuse of prescription medications and, even more important, find ways to curb such activities without adversely affecting the legitimate medical care of millions of individuals who benefit from those medications.[2]

Historical Context

It is useful to recall that this intense policy debate originated more than a century ago, at a time when the most commonly abused drugs were freely available to any willing buyer. In that era in the United States, heroin was sold over the counter as a soothing syrup for colicky babies and cocaine was the reason a then-new beverage invented in an Atlanta pharmacy was called "Coke." Along with opium and its derivatives (including heroin and morphine) and cocaine, alcohol often was mixed into what were called "patent medicines." Buyers—often desperately ill buyers—had no way of knowing what was in the concoctions they used to treat themselves and their families. Indeed, no mechanism existed to protect the public from even the most dangerous substances. It was, literally, the free-market era of "let the buyer beware." The negative, often devastating, consequences of this free market in abusable drugs were so unmistakable that they became politically intolerable by the end of the nineteenth century.

In the first two decades of the twentieth Century, the Progressive Movement focused on the harm caused by this open market in dangerous drugs. Drug control became one of the progressive movement's central concerns, along with the vote for women and an effort to rein in the "trusts" that created business-strangling monopolies. Out of this creative ferment came the Pure Food and Drug Act of 1906 (one of the great achievements of Theodore Roosevelt's administration) and the Harrison Narcotic Act of 1914.

Enactment of these historic laws marked the adoption of a new social contract, which recognized that many of the most widely abused drugs also had important medical uses. Even then, it was recognized that most patients used these medicines in appropriate and safe ways. The new social contract thus affirmed the importance of permitting the use of potentially abusable medications in closely managed medical treatment, so long as the drugs were not used to treat addiction itself. This policy development is recounted in a variety of contemporary records and histories of the evolution of drug policy in the United States and around the world.[3-9] Under the new social contract, morphine (the parent substance from which heroin is made) and cocaine remained available for medical treatment in the United States, but no longer were sold in patent medicines or outside of close medical supervision.

Another important historical fact is that, whereas the early drugs of abuse either were derived directly from plants (such as morphine from the opium poppy and cocaine from the coca leaf) or were simple chemical modifications of those ancient substances (for example, heroin is made by adding two acetyl groups to the morphine molecule), over the course of the twentieth century most new controlled drugs were purely synthetic creations. Among the earliest synthetic agents were the barbiturates, which were followed to market by the stimulants (especially amphetamine and methamphetamine, which were widely prescribed for the first time in the 1930s). More recently, a staggering variety of synthetic agents have been introduced, including the benzodiazepines (which replaced the barbiturates beginning in the 1960s), synthetic opioid analgesics, and synthetic stimulants (such as methylphenidate).

In 1961, the United States joined many other countries in banning the sale and use of the older plant-based drugs such as heroin and cocaine. In 1971, the United States became a signatory to an international treaty covering synthetic controlled substances. The federal Controlled Substances Act (CSA), adopted in 1970, established a "closed" distribution system, that is, one in which every step in drug manufacture and distribution was subject to reporting to and monitoring by federal authorities, and a series of five schedules for all drugs with a recognized potential for abuse was created.[10] The schedules range from Schedule I (for drugs with high abuse potential and no accepted medical use) to Schedule V (for drugs such as paregoric, which have a demonstrated medical use and such minor abuse potential that they can be sold over the counter).

In the 1990s, the picture changed again, as prescription medications assumed a dramatically larger place in the treatment of many medical disorders, sometimes replacing surgery and frequently offering hope for the relief of conditions that previously had been untreatable. In the mental health arena, in which pharmacotherapies had been relatively rare, a new emphasis was placed on use of pharmacologic treatments for the psychotic disorders, mood and anxiety disorders (such as depression and panic disorder), sleep disorders, pain syndromes, and attention-deficit/hyperactivity disorder. As a result, the use of prescribed medications—including controlled drugs—has increased dramatically. Unfortunately, problems with the nonmedical use of these agents have followed a similar arc. This phenomenon has been particularly visible with medications for pain, for which the introduction, widespread use, and subsequent abuse of potent analgesics such as Oxy-Contin have become front-page news.

Since the early twentieth century, the original social contract governing the use of abusable prescribed drugs (as codified in the Harrison Narcotics Act) has worked reasonably well to permit medical treatment while protecting the public from the misuse of potentially dangerous substances. Despite this generally good result, problems with prescription drug diversion and abuse have occurred at every step in the manufacture and distribution process. "Script doctors" and fraudulent patients have contributed, as have hijackings of delivery trucks and armed robberies of pharmacies. Today, Internet pharmacies pose a new danger of unfettered access to potentially dangerous drugs—in many ways re-creating at the beginning of the twenty-first century the chaotic and dangerous situation that existed in the first decade of the twentieth.

DEFINING THE PROBLEM

Accurate use of terminology is essential to understanding and formulating appropriate responses to the nonmedical use of prescription medications. The following terminology is used in this chapter.

Nonmedical use incorporates all uses of a prescription medication other than those that are directed by a physician and used by a patient within the law and the requirements of good medical practice.

Abuse of a medication involves its use in a manner that deviates from approved medical, legal, and social standards, generally to achieve a euphoric state ("high") or sustain an established dependence.

Although not identical, *abuse* and *diversion* are closely related, in that the degree to which a prescribed medication is abused depends in large part on how easily it is redirected (diverted) from the legitimate distribution system.[11]

Addiction to a prescription medication, as with every other form of addiction, involves a complex interplay of biological and environmental factors.[12] Leshner has described addiction as a "disease of the brain," explaining that in vulnerable individuals, repeated self-administration of a drug produces a qualitative change in the way the brain functions. As a result, "the affected individual has an intense need for, and focus on, repeating the drug experience. But there comes a point... at which the drug user becomes an addict. At that point, it appears that a figurative "switch" has been thrown and the individual suffers a significant loss of his or her ability to make free choices about continued use of the drug."[13]

It is important to distinguish addiction from the type of *physical dependence without addiction* that can and does occur within the context of good medical care (as when a patient prescribed an opioid analgesic for pain becomes physically dependent on the medication).[14,15] This distinction is reflected in the two primary diagnostic classification systems used by health care professionals: the *International Classification of Diseases Classification of Mental and Behavioral Disorders,* Tenth Edition[16] of the World Health Organization (WHO), and the *Diagnostic and Statistical Manual of Mental Disorders* of the American Psychiatric Association.[17] According to the World Health Organization, "The development of tolerance and physical dependence denote normal physiologic adaptations of the body to the presence of an opioid."[18]

Determinants of Abuse Potential

Abuse potential has been described as "the relative ease with which a prescribed medication can be extracted or modified to yield the desired psychic effect."[19] For example, certain pharmacologic properties—such as rapid onset and short duration of action, high potency, water solubility, injectibility, and smokability—render some medications intrinsically more abusable than others.

Pharmacologically, the abuse potential of a drug usually is assessed according to (1) the drug's reward-reinforcing effects, as measured by various indicators of liking or "high" in humans and their propensity to vigorous self-administration in nonhuman animals, and (2) the characteristic induction of sensitization when given to laboratory animals on a daily basis. Sensitization occurs when the same dose of a drug induces even greater motor stereotypes and locomotion when tested, even long after withdrawal.[20,21] Although humans and other animals who have not abused alcohol or other drugs often find drugs with high abuse potential to be not only unrewarding, but often adversive, individuals with a history of abuse, those whose "addiction switches" have been turned on previously, are highly skilled in identifying drugs of abuse.

Abuse potential also is related to drug formulation in that formulations designed so as to impede access to the intranasal and intravenous routes of administration generally reduce a drug's abuse potential. Users who smoke or inject their drug are more likely to become dependent than are those who ingest the drug orally or by insufflation.[22]

Medical treatments with controlled substances (that is, drugs with a significant abuse potential) generally seek a relatively slow onset and a steady blood level. In stark contrast, people who abuse drugs seek a brain reward that is associated with rapid onset, rapid offset, and high blood levels. This basic difference in the pharmacodynamics of most medical treatments with controlled substances, and nonmedical abuse has major implications for efforts to promote medical treatment and at the same time reduce nonmedical use. Formulations that produce relatively slow onset and prolonged, relatively steady blood levels are inherently abuse resistant. The problem comes, however, when these formulations can be easily overcome by resourceful drug addicts to produce the rapid onset and high blood levels they seek. The benefits of abuse-resistant formulations are found only when the strategies to produce slow onset and steady blood levels are not easily overcome by highly motivated and often well-informed (thanks today to the Internet) drug abusers.[23] Finally, experience shows that price and availability contribute to the likelihood that a given drug will be abused.[24]

PREVALENCE AND PATTERNS OF NONMEDICAL USE

Among the data sets most widely used to measure the extent of drug abuse in the United States is the National Survey on Drug Use and Health (NSDUH), formerly known as the National Household Survey on Drug Abuse. This annual survey of approximately 46,000 households is the primary source of information on the incidence and prevalence of drug and alcohol use and abuse. In 1979, NSDUH data showed that 30 percent of persons ages eighteen to twenty-five reported ever having abused a prescription drug. By 1989, that figure had declined to 17 percent.[25] A decade later, however, federal data clearly showed a resurgence of the problem.[26,27]

However, neither NSDUH nor other available data sets are adequate to provide a clear and detailed picture of the nature and scope of prescription drug misuse and abuse, or the sources of drugs diverted to such abuse. For example, in using federal data sets, it is difficult to make longitudinal comparisons because of changes over time in survey methodology, the precise wording of the questions, or survey administration. The studies that do ask about use of psychotherapeutics usually group the responses by drug class (such as opioids) rather than reporting results for specific drug products (such as OxyContin). None collect data on specific drug formulations, even though rates of abuse can vary markedly for different formulations of the same drug.

In its report to Congress on diversion of OxyContin®, the General Accounting Office noted that its investigation was hampered by the data on drug abuse and diversion not being "reliable, comprehensive, or timely."[28] Moreover, officials of the Drug Enforcement Administration agreed with the GAO that development of enhanced data collection systems is needed to provide "credible, legally defensible evidence concerning drug abuse trends."[29]

Nor are reliable data available on the number of physicians, pharmacists, and other health practitioners involved—either deliberately or inadvertently—in diverting prescription drugs to nonmedical use. For example, both the AMA (1981) and the DEA (1990) once placed the number of dishonest physicians at less than 3 percent, but such estimates are not based on statistical studies.[30,31] In 2003 testimony before an FDA advisory committee, a DEA official estimated that "1.5 percent to 2 percent of physicians are dishonest, and 5 percent are negligent" in their prescribing of controlled substances[32] but offered no data to support those numbers.

Information compiled by the Federation of State Medical Boards (FSMB) suggests that, overall, the number of actions against physicians for misprescribing controlled drugs is declining (362 actions in 2002, down from 403 actions in 1994).[33] However, most state medical boards do not collect or report case information in ways that allow the cases related to misprescribing to be isolated. Nor are board actions categorized by type of prescribing problem (dishonest, deceived, etc.). Finally, no data set is currently available that can provide any insights into the amount of controlled drugs obtained through Internet pharmacies and other non-standard sources.

Patterns of Nonmedical Use

Clinical experience and limited survey data suggest that three primary patterns characterize most nonmedical use of prescription medications:

1. *Intensive drug abusers* consume prescription drugs nonmedically as part of an established pattern of intensive, compulsive drug use. Many obtain their drugs from the illicit drug market or through illegal activities (such as defrauding a physician, pharmacist, or other health professional).[34]
2. *Polydrug party users* are adolescents and young adults who use prescription medications in combination with other "party drugs" (such as MDMA or GHB) for their psychoactive effects. Users in this category typically are involved in regular but not compulsive use of a variety of substances.[35]
3. So-called *performance enhancers* represent a new pattern of nonmedical use, which involves high school and college students who use prescription stimulants to combat fatigue or enhance performance during periods of high stress, such as exams.[36] Typically, these users obtain their supply through a legitimate prescription or from a friend, usually as a gift; they almost never purchase their drugs from illicit drug markets. Such users do not seek a euphoric effect and many are not involved in the nonmedical use of other drugs.
4. *Quasimedical users* are individuals who use drugs prescribed for themselves or others for purposes or on occasions other than those intended by the prescribing physician but in ways that make use of the medically desirable effects of the drugs (e.g., although used

nonmedically the drugs are not used to get "high"). This pattern may be seen in patients who have inadequately managed pain, as well as patients who choose to treat insomnia and anxiety disorders with appropriate medicines but without benefit of their own prescription. This pattern of nonmedical use occurs when drug abusers use controlled substances to "treat" the adverse effects of alcohol and drug abuse, as when an alcoholic takes a benzodiazepine to combat withdrawal symptoms or a marijuana abuser uses a prescription stimulant to function in the morning after heavy marijuana use.

Each of these patterns is further distinguished by a number of other characteristics. For example, intensive drug abuse usually is associated with adverse consequences, whereas party use may be attended by adverse events but not invariably so, and use for performance enhancement generally does not lead to immediate adverse events. Although the least prevalent, the intensive drug-use pattern is associated with consumption of large amounts of drugs per user. Party users and performance enhancers, although far more numerous, account for a relatively small proportion of all the drug consumed nonmedically. Performance enhancers are engaged in a pattern of use that might be described as "pseudomedical," but their use is unwise and unsafe because it lacks medical supervision, and its long-term consequences are not known.[37]

Sources of Drugs Used Nonmedically

Intensive drug abusers typically obtain their drugs from two types of sources: (1) illicit manufacture and distribution and (2) licitly manufactured drugs that are deliberately redirected ("diverted") from legal channels of distribution. The methods employed in such diversion may involve theft from manufacturers, midlevel distributors, physicians' offices, pharmacies, and other facilities; in fact, armed robberies of pharmacies have become disturbingly common in recent years. Deception of physicians and pharmacists also is common.

Two new sources, involving purchases from Internet pharmacies and prescription drugs illicitly shipped into the United States, have emerged within the past few years, although the magnitude of their contribution to the illicit drug supply is not yet fully understood.

Physicians and Other Health Care Professionals

Smith has classified physicians who are involved in less-than-appropriate prescribing into four groups: deceived, dated, disabled, and dishonest.

Commonly referred to as the "Four Ds," Smith's classification was introduced at a 1980 White House Conference on Prescription Drug Misuse, Abuse, and Diversion.[38] The classification subsequently was incorporated into a seminal policy statement by the American Medical Association[39] and in educational materials disseminated by the Drug Enforcement Administration and others.[40] The classification also applies to nonphysician health care professionals and remains useful today.

In Smith's classification, *deceived practitioners* are victimized by patients who feign physical or psychological problems to obtain drugs, request refills in a shorter period of time than is medically indicated, or alter or counterfeit prescription forms.[41,42] Although any practitioner can be deceived occasionally, some practitioners are frequently manipulated, often because of their own gullibility, discomfort in confronting patients, or false pride.[43,44]

Dated practitioners have failed to keep up with evolving knowledge of pharmacology, differential diagnosis, and the management of chronic pain, anxiety, insomnia, and addiction.[45-47] Dated physicians typically prescribe drugs in excessive quantities or for excessive periods, or for conditions that do not warrant medication therapy or that might be better treated with other drugs.[48]

Disabled or impaired practitioners typically suffer from a medical or psychiatric problem, such as a substance use disorder, depression, dementia, or an Axis II personality disorder, that impairs their ability to practice effectively.[49] Experts have suggested that the lifetime risk of these disorders among physicians and other health professionals is somewhat higher than in the general population for a number of reasons, including ready access to controlled drugs in the course of professional practice.[50]

Dishonest practitioners (commonly referred to as "script doctors") intentionally prescribe controlled drugs for other than medical purposes: for example, in exchange for monetary compensation, sexual favors, or other considerations.[51] Such physicians are not practicing good faith medicine; rather, they are using their medical licenses as a franchise to deal drugs. They constitute the smallest group of physicians who contribute to drug diversion, yet their activities allow a large amount of drugs to be diverted to illicit use, and they bring dishonor on their profession. Leading medical organizations agree that such physicians are not candidates for reeducation or rehabilitation and that they should be prosecuted to the full extent of the law. [52-54]

To the Four Ds classification, Parran (1997) has added two other problematic behaviors, based on his interviews with 974 physicians referred to an educational course on prescribing by the State Medical Board of Ohio.[55] He characterizes these behaviors as "hypertrophied enabling" and "confrontation phobia." *Hypertrophied enabling* refers to a powerful instinct in physicians to do anything medically possible to help their patients. Although this instinct often contributes to heroic efforts to help patients overcome disease, physicians with overdeveloped enabling instincts are easy prey for manipulation. *Confrontation phobia* arises from the tendency of medical school curricula and residency training to emphasize skills in patient interviewing and relationship-building. Such training does not typically involve teaching physicians how to say "no." Parran suggests that "this emphasis on rapport-building techniques to the virtual exclusion of limit-setting skills helps to create the current clinical reality in which physicians feel acutely uncomfortable with conflict and interpersonal confrontation."[56]

Patients

Patients share with physicians a responsibility for appropriate use of prescribed drugs; this responsibility encompasses providing the physician with the best information possible and complying with the treatment plan.[57] However, some patients do not assume their part of this shared responsibility, for reasons that are not always evident to the prescribing physician. For example, a patient may begin to use medications as prescribed, then slowly deviate from the therapeutic regimen. Another patient may not comply as a result of a miscommunication or misunderstanding of the physician's instructions. Still other patients personally follow the regimen prescribed by their physician, but improperly share their drugs with others.[58]

As noted earlier, some patients deliberately abuse controlled drugs, or abuse their relationship with a physician to obtain such drugs. A less widely recognized but potentially more problematic individual is the criminal patient, whose primary purpose is to obtain drugs for resale. Whereas addicted patients seek a long-term relationship with a practitioner, criminal patients shift rapidly from one prescriber (or dispenser) to another. Such "patients" often visit multiple practitioners in a day and travel from one geographic area to another in search of unsuspecting targets. For this reason, they are referred to as "doctor shoppers." Evidence collected by law enforcement authorities demonstrates that such individuals are significant contributors to drug diversion.

Counterfeit Drugs

Until recently, the availability of counterfeit drugs in the United States was thought to be relatively rare. However, federal officials now acknowledge an increase in drug counterfeiting activities worldwide, as well as the emergence of more sophisticated ways to introduce fake products into the U.S. drug distribution system.[59] In fact, FDA officials recently characterized counterfeiting of pharmaceuticals outside the United States as "rampant" and estimated that about 40 percent of prescription drugs in Argentina, Colombia, and Mexico are counterfeit, as are about half of certain drugs in China.[60]

Once drug products enter the United States, they change hands multiple times as they move through the distribution chain. Counterfeit medications thus could enter the distribution chain through unscrupulous secondary wholesalers or unlicensed pharmacies that obtain products lacking a clear "pedigree"—a document that traces the sales history of the product back to the manufacturer. The three wholesale distributors—Cardinal Health, AmerisourceBergen Corporation, and McKesson Corporation—that collectively account for 90 percent of prescription drugs distributed in the United States are exempt from the federal pedigree requirement.[61] Some state boards of pharmacy have complained that for this reason the sales history of many drugs is not readily traced, creating a gap in the drug distribution system. Although the FDA has acknowledged that such a pedigree would be a deterrent to counterfeiting, it has postponed enforcement of this requirement.

Rather than wait for the FDA or the Congress to take action, several states (including Florida, Nevada, and Ohio) have adopted laws and regulations aimed at stopping counterfeit products from entering the supply chain. The National Association of Boards of Pharmacy (NABP) also is moving to update its model practice act to address the situation.[62]

Internet Pharmacies

The volume of Internet drug sales is not known with any degree of certainty. However, federal authorities have estimated that twenty million packages containing pharmaceuticals purchased online enter the United States each year. One mail processing facility in Miami, Florida, handles as many as 150,000 such packages each week.[63]

In congressional testimony, FDA officials have described their growing concern about the safety of prescription drugs purchased on the Internet because of the potential for such drugs to be handled, dispensed, packaged, or shipped incorrectly, as well as the risk that the drugs may be tampered with or counterfeit.[64,65] For example, FDA investigators purchased three commonly prescribed drugs from an Internet site that had been sending "spam" e-mails promoting its products. The drugs purchased were advertised as generic versions of Viagra, Lipitor, and Ambien (because none of the three products had an approved generic version at the time, all the advertised drugs were unapproved for use in the United States). FDA analysts found that the drugs received were fake, substandard, and potentially dangerous.[66] In a joint operation by the U.S. Customs and Border Protection and the FDA, agents seized a random sample of drug packages that arrived at international mail centers in seven U.S. cities and two commercial courier facilities. More than 80 percent of the parcels contained drug products that violated FDA regulations in some way: they were unapproved foreign drugs, or controlled substances, or counterfeits.[67]

The advent of Internet pharmacies raises other challenges as well. Although many Internet pharmacies are legitimate businesses that offer safe and convenient services similar to those provided by traditional neighborhood pharmacies, rogue Internet operations routinely engage in practices that clearly are illegal, such as dispensing drugs without a prescription.[68,69] Still others exploit loopholes in current U.S. laws to engage in "gray area" tactics, such as hiring physicians or others to write "prescriptions" based on a patient-supplied questionnaire, without any direct contact with the patient.[70] Operators of such sites capitalize on the relatively unregulated and borderless nature of cyberspace. Many originate overseas, operating almost completely outside the purview of U.S. authorities.[71]

Pharmacy regulators are struggling to find ways to deal with the presence of Internet pharmacies in general and with Web sites that illegally sell controlled drugs in particular.[72,73] The National Association of Boards of Pharmacy has created a task force to examine the issue, and the Office of National Drug Control Policy has called attention to Internet pharmacies as sources of drugs dispensed outside medical channels and, too often, outside the law.[74]

Smuggling

In its 2006 Annual Report, the International Narcotics Control Board identified smuggling of prescription drugs as "a major threat posed to law enforcement" and urged governments to strengthen national legislation and screen all routes of incoming and outgoing international mail. The Board urged that such screening processes include inspecting the premises of international mail courier companies. It also recommended limiting the number of entry points for parcels to allow for a more effective control of consignments.

INCBN officials further reported that, over the past five years, almost every region of the world has experienced an increase in smuggling activity.

By way of example, they pointed to seizures by Thai authorities of more than a half million diazepam tablets and capsules in 2004 alone. Other benzodiazepines smuggled by mail and seized by authorities included alprazolam shipped from Thailand to the United States and clonazepam shipped from Thailand to the United Kingdom. (All of these substances are controlled under the provisions of the 1971 Convention on Psychotropic Substances and require the express authorization of governments to be shipped across national borders.)

In its report, the INCB concluded that the large size of some the seizures indicates that traffickers are sourcing these substances for distribution on the illicit market. Although some portion of the seized tablets are illegally obtained from licit sources (through theft, falsified trade authorizations, and individual prescriptions, as well as illegal purchases from pharmacies), the INCB warned that significant quantities are provided by counterfeiters of pharmaceutical products, and added: "Counterfeiting narcotic drugs and psychotropic substances has become an important element in supplying illicit markets through illegally operating Internet pharmacies."[75]

OPTIONS FOR CURTAILING NONMEDICAL USE

Traditionally, nonmedical use of prescription drugs has been addressed at one of two potential points of intervention. The first involves *supply reduction* approaches, which are efforts to monitor and control access to the drugs themselves, as well as to delimit the actions of those who are legally empowered to prescribe and dispense them. The second option involves *demand reduction* approaches, which seek to address the underlying causes of prescription diversion and abuse, as by educating the practitioners who prescribe or dispense the drugs. Both supply and demand reduction approaches require extreme care so as not to discourage appropriate medical use.

Supply Reduction Approaches

Former White House counsel Robert Angarola remarked more than a decade ago that, "with the possible exception of nuclear materials, prescription drugs are the most tightly regulated commodity in the world."[76] The observation remains true today. International treaties, federal laws and regulations, and state legal frameworks impose a number of requirements on those who manufacture, distribute, prescribe, administer, or dispense controlled substances.

In general, international treaties address patent, trademark, and scheduling issues, while federal laws are concerned primarily with the approval process for drugs used in medical treatment and with the security of controlled substances between their point of origin and the end user at a retail pharmacy or health care facility. State laws primarily address the practice of medicine or pharmacy, standards of care, and interactions between the medical profession and members of the public.

Several areas exist in which international treaties and federal and state laws overlap or address similar issues. One such area is the scheduling, prescribing, and dispensing of controlled substances.

Federal Food, Drug, and Cosmetic Act

Before reaching the marketplace in the United States, all prescription drugs must be approved by the Food and Drug Administration (FDA) as safe and effective for human use under appropriate medical supervision. This authority is granted to the FDA by the Federal Food, Drug, and Cosmetic Act of 1962 (FFDCA). Under the act, the FDA has authority to regulate the labeling, advertising, and promotion of prescription drugs, and is charged with assuring that the information provided is "truthful, balanced, and accurately communicated."[77] In the past, the agency has used this authority to alert physicians to problems with specific drugs. For example, in response to widespread reports of diversion and abuse of OxyContin, the FDA strengthened the warnings and precautions contained in the labeling of OxyContin tablets, requiring the manufacturer to insert a "black box warning."[78,79]

The FFDCA does *not* grant the FDA authority to regulate medical practice. Because prescribing involves medical decisions, physicians generally are allowed to prescribe for a legitimate medical purpose and in the interest of the patient according to their best judgment.[80] Thus it is lawful and permissible for prescription drugs to be prescribed for other than their labeled or FDA–approved indications, or beyond their recommended doses, if a valid medical reason exists to do so.[81]

Federal Controlled Substances Act

The Controlled Substances Act of 1970[82] is designed to assure both the availability and control of regulated substances. Its requirements parallel the provisions of international treaties to which the United States is signatory. Under the CSA, availability of regulated drugs is accomplished through a system that establishes quotas for drug production and a distribution system that closely monitor the importation, manufacture, distribution, prescribing, dispensing, administering, and possession of controlled drugs.[83] The CSA also established an elaborate system of administrative reporting requirements to track regulated drugs and chemicals from their point of origin to the end user at the retail pharmacy or health care facility. Civil and criminal sanctions for serious violations of the statute are part of the government's control apparatus.

The CSA provides that responsibility for scheduling controlled substances is shared between the FDA and the DEA. In granting regulatory authority to those agencies, Congress noted that both public health and public safety needs are important and that neither takes primacy over the other, but that both are necessary to ensure the public welfare. To accomplish this, Congress provided guidance by specifying the factors that must be considered by the FDA and DEA when assessing public health and safety issues related to a new drug or one that is being considered for rescheduling or removal from control. These factors include the drug's actual or relative potential for abuse, scientific evidence of the drug's pharmacologic effects, if known, and the degree of risk (if any) the drug poses to the public health.

The CSA designates the Attorney General, in consultation with the Secretary of U.S. Department of Health and Human Services, as the official who determines the appropriate schedule for any drug or other substance. (The Attorney General and the Secretary of U.S. Department of Health and Human Services have delegated the authority for making these determinations to the DEA and FDA, respectively.) The factors cited earlier must be used in establishing findings that justify the level at which a particular drug is scheduled. The CSA does *not* limit the amount of drug prescribed, the duration for which a drug is prescribed, or the period for which a prescription is valid (although some states do impose such limits).

Licensed physicians and other health care professionals who wish to prescribe, dispense, or administer controlled drugs must first register with the DEA (and usually also with the state). Such registrations must be renewed periodically and the certificate of registration must be kept available for inspection.[84] Most states have requirements that mirror (and occasionally exceed) the federal rules. Also, as will be discussed, a growing number of states require some form of central reporting of prescriptions issued for certain classes of controlled substances.

State Laws and Regulations

The regulation of professional practice is primarily a state responsibility. State laws, regulations, and policies govern the clinical use of controlled drugs by physicians, nurses, dentists, veterinarians, and other health professionals.[85] The state's interest in regulating standards of care often overlaps the federal government's interest in controlling the prescribing and dispensing of controlled substances.

Virtually every step involved in the practice of medicine, pharmacy, and other health professions (including the prescribing or dispensing of controlled drugs) is governed by state *professional practice acts,* which are administered by licensing boards. Compliance with these acts is monitored (through both routine audits and special investigations) by state inspectors who report to the boards.

Although the exact requirements for prescribing, dispensing or administering controlled drugs differ from state to state, certain features are common to most states. For example, physicians, pharmacists, and other health professionals who prescribe or dispense controlled drugs must be licensed by the state in which they practice, be registered with the DEA, and maintain records of drugs prescribed, dispensed, or administered in a manner that complies with state and federal laws.

To administer their professional practice acts, state legislatures have granted statutory authority to *professional licensing boards* (such as boards of medicine, pharmacy, or nursing) to license and discipline members of their respective professions. Members of the boards typically are appointed by the governor and represent both the group of practitioners governed by the board and the general public. Professional licensing boards have the authority to issue licenses to practice medicine, pharmacy, and other health care professions. The boards also have the authority to review, suspend, or revoke licenses for cause.

In addition to statutes governing professional practice, all states have adopted some version of the federal Controlled Substances Act. Typically, state laws are patterned after the model Uniform Controlled Substances Act (UCSA) prepared by the National Conference of Commissioners on Uniform State Laws.[86] The criminal provisions of the acts are enforced by state and local police agencies, while regulatory departments and licensing boards manage the administrative aspects, such as drug scheduling. State laws may be more, but not less, restrictive than the federal statutes.

Almost half the states have enacted laws that establish *prescription monitoring programs* (PMPs) to facilitate the collection, analysis, and reporting of information on the prescribing, dispensing, and use of controlled substances within a state.[87] Most such programs employ electronic data transfer systems, under which prescription information is transmitted from the dispensing pharmacy to a state agency, which collates and analyzes the information. The older, paper-based monitoring programs (so-called "triplicate prescription programs") are being phased out and currently are in use only in New York and Texas (California repealed its paper-based monitoring program in 2005).

A GAO investigation concluded that PMPs have the potential to help law enforcement and regulatory agencies rapidly identify and investigate activities that may involve illegal prescribing or dispensing of controlled substances, and thus offer regulators "an efficient means of detecting and deterring illegal diversion."[88] However, GAO investigators also found that few states proactively analyze the data collected through PMPs, and only "three states can respond to requests for information within 3 to 4 hours."[89]

In announcing the Bush administration's 2004 National Drug Control Strategy, the Director of National Drug Control Policy endorsed PMPs and announced the availability of funds to help underwrite the costs to states of implementing such programs.[90]

Interventions and Sanctions

Physicians and other practitioners who are not prescribing within customary limits eventually come to the attention of licensing or regulatory authorities, triggering an investigation and—depending on the nature of the infraction—a response ranging from remedial (e.g., referral to an educational program), to rehabilitative (referral to a program treating impaired physicians), to punitive (as when a professional license or DEA registration is suspended or revoked).[91] In relatively rare cases, criminal sanctions also are imposed.

SUCCESSFUL MODELS AND PROMISING INNOVATIONS

In addition to the traditional regulatory and enforcement systems outlined previously, a number of new approaches have been advanced to prevent and curtail nonmedical use.

Research

Alan I. Leshner, PhD, formerly Director of the National Institute on Drug Abuse (NIDA), has written that more research is needed "to identify the drugs and classes of drugs that are being abused; to understand the pathways that lead from use to misuse, abuse, and addiction; and to identify populations most affected."[92] To meet this need, both new and experienced addiction researchers should be encouraged to expand their scope of enquiry to address the nonmedical use of prescription medications. The recent refunding of a prescription drug abuse research grant program offered by NIDA is an encouraging step in this direction.

Professional Education

Physicians and other health care professionals are in a unique position not only to prescribe controlled drugs, but also to identify problems when they occur.[93] To help them fulfill this potential, both the Office of National Drug Control Policy[94] and the American Medical Association[95] have urged that physicians, hospital medical staff organizations, resident physicians, and medical students participate in educational programs to learn (1) the proper prescribing and dispensing of controlled substances, (2) how to address drug-seeking behavior and other irregularities, and (3) how to identify and properly manage drug abuse and addiction. Recently, ONDCP sponsored a Leadership Conference on Medical Education in Substance Abuse to develop consensus on effective strategies to address this need.[96] That physicians need better training in this area seems indisputable.[97,98,99] In a 2001 survey, 46.6 percent of primary care physicians said they find it difficult to discuss prescription drug abuse with patients to whom they prescribe controlled drugs.[100]

To address the situation, a number of state agencies[101] and private sector organizations[102-105] have developed practice guidelines that, although lacking the force of laws or regulations, nevertheless define conduct that is considered to be within the boundaries of acceptable professional practice of medicine, pharmacy, or nursing. For example, in 1998 the Federation of State Medical Boards (FSMB) issued "Model Guidelines for the Use of Controlled Substances for the Treatment of Pain." Developed through a cooperative effort between the FSMB and representatives of state medical boards, the American Pain Society, the American Academy of Pain Medicine, and the American Society of Law, Medicine and Ethics, the model guidelines were distributed to every state medical board with a request that they be considered and adopted as policy. To date, at least twenty-six states have adopted the guidelines in full, and most other states have adopted some or most of the provisions.

Other actions also are under way. For example, the DEA recently announced its intention to work with medical organizations and state medical boards to develop training programs for physicians.[106] The federal Center for Substance Abuse Treatment (CSAT) recently created an interesting model in its buprenorphine training courses, for which the standardized curriculum was designed through a partnership with leading medical experts. Such courses are offered throughout the United States through a similar partnership between the company that distributes buprenorphine and physician groups that provide continuing medical education. In the private sector, prescribing education programs have been developed by task forces and academic centers in Florida,[107] Colorado,[108] Ohio,[109] Tennessee, and Utah.[110]

Finally, Project Mainstream—a collaborative endeavor of the Association for Medical Education and Research in Substance Abuse (AMERSA), the Center for Substance Abuse Treatment (CSAT), and the Health Resources and Services Administration (HRSA)—has used a consensus process to develop detailed guidelines for the knowledge and skills related to prescribing that ought to be taught in medical schools, residency training programs, and through continuing medical education courses. In addition to the guidance for physician education, Project Mainstream has developed similar guidelines for pharmacists, nurses, and other health professionals.[111]

Patient Education

Some patients fail to comply with the therapeutic regimen because of lack of information or failure to appreciate the resulting risks.[112] To address this problem, a number of federal agencies have launched public education initiatives that involve public service announcements for television and radio, as well as distribution of print messages about the dangers of misusing or abusing prescription medications.[113]

The administration's 2004 National Drug Control Strategy announced that ONDCP would collaborate with DEA and FDA to develop public service announcements that appear during Web searches for prescription drugs to alert consumers to the potential danger and illegality involved in purchasing controlled drugs through the Internet.[114]

In the private sector, the National Council on Patient Information and Education (NCPIE) is a leading provider of public education materials on appropriate use of prescription drugs. Various pharmaceutical manufacturers also have developed patient and public education programs.

It is critical to target educational messages to audiences at special risk, such as high school and college students who are actual or potential users of prescription stimulants, opioids, and possibly other drugs for "performance enhancement" or other nonmedical purposes. Precisely because they do not view such activities as constituting drug abuse,[115] this population is not being reached by existing antidrug messages. To be credible, such educational messages must address that the users see few short-term adverse consequences of their nonmedical use. It may be helpful to work with school nurses and college health officials in crafting and disseminating educational campaigns for this population.

Drug Surveillance and Risk-Management Programs

The Food and Drug Administration has initiated a policy under which manufacturers of brand-name drugs that are known or suspected to have abuse potential are asked to develop special programs for postmarketing surveillance and risk management.[116,117] The following examples demonstrate the potential utility of this approach:

Tramadol

The first use of a special postmarketing surveillance system to assess abuse focused on tramadol (Ultram), an analgesic that was introduced in the United States as a nonscheduled medication in 1995. FDA approval of the New Drug Application was contingent on the manufacturer's agreement to develop a system—monitored by an independent steering committee—to detect "unexpectedly" high levels of abuse (the "expected" levels of abuse were calculated from reports from other countries where tramadol was available).

The surveillance system involved systematic collection and evaluation of reports of suspected abuse in high-risk populations (including health care professionals admitted to rehabilitation programs for impaired practitioners) surveyed through a key informant network of addiction specialists, as well as all episodes of abuse reported to the FDA's MedWatch system. Case reports were classified according to the DSM-IV criteria for drug abuse and dependence. In addition, the data were used to identify geographic "hot spots" for more detailed examination and intervention.[118]

Buprenorphine

In a more recent experience with postmarketing surveillance, the FDA accompanied its October 2002 approval of new formulations of buprenorphine (Subutex and Suboxone), an opioid mixed agonist/antagonist, with special requirements for physician training and a postmarketing monitoring system.[119] Approval of the drugs was conditioned on agreement by the manufacturer to develop a comprehensive risk management program that involves close monitoring of drug distribution channels and reports of adverse events, as well as providing the drug in child-resistant packaging.[120]

These steps conform to the recommendations of the GAO, which has concluded that postmarketing surveillance programs can collect timely data about abuse liability for use in devising risk management strategies.[121] In fact, GAO reports have commented favorably on the Researched Abuse, Diversion, and Addiction-Related Surveillance (RADARS) system established by Purdue Pharma LP to "study the nature and extent of abuse of OxyContin and other schedule II and III analgesics" and to implement interventions to reduce diversion and abuse.[122]

Drug Formulations and Delivery Systems

Although a drug's price and availability contribute to its abuse potential, its pharmacokinetic and pharmacodynamic features also are important.[123] In contrast to therapeutic users, those who abuse drugs for their psychic effects prefer formulations that yield rapid onset of effects and high serum levels of medication. This explains why Dilaudid, MS Contin, and OxyContin have a high value in illicit markets: Dilaudid is easily dissolved in a small amount of water and injected, tablets of MS Contin can be crushed to defeat the drugs' controlled-release properties, and OxyContin is twice as potent as morphine and its controlled-release formulation is readily circumvented by drug abusers so that the active ingredient is released all at once.[124]

A number of pharmaceutical manufacturers have developed or are experimenting with methods of modifying their products' formulations or delivery systems to reduce the potential for abuse. For example, the controlled-release delivery system employed in the ADHD drug Concerta contains polymers that react with water to form a sticky matter that cannot be snorted or smoked, and is not easily injected.[125] Such medications have little "street value" and are not often found in the possession of individuals arrested for illicit drug use or distribution. Other manufacturers are experimenting with novel delivery mechanisms, such as osmotic pumps or the transdermal reservoir patch, for example, in which the combination of ingredients provides a measure of resistance to abuse.[126]

On the horizon are compounds that will depend on enzymatic action in the body to convert to, and deliver, their medicinal properties. Published accounts describe such novel delivery systems as able to prevent the extraction of the active ingredient from the bonded adjuvant.[127]

A note of caution is warranted, however: *abuse-resistant* is not synonymous with *abuse-proof*. Experience with sustained-release formulations such as OxyContin has demonstrated that drug abusers are resourceful in overcoming formulations that are designed to release the drug slowly on oral administration. Therefore, it is important that new formulations be tested in ways that replicate the ingenuity of drug abusers if the regulatory authorities are to credit such formulations as real barriers to nonmedical use. Claims that particular formulations can reduce abuse potential need to be documented not only through laboratory studies but also by evidence that the drugs are, in fact, abused less often than comparable drugs by populations of experienced drug abusers. It also is imperative that data on nonmedical use be gathered prospectively and intensively, so that emerging patterns of diversion and abuse can be identified early and appropriate countermeasures taken promptly.[128]

Collaborative Approaches

Many public health, regulatory, and enforcement agencies lack the technical and personnel resources to act promptly on information obtained through prescription monitoring programs, complaints from health care professionals and members of the public, or data acquired through routine examination of prescribing and dispensing records. To maximize the effective use of limited resources, several states have established systems to coordinate investigations of suspected prescribing problems. For example, North Carolina has created a Diversion Investigation Unit within its state police to coordinate investigations and actions against problem physicians and pharmacies. The National Association of State Controlled Substance Authorities (NASCSA) and the National Association of Drug Diversion Investigators (NADDI) have encouraged the formation of such specialized units in many states, and sponsor an informal online information-sharing network to assist in their development.

Given current resource limitations, it appears unlikely that sufficient staff and dollars are available to impose solutions from the public sector alone. Therefore, regulators and enforcement agencies must enlist the help of the private sector—an approach endorsed by the GAO,[129] the Office of National Drug Control Policy,[130] and the Center for Substance Abuse Treatment of the Substance Abuse, and Mental Health Services Administration.[131]

In the private sector, the American Medical Association endorsed collaborative efforts in 1981 in a policy statement (reaffirmed in 1991 and 2001) that called on private-sector organizations to cooperate with public agencies in implementing a series of actions to address prescription drug diversion and abuse.[132] The AMA put its principles into practice by organizing and staffing the informal steering committee on prescription drug abuse, which for a decade served as a central point of information-sharing and cooperation for more than thirty public agencies and private-sector organizations.[133] The steering committee's work at the national level was mirrored in developments at the state level, as exemplified by task forces organized in

Florida, Missouri, Colorado, Ohio, Utah, and other states to share information and coordinate activities.

CONCLUSIONS AND RECOMMENDATIONS

A long-standing dilemma in crafting programs to prevent or curtail the abuse of prescription medications is that a given substance can be both a valuable medication and a drug of abuse.[134,135,136] Historical difficulties in resolving this dilemma have been intensified by the recent introduction of drugs and drug formulations whose potential for abuse is not yet fully understood. For the most part, this is a by-product of the success of medical research, which has found ways to use pharmaceuticals to improve the treatment of many medical disorders.

However, such progress in patient care has come at a cost to public safety. For instance, many of the newer long-acting and sustained-release drug formulations offer clear benefits over immediate-release formulations. To offer such benefits, however, long-acting or sustained-release formulations must contain relatively large amounts of the active ingredient in each dose. Not surprisingly, the feature that makes such formulations attractive to legitimate medical patients and their caregivers makes them highly desirable to drug traffickers and nonmedical users as well.[137]

Further complicating the picture is that, just as the various patterns of nonmedical use have different causes and consequences, prevention and remediation requires entirely different strategies. For example, the intensive drug abuse pattern may be influenced by global strategies involving law enforcement efforts, whereas the performance enhancer's drug supply does not involve drug dealers and is not likely to be affected by law enforcement activities. Performance enhancers and party users are more likely to be influenced by educational programs, whereas intensive drug users are more likely to be affected by changes in formulation that prevent snorting and injecting, since those are the routes of administration that produce the most intense brain reward and are most highly valued by experienced drug abusers. Such changes in formulation are irrelevant to performance enhancers, most of whom ingest the drug orally.

In the coming years it will be essential to carefully evaluate the prevention and remediation strategies currently in use and to encourage the widespread adoption of those found to be most effective. This will involve comprehensive surveillance, not only of entire classes of controlled drugs, but also of specific products and formulations that promise new methods of reducing nonmedical use.

NOTES

1. DuPont RL, chair (2005). *Non-Medical Use of Methylphenidate: Defining the Problem, Creating Solutions—Report of an Advisory Committee to the Institute for Behavior and Health*. Rockville, MD: Institute for Behavior and Health.

2. DuPont RL, chair (2005).

3. Courtwright DT (2001). *Forces of Habit: Drugs and the Making of the Modern World*. Cambridge, MA: Harvard University Press.

4. Goldstein A (2001). *Addiction: From Biology to Drug Policy*, 2nd Edition. New York: Oxford University Press.

5. DuPont RL (2000). *The Selfish Brain—Learning from Addiction*. Center City, MN: Hazelden.

6. Musto D (1999). *The American Disease*, 3rd Edition. New York: Oxford University Press.

7. Stimmel B (1996). *Drug Abuse and Social Policy in America—The War that Must be Won*. Binghamton, NY: The Haworth Press.

8. Nahas GG and Burks TF, eds. (1997). Drug Abuse in the Decade of the Brain. Burke, VA: IOS Press, Inc. National Conference of Commissioners on Uniform State Laws (1994). *Uniform Controlled Substances Act*. Chicago, IL: NCCUSL.

9. Jonnes J (1996). *Hep-Cats, Narcs, and Pipe Dreams—A History of America's Romance with Illegal Drugs*. New York: Scribner.

10. Controlled Substances Act (CSA) (1970). *Controlled Substances Act of 1970 (CFR)*. Public Law No. 91-513, 84 Stat. 1242.

11. Ling W, Wesson DR, and Smith DE (2003). Abuse of prescription opioids. In AW Graham, TK Schultz, MF Mayo-Smith, RK Ries and BB Wilford (eds.) *Principles of Addiction Medicine*, Third Edition (pp. 1142-1144). Chevy Chase, MD: American Society of Addiction Medicine.

12. Vaillant GF (2003). The natural history of addiction. In AW Graham, TK Schultz, MF Mayo-Smith, RK Ries and BB Wilford (eds.) *Principles of Addiction Medicine*, Third Edition (pp. 3-16). Chevy Chase, MD: American Society of Addiction Medicine.

13. Leshner AI (2001). Understanding the risks of prescription drug abuse (Director's Column). *NIDA Notes* 16(3): 1.

14. DuPont RL and DuPont CM (2003). Sedative-hypnotics and benzodiazepines. In RJ Francis and SI Miller (eds.) *Clinical Handbook of Addictive Disorders*, 3rd Edition (pp. 117-132). New York,: Guilford Press.

15. DuPont RL and Gold MS (1995). Withdrawal and reward: Implications for detoxification and relapse prevention. *Psychiatric Annals* 25: 663-668.

16. World Health Organization (WHO) (1996). *Cancer Pain Relief, With a Guide to Opioid Availability*. Geneva, Switzerland: WHO.

17. American Psychiatric Association (APA) (1994). *Diagnostic and Statistical Manual of Mental Disorders, 4th Edition (DSM-IV)*. Washington, DC: American Psychiatric Press.

18. World Health Organization (WHO) (1996), p. 41

19. Ling W, Wesson DR, and Smith DE (2003).

20. DuPont RL and DuPont CM (2003).

21. DuPont RL and Gold MS (1995).

22. Woody GE, Cottler LB, and Cacciola J (1993). Severity of dependence: Data from the DSM-IV field trials. *Addiction* 88: 1573-1579.

23. Coleman JJ, Bensinger PB, Gold MS, et al. (2005). Can drug design inhibit abuse? *Journal of Psychoactive Drugs* 37(4): 343-362.

24. DuPont RL, chair (2005).

25. National Institute on Drug Abuse (1991). *National Household Survey on Drug Abuse: Population Estimates 1990*. Rockville, MD: U.S. Department of Health and Human Services, National Institute on Drug Abuse.

26. Office of Applied Studies (2003). *NHSDA Report: Non-Medical Use of Prescription-Type Drugs Among Youths and Young Adults*. Rockville, MD: Substance Abuse and Mental Health Services Administration, January 16, p. 2.

27. Office of Applied Studies (2005). *2003 Survey Found Over 1 Million People Recently Used Stimulants Non-Medically*. Rockville, MD: Substance Abuse and Mental Health Services Administration, February 4. Available at: www.oas.samhsa.gov/highlights.htm.

28. Government Accountability Office (GAO) (2003). *Prescription Drugs: OxyContin Abuse and Diversion and Efforts to Address the Problem*. Washington, DC: GAO (GAO-04-110), p. 5

29. Government Accountability Office (GAO) (2003), p. 33.

30. American Medical Association (AMA), Council on Scientific Affairs (1981). Drug abuse related to prescribing practices (CSA Rep. C, A-81; Reaffirmed: 1991, 2001). *Proceedings of the House of Delegates of the American Medical Association*.

31. DEA (1990).

32. Woodworth T (2003). *Testimony before the Anesthetic and Life Support Drugs Advisory Committee, September 9, 2003*. Bethesda, MD: U.S. Food and Drug Administration, Center for Drug Evaluation and Research, pp. 63-64.

33. Federation of State Medical Boards of the United States (FSMB) (2002). *Annual Summary of Board Actions (2001). State Medical Boards of the United States, Inc*. Euless, TX: The Federation.

34. DuPont RL, chair (2005).

35. McCabe SE, Knight JR, Teter CJ et al. (2005). Non-medical use of prescription stimulants among US college students: Prevalence and correlates from a national survey (Research Report). *Addiction* 100(1):96-106 [Erratum at 100(4):573].

36. McCabe SE, Knight JR, Teter CJ et al. (2005).

37. DuPont RL, chair (2005).

38. Wesson DR and Smith DE (1990). Prescription drug abuse. Patient, physician, and cultural responsibilities. *Western Journal of Medicine* 152(5):613-616.

39. American Medical Association (AMA), Council on Scientific Affairs (1981).

40. Ling W, Wesson DR and Smith DE (2003).

41. Cohen S (1980). Drug abuse and the prescribing physician. In C Buchwald, S Cohen and D Katz (eds.) *Frequently Prescribed and Abused Drugs: Their Indications, Efficacy and Rational Prescribing* (pp. 179-192). Rockville, MD: National Institute on Drug Abuse.

42. Wilford BB, ed. (1991). *Balancing the Response to Prescription Drug Abuse: Report of a National Symposium.* Chicago, IL: American Medical Association.

43. Ling W, Wesson DR and Smith DE (2003).

44. Parran TV Jr. (1997). Prescription drug abuse: A question of balance. *Alcohol and Other Substance Abuse* 81(4): 967-978.

45. Longo L and Parran TV Jr. (2000). Addiction: Part II. Identification and management of the drug seeking patient. *American Family Physician* 61(8): 2121-2128.

46. Parran TV Jr. (1997).

47. American Medical Association (AMA), Council on Scientific Affairs (1981).

48. Bigby H and Parran TV Jr. (1993). Prescription drug abuse. In J Bigby and H Adger (eds.) *Substance Abuse Education in General Internal Medicine.* Washington, DC: Society of General Internal Medicine, Bureau of Health Professions (HRSA), and Office of Treatment Improvement (ADAMHA).

49. Parran TV Jr. and Grey SF (2000). The role of the disabled physician in the diversion of controlled drugs. *Journal of Addictive Disease* 19(3): 35-41.

50. Ling W, Wesson DR and Smith DE (2003).

51. Ling W, Wesson DR and Smith DE (2003).

52. American Medical Association (AMA), Council on Scientific Affairs (1981).

53. American Medical Association (AMA), Council on Scientific Affairs (1981).

54. American Medical Association (AMA), Council on Scientific Affairs (1981).

55. Parran TV Jr. (1997).

56. Parran TV Jr. (1997), pp. 975-976.

57. Wesson DR and Smith DE (1990).

58. Leshner AI (2001).

59. Rovner J (2003). U.S. Congressional investigation finds counterfeit drug problem growing. *Reuters Health Information*, June 24. Available at: www.medscape.com/viewarticle/457753.

60. Young D (2003). FDA launches new initiative to battle counterfeit drugs. *American Journal of Health-System Pharmacy* 60(17): 1712-1713.

61. Young D (2003).

62. Young D (2003).

63. Grayson C (2004). The crackdown on counterfeit drugs. *WebMD Feature*, October 18. Available at: http://webmd.com/content/Article/95/103350.htm.

64. Government Accountability Office (GAO) (2004). *Internet Pharmacies: Some Pose Safety Risks for Consumers.* Washington, DC: GAO, Report GAO-04-820.

65. Government Accountability Office (GAO) (2004). *Prescription Drugs: Preliminary Observations on Efforts to Enforce the Prohibition on Personal Importation: Statement of Richard M. Stana, Director, Homeland Security and Justice Issues.* Washington, DC: GAO, Testimony GAO-04-839T.

66. Food and Drug Administration (2004). *Media Advisory: FDA Test Results of Prescription Drugs from Bogus Canadian Website Show All Products Are Fake and Substandard.* Washington, DC: FDA, Department of Health and Human Services, July 13. Available at http://www.fda.gov/importeddrugs/chart071304 .html.

67. Grayson C (2004).

68. Government Accountability Office (GAO) (2003).

69. Food and Drug Administration (FDA) (2001). FDA strengthens warnings for OxyContin. *FDA Talk Paper* July 25.

70. Thompson J (2004). A questionnaire does not constitute a patient examination (letter). *Wall Street Journal.*

71. Center on Addiction and Substance Abuse (CASA) (2004). *White Paper on Internet Pharmacy.* New York: CASA.

72. Wilford BB, Smith DE, and Bucher RD (2005). Internet pharmacy: A new source of abused drugs. *Psychiatric Annals* 35(3): 241-252.

73. American Pharmacists Association (APhA) and Canadian Pharmacists Association (CPhA) (2003). *Joint Statement: Pharmacists Across North America Support Call to Address Internet Drug Sales*, May 13. Available at: www.aphanet.org/news/alpha_cphastate.htm.

74. Office of National Drug Control Policy (ONDCP) (2004). *National Drug Control Strategy.* Washington, DC: Executive Office of the President, The White House, pp. 22-35.

75. International Narcotics Control Board (2006). *Annual Report, 2006.* Geneva, Switzerland: United Nations, March 1.

76. Angarola R (1990). The effect of national and international drug control laws on patient care. In BB Wilford (ed.) *Balancing the Response to Prescription Drug Abuse: Report of a National Symposium on Medicine and Public* Policy (pp. 25-33). Chicago, IL: American Medical Association.

77. Government Accountability Office (GAO) (2003), p. 11.

78. Food and Drug Administration (FDA) (2001).

79. Drug Enforcement Administration (DEA) (2002). *Physician's Manual: An Informational Outline of the Controlled Substances Act of 1970.* Washington, DC: U.S. Department of Justice, Drug Enforcement Administration.

80. Federal Register (1975). 15393-94.

81. Federal Register (1983). 2673.

82. Code of Federal Regulations, Title 21, Chapter 2. Controlled Substances Act (CSA) (1970).

83. Drug Enforcement Administration (DEA) (1990). *Physician's Manual: An Informational Outline of the Controlled Substances Act of 1970.* Washington, DC: U.S. Department of Justice, Drug Enforcement Administration.

84. Drug Enforcement Administration (DEA) (1990).

85. Joranson DE and Gilson AM (2003). Legal and regulatory issues in the management of pain. In AW Graham, TK Schultz, MF Mayo-Smith, RK Ries and BB Wilford (eds.) *Principles of Addiction Medicine,* Third Edition (pp. 1465-1474). Chevy Chase, MD: American Society of Addiction Medicine.

86. National Conference of Commissioners on Uniform State Laws (1994). *Uniform Controlled Substances Act.* Chicago, IL: NCCUSL.

87. Government Accountability Office (GAO) (2003).
88. Government Accountability Office (GAO) (2003), p. 15.
89. Government Accountability Office (GAO) (2003), p. 15.
90. Office of National Drug Control Policy (ONDCP) (2004).
91. Wilford BB and Deatsch JH (2001). *Prescribing Controlled Drugs: Helping Your Patients, Protecting Your Practice.* Tampa, FL: University of South Florida School of Medicine.
92. Leshner AI (2001).
93. Schnoll SH and Finch J (1994). Medical education for pain and addiction: Making progress toward answering a need. *Journal of Law, Medicine and Ethics* 22(3): 239-244.
94. Office of National Drug Control Policy (ONDCP) (2004).
95. American Medical Association (AMA), Council on Scientific Affairs (1988). Education regarding prescribing controlled substances (Sub. Res. 76; I-88; Reaffirmed: 1998). *Proceedings of the House of Delegates of the American Medical Association.*
96. Office of National Drug Control Policy (2005). *Report of the Leadership Conference on Medical Education in Substance Abuse, December 1-2, 2004.* Washington, DC: ONDCP, Executive Office of the President. Available at: www.whitehousedrugpolicy.gov.
97. Graham AW and Parran TV Jr. (1992). Physician failure to record alcohol use history when prescribing benzodiazepines. *Journal of Substance Abuse* 4: 179-185.
98. Bigby H and Parran TV Jr. (1993).
99. Longo L and Parran TV Jr. (2000).
100. Leshner AI (2001).
101. Federation of State Medical Boards of the United States, Inc. (1998). *Model Guidelines for the Use of Controlled Substances for the Treatment of Pain* (adopted May 2). Dallas, TX: The Board. Available at: http://www.medsch.wisc.edu/painpolicy/domestic/model.htm.
102. American Academy of Pain Medicine (AAPM) and American Pain Society (APS) (1997). *The Use of Opioids for the Treatment of Chronic Pain: A Consensus Statement. A Policy Document of the American Academy of Pain Medicine and American Pain Society.* Glenview, IL: The Societies.
103. American Pain Society (APS) (1999). *Principles of Analgesic Use in the Treatment of Acute Pain and Cancer Pain, 4th Edition.* Glenview, IL: The Society.
104. New Mexico Board of Medical Examiners (1997). Guidelines on prescribing for pain. *Newsletter Information and Report* 2(1): 1-3.
105. Colorado Prescription Drug Abuse Task Force (1990). *Colorado Guidelines of Professional Practice for Controlled Substances.* Denver, CO: The Task Force.
106. Office of National Drug Control Policy (ONDCP) (2004).
107. Wilford BB and Deatsch JH (2001).
108. Colorado Prescription Drug Abuse Task Force (1990). *Colorado Guidelines of Professional Practice for Controlled Substances.* Denver, CO: The Task Force.
109. Bigby H and Parran TV Jr. (1993).

110. Utah Medical Association (1993). *A Guide to Prescribing Controlled Substances in Utah* (handbook). Salt Lake City, UT: The Association.

111. Project Mainstream, Association for Medical Education and Research in Substance Abuse (2002). *Strategic Plan for Interdisciplinary Faculty Development: Arming the Nation's Health Professional Workforce for a New Approach to Substance Use Disorders; Part I. Evidence Supporting the Strategic Plan.* Providence, RI: The Association.

112. Leshner AI (2001).

113. Zickler P (2001). NIDA scientific panel reports on prescription drug misuse and abuse. *NIDA Notes* 16(3): 4.

114. Office of National Drug Control Policy (ONDCP) (2004).

115. Partnership for a Drug-Free America (PFDFA) (2005). *Partnering with Families: Rx and OTC Abuse Findings.* New York: The Partnership.

116. Government Accountability Office (GAO) (2003).

117. Arfken CL and Cicero TJ (2003). Post-marketing surveillance for drug abuse. *Drug and Alcohol Dependence* 70: S97-S105.

118. Woody GE, Senay EC, Geller A, et al. (2003). An independent assessment of MedWatch reporting for abuse/dependence and withdrawal from Ultram (tramadol hydrochloride). *Drug and Alcohol Dependence* 72(2): 163-168.

119. Comer SD and Collins ED (2002). Self-administration of intravenous buprenorphine and the buprenorphine/naloxone combination by recently detoxified heroin abusers. *Journal of Pharmacology and Experimental Therapeutics* 303: 695-703.

120. Wesson D (2002). Personal communication, November 14.

121. Government Accountability Office (GAO) (2003), p. 6.

122. Government Accountability Office (GAO) (2003), p. 40.

123. DuPont RL, chair (2005).

124. Government Accountability Office (GAO) (2003), p. 29.

125. Alza Corporation (2003). Information for patients taking Concerta or their parents or caregivers (package insert). *Prescribing Information.* Fort Washington, PA: McNeil Consumer and Specialty Pharmaceuticals.

126. DuPont RL and Bensinger PB (2005). Abuse-resistant drug delivery. *Psychiataric Annals* 35(3):253-256.

127. New River Pharmaceuticals (n.d.). *Technology: Conditionally Bioreversible Derivatives.* Available at: http://www.nrpharma.com/company/indiex.htm.

128. DuPont RL, chair (2005).

129. Government Accountability Office (GAO) (2003).

130. Office of National Drug Control Policy (ONDCP) (2004).

131. Clark HW and Bizzell AC (2005). A Federal perspective on the abuse of prescription stimulants. *Psychiatric Annals* 35(3): 260-263.

132. American Medical Association (AMA), Council on Scientific Affairs (1981).

133. Wilford BB, ed. (1991).

134. Leshner AI (2001).

135. Passik SD (2001). Responding rationally to recent reports of abuse/diversion of OxyContin®. *Journal of Pain and Symptom Management* 21(5): 359-360.

136. Drug Enforcement Administration (DEA) (1990). *Physician's Manual: An Informational Outline of the Controlled Substances Act of 1970.* Washington, DC: U.S. Department of Justice, Drug Enforcement Administration.

137. DuPont RL, chair (2005).

FURTHER READING

American Psychiatric Association (APA) (2000). *Diagnostic and Statistical Manual of Mental Disorders (DSM-IV-TR).* Washington, DC: American Psychiatric Press.

Cicero TJ, Adams EH, Geller A, et al. (1999). A post-marketing surveillance program to monitor Ultram® (tramadol hydrochloride) abuse in the United States. *Drug and Alcohol Dependence* 57:7-22.

Croft HA (2005). Physician handling of prescription stimulants. *Psychiatric Annals* 35(3):221-226.

Dodson WW (2000). *ADHD: Overmedicated or Undermedicated?* Denver, CO: Colorado Prescription Drug Abuse Task Force.

Forman RF (2003). Availability of opioids on the Internet (Research letter). *Journal of the American Medical Association* 290(7):889.

Gaul GM & Flaherty MP (2003b). Internet trafficking in narcotics has surged. (From the series "Pharmaceutical Roulette.") *The Washington Post.* October 20, pp. A1, A14.

Gaul GM & Flaherty MP (2003a). U.S. prescription drug system under attack. (From the series "Pharmaceutical Roulette.") *The Washington Post.* October 19, pp. A1, A15.

Government Accountability Office (GAO) (2000). *Internet Pharmacies: Adding Disclosure Requirements Would Aid States and Federal Oversight.* Washington, DC: GAO, Report GAO-01-69.

Jaffe SL (2002). Failed attempts at intranasal abuse of Concerta (letter). *Journal of the American Academy of Child and Adolescent Psychiatry* 41(1):4.

Matthews A & Fields G (2003). Federal agencies seek to curb abuse of potent painkillers. *The Wall Street Journal.* December 3, p. B1.

McCabe SE, Teter CJ, and Boyd CJ (2004). The use, misuse and diversion of prescription stimulants among middle and high school students. *Substance Use and Misuse* 39(7):1095-1116.

Missouri Task Force on Misuse, Abuse and Diversion of Prescription Drugs (1987). *Protecting Your Medical Practice* (handbook). Jefferson City, MO: Missouri Bureau of Narcotics and Dangerous Drugs.

Mitka M (2000). Abuse of prescription drugs: Is a patient ailing or addicted? *Journal of the American Medical Association* 283:1126-1129.

National Institute on Drug Abuse (NIDA) (2001). *Research Report Series: Prescription Drugs/Abuse and Addiction.* April, p. 1.

Office of Applied Studies (2001b). *Summary of Findings From the 2000 National Household Survey on Drug Abuse* (DHHS Publication [SMA] 01-3549). Rockville, MD: Substance Abuse and Mental Health Services Administration.

Stimmel B (1998). Prescribing and the relief of pain. In AW Graham, TK Schultz, BB and Wilford (eds.), *Principles of Addiction Medicine, Second Edition.* Chevy Chase, MD: American Society of Addiction Medicine.

Termin P (1980). *Taking Your Medicine: Drug Regulations in the United States.* Cambridge, MA: Harvard University Press, pp. 12-17.

Chapter 26

Drug Utilization Review: Dealing with Complexity

Thomas R. Fulda
Theodore M. Collins

INTRODUCTION

Drug utilization review (DUR) has been a component of pharmacy practice for decades, but it did not appear on policy radar screens until the late 1960s. In 1967 President Lyndon Johnson directed the establishment of the Task Force on Prescription Drugs to undertake a comprehensive study of the problems relating to the inclusion and cost of drugs under Medicare. The Medicare program to provide health insurance for elderly Americans had been established two years earlier without providing outpatient prescription drug coverage. Prescription drug coverage was omitted from the original Medicare legislation primarily because of concerns about administrative difficulties expected with regard to processing of paper claims and because of concerns about the cost of providing coverage. The lack of such coverage would not be corrected until the passage of the Medicare Prescription Drug, Improvement, and Modernization Act of 2003.

The Task Force on Prescription Drugs described drug utilization review as a "dynamic process aimed first at rational prescribing and the consequent improvement of the quality of health care and second at minimizing needless expenditures."[1] Concerns about rational prescribing and about the cost of prescription drugs reflected in the Task Force Final Report have continued as persistent policy problems ever since.

WHY DRUG UTILIZATION REVIEW?

The enhancement of rational prescribing defined by the Task Force on Prescription Drugs as "prescribing the right drug, for the right patient, at the

531

right time, in the right amounts, and with due consideration for relative costs"[2] provided the impetus for the growing interest, particularly during the 1980s, in DUR. Evidence in the literature began to suggest that drug prescribing was not always rational, and that less-than-appropriate prescribing has significant economic consequences.

A 1995 study by Bates et al. (1995), for example, conducted in a hospital environment over six months found 274 actual and 194 potential adverse drug events (ADEs).[3] Of the ADEs, 1 percent were fatal, 12 percent were deemed life threatening, 30 percent serious, and 57 percent significant. Most important, of the ADEs that were not life threatening, overall 28 percent were considered preventable. Of the life threatening and serious ADEs, 42 percent were preventable. A companion study by Leape et al. (1995) investigated the reasons for these adverse events.[4] It suggested that many of the prescribing errors were due to deficiencies in prescribers' knowledge of the drugs and how to use them. Errors due to this lack of knowledge accounted for 35 percent of the preventable ADEs.

Steadily rising drug expenditures during the 1990s and beyond contributed to growing interest in drug utilization review as a possible tool to help reign in expenditures. Two studies, published five years apart, suggested that the economic consequences of irrational prescribing could be significant. The studies estimated that drug-related morbidity and mortality are responsibility for between $76[5] and $177[6] billion in expenditures. The studies suggested that a significant portion of these expenditures would be due to additional hospitalization of patients.

DUR DEFINED

Drug utilization review (DUR) is "a process to assess the appropriateness of drug therapy by engaging in the evaluation of data on drug use in a given health care environment against predetermined criteria and standards...Criteria are predetermined elements of drug use, supported by FDA–approved labeling, compendia, and the peer reviewed literature, developed by qualified health professionals, against which aspects of quality, medical necessity, clinical outcomes and cost effectiveness of drug use may be compared."[7]

DUR is practiced in a variety of environments, including outpatient pharmacies, hospital pharmacies, and nursing homes. The names given to the drug utilization review process vary. It is drug utilization (DUR) in outpatient pharmacies, drug use evaluation (DUE) in hospitals, and drug regimen review (DRR) in nursing homes. The DUR process begins with the development and application of criteria. Then database reviews are conducted to identify criteria violations. Pharmacists and other health professionals review evidence of criteria violations to determine the need for interventions to correct problems identified. These interventions may, depending on the circumstances, involve counseling the patient, pharmacist contact with the prescriber, and review of the patient's medical record if the patient is hospitalized. The focus of interventions is usually educational rather than punitive in nature. Finally, program reevaluation is necessary to determine the impact of the DUR process on actual drug use.

Given the nature of the DUR process, it should be clear that it is always carried out in an operational, programmatic context. DUR programs are formal, dynamic, and ongoing. DUR may be done prospectively, concurrently, or retrospectively. The environment in which DUR takes place does impact the amount and type of information available for review. Information for review of outpatient prescriptions is usually limited to the information found on the prescription. This includes the names of the patient and the prescriber, the name of the drug, the dosage form, strength, directions for use, and quantity. Diagnosis does not appear on the prescription. In inpatient and nursing home reviews the patient's complete medical record, including diagnosis, may be available.

THE OBRA 1990 MODEL

Probably the high point in the development of DUR policy came with the passage of the Omnibus Budget Reconciliation Act (OBRA) of 1990.[8] This statute required all states to establish a Medicaid Drug Utilization Review (DUR) program by January 1, 1993. These programs were to include prospective and retrospective DURs based on explicit predetermined standards, an offer of counseling of patients by the pharmacists, and educational interventions targeted at common therapy problems. The statute also required each state to establish a DUR board composed mostly of practicing physicians and pharmacists to do such tasks as approve DUR criteria, periodically review such criteria, and design as well as implement interventions. Enhanced matching funds (remember Medicaid is financed jointly by the federal and state governments) were also provided to encourage states to install electronic drug claims processing systems.

Prospective DUR

Prospective DUR had been evolving toward the OBRA model for some time. Initially, pharmacists evaluated drug therapy based on implicit criteria acquired while in school and/or through consulting reference texts available in their pharmacies. With the advent of the use of computers in pharmacies in the 1980s, pharmacists began using prospective DUR software resident on their computers. But these were not necessarily networked, and were usually limited to data in a single pharmacy or at best within the pharmacy chain. By the 1990s, due in no small part to the adoption of electronic drug claims processing equipment encouraged by OBRA 1990, pharmaceutical benefit managers and third party drug insurance programs performed prospective DUR through interactive telecommunication between themselves and individual pharmacies. As a result of the adoption of this technology it became possible to review all prescriptions filled for a given patient wherever they are filled, not just those filled in an individual pharmacy or pharmacy chain.

Using this electronic technology each prescription is reviewed, as part of the drug claims adjudication process, before the prescription is dispensed. OBRA 1990 specifies that these reviews, based on explicit predetermined standards, identify the following types of drug therapy problems:

- Therapeutic duplication
- Drug-drug interactions
- Drug-disease contraindications
- Incorrect dosage
- Incorrect duration of therapy
- Drug allergy interactions
- Clinical abuse and misuse

When pharmacists receive an electronic message alerting them to any of these drug therapy problems several responses are possible. The pharmacist may consult available reference sources, counsel the patient, or consult with the prescriber. As a result the prescription may be dispensed as written, may be changed, or not filled.

Retrospective DUR

Under OBRA 1990 retrospective DUR involves using drug claims processing and information retrieval systems "for the ongoing periodic examination of claims data...in order to identify patterns of fraud, abuse, gross overuse, or inappropriate or medically unnecessary care, among physicians, pharmacists and individuals or associated with specific drugs or groups of drugs."[9] A review of the DUR Annual Reports for federal fiscal year (FFY) 1999, which OBRA 1990 requires the states to submit to the Centers for Medicare and Medicaid Services (the federal agency responsible for administration of the Medicare and Medicaid programs), indicates that most states used retrospective DUR to look for the same types of patient-specific problems identified during prospective DUR reviews.[10] Unlike prospective DUR however, interventions resulting from retrospective reviews usually take the form of letters sent to physicians and pharmacists by drug program administrators. This approach to retrospective DUR was in place before the evolution of prospective DUR to its present electronic form as described previously and before OBRA 1990 was enacted.

LEARNING FROM EXPERIENCE

Implementation of the Medicaid DUR programs provided new opportunities to consider how DUR works in practice and what might be needed to improve its effectiveness. The research that resulted has surfaced a number of issues worthy of consideration by policymakers.

Criteria Problems

Most Medicaid DUR programs rely on drug-specific screening criteria provided by DUR vendors. Until OBRA 1990, DUR criteria were not in the public domain. The statute required that criteria be public and based on three named compendia and the peer reviewed medical literature. Access to criteria by researchers has raised questions about the adequacy of evidence used in developing them and about the lack of consistency in applying the criteria that DUR vendors supplied to the Medicaid programs.

A study by Fulda et al. (2000) documented discrepancies in the listing and clinical significance ratings of drug-drug interactions listed in five leading drug information sources.[11] This review of drug-drug interactions in five drug classes (nonsteroidal anti-inflammatory drugs [NSAIDS], benzodiazepines, beta-blockers, ACE inhibitors, and calcium channel blockers) showed that any given interaction was more likely to be listed in one or two sources than in four or five of them. Disagreements about the clinical significance of particular drug interactions increased as the number of information sources listing them increased. This research suggests the possibility that similar discrepancies may also be present in other drug-specific criteria. It also suggests that to improve DUR performance the strength of evidence supporting these and other drug specific DUR criteria needs to be evaluated.

Research has also documented a lack of consistency in the adoption by Medicaid programs of DUR criteria obtained from vendors.[12] A comparison of 55 drug-drug interaction criteria, obtained from 7 vendors, used in 16 Medicaid programs in 1992 showed that:

- 20 drug-drug interaction criteria involving digoxin were common to the DUR criteria and reference texts listing drugs know to increase serum concentration levels.
- 11 criteria were not mentioned in the reference texts.
- 18 drug-drug interactions mentioned in the reference texts were not included in the criteria.

These studies leave open the question of how many and which drug-specific criteria should be used in prospective DUR and retrospective DUR. Neither the public sector nor the private sector has sought to deal with these criteria issues.

Prospective DUR Performance

Research with regard to the operation of prospective DUR systems has revealed problems with their operation. A study by Chui and Rupp (2000), for example, conducted in forty-one pharmacies, reported that 10.3 percent of prescriptions resulted in the issuance of an alert message, and that 88 percent of these alerts were overridden by pharmacists receiving them.[13] Reasons given for these alert overrides included: that the pharmacist was already aware of the problem; that the pharmacist thought the problem was not clinically significant; or the pharmacist thought that the problem didn't exist.

Another study by Hazlett et al. (2001) found that DUR systems in chain and HMO pharmacies failed to detect sixteen well-known, clinically important drug-drug interaction alerts one-third of the time.[14] The authors indicated that all pharmacies used the same DUR vendor, but suggested that the software installed on pharmacy computers interpreted the data variably among and within software programs. They labeled the performance of these systems as suboptimal, and suggested that programming deficiencies played a part in the suboptimal performance of these systems.

Issues with the quality of alert messages received by pharmacies also contributed to the poor performance of prospective DUR systems. Fulda et al. (2004) suggest "electronic edits are not designed to integrate clinical data and evaluate the appropriateness of pharmacotherapy"[15] They also indicate that the database used to screen prescriptions is limited, that data fields are often incomplete, and that a patient's drug use profile may be incomplete. Still other factors influencing the performance of prospective

DUR systems relate to pharmacist workplace issues. These policy issues will be considered in the following chapter.

Retrospective DUR Performance

Although most Medicaid retrospective DURs continued to focus on identifying drug specific problems, another approach, suggested by the OBRA 1990 statutory language, involves engaging in population-level pattern analysis. Such analyses can be used to identify the prescribing of high cost drugs and their prescribers, compare the use of particular classes of drugs in different facilities (e.g., antidepressants in nursing homes), and monitor adherence to pharmacotherapy recommendations found in clinical practice guidelines for treatment of particular diseases. Lyles et al. (2001) report that this type of pattern analysis "may involve linking drug claims data with databases to access additional information, such as patient diagnosis, to define patterns of treatment for a given condition, or use of a drug product across populations of patients."[16]

Interventions based on retrospective DUR can, as has already been indicated, involve letter interventions with physicians or pharmacists or both. Such interventions may also involve continuing education programs, or academic detailing by peers either by telephone or face-to-face visits.

Evidence from the review of the FFY 1999 DUR Annual Reports indicates that interest in population level pattern analysis is growing among the Medicaid DUR programs, spawned by OBRA 1990.[17] Use of beta-blockers in patients after myocardial infarction and ACE inhibitors in patients with heart failure are examples of the more sophisticated pattern analyses being undertaken by Medicaid DUR programs. Some states are also putting on educational programs and engaging in academic detailing.[18] The review of the Medicaid DUR annual reports for FFY 1999 indicates that no more than twelve states were engaged in population-level pattern analyses. Given the largely duplicative nature of prospective and retrospective DURs when both are focused on the same drug-specific problems, it is surprising that many states continue to engage in drug-specific retrospective DUR.

Evaluating DUR Programs

The 1969 Task Force on Prescription Drugs, which was created to study the coverage of prescription drugs under the Medicare program, reported "There is an urgent need for further research to develop and test various approaches to effective utilization review."[19] When in 1990 Congress enacted the Medicaid DUR program requirements the statute included provisions requiring evaluation of the outcomes of these programs. This legislation also provided for studies of online prospective DUR and for reimbursing pharmacists for patient counseling and intervention to assure appropriate drug therapy. Fiscal constraints limit Medicaid's ability and interest in doing the DUR policy research necessary to make informed decisions about what works.

RETROSPECTIVE DUR

Early evaluations of retrospective DUR were conducted by measuring drug and other health costs before and after interventions. Any change was attributed to the intervention and usually was reported as dramatic savings. Often, no information was provided on research methods. When the methodology was provided, control or comparison groups were seldom used. In the absence of a comparison or control population, changes in utilization resulting from the loss of eligibility, changes in prescribing implemented before the DUR intervention, and many other policy and payment changes would be attributed to the DUR intervention.

DUR programs, for ethical reasons, are reluctant to withhold the intervention if a negative health impact from continuation of the drug-use practice in question is likely. In these circumstances, comparison groups could be identified from other state Medicaid programs not performing the intervention or by using a time-series design, in which multiple measures are taken before and after the intervention. The time-series design controls for various threats to validity and reliability.

Evaluation of RDUR, primarily conducted on Medicaid populations, has shown mixed results. Some researchers reported having a positive impact on targeted inappropriate drug use. Others reported no impact. The diversity of drug issues, interventions, and outcomes measured may account for the discrepancy in results.

Zimmerman et al. (1994) found a DUR letter intervention directed to physicians and pharmacists reduced the long-term use of histamine-2 receptor antagonists without increasing hospitalization rates for GI problems.[20] Brufsky et al. (1998), using an interrupted-time series, showed HMO prescriber education could shift prescribing to cimetidine from other histamine-2 receptor antagonists and reduce costs without increasing GI hospitalizations.[21] In a letter intervention designed to reduce inappropriate dipyridamole use, Collins et al. (1997) found that letters sent to both pharmacists and physicians were more effective than letters sent to only physicians.[22] Both studies used a comparison group. Rascati et al. (1996) evaluated a letter intervention to reduce duplicate antiulcer treatment.[23] Six months after the letters were sent, 47.7 percent of the patients in the experimental group were still on concurrent therapy compared with 64.4 percent of patients in the control group.

The Hennessy et al. (2003) evaluation of six Medicaid DUR programs sharing the same software were unable to identify an effect of DUR letters on the rate of exceptions or on clinical outcomes.[24] Hennessy called for eliminating the Medicaid mandate for DUR as a result of the findings, but this has not happened.

PROSPECTIVE DUR

Fulda et al. (2004) have outlined the problems with online prospective DUR, which include problems with criteria discussed earlier, technical aspects such as duplicate messaging from in-store and online systems, or message text limitations involving how pharmacists interpret and respond to DUR alerts generated by the electronic systems.[25] This review also indicates that published evidence (including one randomized controlled trial and four nonrandomized studies) is inconclusive with regard to the effectiveness of these systems.

Medicaid DUR program reports on "savings" from online prospective DUR often assume claims that are reversed are program savings. A reversal occurs when a claim submitted for payment is backed out of the electronic system. These reversals may result in a savings such as when a drug prescription is not filled or they may not result in savings if the same claim is submitted at a later time. In many cases, these claims are billed at a later date, or another drug is substituted for the drug reversed. Estimated savings reported to the Centers for Medicare and Medicaid Services (CMS) by Medicaid DUR programs in their DUR Annual Report ranged from $500,000 in West Virginia to $22 million in New York.

Kidder and Bae (1999) reported on a CMS–funded study of online prospective DUR by the Iowa Medicaid program.[26] The demonstration of prospective DUR did not show any evidence of measurable impact of the intervention on reducing the frequency of drug problems or on reducing the utilization or expenditures for drugs or other health care services paid by Medicaid. The authors noted that most pharmacies already possess DUR software that screens drug use prior to submitting to Medicaid, so it is likely many problems were identified prior to the Medicaid DUR intervention. The one advantage of prospective DUR conducted by Medicaid programs and other insurers is the access to claims from all pharmacy providers serving a patient. In addition, Medicaid data from other provider types such as hospitals and physicians is available to be used in the DUR evaluation.

DUR UNDER THE MEDICARE DRUG BENEFIT

Title I of the Medicare Prescription Drug, Improvement, and Modernization Act of 2003 contains several provisions that are relevant to this analysis of drug utilization review from a policy perspective. The statute requires that entities providing prescription drugs to Medicare beneficiaries—Part D Providers (PDPs) or Medicare Advantage Plans—have in place the following programs:

1. Drug utilization management programs that include initiatives to reduce costs, when medically appropriate, such as through the use of multiple source drugs.
2. Quality assurance measures and systems to reduce medication errors and adverse drug interactions and improve medication usage.
3. Medication therapy management programs furnished by pharmacists to targeted beneficiaries to assure that drugs are appropriately used to optimize therapeutic outcomes through improved medication use, and to reduce the risk of adverse events, including adverse drug interactions.
4. Programs to control fraud, abuse, and waste.

The implementing regulations for this part of the Medicare drug benefit at Section 423.153 of the Code of Federal Regulations specify that PDPs put in place quality assurance measures and systems for reducing medication errors, reducing adverse drug interactions, and improving medication use. Requirements for drug utilization review, patient counseling, and patient information record keeping are included as part of these quality assurance measures and systems. The CMS indicated in its proposed regulations that in meeting the requirement for DUR, Part D providers should comply with the requirements found in OBRA 1990 as codified in section 456.705 of the Code of Federal Regulations and section 1927(g)(2)(A) of the act. The final regulations indicate that, based on the comments received, OBRA 1990 requirements for DUR patient counseling and patient information "generally describe widely accepted standards of pharmacy practice for both Medicaid and Non-Medicaid patients."[27] Acceptance of these standards is reflected in section 423.153(c) of the Code of Federal Regulations, but they provide no additional detail with regard to what the requirements for DUR will be.

In promulgating its regulations, CMS stated that its final policy concerning drug utilization management, quality assurance, and medication therapy management services is to describe minimum standards "so as to provide plans with flexibility to develop, implement and update their programs and systems to reflect changing best practices and to continue to provide beneficiaries with the best quality prescription drug benefit at the lowest possible cost."[28] CMS recognized the lack of specificity of its requirements for these areas, but indicated that it "expects plans to continually pursue innovative improvements for their programs and systems, and maximize technological advances where appropriate."[29] CMS indicates further that it expects to work with "stakeholders to develop a comprehensive strategy for evaluating plan performance that collectively considers multiple standards and services affecting the cost and quality of drug therapy."[30]

CONCLUSION

It seems fair to suggest that the interest of policymakers in drug utilization review (DUR) resulted from their perception that DUR could contribute to solving two important problems: One was the continuing growth in health care expenditures and prescription drug expenditures in government programs in particular; the other was mounting evidence that prescription drugs are not always used appropriately.

The passage of legislation contributes significantly to progress toward achieving policy objectives. First, the requirements in OBRA 1990 that Medicaid DUR programs be established encouraged the adoption of point-of-sale technology, which significantly impacted prospective DUR and it gave a push toward making patient counseling a standard of pharmacy practice not just for Medicaid patients. Second, the Medicare Prescription Drug, Improvement, and Modernization Act of 2003 has set requirements for quality assurance measures and medication therapy management programs, which may lead Part D providers to take actions that will help improve DUR and create new programs to improve the appropriateness of drug therapy.

Finally, OBRA 1990 increased interest in research about drug utilization review, which has suggested a number of serious deficiencies in how DUR is being practiced. Such research has also failed to establish that DUR does effectively what it is intended to do. Whether these program deficiencies contribute to the findings that DUR is not effective is not known. The experience with OBRA 1990 also suggests that the role of the agencies administering programs created by statute can make a big difference in bringing about enhancements to these programs. Whether the implementation of the provisions of the Medicare Prescription Drug, Improvement, and Modernization Act will result in new, innovative policies to improve the appropriate use of drugs is a question awaiting an answer.

NOTES

1. Task Force on Prescription Drugs (1969). Final Report. February. Washington, DC: U.S. Department of Health Education and Welfare.

2. Task Force on Prescription Drugs (1969). Background Papers: Approaches to Drug Insurance Design. February. Washington, DC: U.S. Department of Health Education and Welfare.

3. D.W. Bates et al. (1995). Incidence of Adverse Drug Events and Potential Adverse Drug Events: Implications for Prevention. *JAMA* 274(1): 29-34.

4. L.L. Leape et al. (1995). Systems Analysis of Adverse Drug Events. *JAMA* 274(1): 35-43.

5. J.A. Johnson and J.L. Bootman (1995). Drug Related Morbidity and Mortality—A Cost of Illness Model. *Archives of Internal Medicine* 155(18): 1949-1956.

6. F.R Ernst and A.J. Grizzle (2001). Drug Related Morbidity and Mortality—Updating the Cost of Illness Model. *J Am Pharm Assoc* 41: 192-199.

7. United States Pharmacopeia Drug Quality and Information Program (1996). *Drug Information Updates,* Volumes 1 and 2. Rockville, MD: United States Pharmacopeia, pp. 72-80.

8. Omnibus Budget Reconciliation Act (1990). PL 101-508. November 5.

9. Omnibus Budget Reconciliation Act (1990).

10. Fulda TR, Collins T, Kuhle J, Devereaux DS, Zuckerman IH (2001). Medicaid Drug Utilization Review Annual Reports for Federal Fiscal Year 1999: Looking Back to Move Forward. *J Am Pharm Assoc* 44(1): 69-74. HCFA Contract 00-0422.

11. Fulda TR, Valuck RJ, Vander Zanden J, Parker S, Byrns P (2000). Disagreements among Drug Compendia on Inclusion and Ratings of Drug-Drug Interactions. *Curr Ther Res* 61: 540-548.

12. U.S. Pharmacopeia Drug Utilization Review Advisory Panel (2000). Drug Utilization Review: Mechanisms to Improve Its Effectiveness and Broaden Its Scope. *J Am Pharm Assoc* 40(4): 538-545.

13. Chui MA, Rupp MT (2000). Evaluation of Online pDUR Programs in Pharmacy Practice. *J Manag Care Pharm* 6(1): 27-32.

14. Hazlett TK, Lee TA, Hansten PD, et al. (2001). Performance of Community Pharmacy Drug Interaction Software. *J Am Pharm Assoc* 41: 200-204.

15. Fulda et al. (2004). Current Status of Prospective Drug Utilization Review. *J Manag Care Pharm* 10(5): 433-441.

16. Lyles et al. (2001). Ambulatory Drug Utilization Review: Opportunities for Improved Prescription Drug Use. *Am Journal of Manag Care* 7(1): 75-81.

17. Fulda et al. (2001).

18. Fulda et al. (2001).

19. Task Force on Prescription Drugs (1969). Final Report.

20. Zimmerman DR, Collins TM, Lipowski EE, Sanifort F (1994). Evaluation of DUR Intervention: A Case Study of Histamine Antagonists. *Inquiry* 31(Spring): 89-101.

21. Brufsky JW, Ross-Degnan D, Calabrese D, et al. (1998). Shifting Physician Prescribing to a Preferred Histamine-2-Receptor Antagonist. *Medical Care* 36(3): 321-331.

22. Collins TM, Mott DA, Bigelow WE, Zimmerman DR (1997). A Controlled Letter Intervetion to Change Prescribing Behavior: Results of a Dual-Targeted Approach. *Health Serv Res* 32(4): 471-489.

23. Rascati KL, Okano GJ, Burch C (1996). Evaluation of Physician Intervention Letters. *Medical Care* 34(8): 760-766.

24. Hennessy S, Strom BL (2003). The Ineffectiveness of Retrospective Drug Utilization Review. *LDI Issue Brief* 9(1):1-4.

25. Fulda et al. (2004).

26. Kidder D and Bay J (1999). Evaluation Results from Prospective Drug Utilization Review: Medicaid Demonstrations. *Health Care Financing Review* 20(3): 107-118.

27. U.S. Department of Health and Human Services (2005). Medicare Program: Medicare Prescription Drug Benefit Notice: Action: Final Revision Rules and Regulations. *Federal Register* 70(18): 4193-4585.

28. U.S. Department of Health and Human Services (2005).

20. U.S. Department of Health and Human Services (2005).

30. U.S. Department of Health and Human Services (2005).

FURTHER READING

Hanlon, Joseph T. et al. (2002). Use of Inappropriate Prescription Drugs by Older People. *Journal of the American Geriatric Society* 50(1): 26-34.

Monane, Mark et al. (1998). Improving Prescribing Patterns for the Elderly Through an Online Drug Utilization Review Intervention. *Journal of the American Medical Association* 280(14): 1249- 1252.

Chapter 27

Pharmaceutical Care and Payment for Medication Management Services

Dale B. Christensen

INTRODUCTION

This chapter addresses policy issues regarding payment for pharmacist services. Different methods of payment for pharmacists services have slowly evolved, reflecting, and usually lagging behind, changes in pharmacist practice patterns. The chapter has three parts: First, what pharmacists do that justifies compensation is defined. Second, different approaches to compensation for professional and medical services generally, and particularly for pharmacists, are described. Third, old and new methods of compensation in the context of changing practice patterns are reviewed to better understand the future. In each case, important policy change "mileposts" are addressed.

PHARMACIST CONTRIBUTIONS TO HEALTH CARE: THE PAST, PRESENT, AND FUTURE

Terminology can be confusing. What are value-added pharmacist services? What are cognitive services, pharmaceutical care, and medication therapy management services? How did they evolve, and what is to come? Each of these terms describes drug-related services that are focused on the patient, and are not dispensing-related. The nuances of different definitions will be described later. First, let's take a retrospective look at the profession of pharmacy to better understand how these services—by whatever name—evolved.

The history of the profession of pharmacy is fascinating in how it has and continues to evolve over time in response to its environment. Historically, pharmacists were recognized as gatherers and compounders of herbal and medicinal supplements used to mitigate or cure disease. It can be argued that the source of their societal value was their knowledge about medicinal products and their ability to gather and assemble those that were pure and of known strength. However, beginning in the first half of the twentieth century, their role changed with the emergence of the pharmaceutical industry. They increasingly became distributors of drug products rather than compounders, with the attendant responsibility to ensure that a physician's prescription was safely and accurately assembled.

In the nineteenth century the focus of pharmacist education changed, to an emphasis on understanding much more about natural and particularly about manufactured drug products. The focus of pharmacist education changed again over the latter half of the twentieth century, as pharmacists received additional training in pharmacology and therapeutics. In practice, they increasingly assumed formal or informal roles as a drug therapy knowledge resource to the prescriber, starting in hospital and managed-care settings.

The decades of the 1970s and 1980s marked the explicit recognition of enhanced pharmacist services. Prior to that time, such services were provided in the community by some professionally oriented pharmacists or by clinical pharmacists rounding with attending physicians on hospital floors. Early studies began to show that provision of services directed at addressing drug-related problems added value to health care delivery in these settings.

During the most recent thirty years, several important milestones cumulatively set the stage for the clinical practice roles that pharmacists assume today. One was the report of the Study Commission on Pharmacy in 1975.[1] This report, commissioned by the American Association of Colleges of Pharmacy, was a comprehensive examination of pharmacy as a profession. It defined pharmacy as a knowledge system that produces a service. The commission recommended that the profession move to meet the health care system's unmet needs, which involve drugs and drug information, and issued specific recommendations with respect to professional educational objectives, curricular restructuring, the faculty, and credentialing. These recommendations called for greater emphasis in pharmacy education on the behavioral and social sciences and an establishment of a small body of "clinical scientists." This report became an important blueprint for revisions in schools of pharmacy curricula.

Many schools began to offer the doctor of pharmacy (Pharm.D) degree as an add-on degree to the bachelor of science degree in pharmacy for clinically oriented pharmacists. In 1992, a majority of pharmacy schools in the United States voted to adopt the PharmD as the sole entry-level degree, following the lead of a few schools (notably in California) who had done so years earlier. Today, a minimum of two years of pre–pharmacy college training is required, followed by three years of professional courses, and a clinical clerkship year.

A series of conferences were held to discuss and position the profession of pharmacy for the future. Hepler and Strand (1990) defined *pharmaceutical care services* (PCS) as the obligation of pharmacists to provide drug-related care to patients in collaboration with other health professionals to achieve optimal drug therapy.[2] Pharmacists subsequently have used the term to describe a variety of patient-centered, nondistributive activities. Another term, *cognitive services* also emerged at about this time. Cognitive services (CS) have been defined as "... those services provided by a pharmacist to, or for a patient or health care professional that are either judgmental or educational in nature"[3,4] Under this definition, *cognitive services* is the broader term that encompasses patient-focused pharmaceutical care services, but may include other nondistributive services.

In 1990, the Omnibus Budget Reconciliation Act (OBRA-90) legislation contained several provisions that expanded the professional obligations of pharmacists when serving Medicaid recipients. These included a requirement that pharmacists "offer to counsel" patients when dispensing new prescriptions and to maintain and review patient drug profiles prior to dispensing as a component of prospective drug use review (DUR) responsibilities. OBRA-90 also authorized demonstration programs to determine the value of computer-based drug problem alert systems based on submission of prescription records, and also authorized a project to pay pharmacists for performing a particular form of cognitive services: drug problem identification and resolution services, including the decision not to dispense a prescription when the patient's safety may be harmed.

Although most state boards of pharmacy did not have patient counseling regulations in place prior to 1990, they adopted them soon after passage of this act. This meant that the standards for Medicaid recipients were, in effect, applied to the general public. This serves as a good example of how a policy applicable to government-sponsored health program can become applicable to all citizens.

By the mid-1990s, pharmacists' performance of CS or PCS had been developed, documented, and reported in many institutional or specialty clinics (e.g., hospitals, HMOs, and academically affiliated medical clinics).[5-10] Within community practice settings, reports of cognitive services performance were less frequent and involved small numbers of volunteering pharmacies who documented activities for relatively short periods of time.[11-13]

In the late 1990s, the findings of the pharmacist CARE project were published.[14,15] This was a Health Care Financing Administration (HCFA) sponsored cognitive services demonstration project. It tested the simple hypothesis that providing community pharmacies additional compensation for each drug problem identified and addressed would lead to more problems being detected, and would be at least cost-neutral. The study found that a financial incentive was indeed associated with significantly more, and different types of, cognitive services performed by pharmacists as compared to control pharmacies who documented services but were not compensated. Pharmacists documented some type of drug therapy problem in 1 percent to 4 percent of all prescriptions dispensed, with higher documentation rates occurring in pharmacies with compensation. The most common type of problem found and service performed involved patient drug-taking behavior, such as drug-taking noncompliance and patient misunderstanding of drug-use instructions. The next most frequently reported were problems involving combinations of drugs taken by patients, such as therapeutic duplication. Drug therapy changes initiated by pharmacists (except add-drug therapy) were estimated to have saved an additional $10 per 1,000 prescriptions dispensed (in 1995 dollars), or enough to cover the reimbursement amount for all CS performed, whether or not they resulted in drug therapy change. These findings affirmed the hypothesis that efforts to encourage CS interventions not only improve the quality of drug therapy but that they can be at least cost-neutral, based on drug usage alone.

Beginning in 1996, the American Pharmacists Association launched a project to develop a taxonomy of pharmacist services.[16] It used an expert panel to differentiate services into four domains: patient care, drug distribution and dispensing, management activities, and public health activities. The Pharmacy Practice Activity Classification was subsequently adopted by most of the major pharmacy professional associations, and was used later as a blueprint for justifying patient care activities eligible for compensation.

Present

In general, pharmaceutical care services that are directed to patients may be differentiated into three components: disease-state focused, polypharmacy focused, and drug-problem focused. (See Figure 27.1.) Each is briefly described in the following sections.

Prescription-Related Medication Problems Detected at the Time of Dispensing

This service is focused on identifying and resolving potential medication therapy problems at the time of dispensing. It involves identifying problems

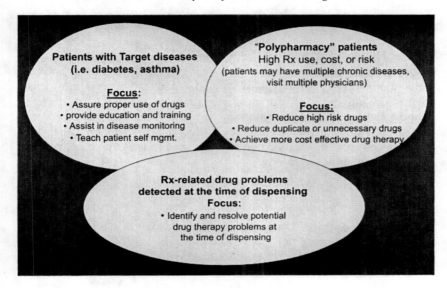

FIGURE 27.1. Models of medication therapy management programs involving pharmacists.

with the medication or patient's medication regimen where "the rubber meets the road"—at the point of dispensing. Examples include a patient who presents a prescription that conflicts with an existing drug a patient may be taking, as reflected on the patient's drug profile; a prescription with an unusually high or low dose; a drug to which the patient is allergic; or a drug that is not covered by a patient's insurance plan. The service involves documenting each specific medication problem that occurs, the activities undertaken to resolve the problem, and the results of the intervention, including changes to medication therapy.

Disease-Specific Medication Therapy Management

This service is focused on specific chronic disease states in which medication therapy is an important key to management of the disease and to avoiding adverse and costly consequences. Examples include diabetes, asthma, hypertension, and lipid management. In this case, the focus is primarily on behavioral aspects of therapy. The pharmacist is a coach and source of information to the patient regarding such matters as disease management goal setting, medication therapy, and diet and exercise.

Polypharmacy Patient Medication Therapy Management

The old saying that 20 percent of the population will generate 80 percent of the problems, resources, and costs is generally true for patients and their medication therapy. The polypharmacy patient education approach focuses on the "low hanging fruit": patients with complex medication therapies that are best managed by a medication therapy expert (i.e., pharmacist) in collaboration with the patient's physician. Proper management of drug therapy has been shown to lower total overall costs, and to lead to better quality of care and health outcomes.

Future

A sentinel event for pharmacists was the passage of the Medicare Prescription Drug, Improvement, and Modernization Act (MMA) of 2003, administered by the Centers for Medicare and Medicaid Services (CMS).[17] The pharmacy community generally agrees that the quality assurance provisions of the act sent an important policy message. The MMA essentially states that merely providing prescription drug products to recipients is not enough. Quality assurance programs are needed to ensure patients use needed prescription drugs appropriately to maintain or improve health. Prescription drug program (PDP) sponsors and Medicare Advantage (MA-PD plans) under the act must have a quality assurance plan that includes:

- a cost-effective drug utilization management program including incentives to reduce costs when medically appropriate,
- quality assurance measures and systems to reduce medication errors and adverse drug reactions (ADRs) and improve medication use,
- a medication therapy management program, and
- a program to control fraud, waste, and abuse.

A medication therapy management (MTM) program must, in turn, have elements that will promote:

- enhanced patient understanding and promote appropriate use of medications and reduce the risk of potential adverse effects from medications through education and counseling;
- increased adherence with medications via medication-refill reminders, special packaging, or other compliance programs; and
- the detection of adverse drug events and patterns of overuse and underuse of prescription drugs.

Another policy decision was to require that MTM programs be directed not to all patients, but rather to those patients presumably most in need of these services. According to regulations, MTM programs are to be targeted at beneficiaries with multiple chronic diseases, who are taking multiple Part D covered drugs, and are likely to incur annual costs that exceed a certain level (set at $4,000 annually for 2006-2007). PDP sponsors must specify the nature of such programs in their applications to CMS. In 2005, the CMS offered little guidance as to the nature and breadth of MTM programs, other than to ask sponsors to clearly state the target population for MTM services. However, CMS is expected to tighten MTM requirements over time, based on reported PDP experiences and best practice models. Health professionals, including pharmacists, are to be fairly compensated for providing MTM services, with compensation coming from the PDP sponsor, not CMS.

MEASURING THE "PRODUCT" OR THE "WORTH" OF PHARMACEUTICAL CARE

Past

It has been asserted that the rationale for providing medication therapy management services is the resolution of actual or potential drug therapy problems.[18] A number of different schemes exist for classifying drug therapy problems. A common one is the "reason for intervention" codes used by the National Council for Prescription Drug Programs as part of the electronic standard for prescription drug transactions.[19] One version for categorizing potential drug therapy problems/reasons for intervention is the following:

- Medical indication: needs drug therapy, or unnecessary drug therapy
- Drug efficacy: suboptimal drug, or insufficient dose or duration
- Drug safety adverse drug event, or drug interaction, or excessive dose/duration of therapy
- Drug-taking compliance: drug overuse, drug underuse, or inappropriate administration or technique
- Other: health problem or other[20]

The structure-process-outcome framework, developed by Donabedian (1988) provides a useful framework for measuring the quality of pharmaceutical care services.[21] Structural characteristics include elements such as pharmacist credentials (e.g., PharmD degree, specialized residencies, recognized specialty designation, prior patient management experience) and being recognized as a partner in collaborative practice agreements with physicians. Process measures refer to the activities pharmacists perform, including assessing the patient's need for drug therapy and drug regimen, identifying potential drug related problems and resolving them, and communicating with the patient. Outcome measures are the end result of process activities, and define, in a real sense, the worth of the pharmaceutical care service. Outcomes can be further differentiated into intermediate outcomes or "process outcomes" and final end result outcomes.

Outcomes can be defined in multiple ways. An excellent framework is the economic, clinical, and humanistic outcomes (ECHO) model, which depicts the value of a pharmaceutical service as a combination of traditional clinical-based outcomes with measures of economic efficiency and quality.[22] Economic outcomes consider the impact of the service expressed in economic terms, often related to medical-care utilization. Common approaches include cost minimization, cost-benefit, and cost-effectiveness analysis. Economic outcomes are often expressed as drug or total medical care costs per member per month (PMPM). Clinical outcomes refer to surrogate measures of disease status that are potentially influenced by drug therapy or by drug-related information and advice provided by a health professional. Examples include hypertension: systolic and diastolic blood pressure; diabetes: hemoglobin A1c; hypercholesterolemia: high-density lipoprotein (HDL), low-density lipoprotein (LDL), total cholesterol; and asthma: peak expiratory flow rate, and number of breathing difficulty episodes. Humanistic outcomes relate to dimensions of patient health status, functional activities of daily living, or health-related quality of life, and also to patient satisfaction with provider services. One commonly used general health status measure is the Medical Outcomes Study short form 36 or 12 (SF-36, SF-12), which include measures of physical and social functioning. Other, more disease-specific health status measures are available, and may be more sensitive to the impact of medication therapy management services.

Contributions of Pharmaceutical Care:
Review of the Evidence

Literature reviews over the past decade reflect the progression of the pharmacy profession in documenting and evaluating PCS models of care across different settings and disease states.[23-27] Early studies were descriptive and often lacked a control or comparison group, involved small numbers of patients, had short follow-up periods, or evaluated process of care but not outcomes. More recently, evaluative studies of PCS have exhibited stronger research designs. Together,they make a compelling case that pharmacist services contribute qualitatively to processes and outcomes related to patient care, and that such services are often at least cost neutral if not cost saving.[28-37]

In a systematic review of published evaluative studies of pharmacist professional services that included an economic evaluation, Schumock et al. (2003) found that, on average, pharmacist service programs generated a savings-to-cost ratio of 4.68 to 1.[38] In a cost-effectiveness analysis model of pharmaceutical care services under a Medicare drug benefit program, Etemad and Hay (2003) estimated that such a benefit would be highly cost-effective at $2,100 per life year saved.[39]

BASES FOR PAYMENT OF PROFESSIONAL SERVICES, INCLUDING PHARMACEUTICAL CARE

Product-Based Reimbursement

Historically, the basis for payment of pharmacists' services has been the drug product and a dispensing fee. The drug product was typically subject to a percent markup to cover the cost of acquisition, storage, and overhead costs such as inventory management. The professional fee was a flat amount meant to compensate pharmacists for their expertise and time in preparing the prescription and related overhead costs. The Medicare and Medicaid Amendments to the Social Security Act of 1965 solidified this approach as the basis for compensating pharmacists for dispensing prescriptions. Medicaid reimbursement policies and interpretive guidelines became the basis for private sector third party programs as well. Over time the allowable percent markup on multisource prescription drugs was capped by federal or state Medicaid "maximum allowable cost" limits. Prescription dispensing fees were also adjusted to reflect, in part, changes in the community pharmacies' average cost to dispense a prescription, and the marketplace.

Several variants of this formula exist. Some state Medicaid programs have allowed different dispensing-fee levels depending on type of pharmacy or pharmacy prescription volume. For example, providing lower volume pharmacies with higher dispensing fees was considered a fair way to compensate them for their higher operating costs and thereby maximize pharmacy participation in the Medicaid program and patient access to prescriptions. Pharmacies providing prescriptions to nursing homes sometimes receive higher dispensing fees for the additional services or product packaging provided. Another variant is to charge a different dispensing fee based on the type of product dispensed. For example, providing a higher dispensing fee for generically available drugs is seen as one way to encourage pharmacists to initiate efforts to dispense lower-cost generic drugs to patients when permitted.

In 1991, the OBRA-90 Act essentially froze dispensing fees under Medicaid programs as a cost-savings measure. In the meantime, market consolidation among third party programs and pharmaceutical benefits managers (PBMs) created an oligopoly situation in many regions, resulted in lower dispensing fees offered to pharmacists to participate in third party programs. Medicaid thus became the highest paying third party prescription program in many states. Dispensing fees became unfrozen in later budget reconciliation acts, and state Medicaid programs began to embrace alternatives to controlling drug costs, such as prior authorization and, more recently, preferred drug lists. They also began exploring methods and incentives to engage prescribers and pharmacists in cost-savings activities.

Reimbursement for Pharmacist Professional Services Unrelated to Dispensing

Compensation for pharmacist cognitive services has a more recent history, and is only gradually gaining acceptance. It has slowly emulated the medical profession compensation model.

Within the medical and dental professions the service fees vary according to the type of service provided and the time to perform the service. The fee depends on the service's underlying value to the purchaser, which is in turn a function of the technical nature of the service, and number and exclusivity of providers with the technical skills to provide the service. Thus, highly specialized physicians, dentists, attorneys, and others are able to command higher fees for their services.

A question often asked by third party program administrators is, "Why should I pay for a 'cognitive service'? Isn't it just part of the dispensing obligations of a pharmacist?" In answering this question, a distinction must first be made between what is expected from a pharmacist as part of a dispensing fee, and what might be expected from a value-added dispensing-related cognitive service. Most state pharmacy practice acts require pharmacists to maintain and review patient drug profiles as part of quality assurance activities associated with dispensing. The pharmacist has a duty to catch errors that, if undetected, would render harm to a patient, but not necessarily to intervene in an attempt to optimize therapy or to render a more cost-effective choice.[40] Admittedly, the line separating these two functions can be characterized as a gray zone.

Two examples help illustrate this difference.

Example 1: A prescription is written for an eighteen-month-old child for Keflex 500mg TID. This results from an initial physician visit with a diagnosis of acute otitis media. As part of a minimal dispensing service the pharmacist might check for allergies and suggest a lower dosage for this infant. A value-added service, on the other hand, might involve the pharmacist questioning the use of this or any other second-line antibiotic for otitis based on current practice guidelines suggesting that most episodes of acute otitis media respond spontaneously. The pharmacist might suggest palliative care or at least a lower-cost generic version if the prescriber still wanted antibiotic therapy.

Example 2: A patient presents a prescription for Nexium, a Tier 3 (highest copay) drug under many insurance plans. As part of a basic dispensing service, the pharmacist determines that the prescribed drug poses no problems in terms of dosage or of interactions with other drugs the patient is taking, then dispenses it as written for a $40 patient copayment. As a value-added service, the pharmacist informs the patient that a close therapeutic alternative is available. The pharmacist checks with the prescriber, who authorizes a different proton pump inhibitor that is a Tier 2 preferred drug under the plan ($20 copayment). The pharmacist might further inform the patient that Prilosec OTC is available, for an even greater savings.

Other Forms of Service-Based Reimbursement

Heretofore we have identified two forms of reimbursement: markup based on product cost, and service fees based on skill or time (time-based reimbursement; relative value system). Capitation is another form of service-based reimbursement involving a negotiated monthly fee per eligible person (per member per month, PMPM). Auto and health insurance are examples. In the health insurance sector, it is common to quote rates for medical care coverage as a PMPM rate. As with auto insurance, these rates may be further adjusted according to age, risk, or experience to reflect the risk of higher future medical care costs. Insurers, in turn, sometimes share the risk by contracting with medical service provider organizations such as HMOs. Whoever assumes the risk must be reasonably sure they can prevent unnecessary use of resources. Often, risk corridors are established wherein any losses above the first, say, 5 to 10 percent, is shared equally between the parties. In prescription drug programs, risk sharing under capitation with pharmacists has been tried but has not been successful, in large part because of the limited control pharmacists have over the selection and cost of prescribed drugs dispensed.

Each compensation method has its own economic incentives and disincentives. Under compensation based on a percent markup (such as in the sale of OTC products), a seller has a financial incentive to maximize the sale of products with high unit costs. A fee-for-service system (such as prescription dispensing fees) provides no particular economic incentive to use higher priced drugs, but does provide an incentive to increase the volume of prescriptions dispensed. Under time-based reimbursement, a provider maximizes revenue by increasing the amount of billing time, or billable hours. Capitation-based reimbursement provides incentives to provide fewer or lower-cost services while still meeting contractual service obligations.

Present/Future

Newer forms of reimbursement affecting physicians and, increasingly, pharmacists include paying for results (e.g., "pay for performance"), and resource-based relative value system (RBRVS) payment.

Paying for results implies an outcomes-based approach to payment rather than a process-based system. The shift away from the time-honored traditional practice of paying for services to paying for outcomes is a recent phenomenon and reflects an industry-wide concern about rising health care costs. Outcomes may or may not be specifically defined, but usually have a cost-lowering or cost-containment element.

An example in pharmacy is compensation for pharmacist cognitive services that are specifically focused on making changes in drug therapy that result in lower drug costs without affecting quality. Cognitive service fees tied to initiating an action that results in a change in a prescription from a Tier 3 to a lower tiered drug is one example. Another example is a plan that compensates pharmacists when a cognitive service is performed that has an estimated or actual impact on either drug costs or use of medical services.

A documentation billing system for pharmacist cognitive services exists in the form of professional pharmacy services codes that are part of the National Council for Prescription Drug Programs (NCPDP) electronic prescription processing system (version 5.1). The NCPDP is a standard-setting body for the electronic transmission of prescriptions. Codes were expanded to accept cognitive or value added dispensing services several years ago. This coding system is based on a [reason for intervention] ? [intervention activities] ? [results] framework. To date, few major health insurers compensate pharmacists for these services directly, hence it has not heretofore been used much in practice.

One private sector firm, Outcomes Pharmaceutical Health Care has developed a documentation and service billing system that is built on the NCPDP model and compensates pharmacists for providing these value-added services but also evaluates them as to their potential impact on health care costs.[41] A unique feature of this program is that it guarantees to the third party payer that the charges for these services will not exceed the estimated cost-savings impact.

The principle behind a RBRVS system is that compensation is based on a number of factors, such as complexity of the patient case, level of expertise required in performing the service, and time involved.

Physicians typically bill for medical services using current procedure terminology evaluation and management codes (CPT E&M). Basically, this is a service-based (as opposed to an outcomes-based) coding and reimbursement system. This system is of interest to pharmacists because many of the clinical services performed by pharmacists would seem to fit under this coding structure.

A little-known section of the Health Insurance Portability and Accountability Act of 1996 (HIPAA) requires standardization in the use of electronic data interchange transactions for health care professional services claims, including pharmacist services. This requirement provided the impetus to systematically examine coding systems used in pharmacy for services of all type. Beginning in 2003, several pharmacy professional organizations formed an advisory panel to address the issue. The American Medical Association's Health Care Professionals Advisory Committee (HCPAC) is responsible for maintaining current procedure terminology codes (CPT) for health professional billings. The Pharmacist Services Technical Advisory Coalition (PSTAC), as the advisory panel became known, was formed to advise HCPAC on whether existing or new CPT codes for MTMS should be used. In 2005, an agreement was reached on the first version of professional service codes applicable to pharmacists providing drug-related, nondispensing services beginning January 1, 2006. Codes and guidelines have been established to report the provision of face-to-face patient assessment and intervention as services by a pharmacist.

0115T	MTM service(s) provided by a pharmacist, individual, face-to-face with patient, initial 15 minutes, with assessment, and intervention if provided;
0116T	subsequent encounter
+0117	Teach additional 15 minutes (List separately in addition to code for the primary service)

These are temporary codes. Adoption of equivalent CPT codes awaits further review and consideration by the AMA's HCPAC. Among the factors they will consider is pharmacist and payer experience in using these codes, including how widely they are used.

As these codes (or equivalent CPT codes) are used for payment for MTM services, pharmacy leaders expect that they will be adopted as a basis for compensation of MTM services to other populations, such as Medicaid program recipients and persons enrolled in private sector health plans. Pharmacy computer system vendors are expected to develop "crosswalks" from existing professional service coding systems to applicable "T" or CPT codes using the same format as physicians use (i.e., CMS 1500 forms).

Proposed Compensation Mechanisms Based on Different Types or Levels of Cognitive Services

An ideal compensation model for pharmacist providers of clinical (i.e., nondispensing) services of all type, including MTM services, would recognize specific value added services, and would have built in incentives to perform services designed to optimize desirable outcomes. Given the diverse nature of nondispensing services, tiers should be used. Briefly, I suggest the following approach.

Compensation Level 1

Dispensing fees should vary according to the complexity and needs of the prescription dispensed for a patient.

Examples and Rationale. New versus refill prescriptions. New prescriptions require more professional time than refills. A pharmacist must spend additional time to check the drug profile for incompatibilities, and address third party payment requirements. Furthermore, patients with new prescriptions have a greater need for drug-use instruction and advice. New prescriptions should therefore receive a higher dispensing fee than refills.

Patients receiving particular drugs. A patient who receives a nonoral dose form, such as a topical ophthalmic or inhaler, requires special instruction to ensure optimal drug response. Prescriptions for these products (especially as new prescriptions) should receive a higher dispensing fee than new prescriptions for other drug products.

Compensation Level 2

Patients with potential drug-related problems identified *at the time of dispensing* should be compensated an additional drug problem resolution fee. This fee should vary according to the complexity, time involved, and estimated cost avoidance.

Examples and Rationale. In most community settings, approximately 8 percent of all prescriptions presented for dispensing incur some type of flag based on a computer-generated review of previously dispensed prescriptions. Examples include early or late refill, drug-drug interaction, therapeutic duplication, or drug-allergy interaction. In most community pharmacy practice settings today these alerts are too frequently ignored by pharmacists, either because they are deemed false positive signals or because of workplace demands to process the next prescription waiting in line as soon as possible, or both. In this manner, the flat dispensing fee system prevalent in practice today serves as an economic disincentive to provide these services. If a "pay for problem resolved" compensation system were adopted in addition to a modified dispensing fee, pharmacists would have economic incentives to not only respond to computer generated alerts but also to investigate other problems not identifiable by a computer algorithm, such as patient noncompliance or communication difficulty. This system has been successfully demonstrated in practice, both in the public and private sectors. One example is the pharmacist CARE project in Washington State, wherein pharmacists who were compensated in this manner were shown to consistently identify more problems than control group (usual care) pharmacies, and that the savings from drug costs alone would have covered the costs of pharmacist compensation for cognitive services, even if no change in drug costs occurred. In the private sector a working example is the previously described Outcomes Pharmaceutical Health Care approach.

The compensation mechanism should be based on a fixed or graduated fee for every potential drug therapy problem detected and resolved, even if such intervention results in no change in therapy but drug therapy advice to the patient. A graduated fee system should be used based on the seriousness or complexity of the problem, and the time involved to resolve it.

Compensation Level 3

Pharmacists who provide *retrospective comprehensive drug regimen review services* to patients at highest risk for medical errors, suboptimal drug therapy, or costly care should be compensated based on services provided that optimize patient drug therapy and ensure appropriate patient use.

Examples and Rationale. Patients at higher risk of adverse consequences of drug therapy include patients with specific disease states for which appropriate drug use is critical, such as heart disease, asthma, and diabetes. Furthermore, patients with multiple disease states and receiving multiple prescriptions are at high risk. Finally, patients taking some prescriptions are at higher risk merely because of the toxicity or narrow therapeutic window of the drug involved (e.g., methotrexate, oncolytic agents, and HIV drugs). A compensation system focused on these patients would maximize the opportunity for benefits, while minimizing unnecessary care.

The MTM provisions of the MMA of 2003 explicitly target these patients as candidates for focused review. Reviews would be retrospective in nature, and preferably would be performed separately from dispensing activities. Pharmacist services would involve a scheduled 1:1 conference with a targeted patient, taking a medication history, reviewing the drug profile, contacting the prescriber for any potential drug problems, explaining any changes in drug therapy to the patient, new or reinforced instructions for use, and monitoring and follow-up. Services would be billable by either a prescriber or pharmacist as a recognized "T" code or CPT E&M code as noted previously.

Compensation Level 4

Specialty care patients who need frequent dosage adjustment and monitoring

Examples and Rationale. At first glance this category would seem to be a subset of the previous level. However, certain patients with chronic diseases require additional specialized services. Examples include patients on anticoagulation therapy, new diabetic patients needing training, end-stage renal disease patients, and patients with HIV disease. This is a disease management service model. Compensation could be based on a resource-based, relative value, fee-for-service system similar to that now used by physicians (e.g., higher CPT E&M codes), or could be on a fee-per-patient (capitated) system.

A common thread among levels of this proposed compensation plan is that it focuses on patients for whom extra instruction or monitoring of drug therapy is needed and is likely to have a payoff in terms of better health outcomes. Moreover, it better aligns incentives in the direction of providing services appropriate to need to achieve the best levels of cost-effective drug-related therapy.

SUMMARY

We live in interesting times. The profession of pharmacy is on the brink of substantially changing the focus of its activities away from mere provision of drug products to embracing roles that include offering advice on the choice of drugs patients receive, instructing patients regarding appropriate use, and monitoring the results of drug therapy. This chapter has focused on the past, present, and future of pharmacists in nondistributive roles, with an emphasis on compensation for services. Recent developments in health care policy, including the MTM provisions of the MMA of 2003, are unfolding, and they provide a basis for a change in the practice environment for pharmacists in the United States. Finally, I propose four pharmaceutical service compensation policies that, together, would align incentives to achieve cost-effective drug use and disease management for patients.

NOTES

1. Millis JS (1976). Looking ahead—The report of the Study Commission on Pharmacy. *Am J Hosp Pharm* 33(2):134-138.

2. Hepler CD, Strand LM (1990). Opportunities and responsibilities in pharmaceutical care. *Am J Hosp Pharm* 47: 533-542.

3. Kusserow RP (1989). *Medicare Drug Utilization Review.* Inspector General (Office of Analysis and Inspections). Washington, DC: U.S. Department of Health and Human Services.

4. Christensen DB, Fassett WE, Andrews GA (1993). A practical billing and payment plan for cognitive services. *Am Pharm* NS33(3): 34-40.

5. Dager WE, Branch JM, King JH, White RH, Quan RS, Musallam NA, Albertson TE (2000). Optimization of inpatient warfarin therapy: Impact of daily consultation by a pharmacist-managed anticoagulation service. *Ann Pharmacother* 34(5): 567-572.

6. Willey ML, Chagan L, Sisca TS, Chapple KJ, Callahan AK, Crain JL, Kitenko LE, Martin T, Spedden KD (2003). A pharmacist-managed anticoagulation clinic: Six-year assessment of patient outcomes. *Am J Health Syst Pharm* 60(10): 1033-1037.

7. Christensen DB, Campbell WH, Madsen S, Hartzema AG, and Nudelman PM (1981). Documenting outpatient problem intervention activities of pharmacists in an HMO. *Med Care* 9: 104-117.

8. Chenella FC, Klotz TA, Gill MA, et al. (1983). Comparison of physician and pharmacist management of anticoagulant therapy of inpatients. *Am J Hosp Pharm* 40:1642-1645.

9. Gray DR, Garabedian-Ruffalo SM, Chretien SD (1985). Cost-justification of a clinical pharmacist-managed anticoagulation clinic. *Drug Intell Clin Pharm* 19(7-8): 575-580.

10. McKenney JM, Witherspoon JM (1985). The impact of outpatient hospital pharmacists on patients receiving antihypertensive and anticoagulant therapy. *Hosp Pharm* 20(6): 406, 409-11, 415.

11. Rupp MT, DeYOung M, Schondelmeyer SW (1992). Prescribing problems and pharmacist interventions in community practice. *Med Care* 30(10): 926-940.

12. Knowlton CH, Knapp DA (1994). Community pharmacists help HMO cut drug costs. *Am Pharm* NS34(1): 36-42.

13. Dobie RL III, Rascati KL (1994). Documenting the value of pharmacist interventions. *Am Pharm* NS34(5): 50-54.

14. Christensen DB, Neil N, Fassett WE, Smith DH, Holmes G, Stergachis A (2000). Frequency and characteristics of cognitive services performed by pharmacists in response to a financial incentive. *J Am Pharm Assoc* 41: 609-17.

15. Smith DH, Fassett WE, Christensen DB. Downstream cost changes associated with the provision of cognitive services by pharmacists: Data from the Washington CARE project. *J Am Pharm Assoc* 39: 650-657.

16. Maine LL (1998). Pharmacy practice activity classification. *J Am Pharm Assoc* 38(2): 139-148.

17. Medicare Prescription Drug, Improvement, and Modernization Act of 2003. PL 108-173.

18. Cipolle RJ, Strand LM, Morley PC (1998). *Pharmaceutical Care Practice*. New York: McGraw-Hill.

19. Pharmacy Quality Alliance (2006). Quality measures for patient safety. November 20. Available at: http://www.pqaalliance.org/files/PatientSafetyFINALwDINov20.doc.

20. Farris KB, Kumbera P, Halterman T, Fang G (2002). Outcomes-based pharmaceutical reimbursement: Reimbursement of cognitive services. *J Managed Care Pharm* 5: 383-389.

21. Donabedian A (1988). The quality of care: How can it be assessed? *JAMA* 260(12): 1743-1748.

22. Kozma CM, Reeder CE, Schulz RM. (1993) Economic, clinical, and humanistic outcomes: A planning model for pharmacoeconomic research. *Clin Ther* 15(6): 1121-1132.

23. Tully MT, Sexton EM (2000). Impact of pharmacists providing a Rx review and monitoring service in ambulatory care or community practice. *Ann Pharmacother.*

24. Plumridge RJ, Wojnar-Horton RE (1998). Review of the pharmacoeconomics of pharmaceutical care. *Pharmacoeconomics* 14: 175-189.

25. Kennie NR, Schuster BG, Einarson TR (1998). Critical analysis of the pharmaceutical care research literature. *Ann Pharmacother* 32(1): 17-26.

26. Beney J, Bero LA, Bond C (2000). Expanding the roles of outpatient pharmacists: Effects on health services utilisation, costs, and patient outcomes. Cochrane Database Syst Rev (3):CD000336. Review.

27. Singhal PK, Raisch DW, Gupchup GV (1999). The impact of pharmaceutical services in community and ambulatory care settings: Evidence and recommendations for future research. *Ann Pharmacother* 33(12):1336-1355.

28. Chrischilles EA, Carter BL, Lund BC, Rubenstein LM, Chen-Hardee SS, Voelker MD, Park TR, Kuehl AK (2004). Evaluation of the Iowa Medicaid pharmaceutical case management program *J Am Pharm Assoc* 44(3): 337-349.

29. Carter BL, Chrischilles EA, Scholz D, et al. (2003). Extent of services provided by pharmacists in the Iowa Medicaid Pharmaceutical Case Management program. *J Am Pharm Assoc* 43: 24-33.

30. Bluml BM, McKenney JM, Cziraky MJ (2000). Pharmaceutical care services and results in project ImPACT: Hyperlipidemia. *J Am Pharm Assoc* 40(2): 157-165.

31. Christensen DB, Neil N, Fassett WE, et al. (2000). Frequency and characteristics of cognitive services performed by pharmacists in response to a financial incentive. J Am Pharm Assoc 41: 609-617.

32. Carter BL, Malone DC, Billups SJ, et al. (2001). Interpreting the findings of the IMPROVE study. *Am J Health Syst Pharm* 58:1330-1337.

33. Malone DC, Carter BL, Billups SJ, et al. (2000). An economic analysis of a randomized, controlled, multicenter study of clinical pharmacist interventions for high-risk veterans: The IMPROVE study. *Pharmacotherapy* 20(10):1149-1158.

34. Weinberger M, Murray MD, Marrero DG, et al. (2002). Effectiveness of pharmacist care for patients with reactive airways disease: A randomized controlled trial. *JAMA* 288(13): 1594-1602.

35. Cranor CW, Christensen DB (2003). The Asheville Project: Short-term outcomes of community pharmacy diabetes care program. *J Am Pharm Assoc* 43: 149-159.

36. Cranor CW, Bunting BA, Christensen DB (2003). The Asheville Project: Long-term clinical and economic outcomes of community pharmacy diabetes care program. *J Am Pharm Assoc* 43:173-184.

37. Stergachis A, Gardner JS, Anderson MT, et al. (2002). Improving pediatric asthma outcomes in the community setting: Does pharmaceutical care make a difference? *J Am Pharm Assoc* 42(5): 743-752.

38. Schumock GT, Butler MG, Meek PD, et al. (2003). Evidence of the economic benefit of clinical pharmacy services: 1996-2000. *Pharmacotherapy* 23(1): 113-132.

39. Etemad LR, Hay JW (2003). Cost-effectiveness analysis of pharmaceutical care in a Medicare drug benefit program. *Value in Health* 6: 425-435.

40. Christensen DB, Fassett WF, Andrews GA (1993). A practical billing and payment plan for CS. *Am Pharm* NS33: 34-40.

41. Farris KB, Kumbera P, Halterman T, Fang G (2002). Outcomes-based pharmacist reimbursement: Reimbursing pharmacists for cognitive services part 1. *J Manag Care Pharm* 8(5): 383-393.

Chapter 28

Patient Compliance

Jon C. Schommer
Reshmi L. Singh

The purpose of this chapter is to review patient compliance within a public policy context. To accomplish this goal, we will present evidence regarding the clinical and economic importance of compliance with medication regimens. Next, we will describe how compliance has been viewed historically and then provide insight about how compliance is being viewed today. The roles of various health care stakeholders will be summarized, followed by a review of selected policy trends in the area of compliance. Finally, we will conclude the chapter with some ideas for policy options regarding compliance for various health care stakeholders and our recommendations for the future. Our guiding assumption for this chapter is that even though compliance with self-administered medications depends on individual patient choices, important public policy considerations can help improve compliance through their effects on health care systems and health service delivery processes.

CLINICAL AND ECONOMIC IMPORTANCE OF COMPLIANCE

Estimates show that more than half of all prescriptions filled each year in the United States may be taken incorrectly.[1] The clinical and economic impacts of noncompliance with medication regimens are astounding. For example, one-sixth of all hospital admissions, one-fourth of nursing home admissions, one-fourth of all malpractice suits, and millions of medical emergencies each year are attributable to medication compliance problems.[2-7] Noncompliance with medication therapies also may be the root cause of half of all therapeutic failures.[8] It is estimated that nearly two million hospital admissions annually can be linked directly to noncompliance, and that 125,000 Americans die needlessly each year simply because they fail to take their medications as prescribed.[9,10] A 1992 study estimated that failure of patients to have prescriptions filled results in "a shortfall at the pharmacy counter of about 140 million prescriptions worth $2.8 billion." These estimates were based on interviews with two thousand consumers, of whom 8.7 percent reported failure to have an initial prescription filled.[11]

In 1993, the Task Force for Compliance[12] estimated that the total cost of noncompliance to the American economy was almost $100 billion annually. Of this amount, the yearly cost of reduced worker productivity and absenteeism due to noncompliance was $50 billion, yearly costs for hospital admissions due to noncompliance were $25 billion, and costs related to premature deaths of working citizens and added treatment costs for ambulatory patients was $20 billion annually.

In 2003, the World Health Organization (WHO) released a report and concluded that in developed countries, compliance rates for patients suffering from chronic conditions average only about 50 percent, but that in developing countries, compliance rates are even lower due to the paucity of health resources and inequities in access to health care.[13] Compliance was viewed as the "single most important modifiable factor that compromises treatment outcome," and poor compliance was viewed as "the primary reason for suboptimal clinical benefit. It causes medical and psychosocial complications of disease, reduces patients' quality of life, and wastes health care resources. Taken together, these direct consequences impair the ability of health care systems around the world to achieve population health goals."[14] Furthermore, the WHO report suggested that, in addition to characteristics of the disease and treatment regimens, attributes of the health care system and service delivery processes also have an influence on patient compliance.[15] Therefore, noncompliance can be viewed as a pubic health and public policy issue to the extent that policy can affect health care systems and service delivery processes.

So far in this chapter, the clinical and economic importance of compliance has been presented in terms of populations as a whole. In addition to that perspective, a body of evidence exists that shows that noncompliance has clinical and economic costs for specific diseases, specific drug classes, and specific patient populations as well. A few examples of this type of evidence regarding the clinical and economic impact of noncompliance are outlined in the next paragraphs.

As these studies are considered, it should be noted that differences exist in the nature of outcomes associated with noncompliance among different drug product classes due to the differences in the nature of the diseases being treated. Also, researchers who conducted these studies used different measures of noncompliance, different time horizons for their evaluations, and different data collection techniques for studying the effects of noncompliance on clinical and economic outcomes. These differences result in wide variation in estimates. Nonetheless, the results further reveal the impact that noncompliance can have on patient care outcomes.

The National Council on Patient Information and Education provided a comparison of selected outcomes for patients categorized as having "good" versus "poor" compliance.[16] They reported that patients with good compliance achieved a 39 percent drop in blood cholesterol compared to only an 11 percent drop for patients with poor compliance. For patients taking antidepressant medications, 90 percent of patients who took 90 percent of doses improved compared to none of the patients who took less than 80 percent of the prescribed doses showing improvement.

A study by McCombs et al. (1994) showed that 86 percent of new antihypertensive drug therapy patients interrupted or discontinued purchasing any form of antihypertensive medication during the first year of treatment. Patients with interrupted antihypertensive therapy consumed an additional $873 per patient in health care during that first year, not counting a reduction in prescription drug cost ($281). Increased costs primarily were due to increased hospital expenditures of $637.[17]

Col et al. (1990) studied elderly patients admitted to an acute care hospital to determine the percentage of elderly hospital admissions due to noncompliance with medication regimens or adverse drug reactions. They reported that 28 percent of the admissions were drug related (17 percent due to noncompliance plus 11 percent due to adverse drug reactions). They also reported that 33 percent of their study subjects admitted to having a history of noncompliance.[18]

In a study of patients with schizophrenia or schizoaffective disorder, Svarstad et al. (2001) reported that 31 percent used medications irregularly. During their twelve month study period, irregular users had significantly higher rates of hospitalization than regular users (42 percent versus 20 percent), more hospital days (sixteen days versus four days), and higher hospital costs ($3,992 versus $1,048). Irregular medication use was one of the strongest predictors of hospital use and costs even after the analysis controlled for diagnosis, demographic characteristics, baseline functioning, and previous hospitalizations.[19]

Kennedy and Erb (2002) utilized the Disability Supplement and the Disability Followback Survey, which are special supplements to the National Health Interview Survey, as their data source for their study. They focused their analysis on the population of 1.3 million adults with disabilities who reportedly did not take their medications as prescribed because the cost of the medication was so high that they did not get their prescription filled, did not fill their prescription completely, did not refill their prescription, or used their medicine less often than prescribed because of the high cost. They reported that more than half of this group identified one or more potentially serious and costly health problems that they attributed to noncompliance. Severe disability, poor health, low income, lack of insurance, and a high number of prescriptions increased the odds of being noncompliant as a result of cost of therapy.[20]

The examples just outlined provide evidence that noncompliance presents important clinical and economic challenges for individuals and society. Noncompliance may be the most important factor that compromises the ability to achieve the full potential from medications. Noncompliance causes medical and psychosocial complications of disease, reduces patients' quality of life, and wastes health care resources.[21] It is a well-documented problem, but yet is not fully understood. The next sections will describe how compliance has been viewed historically, and also will provide insight about how compliance currently is being viewed.

THE HISTORY OF COMPLIANCE AS AN IDEOLOGY

Hippocrates has been attributed with stating, "Keep a watch also on the faults of the patients, which often make them lie about the taking of things prescribed." Although noncompliance with prescribed medication regimens may have been occurring for ages, physicians did not obtain many truly effective medications, such as antibiotics, to treat diseases until after World War II. Only then did it become as important for physicians to make sure that the medications they prescribed were actually consumed by patients as it was to make sure that the medications were properly selected.[22] A body of research developed in this area, and by the late 1970s an accepted definition of compliance emerged as "the extent to which the patient's behavior (in terms of taking medications, following diets, or executing other lifestyle changes) coincides with medical or health advice."[23] This definition of compliance assumes that physicians serve as an agent of the patient and make decisions on behalf of the patient that the patient is expected to follow. Patients are viewed as not having sufficient expertise to make such decisions and must rely on their physicians' training and experience. Noncompliance with such expert advice is assumed to lead to suboptimal clinical and economic outcomes for patients and for society.

Within this view of compliance (i.e., not following a doctor's orders), the misuse of medication has been classified as errors of omission or errors of commission. Errors of omission include such things as failure to purchase initial or refill prescriptions.[24,25] One study estimated that 7 percent of patients fail to have an initial prescription filled and 32 percent fail to purchase therapeutically necessary refills.[9] Errors of omission also include underuse of prescribed medications, such as taking less medicine than the health care professional prescribed, taking it less frequently than prescribed, taking medicine "holidays," or not taking it at all.[26,27] As an example of underuse, a compliance study showed that 50 percent of arthritis patients and 76 percent of hypertension patients inadvertently missed an occasional dose of their regular maintenance medications.[28]

Another error of omission is stopping a medication too soon. As to how many patients stop taking their medication too soon, a study showed that 15 percent of patients who were taking a medication terminated their therapy prematurely.[29] The most frequent offenders included younger patients, patients with better educations, those living in large urban areas, and those coping with new medical problems.[30]

Four errors of commission that commonly occur are: (1) overuse, (2) sharing, (3) mistakes in dose timing, and (4) self-regulating. Overuse is a problem since it can lead to increased incidence of adverse effects and avoidable hospitalization.[31] Sharing medications is another error of commission. One study showed that about 10 percent of the patients who were prescribed sedatives shared these medications with others.[32] An example of making mistakes in dose timing was revealed by one study in which more than 75 percent of the diabetic patients failed to administer insulin injections within 30 minutes of the prescribed times, in spite of being aware of the importance of proper timing for blood sugar control.[33] The "self-regulating" problem occurs when patients change dosages on their own. In one study, 42 percent of patients with epilepsy self-regulated doses by raising or lowering dosages or simply skipping dosages intentionally.[34]

This traditional view of compliance/noncompliance tends to place blame on patients for not following directions that were given to them. More recently, a focus has been placed on the need for patients to be supported, and not blamed, for noncompliant behaviors. This newer approach to understanding and achieving compliance with medication therapies is outlined next.

CONTEMPORARY IDEOLOGY OF COMPLIANCE

Much of the early compliance research placed undue emphasis on the power of physicians as sole decision maker and neglected to acknowledge the existence of more universal forms of obtaining care and advice, such as self-management and relying on family, friends, neighbors, and others for making health behavior choices.[35] Since the 1980s, the compliance concept has evolved and more emphasis has been given to (1) practitioner-patient communication, (2) practitioner-patient relationships, and (3) practitioner-patient partnerships as ideologies for patient compliance.

Practitioner-Patient Communication

During the 1980s and 1990s, researchers revealed evidence that compliance with a medication regimen was primarily determined by the nature and quality of practitioner-patient communication.[36-39] Improved communication between a practitioner and patient has been shown to increase patient knowledge and recall, patient satisfaction, genuine informed consent, patient compliance behaviors, and speed of recovery from illness.[40] It appears that in addition to increasing understanding of treatment regimens, practitioner-patient communication helps improve patients' understanding about the rationale and importance of a medication regimen.[41] Thus, communication between practitioners and patients about medication regimens can not only help patients understand how to use those medications appropriately, but also can help provide patients with the motivation necessary for compliance.

Roter (1995) outlined eight principles related to communication with particular relevance to patient compliance. First, the patient's perspective of his or her medical condition and its treatment should be considered and respected. Second, practitioners should take care to make sure that a medication is not prescribed only as an expediency or as an attempt to satisfy or placate the patient. Third, the diagnostic and treatment rationale for prescribed medications must be provided to the patient. Fourth, practitioners should negotiate a plan and anticipate problems and relevant solutions. The likelihood of compliance is enhanced when patients' preferences and concerns can be accommodated through individualized tailoring. Fifth, practitioners' expertise should be shared with patients in such a way that the information is both relevant and useful to patients. Simply giving information is not enough. Asking what a patient knows and responding appropriately allows for a tailored approach. Sixth, communication should have both cognitive and emotional significance. Patients need factual information (cognitive significance), but they also need information that will reduce uncertainty and anxiety (emotional significance) so that they can be better prepared to successfully use the agreed-upon medication regimen. Seventh, compliance monitoring should be asked about during every interaction, but in a nonjudgmental and nonthreatening manner. It is best to ask patients about what medications they are taking, what dose and schedule they are following for each, and if they experienced any problems, and then to use this information as a practitioner to determine compliance problems. Finally, the eighth principle is to use a collaborative process for identifying and resolving problems when compliance difficulties are uncovered.[42]

Practitioner-Patient Relationships

Researchers also have discovered that successful communication between practitioners and patients requires professional relationships between these parties.[43] Simple information giving will not achieve compliance for patients who continually need to make decisions about how they take their medications. Their perceptions and the social environment in which they live have been shown to have great impact on their decision making regarding compliance behaviors.[44] A practitioner may view a patient's noncompliant behavior as irrational, but such behavior may be a very rational action when viewed from the patient's point of view. Patients do not perceive taking medications entirely in terms of obeying orders from their physician. Instead, they often compare the costs and benefits as they perceive them within the contexts and constraints of their everyday lives and needs. Furthermore, what appears to be noncompliance from a medical perspective may actually be a way for patients' to exert a measure of control over their medical disorder.[45]

In order to provide a social context for patients' decision making, open and cooperative physician-patient relationships have been shown to be helpful for improving the medication use process.[46] According to Donovan and Blake (1992), the key to improving rates of compliance is "the development of active, co-operative relationships between patients and doctors. For this to be successful, doctors will need to recognize patients' needs and constraints, and to work with patients in the development of treatment regimes. For their part, patients will need to make more explicit their needs and expectations, and particularly how they reach their decisions about their treatments."[47]

Research reported by Bultman and Svarstad (2000) provides support for the importance of practitioner-patient relationships in terms of communication style and patient satisfaction. They found that *initial* communication between physician and patient positively influenced patients' knowledge and initial beliefs about their medication. However, it was the *follow-up* communication style (collaborative/participative) and also patients' *satisfaction* with their overall treatment experience that were predictive of compliance with medication regimens.[48]

Another study, reported by Ciechanowski et al. (2001), used attachment theory as a way to study interpersonal relationships. This theory proposes that the quality of early caregiving influences how an individual perceives and engages in subsequent relationships.[49] A "dismissing" style is one of independence and self-sufficiency because the health care practitioner had been unresponsive or even neglectful of the patient. They reported that patients with diabetes who exhibited "dismissing attachment" had significantly poorer compliance with their treatment than patients who had more attached relationships, regardless of the quality of the communication.[50]

Kerse et al.(2004) studied the effects of physician-patient relationships on medication compliance. They operationalized these relationships in terms of continuity of care, trust in the physician, concordance, and patient enablement. They found that patients who reported high levels of concordance (bidirectional, negotiated agreement) with their physician were one-third more likely to be compliant in taking medications that were prescribed during a medical consultation visit. In contrast, continuity of care, trust in the physician, and enablement were not consistently or not independently related to compliance with medications.[51]

Collectively, these studies suggest that communication and relationships are important for understanding patient compliance. However, it also appears that communication and relationships are not in themselves sufficient for optimizing compliance.[52] The notion of concordance, also referred to as the "taking of medicines based on a partnership," has emerged [53-55] as a vital component for patient compliance and will be discussed next.

Practitioner-Patient Partnerships

It appears that the consideration of both practitioner-patient communication and also practitioner-patient relationships has provided a richer conceptualization for patient compliance. However, the concordance (partnership) concept goes beyond just information exchange and relationships. Concordance is "an agreement reached after negotiation between a patient and health care professional that respects the beliefs and wishes of the patient in determining whether, when and how medicines are to be taken. Although reciprocal, this is an alliance in which the health care professional recognizes the primacy of the patient's decisions about taking the recommended medications."[56] Although practitioners have professional expertise, the concordance (partnership) approach assumes that patients alone know their goals and priorities, preferred medication side effect/benefit trade-offs, lifestyle resources and constraints, skills for evaluating their regimen, and likely self-care they will engage in.[57] Thus, patient compliance no longer is viewed as solely following a doctor's orders, but rather is reflective of the practitioner's ability to "assess and respect patient expertise, giving the patient much more control than in the traditional medical model."[58] Patient compliance is no longer defined only by patient behavior, but also is defined by the health care practitioners' behaviors in assessing and respecting their patients' expertise and desires.

Under this view of compliance (also referred to as concordance), agreement between practitioner and patient should be sought with respect to treatment goals and selecting a medication regimen.[59] The emphasis is on preparing patients to monitor and evaluate their regimens as a foundation for future regimen decisions.[60] Behavioral change is no longer placed exclusively on the patient, but rather it is the practitioner who must often change behaviors in order to come into compliance (concordance). In fact, medication compliance may not even be the primary treatment goal under the concordance concept. Instead, the primary goal might be the continual monitoring and evaluation of treatments as a disease or condition evolves for the patient. This approach allows for flexibility and alterations to treatment regimens in light of the patient's experiences with medications and disease progression.

Such a change in how patient compliance is viewed and conceptualized does not make it easier to achieve, however. Health practitioners have a set of beliefs about the appropriateness of particular medications and about how they should be used based on a biomedical model.[61] These beliefs are shaped by professional training, experience, and scientific evidence. The patient has a different, but equally cogent and valid set of ideas about their own illness, medicines in general, and the medications they are prescribed in particular. These are based on their preferences, beliefs, priorities, and life experiences.[62] Whether to take a medication or not is ultimately the choice of the patient. A successful prescribing process will be characterized by agreement between the practitioner's and patient's opinions. This agreement is not easily reached, but without addressing these issues desired treatment outcomes will not be achieved.[63]

In light of the current ideology of patient compliance, what role can policy play in maximizing the outcomes that are desired from using medication therapy? In the remaining parts of this chapter, we address this question by summarizing roles that various health care stakeholders have served in the past, and by reviewing selected policy trends in the area of compliance. We then conclude the chapter with some ideas for policy options regarding compliance for various stakeholders and our recommendations for the future.

ROLES IN COMPLIANCE

Government

In the 1970s, health policy debate focused on whether government or the medical profession should control the health care system.[64] It appears that these two forms of centralized control were both less promising than allowing more decision-making authority for patients and their agents. There was a deprofessionalization and a depoliticization of health care decision making, which opened up opportunities for more consumer choice within the system.[65] Throughout the 1980s, government regulation was focused on efficiency and equity issues within the policy domain.[66] This approach resulted in deregulation of industries and also the expansion of decision-making authority and choice for health care consumers and their agents.

Since patient compliance is rooted in individual choice, few government policies are devoted to this issue directly. However, in November 1990, the Office of the Inspector General of the Department of Health and Human Services released a report in which they concluded that "clinical pharmacy services add value to patient care ... not only improvements in clinical outcomes and patient compliance, but also reductions in health care utilization costs associated with adverse drug reactions.[67] In light of this report, Congress passed legislation that mandated that pharmacists offer to counsel all Medicaid patients starting in 1993. Most states quickly extended the provision to cover all patients.

Another example of government action for improving compliance was to develop an Action Plan for the Provision of Useful Prescription Medicine Information as a result of a collaborative process mandated by Congress (Public Law 104-180, which was passed on August 6, 1996). This required the Secretary of Health and Human Services to organize a committee to develop a plan to improve oral and written communication to patients about prescription medications. A primary reason for this government action was to improve appropriate medication use in order to improve quality of life for Americans and to reduce waste that is created by the suboptimal use of medications.

These government actions were rooted in the communication and information view of patient compliance, which assumes that information can enhance patient understanding of medication regimens and, thus, compliance.

Payers

As more decision-making authority and choice were being transferred to patients and their agents in the U.S. health care system, payers were afforded opportunities to develop policies that would help empower patients to comply with medication regimens. From a cost savings and waste reduction standpoint, it was in the payers' interest to develop patient compliance and disease management programs to help assure that prescribed medications were used appropriately.

Some examples of these policies include the eighth Report of the Joint National Committee on Prevention, Detection, Evaluation and Treatment of

High Blood Pressure, which called noncompliance the "most significant problem in hypertension control" and made explicit recommendations for health professional action to improve compliance.[68] Another example is the Teach Your Patients About Asthma: Clinician's Guide, which was designed by the National Heart, Blood, and Lung Institute to improve treatment understanding and compliance. It contained instructions for developing a patient/practitioner partnership and a mutually agreeable treatment plan for teaching patients about their medications.[69]

Programs such as these incorporated components of practitioner-patient communication and also relationship building. A shortcoming from these programs typically has been a "one size fits all" approach since they did not incorporate very many of the concordance principles outlined earlier in this chapter through which a more patient-centered approach would be taken.

Pharmaceutical Manufacturers

It is in the interest of pharmaceutical manufacturers to not only have their products prescribed by physicians, but also to have them taken as directed by patients. Appropriate use not only increases the likelihood of desirable outcomes, but also contributes to long-term use by patients with chronic conditions, resulting in greater product sales. Pharmaceutical manufacturers have focused on disease-related factors and therapy-related factors as ways to help contribute to better patient compliance with therapy. Some disease-related factors that can affect compliance include the severity of symptoms, level of disability (physical, psychological, social, and vocational), rate of progression, and the availability of treatments.[70] For example, a chronic condition such as high blood pressure often does not have detectable symptoms and may not cause detectable disability to patients during the early stages of the disease. Manufacturers of products that are used to treat high blood pressure have tried to improve compliance with these medications through educational campaigns for patients and practitioners, reminder programs, and public awareness campaigns. Disease management programs also were developed in collaboration with payers of health care services in an effort to improve compliance by patients with such diseases.

Therapy-related factors that can affect compliance include the complexity of the medication regimen, duration of the treatment, previous treatment failures, frequent changes in treatment, the immediacy of benefits, side effects, and the availability of medical support to deal with them.[71] Manufacturers have developed various drug combinations, dosages, dosage forms, and packaging options to help make it possible to individualize medication regimens for patients so that it will be easier for these patients to comply with their therapies. Manufacturers also have provided research support for investigations in this area. Through this support they have contributed to the evolving understanding of patient compliance. An example of this is the often cited report from the Task Force for Compliance.[72]

A limitation to the policies developed by manufacturers is that educational campaigns, promotional campaigns, public awareness campaigns, disease management programs, and the development of new drug combinations, dosage forms, and packaging options do not always have patient compliance as the primary goal for such activities. Increasing sales, obtaining market share, obtaining preferred formulary placement, and extending patent power in the marketplace are driving forces behind these decisions as well.

Practitioners

Health care practitioners have not always been trained in patient-centered care, and patients are still seeing practitioners from that era. Many of these practitioners have changed their practices into more patient-centered ones, but some still hold to the more traditional medical model of care. More recently, practitioners have been trained in patient-centered care and are applying these techniques to problem of patient compliance.

Professional associations often have written policies about patient compliance that reflect a profession's view of the practitioner's role. For example, the American Pharmacists Association has a policy that states, "pharmacists are responsible for assisting patients to become active, informed decision makers regarding compliance with their prescribed therapeutic plans."[73] Further policy states that "the pharmacist is responsible for initiating pharmacist-patient dialogue and assessing the patient's ability to comprehend and communicate so as to optimize the patient's understanding of and compliance with drug therapy."[74] Practitioners usually agree with such policies, but are faced with barriers in their everyday practice, such as not having enough time to communicate with every patient or not having financial incentives for providing such services for patients.

Patients

Most patients have the desire to use medications appropriately in order to feel better and to live healthier lives. However, they often do not purchase prescribed medications, or they discontinue them prematurely because they are confused about why they are taking a particular medication, don't think that they need the medication, don't think that the medication will work, think that they will experience a side effect, don't think that they can afford the cost, or simply do not want to take it because it reminds them that they have a disease.[75,76]

Organizations such as the American Association of Retired Persons (AARP) devote resources to helping their members understand policy issues related to health care and provide a collective voice for their concerns. Many of the public policy issues of concern are related to the costs of health care and government programs that affect the delivery of health care. Within this focus of concern, the use of prescription drugs has been an important consideration for organizations that represent patients' interests.

Organizations such as AARP have developed information and brochures to help empower patients as they interact with their health care practitioners. Some of these can be used to help patients prepare for these interactions and also be used during the visits to remind patients about what to ask and what to tell their practitioners to make the interaction more patient-centered. In addition, public campaigns have been developed to help patients learn about compliance-enhancing products and services that are available. Numerous medication-compliance aids are available from various companies. A visit to a local pharmacy or a visit to Internet sites will reveal the many compliance aids that are designed to help patients sort their medications and to help them remember to take their medications at the right times.

Medication policy issues of concern to patient groups have been related mostly to how to be empowered in their interactions with health care practitioners and also how to be able to manage their medication therapies, particularly if the therapies are numerous and complicated. A frustration for patients has been that they often are not certain about the reason a prescribing decision was made on their behalf and struggle with deciding about whether the potential benefits of the medication outweigh the potential risks and costs of the therapy.

POLICY TRENDS IN COMPLIANCE

Before we conclude the chapter with a description of future policy options, we have selected a small number of policy trends that are likely to affect patient compliance in the future. These trends include: (1) direct-to-consumer advertising for prescription drugs, (2) Medicare and Medicaid, (3) information technology, and (4) continuous quality improvement applied to health care systems.

Direct-to-consumer advertising (see also Chapter 19) for prescription drugs was approved by the Food and Drug Administration in the United States and has resulted in more informed and more assertive patients during physician visits.[77] Five percent of American adults receive a prescription each year because they asked for the product based on an advertisement that they saw or heard.[78] These patients want to try the medication to see if it will work, and most of the time report that the result is what they expected.[79,80] This patient-initiated process results in more compliance with the medication regimen since the patient "believes" in the product.[81] However, it appears that the patients who are initiating such prescribing already tended to be relatively compliant with their therapies.[82] What is not known is the effect that direct-to-consumer advertising might have on patients who had not been compliant with their therapies due to not believing that they needed their medication.

Another policy trend is changes in Medicaid and Medicare programs. Both programs now provide prescription drug payment for patients who are eligible to participate in these programs. Over half of all prescriptions dispensed in the United States are likely to be paid for through these programs. Due to financial pressures, it is likely that restrictions will be placed on individual choice regarding therapies. For example, formulary restrictions, prior authorization restrictions, caps, and negotiated prices are likely to be used for these programs, and the effects of these decisions rooted in financial concerns could affect patient compliance behaviors. On the other hand, these policies also require that "medication therapy management services" would be provided to patients in these programs so that appropriate drug utilization could be maximized for patients. It is likely that patient compliance will be an important component of such services.

A third policy trend we selected for discussion is information technology (See also Chapter 30). In light of the trends that have placed the patient as the center of care, a new health care consumer has emerged who wants information, choice, and service as part of the health care experience.[83] Informed and engaged in their own care, these patients have the ability to work collaboratively with their health care practitioners to better focus treatment plans on their needs and avoid medical mistakes. Such an approach elevates health information to a position as important to care as a medication, a lab test, or a medical procedure. Information guides patient decisions, changes patient behaviors, and often can help patients reach treatment outcomes. Without information, patients can do themselves harm, overlook effective therapeutic plans, and undermine the best-designed therapeutic plans.[84] When information is seen as care, it triggers new standards of quality, new expectations, and becomes a reimbursable health care service. Such a focus opens the door for information technologies to help increase the convenience of information, the quality of information, and the integration of information to match the health situation, the health system, and the patient.

A final trend we would like to present is the notion of continuous quality improvement and how it can be applied to health care systems as a way to improve patient compliance. The continuous quality improvement perspective holds that patients' experiences should serve as the fundamental source for the definition of health care quality.[85] Berwick developed ten rules as a framework for the enhancement of health care delivery systems that are quite similar to the current ideology of patient compliance outlined earlier. As this approach is adopted in health care, it is likely that opportunities for enhanced patient compliance will become available. Table 28.1 summarizes Berwick's rules for continuous quality improvement in health care.

TABLE 28.1. Continuous quality improvement applied to health care systems. (Adapted from Berwick's 10 Rules.[85])

Traditional (medical-centered) approach	Continuous quality improvement (patient-centered) approach
Care is based primarily on health care visits.	Care is based on continuous healing relationships.
Professional autonomy drives variations in care plans.	Care is customized according to patients' needs and values.
Professionals control care.	The patient is the source of control.
Information is a record.	Knowledge is shared freely. Information is a treatment.[83]
Decision making is based on a practitioner's training and experience.	Decision making is based on evidence and on patient's desires.[53-55]
"Do no harm" is an individual practitioner's responsibility.	Patient safety is a health system property.
Secrecy is necessary.	Transparency is necessary.
The system reacts to needs.	Needs are anticipated.
Cost reduction is sought.	Waste is continuously decreased.
Preference is given to professional roles over a coordinated system.	Cooperation among practitioners is a priority for exchanging information within a coordinated system.
Focus is on patient compliance which is the extent to which a patient's behavior coincides with medical instructions for taking medicines.[22]	Focus is on concordance which is the extent to which an agreement is reached after negotiation between a patient and health care practitioner that respects the beliefs and wishes of the patient in determining whether, when and how medicines are to be taken.[53]

POLICY OPTIONS FOR COMPLIANCE

In this chapter, we established that patient compliance is a primary determinant of treatment success. We traced the development of compliance as an ideology, described the roles that various health care stakeholders have played in the area of patient compliance, and highlighted some health care trends that might affect patient compliance in the future. Now, we would like to conclude the chapter with ideas for policy options that stakeholders can use to contribute to patient compliance in the future.

Government

Policymakers can impact patient compliance through the decisions they make regarding health care system and health care delivery policies. As these decisions are made, the important effects of patient compliance can and should be considered. For example, patient compliance should be viewed as an important modifier of health system effectiveness.[86] When health programs and systems are evaluated, resource utilization and efficacy of interventions under controlled trials are often utilized as the relevant metrics. However, consideration should be given to how compliance could affect the success or failure of programs and systems. It is possible that interventions that improve patient compliance would be the best investment for tackling chronic conditions effectively.[87]

Payers

Entities that coordinate the payment of health care typically are organized into complex systems. In developed countries, such as the United States, a shift in disease burden from acute to chronic diseases has occurred. This shift has rendered acute-care models of health service delivery inadequate to address the health needs of the population.[88] A need exists for these systems to evolve so that they can address the treatment of chronic conditions over long periods of time. A number of changes could be made to help in this regard. For example, current financial incentives often are based on maximization of short-term returns and also tend to be compartmentalized between competing departments within the system. A long-term, integrated approach could help develop incentives that would be more in line with patient-compliance-enhancing strategies. Such changes could result in appointment lengths, fee structures, resource allocation, continuity of care, information sharing, communication patterns, and practitioner-patient partnerships that result in compliance enhancing rather than compliance reducing environments.

Pharmaceutical Manufacturers

As developers and promoters of drug products, pharmaceutical manufacturers collect, analyze, and disseminate vast amounts of information about their products. Even though the information required by the U.S. Food and Drug Administration is still primarily related to safety and efficacy under controlled clinical trial conditions, a need exists for both premarketing and postmarketing information about the effectiveness of these products under naturalistic conditions. An important contribution to patient compliance with these products would be the sharing of premarketing and postmarketing studies that help practitioners and patients understand the relative advantages of drug products in terms of how these products can be tailored to individual needs and desires.

Some of this information is being disseminated through direct-to-consumer advertising and through evidence submitted to formulary decision makers as they consider the preferential placement of medications onto formulary lists. However, more transparent and thorough dissemination would benefit society and individuals, and, in the long run, could help pharmaceutical manufacturers' self-interests through the effect that such information could have on patient compliance with the medications.

Practitioners

Health care practitioners can have a significant impact on patient compliance if they change their behaviors from being medical-centered to being more patient-centered. The development of active, cooperative relationships between practitioners and patients in which an agreement about how medications are to be taken is reached that respects the beliefs and wishes of the patient is not an easy task. Models for educating and training health care practitioners are embracing the patient-centered approach and also are embracing models of practice that are collaborative with patients and integrated among the whole health care team. What appears to be lacking is the suitable practice environment in which such a patient-centered approach can be applied. Many practitioners work in environments that are more conducive to treating acute conditions and one-time services, and less conducive to treating the more commonly encountered chronic-care patient.

Patients

Patients will likely be the determining factor in how patient compliance evolves over the next decades in the United States. If patients become active participants in making treatment decisions and solving problems, the health care system is likely to change in concert. However, if patients deem the costs of such involvement to be too high, they may settle for a less participative role in the health care system. They may accept an impersonal system and use alternative systems for obtaining information. As in the past, they may passively accept health care practitioner's advice and decide later about whether or not to follow that advice.

We believe that in light of information technology, changes in health care practitioner training, and emerging characteristics of new generations of patients (e.g., baby boomers, Generation X, Millennials), patients will take on active roles in their health care decision making. These trends open up new doors for improving patient compliance through communication, relationships, and partnerships.

SUMMARY

Noncompliance with medication therapies may be the most important factor that compromises the ability to achieve the full potential from medications. Noncompliance causes medical and psychosocial complications of disease, reduces patients' quality of life, and wastes health care resources. Although compliance with self-administered medications depends upon individual patient choices, important public policy considerations can help improve compliance through their effects on health care systems and health service delivery processes.

As health care stakeholders develop and implement policies, attention should be paid to how those policies and their implementation will affect the ability for practitioners and patients to come to agreement with respect to treatment goals and selecting a regimen. Emphasis should be placed on preparing patients to monitor and evaluate their regimens as a foundation for future regimen decisions. Compliance with medication therapies is as much dependent on practitioners' behaviors as it is on patients' behaviors. A successful medication-use process will be characterized by agreement between the practitioner's and patient's opinions. This agreement is not easily reached, but without addressing these issues, desired outcomes will not be achieved. Policy development and implementation that either enhance or deter these practitioner-patient partnerships are important considerations for patient compliance with medication therapies.

DISCUSSION QUESTIONS

1. Of the evidence provided in this chapter regarding the clinical and economic impact of noncompliance with medication therapies, which were the most surprising to you? Why?
2. Do you agree that noncompliance with medication therapy is the "single most important modifiable factor that compromises treatment outcome"? What are some other factors that have an impact on treatment outcome?
3. Discuss the impact that practitioner-patient communication can have on compliance.
4. Discuss the impact that practitioner-patient relationships can have on compliance.
5. Discuss the impact that practitioner-patient partnerships (concordance) can have on compliance.
6. If you were asked to choose only one policy change in order to affect patient compliance, what would that policy change be?

NOTES

1. Cramer J et al. (1989). "How Often is Medication Taken as Prescribed?" *Journal of the American Medical Association* 261 (June): 3273-3277.

2. Cramer J et al. (1989).

3. National Council on Patient Information and Education (1991). "October is Talk About Prescriptions Month." *Talk About Prescriptions Month Newsletter.* Washington DC: National Council on Patient Information and Education.

4. National Council on Patient Information and Education (1990). *Talk About Prescriptions Month Newsletter.* Washington DC: National Council on Patient Information and Education.

5. Peck C and N King (1982). "Increasing Patient Compliance with Prescriptions." *Journal of the American Medical Association* 248 (December): 2874-2877.

6. Perrin FV (1988). "Improving Communication with Your Patients." *Drug Topics* May 2: 48, 50, 52, 54, 56.

7. Office of the Inspector General (1990). *Medication Regimens: Causes of Noncompliance.* Washington, DC: U.S. Department of Health and Human Services.

8. American Pharmaceutical Association (1990). "When Adults Take Medicine: Improper Use a National Health Problem." *Pharmacy Update* October 1: 5-6.

9. Sullivan SD, DH Kreling, and TK Hazlet (1990). "Noncompliance with Medication Regimens and Subsequent Hospitalizations: A Literature Analysis and Cost of Hospitalization Estimate." *Journal of Research in Pharmaceutical Economics* 2(2): 19-33.

10. Schering Laboratories (1987). "The Forgetful Patient." Schering Report IX. Kenilworth, NJ: Schering Laboratories.

11. Schering Laboratories (1992). "Improving Patient Compliance: Is There a Pharmacist in the House?" Schering Report XIV. Kenilworth, NJ: Schering Laboratories.

12. The Task Force for Compliance (1993). *Noncompliance with Medications: An Economic Tragedy with Important Implications for Health Care Reform.* John Hawks, Task Force Director. Baltimore, MD: The Task Force for Compliance.

13. World Health Organization (2003). *Adherence to Long-Term Therapies: Evidence for Action.* Geneva, Switzerland: World Health Organization.

14. World Health Organization (2003).

15. World Health Organization (2003).

16. National Council on Patient Information and Education (1990).

17. McCombs JS, MB Nichol, CM Newman, and DA Sclar (1994). "The Costs of Interrupting Antihypertensive Drug Therapy in a Medicaid Population." *Medical Care* 32(3): 214-226.

18. Col N, JE Fanale, and P Kronholm (1990). "The Role of Medication Noncompliance and Adverse Drug Reactions in Hospitalizations of the Elderly." *Archives of Internal Medicine* 150(4): 841-845.

19. Svarstad BL, TI Shireman, and JK Sweeney (2001). "Using Drug Claims Data to Assess the Relationship of Medication Adherence with Hospitalization and Costs." *Psychiatric Services* 52(6): 805-811.

20. Kennedy J and C Erb (2002). "Prescription Noncompliance due to Cost Among Adults with Disabilities in the United States." *American Journal of Public Health* 92(7): 1120-1124.

21. World Health Organization (2003).

22. Haynes RB (1979). Introduction. In RB Haynes, DL Sacket, and DW Taylor (eds.), *Compliance in Health Care* (pp. 1-10). Baltimore, MD: Johns Hopkins University Press.

23. Haynes RB (1979).

24. Schering Laboratories (1987).

25. Rogers PG and WR Bullman (1995). "Prescription Medication Compliance: A Review of the Baseline of Knowledge—A Report of the National Council on Patient Information and Education." *Journal of Pharmacoepidemiology* 3(2): 3-36.

26. Schering Laboratories (1987).

27. Rogers PG and WR Bullman (1995).

28. Schering Laboratories (1987).

29. Schering Laboratories (1987).

30. Schering Laboratories (1987).

31. Schernitzki P, JL Bootman, J Byers, et al. (1980). "Demographic Characteristics of Elderly Drug Overdose Patients Admitted to a Hospital Emergency Department." *Journal of the American Geriatric Society* 28: 544-546.

32. Bush PJ et al. (1984). "Use of Sedatives and Hypnotics Prescribed in a Family Practice." *Southern Medical Journal* 77(June): 677-681.

33. Glasgow R et al. (1987). "Self-Care Behaviors and Glycemic Control in Type I Diabetes." *Journal of Chronic Disease* 40: 399-412.

34. Conrad P (1985). "The Meaning of Medications: Another Look at Compliance." *Social Science and Medicine* 20: 29-37.

35. Trostle JA (1997). "The History and Meaning of Patient Compliance As an Ideology." In DS Gochman (ed.), *Handbook of Health Behavior Research II: Provider Determinants* (pp. 109-124). New York: Plenum Press.

36. Morse EV, PM Simon, M Coburn, et al. (1991). "Determinants of Subject Compliance Within an Experimental Anti-HIV Drug Protocol." *Social Science and Medicine* 32: 1161-1167.

37. Manson A (1988). "Language Concordance as a Determinant of Patient Compliance and Emergency Room use in Patients with Asthma." *Medical Care* 26: 1119-1128.

38. Svarstad BL (1986). "Patient-Practitioner Relationships and Compliance with Prescribed Medical Regimens." In L Aiken and D Mechanic (eds.), *Applications of Social Science to Clinical Medicine and Health Policy* (pp. 438-459). New Brunswick, NJ: Rutgers University Press.

39. Svarstad BL (1987). "The Relationship Between Patient Communication and Compliance." In *Topics in Pharmaceutical Sciences*. The Hauge, the Netherlands: Elsevier Publishers.

40. Ley P (1988). "The Benefits of Improved Communication." In P Ley, *Communicating with Patients* (pp. 157-171). London: Croom Helm.

41. Roter D and J Hall (1992). *Doctors Talking with Patients/Patients Talking with Doctors: Improving Communication in Medical Visits.* Westport, CT: Auburn House.

42. Roter D (1995). "Advancing the Physician's Contribution to Enhancing Compliance." *Journal of Pharmacoepidemiology* 3(2): 37-48.

43. Donovan JL and DR Blake (1992). "Patient Non-Compliance: Deviance or Reasoned Decision-Making?" *Social Science and Medicine* 34(5): 507-513.

44. Donovan JL and DR Blake (1992).

45. Conrad P (1985). "The Meaning of Medications: Another Look at Compliance." *Social Science and Medicine* 20(1): 39-37.

46. Donovan JL and DR Blake (1992).

47. Donovan JL and DR Blake (1992).

48. Bultman DC and BL Svarstad (2000). "Effects of Physician Communication Style on Client Medication Beliefs and Adherence with Antidepressant Treatment." *Patient Education and Counseling* 40: 173-185.

49. Ciechanowski PS, WJ Katon, JE Russo, and EA Walker (2001). "The Patient-Provider Relationship: Attachment Theory and Adherence to Treatment in Diabetes." *The American Journal of Psychiatry* 158(1): 29-35.

50. Ciechanowski PS, WJ Katon, JE Russo, and EA Walker (2001).

51. Kerse N, S Buetow, A Mainous, et al. (2004). "Physician- Patient Relationship and Medication Compliance: A Primary Care Investigation." *Annals of Family Medicine* 2(5): 455-461.

52. Kerse N, S Buetow, A Mainous, et al. (2004).

53. Chewning B, L Boh, J Wiederholt, et al. (2001). "Does the Concordance Concept Serve Patient Medication Management?" *The International Journal of Pharmacy Practice* June: 71-79.

54. National Prescribing Centre (2006). Medicines Partnership. Available at: http://www.npc.co.uk/med_partnership/index.htm.

55. Chewning, B and B Sleath (1996). "Medication Decision-Making and Management: A Client-Centered Model." *Social Science and Medicine* 42(3): 389-398.

56. Chewning B, L Boh, J Wiederholt, et al. (2001).

57. National Prescribing Centre (2006).

58. Chewning B, L Boh, J Wiederholt, et al. (2001).

59. Chewning, B and B Sleath (1996).

60. Chewning B, L Boh, J Wiederholt, et al. (2001).

61. National Prescribing Centre (2006).

62. National Prescribing Centre (2006).

63. Chewning, B and B Sleath (1996).

64. Havighurst CC (1986). "The Changing Locus of Decision Making in the Health Care Sector." *Journal of Health Politics, Policy and Law* 11(4): 697-735.

65. Havighurst CC (1986).

66. Panel on the Government and the Regulation of Corporate and Individual Decisions (1980). *Government and the Regulation of Corporate and Individual Decisions in the Eighties.* Englewood Cliffs, NJ: Prentice-Hall, Inc.

67. Kusserow RP (1990). The Clinical Role of the Community Pharmacist. Report of the Office of the Inspector General. Washington, DC: U.S. Department of Health and Human Services.

68. Rogers PG and WR Bullman (1995).

69. Rogers PG and WR Bullman (1995).

70. World Health Organization (2003).

71. World Health Organization (2003).

72. The Task Force for Compliance (1993).

73. American Pharmacists Association (1993). "Patient Compliance: Pharmacists' Responsibilities." *American Pharmacy* July NS33(7): 55.

74. American Pharmacists Association (2002). "Pharmacist/Patient Communication." *Journal of the American Pharmacists Association* NS2(5) (Suppl. 1): 563.

75. The Task Force for Compliance (1993).

76. American Association of Retired Persons (1992). *A Survey on the Need for a Prescription Drug Benefit Under the Medicare Program.* Washington, DC: AARP.

77. Schommer JC, RL Singh, RA Hansen (2005). "Distinguishing Characteristics of Patients Who Seek More Information or Request a Prescription in Response to Direct-to-Consumer Advertisements." *Research in Social and Administrative Pharmacy* 1(2): 231-250.

78. Schommer JC, RL Singh, RA Hansen (2005).

79. Schommer JC, RL Singh, RA Hansen (2005).

80. Glasgow C, JC Schommer, K Gupta, K Pierson (2002). "Promotion of Prescription Drugs to Consumers: Case Study Results." *Journal of Managed Care Pharmacy* 8: 512-518.

81. Weissman JS, D Blumenthal, AJ Silk, et al. (2003). "Consumers' Reports on the Health Effects of Direct-to-Consumer Drug Advertising." *Health Affairs* February 26 (Suppl. Web Exclusives): W3, 82-95.

82. White HJ, LP Draves, R Soong, C Moore (2004). "Ask Your Doctor! Measuring the Effect of Direct-to-Consumer Communications in the World's Largest Healthcare Market." *International Journal of Advertising* 23: 53-68.

83. Kemper DW and M Mettler (2002). *Information Therapy.* Center for Information Therapy. Boise, ID: Healthwise, Incorporated.

84. Kemper DW and M Mettler (2002).

85. Berwick DM (2002). "A User's Manual for the IOM's 'Quality Chasm' Report." *Health Affairs* 21(3): 80-90.

86. World Health Organization (2003).

87. World Health Organization (2003).

88. World Health Organization (2003).

Chapter 29

Electronic Technology

Gordon Schiff
Bill G. Felkey

INTRODUCTION

Electronic information technology is such an integral factor and force in our medication use and policy environment that it is difficult to isolate and package the topic in a separate chapter. The need for high quality information is acute, and information management is a common denominator that permeates all disciplines and specialties. An even greater challenge is presenting a snapshot of the state of the art given its dynamic nature and uneven implementation. Given all the hype and failed promises, presenting a balanced view likewise represents a formidable challenge. A final difficult task, but one we eagerly will attempt, is to bring together a more unified and collaborative perspective from our two different vantage points—medicine and pharmacy, two disciplines whose professional activities and information databases have historically been more disconnected than shared. This has been true despite both professions sharing similar patient-focused missions, both with strong emphases on safe and effective medication use.

Given these challenges, only a high-level overview, one that attempts to give big-picture lessons and perspectives yet is grounded in clinical realities can best serve the readers of this book. Thus, we will focus less on particular technologies, and more on broad trends, issues, and insights. Coming at the end of this book's journey through the various aspects of our pharmaceutical care system, this chapter will both draw upon issues raised by these pharmacy policy topics generally as well as point to the specific impact of electronic information technology on pharmacy policy formation. The chapter reflects our strong view that information technology will play a major role in shaping how policy is going to be developed, implemented, and integrated into myriad clinical care settings. What directions the policy and application of these tools will take is an uncertain and contentious fore-cast—one that will require thoughtful and informed choices. Because those choices will need to be first and foremost based on the needs of the patients and their practitioners, to the greatest extent possible, we will be focusing on clinical applications of computer technology and how it can make health care more efficient and effective.

New technologies are emerging at a rapid pace, making it very difficult to make accurate predictions about how a technologically transformed health care landscape will look, even five years into the future. Yet at the same time, progress in the actual implementation of available technologies has been slow and limited, with many false starts and barriers to adoption, which we will touch on in this chapter. Rapid technologic change makes the formulation of policy and regulations very challenging when the discovery and policy formation process takes place over longer time frames. Policy and regulatory documents that are produced, targeting a technology field where quick obsolescence is the rule, may no longer be relevant when they are enacted. Therefore, understanding technology and information princi-ples will assist regulators no matter how quickly the specific features and benefits of new technologies emerge.[1,2]

One of the most basic concepts to understand is the purpose of informa-tion and technology. At the most fundamental level, information has the purpose of reducing uncertainty during decision making. Technology has two primary impacts as it relates to the work of human beings: it can either be used to enhance the work of a human being or replace work done by hu-mans.[3] Depending on the policy context and methods used for the imple-mentation of a specific type of hardware or software solution, these two purposes for technology may conflict, or even produce synergies. Much of the historical introduction of new labor-saving technologies have been experienced as a threat to workers and their jobs, and thus met with resis-tance.[4,5] We believe that positively involving health care practitioners, par-ticularly physicians and pharmacists, to creatively use these tools and inno-vations to enhance the quality of the care they deliver should be the most important goal of their introduction. Even those who consider cost savings to be their primary aim will be missing the real opportunities for savings that can be achieved by a broader quality-directed focus rather than a nar-row labor cost-cutting focus. Health care providers must be supported to take the offensive, fully cognizant of the problems of the status quo and the need for change—to take the initiative to use the often misdirected potential of this powerful tool for improving the way medications are used.[6]

FIVE ROLES FOR HEALTH CARE/
MEDICATION TECHNOLOGY

Experience in patient safety and quality improvement have identified a number of complementary potentials for information technology for preventing errors and adverse events as well as facilitating earlier recognition and reporting of problems.[7] First and foremost is the need "to decrease reliance on human memory."[8] Leaders in the field of evidence-based medicine believe that the complexity of practice is such that it has exceeded the capacity of the unaided human mind.[9] Clearly computer and information technology are key to overcoming this limitation. As we will see in our discussion of clinical decision support—the epitome of this type of memory-aiding information delivery—the more electronic medication-related information can be delivered in a timely way, customized with a high degree of specificity for the particular patient and clinical situation, the more likely it will be used and useful.

A second related, basic function of information and electronic technology is to improve communication among caregivers. One major requirement is to improve communication between physicians, pharmacists, and patients. Care can thereby be radically transformed by information technology. At the most basic level, communication about a patient's medicines requires everyone to be "working off the same page," which requires creation of a single shared medication profile, initially, and eventually a shared, comprehensive electronic medical record. This is needed to replace what currently can be more than a dozen different "medication profiles" for a particular patient. These often "unreconciled profiles" might include: (1) the list in the retail pharmacy computer, (2) outpatient physicians' (primary care and specialists) notes and orders, (3) multiple conflicting inpatient profiles including handwritten and computerized orders, (4) the nursing MAR (medication administration record), (5) electronic dispensing cabinet (e.g., Pyxis) profiles, (6) anesthesia records, (7) discharge prescriptions, (8) the patient's "brown bag" of assorted medications and alternative/herbal remedies he or she may or may not be taking, (9) handwritten medication pocket cards, (10) aggregated pharmacy benefit insurance claims (that pool transactions from multiple sources), (11) Web-based (provider or patient maintained) profiles, (12) OTC drug or grocery store or mail-order purchases, not to mention medications borrowed from relatives or "free samples" acquired from a variety of sources. Thus an essential focus of communication-enhancing technologies must be the unification and simplification of these paper and electronic "records, which represents a modern-day and worsening Tower of Babel with few of these systems able to 'talk' to each other."[10]

A third, broad category of technology functions are those deployed to more reliably ensure the carrying out of simple repetitive tasks that, because of their very nature (the tasks and the people), humans do not always perform reliably. Technology will be needed to overcome current human workflow limitations, whether due to frequent interruptions or distractions, lack of time for repeated manual checks, or lack of interest due to their sheer volume or boring nature (recording detailed information about medication administration, teaching the same diabetes program over and over, etc.). These activities are often good candidates for reengineering with new technologic tools. Bar coding is an example of a tool that can function in this way. Unlike in supermarkets or factory inventory control, this relatively simple technology is in its infancy in health care and may be trailing industries such as banking and finance by as much as ten years.[11]

A fourth, often more subtle and unrecognized function for information technology is to provide more evidence-based practice standards, a lack of which results in questionable practice variation. This concept takes us beyond merely timely delivery of needed bits of information. Many aspects of medication use are highly individualized, which is good if this is based on individual patient characteristics (and the essence of the promise of the pharmacogenomic revolution). However, if variations instead stem from a lack of clear standards, personal preferences based on insufficient or contradictory evidence, or worse yet, irrational factors or impulses (colorful, musical, or titillating ads), then drug therapy can be irrational at best, and wasteful and potentially dangerous at worst. Implementing practice standards can both help expose the lack of or arbitrariness of decision-making rules, force organizations to collectively and prospectively grapple with treatment guidelines, and provide the vehicle for delivering this content at the point of care, once the experts and researcher define appropriate practices.[12,13] This is at times is mistakenly considered to be "cookbook" medicine. Rather, it is a trail that needs to be blazed, where all can more safely and securely travel, with the practitioner and patient free to wander off of it and their own risk (while hopefully taking appropriate precautions).

This leads us to our fifth area, in which modern information technology has an important role to play—monitoring and surveillance. We need to do a much better job monitoring both the individual patient's response to interventions and in aggregating and analyzing large-scale epidemiologic data. Never before has it been possible to evaluate the results of the drug-taking "experiment" (which is in its essence what each administration of a foreign chemical, otherwise known as a "drug," actually is) on such a large scale. Linking large insurance claims databases with outcomes databases (e.g., of subsequent hospitalizations or laboratory records) is the basis of the emerging discipline and function of pharmacoepidemiology. Simple questions would be answered, such as how many patients persist in taking a chronic medication after six or twelve months (surprisingly few it turns out), or examination of more varied health outcomes (often requiring complex risk adjustments for analysis of these observational databases), or evaluating long-term, drug therapy outcomes (most clinical trials seldom look beyond a few weeks or months).[14] Learning from such outcomes data and using this feedback to change practice is essential for improving the use and safety of drugs, yet it has received relatively scant support from policymakers (except briefly after periodic, public disclosures of "unanticipated" toxicities that thousands or even millions of people have been subjected to).

The consumer-electronics industry, has developed and marketed "outcomes monitoring" technologies that can capture and transmit data such as blood pressure readings, blood glucose measurements, and electrocardiograms online, providing real-time feedback and monitoring to the health care system. These "home-health" parameters need to be combined with laboratory data, as lab data is yearning to be electronically linked to medication data. When these two sets of data are cross-linked, new, more reliable and transforming levels of clinically relevant functionality will emerge (see Table 29.1).[15] In this way we can apply evidence-based reasoning to clinical decision making in a way that provides ongoing evidence that improves practice as a by-product of rendering the care and receiving the feedback that helps us evaluate how each patient has responded to interventions. In effect, every patient can benefit from each patient who has gone before, and each patient is contributing to better care for the next. Moreover, we can respond to patient problems that arise before they require emergency room visits, hospitalization, or lead to more serious adverse outcomes.

Thus, we are entering a time when we can become highly connected and interconnected in ways that transform our current health care systems, ways unimaginable in a paper-based system. In this scenario, health care ultimately becomes a closed-loop system with online, real-time connectivity driving appraisal, intervention, and evaluation of outcomes with long-term monitoring supported by a technology-driven system.[16]

LEARNING FROM EXPERIENCE—WHERE WE ARE TODAY: WHAT ARE ISSUES, QUESTIONS TO CONSIDER

To understand where we are today and how we got here, selected key events and trends occurring during that past decade that have played major roles in shaping the current situation and policy issues will be highlighted and summarized. For each, we describe the experience and briefly comment on its relevance for current and future clinical care and technology deploy-

TABLE 29.1. Benefits of linking laboratory and pharmacy data.

Core function	Ways automated lab-pharmacy linkages can help
Drug selection	1. *Lab contraindicates drug:* Automatic alerts to prevent inappropriate prescription or administration 2. *Lab suggests indication for drug:* Alerts clinicians of patients whose regimen is missing an indicated medication
Dosing	3. *Lab affecting drug dose:* Automates adjustment of dosing for patients with preexisting risks such as renal insufficiency 4. *Drug requiring lab for titration:* Feedback of INR or anticonvulsant drug levels to automate intelligent dose adjustments
Monitoring	5. *Abnormal lab signaling toxicity:* Screen for changes in lab parameters that are relevant for that drug, such as liver abnormalities for patients on TB Rx 6. *Drug warranting lab monitoring for toxicity:* Oversee regular monitoring of electrolytes, or CBC for patients on drugs that
Lab interpretation	7. *Drug influencing or interfering with lab:* Can avoid false positive misinterpretation of abnormal resulting from drug interference in vivo or in vitro 8. *Drug impacting on response to lab:* Alerts that remind of prior Rx of same abnormality
Improvement	9. *Drug toxicity/effects surveillance* by monitoring for new drug-lab associations (eg liver abnormalties w/ a new drug) 10. *Quality oversight* by signaling outliers

Note: Electronic linkage of pharmacy data with laboratory data represents a powerful illustration of the potential for information technology, when more fully and creatively deployed, to transform pharmacotherapy delivery and quality. *Source:* Adapted from Schiff, G.D. et al. (2003). Linking laboratory and pharmacy: Opportunities for reducing errors and improving care. *Arch Intern Med* 163(8): 893-900.

ment. For more experienced readers who have lived through many of these events (or in some cases directly participated), we believe that placing these puzzle pieces can help put together the "big picture" of how the landscape appears today and may move in the future. For novices, we believe that knowledge of these events and trends will help establish a baseline from which to weigh the daily news, fads, claims, and disasters. At the end of this section we pose seven questions to challenge you to delve much more deeply into these events to ponder even more profound questions. We leave these questions for you to consider and investigate further, questions begging for more detailed historical and policy research that has yet to be undertaken.

Patient Safety: Medication Overdose of Betsy Lehman and the IOM Publication of To Err Is Human

Although a single patient or book can hardly be responsible for reshaping our understanding of medical and medication errors, it would be impossible to exaggerate the importance and impact of the national patient safety movement that arose in relation to the overdose of Betsy Lehman and the publication of *To Err Is Human*. *Boston Globe* reporter Ms. Lehman received a fourfold cyclophosphamide overdose when the ambiguous regimen instructing "cyclophosphamide dose 4 grams/square meter (of body surface area) over 4 days" was given *each* of four days. Mirroring the cultural shift that permeated the Institute of Medicine (IOM) report—that errors should be opportunities to learn and change, not to find fault and blame—a whole new national patient movement was born, seeking tools to prevent medication errors.[17] Today, if you ask any health care system CEO to list his or her strategic priorities, patient safety will be mentioned. These events and imperatives have helped create much of the impetus for study and deployment of computerized physician order entry (CPOE). The IOM report, along with the two follow-up IOM reports that built on *To Err Is Human (Crossing the Quality Chasm: The IOM Health Care Initiative* and *Patient Safety: Achieving a New Standard for Care),* emphasized information technology and computerized prescribing and decision support (that intelligently programmed could stop dead in its tracks such an overdose) and captured the attention of both the public, academics, and policymakers.[18,19,20,21]

Pioneering Clinical Information and Order Entry Systems: Clinical Information System Development and Research at Institutions Such As Brigham and Women's Hospital, Regenstrief, and LDS Hospital

A series of studies performed at a number of academic institutions that thoughtfully implemented computer order entry during the 1990s showed how CPOE can (1) decrease errors (work by David Bates and Lucian Leape at Harvard's Brigham and Woman's Hospital shows that errors can be decreased up to 80 percent,[22] (2) improve antimicrobial ordering appropriateness or detect adverse drug events (studies by David Classen in Utah LDS Hospitals),[23,24] or (3) assist in monitoring patients on medications (by triggering "corollary orders")[25] or ensuring prevention guidelines are followed (as demonstrated in studies by Clem McDonald, Bill Tierney, Mick Murray, and Marc Overhage at Reginstreif in Indianapolis).[26]This evidence helped others to desire and purchase their own large clinical information systems. Although systems such as those at Brigham, Regenstrief, LDS, and Vanderbilt Medical Center were typically homegrown and their design and implementation was led by academic clinicians, they helped spur a demand and marketplace that was filled by commercial vendors. These commercial systems were more often developed, marketed, and implemented in a less clinician-led and less flexible fashion. These academic pioneers continue to refine the features of their unique systems, and have, with funding assistance of organizations such as the Agency for Healthcare Research and Quality (AHRQ), continued to shape directions for functionality of large information systems.[27]

Federal Initiatives: National Committee on Vital and Health Statistics (NCVHS) Initiatives for National Health Information Infrastructure (NHII) and the Establishment of Office of the National Coordinator for Health Information Technology (ONC)

The appointment of David Brailer as National Coordinator for Health Information Technology, U.S. Department of Health and Human Services (HHS), marked a turning point for federal government's recognition and support for development of a health information technology infrastructure. It built upon on earlier and ongoing initiatives by the National Committee on Vital and Health Statistics (NCVHS) for developing a the National Health Information Infrastructure (NHII). The Office of the National Coordinator for Health Information Technology (ONC), established in 2004, is charged with ensuring coordination of HHS information technology (IT) programs and accelerating the sluggish and uneven progress in adoption of information technologies.[28]

Two ambitious goals immediately announced were widespread adoption of electronic health records (EHRs) within ten years and "interoperability" improvements so that clinicians, patients, and pharmacists can easily exchange health information using advanced and secure electronic communication. This stepping up to the plate by the federal government represents an acknowledgment, even by more market-oriented Republican leaders, that the market alone is not sufficient to deliver needed progress. The United States is in fact falling behind other countries such as the UK (where virtually all prescriptions are already written electronically),[29] and Sweden, the

Netherlands, and Denmark (where most physicians are using electronic medical records).[30] A Leadership Panel report to the ONC (building on the recommendations of another IOM report, *Patient Safety: Achieving a New Standard for Care*) recommended as a key imperative that the federal government should act as "leader, catalyst, and convener" of the nation's health information technology effort.[31] A series of multimillion dollar awards have recently been launched by HHS to develop a nationwide health information network.[32]

Privacy and Security: Health Insurance Portability and Accountability Act (HIPAA)

The U.S. Health Insurance Portability and Accountability Act (HIPAA) was not originally about information technology or privacy, but rather was designed to protect health insurance coverage for workers and their families when they changed or lost their jobs. It was passed in 1996, in the wake of the of the failure of the more sweeping Clinton health plan, as a modest "incremental" bipartisan reform to address insurance "portability" for workers whose health insurance is (as most private health insurance is) tied to their employment. Few anticipated the firestorm that would be triggered by a series of secondary provisions designed to facilitate its implementation.[33]

These provisions, successively "rolled out" over the past five years, initially were designed to streamline and standardize electronic insurance claims (electronic transactions standards). Opening this electronic standard Pandora's box made evident the need for uniform level of protection of all health information that is housed or transmitted electronically and led to development of further complex and controversial rules (privacy rule, security rule) that took nearly a decade to officially go into effect.

Various health care providers have objected to the added burdens imposed in implementing these patient-confidentiality protections, and the debate has on the other side activated patient advocacy groups with extreme privacy/disclosure fears. Nonetheless, the discussions have played an important role in focusing attention and correcting the previously lax (or in many states and institutions, nonexistent), contradictory hodgepodge of existing rules and practices. The most controversial "rule"—the Unique Identifiers Standard—remains without resolution. Although the ability to reliably identify and track the health information of a patient critically depends on being able to uniquely identify that patient, the lack of agreement on how to do this illustrates the lack of trust by some consumer groups and the significant challenges still ahead on how to both protect and make accessible sensitive health information (e.g., patients' HIV or psychiatric medications).[34]

The following quote is taken from a 2004 NCVHS document, and it aptly describes the stalled situation related to unique patient identifiers:

> Plans for a unique patient identifier have been sidelined, primarily due to privacy and confidentiality concerns. The need for this identifier was recognized in the HIPAA legislation passed in 1996, and that need persists today. The full benefits of administrative simplification will not be realized until standard patient identifiers are established. The lack of a unique patient identifier seriously limits the linkage of clinical records across care settings and health plans and impedes the identification and analysis of care episodes that span settings, providers or health benefit coverage arrangements. It also impedes electronic data exchange among clinicians who share responsibility for a patient's care and with patients in the context of a Personal Health Record.[35]

Highly Publicized Electronic Order Entry Information System Adoption Failures and Issues of Error Introduction Coming from Technology That Was Designed to Reduce Errors: Cedars Sinai, University of Pennsylvania, Journal of the American Medical Association Study

Publication of these headline-grabbing experiences served as a lightning rod and shorthand for the failings and critics of electronic systems and CPOE. In fact, the story behind the headlines for these (and other failed) experiences was considerably more complex, and contained more lessons about *how* to (and how not to) implement computer provider order entry rather than *whether* to do so. At Cedars Sinai Hospital, a 20 million dollar customized IT installation featuring a customized Web-based CPOE application was suspended in January 2003, shortly after it went live, due to physician complaints that it slowed their work flow. Because of fears of repeating this failure, CPOE still (now three years later) has not been restarted at Cedar Sinai. A postmortem revealed that eleventh-hour resistance and threats from a minority of affiliated physicians resulted in the CEO backing down from the implementation of the system.[36,37]

At the University of Pennsylvania, patient safety interviews with house staff led medical sociologist Ross Koppel to unexpectedly uncover twenty-two types of errors that residents experienced in their use of the hospitals' electronic ordering system.[38] These errors "facilitated" by their CPOE system were of two types: (1) information errors and (2) human-machine interface flaws. Information errors resulted from fragmentation of data and information, or from circumstances in which a failure to fully integrate a hospital's multiple computer and information systems occurred. For example, physicians were ordering the wrong medication dose of a drug because the CPOE system displayed pharmacy warehouse information that they misinterpreted as being clinical-dosage guidelines rather than just the formulations in stock. They also described human-machine interface flaws that stemmed from technology design that does not "articulate well within the work flow within the organization."[39] In the Pennsylvania system, up to twenty screens were at times needed to view the totality of just one patient's medications, thereby increasing the risk of selecting a wrong medication.[40]

In fairness, the system studied was an older system that has subsequently been replaced.[41] But their experience illustrates the need for continuous monitoring and fixing that must be aggressively undertaken as part of any well-managed technology installation, and it showed that such processes were far from ideal in this university site. Unfortunately, this is the reality for many sites with less flexible/responsive commercial installations, and the findings resonated with frustrations providers were experiencing elsewhere.

PDA–Based Information and Prescribing: Failure of First Generation of CPOE Applications: Success of Drug Knowledge Databases

In the late 1990s and early 2000s, as many physicians began using personal digital assistants (PDAs) for personal date book and address book functions, great hope existed that the PDA would replace the paper prescription pad and serve as the perfect vehicle for moving to electronic prescribing. As this low cost and seemingly physician-friendly technology spread, multiple vendors (iScribe, Allscripts, PocketScript, ePhysician ePad) poured tens of millions of dollars into ultimately a failed effort to develop widely used PDA prescribing applications. These efforts faltered around the "business model" (payment for the hardware, networks, database maintenance) and limitations in the handheld hardware (problems with screen size, connectivity with pharmacies and other clinical data, data security).[42]

Although continuing attempts have been made to resurrect PDA prescribing, desktop electronic prescribing appears to be a more viable approach.[43] The larger-form factor (device/screen size) of a desktop monitor compares favorably to the small-form factor of the PDA screen, thus the greater information real estate of the desktop is driving usability in actual practice environments. On the desktop or notebook computer screen, the ability to see a synopsis of information that might take more than ten screen changes to cover on the PDA makes the larger area the clear choice. On the other hand, when a workstation is unavailable or inconvenient, the ability to connect to systems using more portable technology is possible and may be necessary. Thus, an array of one to three information appliances may be employed by prescribers. Typically these would be a stationary workstation, a notebook/tablet/subnotebook computer and a smartphone. [44]

In marked contrast to the failures of handheld electronic prescribing, has been the huge success of PDA drug references such as Epocrates (other examples include Lexi-Drugs, and Medical Letter Handheld Edition). A survey of internists by the American College of Physicians found that more than 80 percent of handheld owners used their devices to access drug information. [45] A Harvard survey of Epocrates users found that users reported that Epocrates Rx saves time during information retrieval, is easily incorporated into their usual workflow, and improves drug-related decision making. Users also perceived that it reduced the rate of preventable adverse drug events. [46]

Business Initiatives: The Leapfrog Group for Patient Safety: Private Purchasers Coalition Push Electronic Prescribing

In 2000 the Leapfrog Group, a coalition of nearly two hundred Fortune 500 corporations and other purchasers of health care, launched its initiative to improve health care quality and safety. [47] The initiative focused on three key areas for improvement: steering patient referrals for procedures to higher quality/more experienced hospitals, ICU physician staffing with critical care specialists, and, most important, computerized physician order entry. By putting the most powerful purchasers in the county on record encouraging CPOE, a tremendous impetus was added to the movement to CPOE. This "urging" was backed up by a multipronged effort to give added weight to these recommendations, including publicly publishing on their Web site how well each hospital (in targeted geographic areas) performed on their CPOE report card, as well as creating financial incentives to reward (or in some cases punish) institutions based on their scores. These incentives are based on the firm belief by Leapfrog that purchaser incentives and rewards are the key to improved quality (an assumption that some such as Don Berwick have questioned). [48] Thus, Leapfrog is behind the growing movement for pay for performance. Both political and financial pressures such as these are intended to accelerate progress to CPOE as well as fuel the growth of electronic medical records and data aggregation in clinical data repositories (CDRs), which will be produced as a by-product of health care providers (physician practices, hospitals) rendering care to comply with reporting requirements.[49,50] (See Exhibit 29.1.)

PROBLEMS AND CONTRADICTIONS IN ELECTRONIC SOLUTIONS

In this section we will briefly touch upon a number of formidable (but we believe, in theory, surmountable) problems that are pervasive in our current health care IT environment. We raise these here not because they are inherent, nor in the right environment unable to be largely overcome, but because they are challenges that are essential for policymakers to understand and grapple with. Ultimately, the success of IT solutions, and more fundamen-

---

EXHIBIT 29.1. Questions to ask/raise about technology milestone developments

1. What is the "real story" (what patient safety experts term the "second story") behind each of these developments: what really happened, who made it happen and how, what were the behind-the-scenes financial supports and barriers?
2. What has been the lasting impact resulting from each of these developments, and why?
3. Where and what is the data (over time) to better support, characterize, understand their role in the improvement of current and future systems?
4. Why have these not created more accelerated impact/implementation: what have been the barriers, sidetracks, miscues, and controversies?
5. How can stakeholders more fully learn from these events, to more expeditiously and efficiently apply these lessons to remedies to the current and future problems?
6. What are the most obvious and even more subtle mistakes we can learn from, to do differently/better if are to "do it again"? To what extent are we succeeding or failing to learn lessons from these mistakes and why?
7. What are the deeper lessons yet to be learned and what unfinished business remains?

tally the future quality of health care in general, hinges on how effectively they are addressed.

Exceedingly Expensive

IT solutions are costly and often end up costing much more than initial estimates, which are already in the tens of millions for many hospitals and hundreds of thousands of dollars for office practices. Not only do projects often go "over budget," but many hidden costs exist that are rarely accounted for up front. These include cost of maintenance, training, transition disruptions, loss of efficiencies for various members of the team (often the most expensive team members, namely clinicians, even though overall efficiencies for the organization exist), uncovering previously hidden problems that can no longer be ignored and ultimately require fixing (although this is obviously also a plus).

Misguided Technical "Fixes" for More Fundamental Problems

Health care organizations are dysfunctional in myriad ways that have been both well documented and are poorly understood. Problems such as poor communication; department-by-department "silo" behaviors with misaligned and conflicting priorities; complex processes suboptimized for smooth, error-free handoffs; and lack of standardized processes for everything from simple documentation to how surgery is performed. Computerizing this chaos will not solve these problems and can even make them worse. At a larger system level, the U.S. health system is costly and inefficient due to these same dysfunctions, in addition to poor coordination and fragmentation between institutions, as well as a wasteful and patchwork (with many holes) insurance financing system. Adding computers and new technology will add cost but will not remove these more deeply rooted problems. It can even distract us from addressing them. Thus, automating a chaotic system without reengineering it will simply result in an acceleration of speed with which the chaos occurs.

Suboptimal and Often Poor Design

Issues such as human-machine interface factors in screen design, inadequate hardware and software integration, problems with scalability (works fine small scale, but glitches when deployed on larger scale), and poor integration into work flow are ubiquitous. Many applications are designed with insufficient input from knowledgeable frontline staff. Worse yet, the process of iteratively debugging problems in design and improving work flow is often shortchanged in the name of "standardization."

Response Time, Downtime, Crashes, Viruses, and Hardware Failures

By definition these problems, when they occur, are almost always "unexpected," yet they should be anticipated during every implementation and throughout the application use cycle. Organizations have varying IT protections and processes to deal with these issues, but it would be impossible to calculate the enormous collective impacts and costs of these failures on clinicians trying to do their jobs. Past problems are often written off as "we've licked those" while new failures are rationalized as "unanticipatable surprises."

Deferred Improvement and Waiting for the Computer

We have watched as problem after problem within our organizations are placed on the "back burner," awaiting the new computer system/solution to be implemented, deferring action for months or years, unjustifiably exposing patients to risks and staff to a message of complacency. Many of these problems indeed can be more effectively tackled by new computer functionality (such as CPOE to prevent dosing errors, or drug allergy mishaps). But institutions will need a more thoughtful and critical approach to strike a balance between waiting versus improving now. Often these deferred improvements are misunderstood or miscommunicated as being amenable to a simple computer fix, when in fact they are complex problems, addressable only by interactive vendor upgrade cycles, small process improvement by the end users, and testing and feedback by all stakeholders.

Losses in Clinician Time and Efficiency

Computers can and often do save time, but not always. For example, implementation of electronic health records in outpatient primary care practices (especially those that include computer documentation) invariably slows or impairs productivity from 15 to 50 percent during its initial stages.[51,52] Studies on time impacts, once beyond the initial implementation and learning stages, as well as transferring all patients to a new system (each patient in effect a new patient for weeks to months) have had mixed results.[53] But in our view, many functions could and need to be markedly improved to speed clinician entry, navigation, and display data into a much better organized view.

Poor Interconnectivity, Particularly Between Pharmacy and Prescribers

One recent survey from the *KLAS CPOE Digest* found that in 36 percent of hospitals using CPOE, the prescription could not be electronically entered into their own pharmacy computer electronically because the pharmacy and CPOE computers could not talk to one another.[54] Instead, the electronically ordered prescriptions had to be printed out on paper and then be manually reentered by the pharmacist! This near farcical situation pales in comparison to this being the rule rather than the exception in most settings (VA and Kaiser are notable exceptions).[55,56,57] Not only is such double entry inefficient, but it is more error-prone and squanders opportunities for joint electronic decision support and two-way communication between pharmacist and physician. And, at the pharmacy end, it means that pharmacists rarely have access to important clinical data such as diagnoses or laboratory results. Looking at the bigger picture, as a nation we are spending hundreds of millions dollars per year on proprietary clinical IT systems that do not talk to one another.[58]

Volatile, Vendor-Driven Marketplace

Clinicians purchasing electronic medical record systems frequently find themselves at the mercy of various commercial IT vendors, who often have placed sales/marketing ahead of reliable and long-term support. Systems are often oversold with hype and claims that do not match the performance they actually deliver. And because these systems can rarely exchange data with other systems, even importing basic lab data can represent a major interfacing challenge.[59] Many physicians who have purchased prescribing systems/modules from one of the hundreds of current vendors have experienced or risk losing their data and their time investment as companies disappear or are merged with the competitors.[60]

Insufficient "Marketplace Memory" of Failed Implementations

Other than word of mouth and an occasional newspaper or journal article, no systematic, publicly administered and accessible repository collecting and analyzing of failures, both small and large, exists. Vendors come and go, systems are purchased with great fanfare and then quietly abandoned, in what might be considered a conspiracy of silence. (Institutions' executives may be too embarrassed to admit costly mistakes, and IT companies try to avoid bad publicity.) This is unfortunate, because the great promise of IT can be realized only by learning from these negative experiences.

Underdeveloped Mechanisms for Continuous Learning and Revision

Here we are referring not to the dramatic failures noted previously, but rather to the necessity for software development and system implementation to be an ongoing process of testing, feedback, revision, and reassessment. This basic quality cycle and formation of user-accessible knowledge bases is often absent, or has such long delay loops ("annual product releases") that it is useless for rapidly responding and learning from actual experience. One would have hoped that this treasure of free product improvement suggestions would be nourished and quickly responded to by vendors. But this seems rarely the case in systems other than the home-grown academic pioneering systems mentioned previously. Perhaps this is why progress is so much slower and outcomes less uniformly successful than published results.

Unstandardized, Untested Clinical Decision Support Rules That Offer Poor Signal to Noise Ratios

Although many pharmacy and CPOE systems have their own or third party "starter sets" for clinical alert rules (e.g., which drugs require renal dosing adjustments), each hospital finds itself reinventing the wheel in deciding which alerts need to be programmed and at what thresholds they should be triggered (e.g., at what creatinine clearance should renal impairment calculation of the dose of drugs be adjusted and how). Pharmacies are familiar with the overload of drug-drug interactions, "flags" that interrupt their workflow (many of which are false positive alarms). Many pharmacists find such warnings so disruptive and unhelpful that they either turn off the alerts entirely or reduce the "level" of interaction severity to exclude all but the most severe. Currently no group is creating, sharing, and testing standardized rules or alerts. Even when standard sets of alerts are offered by an information-content vendors (e.g., First Databank), the "rules" are proprietary, and many institutions and systems refuse to use them without customization generated by local health system committees.[61]

Large-Scale Errors

CPOE and pharmacy automation have been proven to reduce errors in a number of settings, but growing evidence suggest that these technologies can also introduce errors. Reports of automated filling equipment (robots) being filled with the wrong medication occurs too frequently. These errors then will result in medication errors not just for a single patient but for dozens of patients. Pick-list errors (choosing the wrong patient's name or drug on a pull-down menu), or dosing confusion related to formulations stocked by pharmacy (versus recommended for routine dosing) have been reported from a number of institutions. Another factor that contributes to errors involves technology-fostered complacence, for example, a nurse stopping manual procedures that assure that the correct drug is administered and simply trusting the automated cabinet to dispense the correct dose.[62] More profoundly, it has been claimed that many errors related to complex IT systems can be exceptionally difficult to discover and repair, and the usual human capabilities to troubleshoot in times of crisis can be overwhelmed by complex technological failures.[63,64]

Overreliance on Information from the Computer Rather Than from the Patient

For the many circumstances in which a patient cannot recall the names of prescribed medications, the computer is invaluable, even lifesaving. But exclusive reliance on information from the database, rather than listening to what the patient is trying to tell us ("yes I got that medicine, but I never took it" or "I've been taking my wife's meds"), is dangerous. Studies from Harvard's Brigham's outpatient clinics, venue of some of the best designed programs, suggest that only 70 percent of patient's drugs accurately appear on their computerized medication lists.[65] Will we as professionals be so distracted by the computer terminal that we will compromise our listening skills, or become more dismissive of what patients have to say?

Inability to Streamline Medication Reconciliation

Although the Joint Commission on Accreditation of Healthcare Organizations (JCAHO) established January 1, 2006, as the date organizations must "reconcile" various patients medication lists (i.e., attempt to sort out the list of different medication profiles we list in the first section of this chapter), existing information technology systems were and still are not ready for the task. They do not have the capability to aggregate all of the disparate sources of medication data (mainly due to the disparate data residing in "noninteroperable" silos), and also lack sophisticated tools to help providers match up, sort through, and make decisions on which meds to continue and which to discontinue.

From Information Dearth to Information Overload

The sheer volume of information stored in the computer that is now accessible is overwhelming. Without well-designed filter and display tools, more and more information risks being "lost" in a sea of less important data. As serious as information overload is presently, imagine the magnitude of this problem as the number of inputs grows exponentially in ways we describe in the next section of this chapter.

A VISION OF FUTURE POSSIBILITIES AND CHALLENGES POLICYMAKERS WILL FACE

Regardless of the bumps in the road, the continuing development and introduction of health care technology can't be slowed down. What follows is both a "gee whiz" illustration of "future" technologies and applications, and a taste for how emerging technology will continue to create new issues that policymakers are likely to face. These functions are not just theoretical ideas on some distant horizon, but are technologies already available today, and most are being tested in human subjects in early adopter organizations. Thus, the future is closer than we think. As with past technology development and implementation we will have to sort out the benefits and risks, especially with regard to the cost-effectiveness of such tantalizing technologies. Particularly with technologies that point toward newer and higher levels of monitoring and interconnectivity, we will also have to sort out and balance their appropriateness with due consideration of privacy rights for the individual and the human elements of health care interactions.

Consumer-Driven, Internet-Based Health Technologies

Although only in existence for barely two decades, it is difficult to imagine what the world was like before the Internet. The current Internet protocol (IP) address for each computer on the Internet allows for 4.3 billion discrete machine addresses, and two-thirds of those addresses are already being utilized. The next version of this protocol is currently being implemented and will allow 3.4×10^{66} devices to be interconnected globally. This will allow each of the 6.5 billion humans on the planet to employ up to 5×10^{67} discreet Internet addresses for their personal and professional use.[68]

This number of available machine addresses will be so large that we could potentially assign an address and connect every car, every cell phone, every watch, every appliance, and every other conceivable health-care-related device on the planet to one another. Consider how health care will potentially utilize this level of ubiquitous, pervasive connectivity. We recommend that you digest each scenario and reflect on how current policy and regulation will be challenged to deal with these capabilities in everyday, mainstream practice.

Consider the elderly patient whose heart condition can be monitored continually through a device that resembles a watch. The device uses a combination of cellular and GPS connectivity. A patient is taking a walk by himself on a path in the woods near his home when his heart stops beating properly. His brain loses oxygen and he collapses, alone in the woods. The instrument, which is already available today, would alert a monitoring center that he has collapsed and would transmit exactly how his heart has stopped beating properly. An implanted, wirelessly controlled defibrillator would be remotely activated to attempt to revive the patient. First responders would also be dispatched to the exact place where he had collapsed, and his current medical record would be communicated and accessible on their mobile care information appliances.

Internet transportation technology could protect public health by avoiding traumatic motor vehicle accident injury. Imagine dozens of vehicles are driving along an interstate. Just over the hill from a car you are driving traffic speed has slowed down to less than five miles per hour due to a road construction project. Through Internet connectivity this occurrence would be tracked, and your vehicle would start responding to the situation ahead before your vehicle tops the hill.

Now imagine that a patient with heart failure steps on a digital scale before entering her shower. Her five pound weight gain (increased within twenty-four hours from heart failure related edema) would trigger an intervention procedure to address the potential precipitating factors and take appropriate action. More sophisticated implanted devices whose purpose ranges from assistance in the location of Alzheimer's patients, regulation of reproductive systems, neuromuscular strengthening, hunger control, pain control, and drug delivery will present additional therapeutic alternatives. Genomic levels of technology will bring about even more complicated and fantastic possibilities for consideration.

A Reengineered Vision for Patient Encounters

We envision that many of the previously mentioned measurement and communication technologies will obviate the need for office or emergency room visits (by some estimates up to three-fourths could be eliminated).[69] For those clinician-patient visits that do need to occur, new technologies offer the promise of reengineering patient encounters. Simply walking up to the reception desk will check the patient into the clinic, and capture all insurance and self-recorded (at home or touch screens in the physician's office) subjective data, chief complaint, relevant history, and functional measures.

As health care providers enter the patient exam room, a radio frequency identification (RFID) chip in their name badges will activate a door scanner to track their location in the office, the total time of the encounter (to estimate the service intensity of the visit). Physician and patients working together on the "same side of the screen" will collaborative work together using touch screens as a canvas to "paint" a picture of the patients' problems, medications, and facilitate making and recording of joint medical decision making. Documentation and billing considerations will thus take place as a by-product of rendering care through digital systems.

An emerging form of medical record called the continuity of care record (CCR) will allow the linking of multidisciplinary activities and encounters across offices and hospitals.[70] Closed-loop systems (online and real-time) will engage patients in their own self-care management. Patients will be told what and how to do self-care management procedures such as blood glucose monitoring and insulin administration. Measurement of relevant outcomes will occur at appropriate intervals, and interventions will take place using lower cost, lower intensity means for achieving desired results in chronic conditions at the patient and population level.[71]

Clinical performance will be measured and referenced to counterpart providers in comparable group practice facilities so that providers can learn how their efficiency and effectiveness compares with their peers. It has been demonstrated that providers are frequently motivated by a desire to perform at a level commensurate with relevant peers. No reward or punishment has been needed in the past, only feedback and performance improvement assistance will help achieve desired outcomes.

Reengineering Medication-Use Processes

Technology oversight of the medication-use process and patient safety metrics will also combine several technologies. Bar codes, wireless connectivity, RFID product authentication, and real-time feedback during the point-of-administration component of medication delivery will help reduce errors and provide additional evidence-based resources to analyze breakdowns when they occur. From the moment a medication order is conceptualized in the mind of a prescriber to the pushing of the syringe into the intravenous port of the patient, rules engines will be integrated into each step of the process.

When it is not cost-effective for pharmacy departments to operate twenty-four hours a day, robotics will dispense medications for emergency departments that are operating twenty-four hours a day. Selection of the prescribed medication, labeling, insurance adjudication, and videoconferencing for counseling will take place at dispensing kiosks located in the waiting area of the emergency department. Prescription containers can be handed to the patient appropriately labeled, and then inspected remotely to assure all aspects of the process are done appropriately. Checking prior to dispensing of medication, currently a laborious manual final step by pharmacists, can be accomplished with enormous efficiencies with throughput speeds of nearly four hundred prescriptions per hour per pharmacist with new scanning and barcode technologies (personal communication McKesson automation specialist).

Medication regimen adherence will become more of a closed-loop system. Systems that are matched appropriately for each patients' needs will tell patients what medications should be taken, indicate which medications have been taken, regimen complexity will be reduced by appropriate prompting and organization, and refills for chronic medication will be staged for dispensing in a just-in-time manner. Since elderly patients who live alone could potentially take a fall in a bathroom and break a hip, dispensing devices will also alert caregivers that a potential problem may be taking place at the patient's residency when the device dispensing medication has not been accessed for a predetermined period of time.

Other Potentials for Telemedicine

Telemedicine, telepharmacy, and telenursing offer the promise of helping manage critical shortages of medical disciplines and specialties. The initial focus of these services will address rural coverage, bottlenecks, and acute shortages of specialties such as medical intensivists or disaster relief manpower demands when they take place. Increasingly, telecommunication, and central processing where appropriate, can potentially fill voids in our health care system nationally. Physically impaired health care providers will be able to make contributions without leaving their homes, and those who have withdrawn from full-time practice will still be able to provide care remotely. Health care providers who have aged to the point that fine muscle control needed to perform surgical procedures is a problem can be available to make other contributions, including supervising other surgeons and surgical robots.

Issues Related to Access, Ownership, and Protection of Health Information Technology

Patients are supposed to be legal owner's of the information contained in their medical records. Currently, few would say they feel they own and control this information. The pivotal nub is how to ensure instantaneous access to this information by patients and their designated caregivers, while protecting it from a panoply of undesirable misuses and unauthorized activities. Dilemmas about whether and how to safely communicate health information, such as lab test results, using e-mail are being struggled with.[72] In the meantime, challenges for using electronic forms of communication with patients that contain protected health information are being dealt with by encrypted e-mails. Results from laboratory tests, current drug profiles, scheduling software, and access to health information libraries can all be accessed through Internet browsers when available, but secure forms of communication are required now and in the future.

Health system intranets allow data to be transferred with minimal risk because its connection to the Internet is protected by one or more layers of firewalls. These serve as an electronic no-man's-land between networks and consist set of security-related programs, which protect a network from unauthorized users from other networks. Firewalls can determine whether to forward messages between the PC or internal network and the Internet. Mobile users can get remote access to private networks that have firewalls by using secure log-on procedures and authentication certificates (usually consisting of continuously generated random number keys on keychain display that users carry and type in along with passwords, a process called virtual private networking, or VPN).

Providing access to electronic medical records and the data they contain will require some form of patient consent. One model is the banking industry's ATM card. Patients can carry a health ATM card that will contain a RFID chip supplemented by a biometric fingerprint or iris scanned authentication.

CONCLUSION: FUTURE CHALLENGES

New information technologies will continue to be introduced into health care organizations at a rapid pace. No guarantee exists, however, that they will be optimally designed or that the many millions of dollars invested will be well spent. In this chapter we have presented the perils and promises, and will conclude by summarizing key issues that policymakers will inevitably be facing as they grapple with issues of design and direction of IT implantation.

Globalization of Information and Standards

Because the Internet knows no international boundaries, nor does it (unless highly restricted) limit access to information, exposure to diverse individuals and thinking that may be unsupported by any scientific evidences is a daily reality. What will be the implications for policymaking as this Internet connectivity matures in every aspect of health care? Will an indication for a medication that is approved in Italy need to be considered globally because prescribers will be informed of this information in other countries? Will knowledge workers addressing health care issues through telecommunication channels anywhere in the United States require licensure in every state in which they assist patients?

Integrating Technology with Policies Organizational Practices, Culture, and Work Flow

New technology is rarely "plug and play." One of the repeated lessons of the past is that technology implementation depends more on the people, policies, practices, and politics, than it does on the technology. Although this truism has been written so often it could be considered trite to merely repeat it, we have only a few clues about how to implement more policy-oriented applications. For example, to be effective, computer-delivered decision support requires attention to how physicians and pharmacists work with and react to the technology and how it is implemented. These principles illustrate not only what it is required to successfully implement such real-time alerts and reminders, but also broader lessons applicable to any IT endeavors (see Exhibit 29.2).[73]

EXHIBIT 29.2. Ten commandments for effective clinical decision support: Making the practice of evidence-based medicine a reality

1. *Speed Is Everything.* Speed is a parameter that users value most; cannot slow them down.
2. *Anticipate Needs and Deliver in Real Time.* It's not sufficient to have buried information, must bring it to user at time needed.
3. *Fit into the User's Workflow.* Stand-alone guidelines that need to be manually looked up, rarely get used.
4. *Little Things Can Make a Big Difference.* Developers must make it easy for clinicians to do the right thing.
5. *Recognize that Physicians Will Strongly Resist Stopping.* Clinicians strongly resist warnings to not carry out actions they have decided upon, unless offer easy and acceptable alternatives.
6. *Changing Direction Is Easier than Stopping.* Easier to get prescribers to give a lower dose or less frequent or shorter duration regimens than stopping entirely.
7. *Simple Interventions Work Best.* If intervention can't fit on a single screen, clinicians won't be happy about using it.
8. *Ask for Additional Information Only When You Really Need It.* Although often temping to request additional information from clinician, this should avoided unless absolutely essential to minimize risk of noncompliance.
9. *Monitor Impact, Get Feedback, and Respond.* If clinicians are ignoring alerts (e.g., less than 50 percent of the time an alert sounds), reassess their prudence/design.
10. *Manage and Maintain Your Knowledge-Based Systems.* Clinicians need to constantly monitor alert frequency and responses over time (what if suddenly starts triggering ten times per day?) and keeping knowledge updated; the work to do is frequently underestimated.[75]

Protecting Privacy, Confidentiality, and Security

Policymakers have a duty to protect the public's legally mandated basic rights. These rights include the rights to privacy, confidentiality, and security. Privacy is the legal right to be left alone. Confidentiality is both an ethical principle and a legal right that health professionals will hold secret all information relating to a patient, unless the patient gives consent permitting disclosure. Security provides freedom from risk for patients by adopting measures that prevent unauthorized access to patients' health information. Dramatic security breaches continue to fuel worst fears of privacy zealots. How to best move beyond these dilemmas is a fundamental unresolved challenge.

Achieving Standardization

Health care IT specialists can be overheard to say, "The nice thing about information technology standards in health care is there are so many to pick from." Additional layers of technology called middleware are necessitated because of the lack of standards that allow information layers and hardware to become effectively integrated. Point-to-point interfaces and interface engines could be virtually eliminated if we could agree upon standardization of systems within health care. The private-sector risks enforced imposition of standards by the government, and ultimately international harmonization will become equally important.

Dealing with Information Overload

With more than one billion health care related Web pages, thousands of articles being published in the biomedical literature every week, and hundreds of information alerts preloaded into every clinical system, prioritization and filtration of information is necessary. The sophistication present in most systems allows information to travel for delivery in equal valence (i.e., it has not been filtered for significance to the patient care process). Systems will need to be designed so that important information is emphasized, and less important information is searchable upon demand. New ways to filter and organize information will be a necessity.

Balance and Optimizing Public versus Private Investments

The debate over how much the infrastructure needs to be supported by public funds (similar to the public roadway system) versus allowing the process and innovation to be driven by private capital is an ongoing tension that will shape technology development in profound and unpredictable ways. One recent example particularly germane to drug prescribing, financing, and usage in the United States is the Medicare Modernization Act of 2003. This act makes the U.S. government the largest purchaser of medications in the country. The act contains numerous references and requirements related to electronic transactions and computerized prescribing, which are likely to accelerate the transition to electronic prescribing. An entire IT industry is now developing just to carry out the electronic eligibility, copay, and transaction logistics necessitated by the complex financial requirements of this act. The requirement for competing private pharmaceutical benefits management firms to administer this coverage is contributing to confusion and complexity and stands in contrast to past public sector drug coverage (Medicaid) and systems in other countries, both of which have been the source of rich pharmacoepidemiologic data that risks being fragmented in such a privately administered system.

Achieving Substantial Leaps in Ease of Use and Maintenance of Systems

Pilot studies are underway to test a new generation of chronic disease management programs, electronic medical records, and order entry systems.[74] Research is urgently needed on enhancing the creation and design of computer applications that actually promote exemplary practice activities. The "look and feel" created by computer screens that have been designed to support patient care processes can either enhance or alternatively confuse those end users who employ these applications in their practice. When vendors create these applications for use in health care, less of a priority should be placed on having each vendor's product present radically different product designs. Again these design differences can create confusion on the part of users that may subsequently cause increased errors. We need more research that studies the use of design principles in software that could actually promote and facilitate better patient appraisal, interventions, evaluation, and monitoring. This could be done by guiding end users appropriately through the software management of evidence-based protocols. Advancing our knowledge about this important and practical aspect of information technology could go a long way toward timely, context-sensitive support of all patient care processes.

Interoperability and Interconnectivity

Information transfer across the span of a room or the country continues to be a problem. Standardization will address some of this problem. The creation of data warehouses and clinical data repositories will facilitate better telecommunication within a system or enterprise. A great deal more effort in both horizontal and vertical transfer of protected health information is required. Other industries, such as banking and finance, can be used as models and potentially their infrastructure could be employed to resolve interoperability and interconnectivity issues in health care. "Web services" represents an important approach currently being developed and deployed using XML (extensible markup language) as a standard means of inter-operating between different software applications, running on a variety of platforms and/or frameworks. Web services are characterized by their great interoperability and extensibility and can be combined in a loosely coupled way in order to achieve complex operations.[75]

NOTES

1. Mosley-Williams, A. and C. Williams (2005). Computer applications in clinical practice. *Curr Opin Rheumatol* 17(2): 124-128.

2. Detmer, D.E. and C. Safran (2005). *AMIA's White Paper Policy Series on Timely Issues in Informatics. J Am Med Inform Assoc* 12(4): 495-.

3. Felkey, B.G. and K.N. Barker (1996). Technology and automation in pharmaceutical care. *Journal of the American Pharmaceutical Association* NS36(May): 309-314.

4. Schiff, G.D. and N.I. Goldfield (1994). Deming meets Braverman: Toward a progressive analysis of the continuous quality improvement paradigm. *Int J Health Serv.* 24(4): 655-673.

5. Sclove, R.E. (1995). *Democracy and Technology.* New York: Guilford Press.

6. Schiff, G.D. and T.D. Rucker (1998). Computerized prescribing: Building the electronic infrastructure for better medication usage. *JAMA* 279(13): 1024-1029.

7. Bates, D.W. and A.A. Gawande (2003). Improving safety with information technology. *N Engl J Med* 348(25): 2526-2534.

8. Kohn, L.T., J.M. Corrigan, and M.S. Donaldson (Eds.) (2000). *To Err is Human: Building a Safer Health System.* Institute of Medicine. Washington, DC: National Academy Press.

9. Sackett, D.L. (1998). *Evidence-based medicine. Spine* 23(10): 1085-1086.

10. Rozich, J.D. and R.K. Resar (2001). Medication safety: One organization's approach to the challenge. *JCOM* 8(10): 27-34.

11. Sodorff, M.M. and C.T. Galusha (2004). Impact of point-of-care barcode technology on medication error prevention. *Advances in Pharmacy* 2(2): 168-174.

12. ASHP Council on Professional Affairs (1993). ASHP guidelines on preventing medication errors in hospitals. *AJHP* 50(2): 305-314.

13. Manthous, C. (2004). Leapfrog and critical care: Evidence- and reality-based intensive care for the 21st century. *Am J Med* 116(3): 188-193.

14. Avorn, J. et al. (1998). Persistence of use of lipid-lowering medications: a cross-national study. *JAMA* 279(18): 1458-1462.

15. Schiff, G.D. et al. (2003). Linking laboratory and pharmacy: Opportunities for reducing errors and improving care. *Arch Intern Med* 163(8): 893-900.

16. Garg, A.X. et al. (2005). Effects of computerized clinical decision support systems on practitioner performance and patient outcomes: A systematic review. *JAMA* 293(10): 1223-1238.

17. Conway, J.B. (2004). Developing a strategic plan: Leadership for organizational change. *Psychiatr Serv* 55(3): 259-260.

18. Kohn, L.T., J.M. Corrigan, and M.S. Donaldson (Eds.) (2000).

19. Institute of Medicine (2001). *Crossing the Quality Chasm: A New Health System for the 21st Century.* Washington, DC: National Academy Press.

20. Aspden, P. (2004). *Patient Safety: Achieving a New Standard for Care.* Washington, DC: National Academy Press.

21. Leape, L.L.M. and D.M.M. Berwick (2005). Five years after *To Err Is Human:* What have we learned? *JAMA* 293(19): 2384-2390.

22. Bates, D. et al. (1998). Effect of computerized physician order entry and a team intervention on prevention of serious medication errors. *JAMA* 280(15): 1311-136.

23. Classen, D. et al. (1997). Adverse drug events in hospitalized patients. Excess length of stay, extra costs, and attributable mortality. *JAMA* 277(4): 301-306.

24. Evans, R. et al. (1992). Prevention of adverse drug events through computerized surveillance. *Proc Annu Symp Comput Appl Med Care*: 437-441.

25. Overhage, J.M. et al. (1997). A randomized trial of "corollary orders" to prevent errors of omission. *J Am Med Inform Assoc* 4(5): 364-375.

26. Overhage, J.M. et al. (2001). Controlled trial of direct physician order entry: Effects on physicians' time utilization in ambulatory primary care internal medicine practices. *J Am Med Inform Assoc.* 8(4): 361-371.

27. Shojania, K.G. et al. (Eds.) (2001). *Making Health Care Safer: A Critical Analysis of Patient Safety Practices.* Evidence-Based Practice Center. Rockville, MD: Agency for Healthcare Research and Quality.

28. Brailer, D.J. (2005). Interoperability: The key to the future health care system. *Health Affairs* W5(19). January. Available at: http://content.healthaffairs.org/cgi/content/full/hlthaff.w5.19/DC1.

29. Doolan, D.F. and D.W. Bates (2002). Computerized physician order entry systems in hospitals: Mandates and incentives. *Health Affairs* 21(4): 180-188.

30. Brookstone, A.B. and C. Braziller (2003). Engaging physicians in the use of electronic medical records. *Electronic Healthcare* 2(1): 23-27.

31. Aspden, P. (2004).

32. U.S. Department of Health and Human Services (2005). News Release: HHS Awards Contracts to Develop Nationwide Health Information Network. November 10. Available at: http://www.hhs.gov/news/press/2005pres/20051110.html.

33. Annas G. (2003). HIPAA regulations: A new era of medical-record privacy? *N Engl J Med* 348(15): 1486-1490.

34. Poon, E.G. et al. (2004). Overcoming barriers to adopting and implementing computerized physician order entry systems in U.S. hospitals. *Health Affairs* 23(4): 184-190.

35. Workgroup on Quality, National Committee on Vital and Health Statistics (2004). *Measuring Health Care Quality: Obstacles and Opportunities.* Washington, DC: U.S. Department of Health and Human Services.

36. Connolly, C. (2005). Cedars-Sinai doctors cling to pen and paper. *Washington Post.* March 21, p. A01.

37. Poon, E.G. et al. (2004).

38. Koppel, R. et al. (2005). Role of computerized physician order entry systems in facilitating medication errors. *JAMA* 293(10): 1197-1203.

39. Patton, S. (2005). The right dose of technology helps the medicine go down. *CIO Magazine.* November 1. Available at: http://www.cio.com/archive/110105/health_care.html.

40. Koppel, R. et al. (2005).

41. Bates, D.W. (2005). Computerized physician order entry and medication errors: Finding a balance. *J Biomed Inform* 38(4): 259-261.

42. Galt K.A., A.M. Rule, W. Taylor, M. Siracuse, J.D. Bramble, E.C. Rich, W. Young, B. Clark, and B. Houghton (2005). Impact of personal digital assistant devices on medication safety in primary care. *Advances in Patient Safety* 3: 247-263. Agency for Healthcare Research and Quality, Rockville, Maryland.

43. Waitman, L.R. et al. (2003). Enhancing computerized provider order entry (CPOE) for neonatal intensive care. *AMIA Annu Symp Proc:* 1078.

44. Gray, M.D. and B.G. Felkey (2004). Computerized prescriber order-entry systems: Evaluation, selection, and implementation. *AJHP* 61(2): 190-197.

45. Adatia, F. and P.L. Bedard (2003)."Palm reading": 2. Handheld software for physicians. *Can Med Assoc J* 168(6): 727-734.

46. Rothschild, J.M., T.H. Lee, T. Bae, and D.W. Bates (2002). Clinician use of a palmtop drug reference guide. *J Am Med Inform Assoc* 9(3): 223-229.

47. The Leapfrog Group (2004). Fact sheet: Computer physician order entry. Washington, DC: AcademyHealth. Available at: http://www.leapfroggroup.org/media/file/Leapfrog-Computer_Physician_Order_Entry_Fact_Sheet.pdf.

48. Galvin, R. (2005). Interview: "A Deficiency Of Will And Ambition": A Conversation With Donald Berwick. *Health Affairs* Jan-Jun (suppl. Web exclusive): w5.1-w5.9. Available at: http://content.healthaffairs.org/cgi/content/abstract/hlthaff.w5.1v3.

49. McDonnell, P.J. (2003). Overview of medication errors in pharmacy practice. *Pharmacy Times.* Available at: https://secure.pharmacytimes.com/lessons/200304-01.asp.

50. Kim, K. (2005). Clinical data standard in healthcare: Five case studies. *ihealthreports* July. California HealthCare Foundation. Available at: http://www.chcf.org/documents/ihealth/ClinicalDataStandardsInHealthCare.pdf.

51. Overhage et al. (2001).

52. Ash, J.S. et al. (2003). Implementing computerized physician order entry: The importance of special people. *Methods Inf Med* 69(2-3): 235-250.

53. Stavri, P.Z. and J.S. Ash (2004). Some unintended consequences of information technology in health care: The nature of patient care information system-related errors. *Int J Med Inform* 11(2): 104-112.

54. Ondo, K. (2004). CPOE grows but still has a way to go. *KLAS CPOE Digest.* Healthcare Informatics. Available at: http://www.healthcare-informatics.com/newsclips/newsclips03_4_04.htm.

55. Rolland, P. (2004). Occurrence of dispensing errors and efforts to reduce medication errors at the Central Arkansas Veteran's Healthcare System. *Drug Safety* 27(4): 271-282.

56. Lansky, D. (2002). Improving quality through public disclosure of performance information. *Health Affairs* 21(4): 52-62.

57. Scott, J.T. et al. (2005). Information in practice. *BMJ* 331: 1313-1316.

58. Kleinke, J.D. (2001). The price of progress: Prescription drugs in the health care market. *Health Affairs* 20(5): 43-60.

59. Schiff, G.D. et al. (2003).

60. Bobb, A. (2004). Computerized entry systems may have limited impact on patient harm. News-Medical.Net. April 12. Available at: http://www.news-medical.net/?id=426.

61. Shah, N.R., A.C. Seger, D.L. Seger, et al (2006). Improving acceptance of computerized prescribing alerts in ambulatory care. *J Am Med. Inform Assoc* 13: 5-11.

62. Barker, K.N. et al. (2002). Medication errors observed in 36 health care facilities. *Arch Intern Med* 162(16): 1897-1903.

63. Barker, K.N. et al. (1998). White paper on automation in pharmacy. *Consultant Pharmacist* 13(Mar): p. 256, 261, 265-266, 268, 274-276, 279, 283-284, 286, 289-290, 293.

64. Nemeth, C. and R. Cook (2005). Hiding in plain sight: What Koppel et al. tell us about healthcare IT. *Journal of Biomedical Informatics* 38(4): 262.

65. Tsurikova R, L. Volk., L. Pizziferri, M. Lippincott, A. Kittler, T. Wang, J. Wald, D.W. Bates (2005). Increasing medication list accuracy in the electronic health record. *J Gen Intern Med* 20(Suppl 1): p. 203.

66. Waitman, L.R. et al. (2003).

67. Brookstone, A.B. and C. Braziller (2003).

68. *Wikipedia* (2006). s.v. "IPv6." Available at: http://en.wikipedia.org/wiki/IPv6.

69. Risser, D.T. et al. (1999). The potential for improved teamwork to reduce medical errors in the emergency department. The MedTeams Research Consortium. *Ann Emerg Med* 34(3): 373-383.

70. Tessier, C. and C.P. Waegemann (2003). The continuity of care record. Organizations unite to create a portable, electronic record for use at transfer points in patients' care. *Healthc Inform* 20(10): 54-56.

71. Williams, C.T. (2005). Inside a closed-loop medication strategy. *Comput Inform Nurs* 23(1): 55-56.

72. Schiff, G.D. (2005). Introduction: Communicating critical test results. *Jt Comm J Qual Patient Saf* 31(2): 61, 63-55.

73. Bates, D.W., G.J. Kuperman, S. Wang, et al (2003). Ten commandments for effective clinical decision support: Making the practice of evidence-based medicine a reality. *J Am Med Inform Assoc* 10: 523-530.

74. Neville, D. et al. (2004). *Towards an Evaluation Framework for Electronic Health Records Initiatives: Final Report*. St. John's, Newfoundland: Newfoundland and Labrador Centre for Health Information.

75. Berners-Lee, T. (Ed.) (2006). Web Services Activity Statement. Cambridge, MA: World Wide Web Consortium.

Chapter 30

Health Care Systems and Health Insurance from a European Perspective

Marion Schaefer
Katja Borchardt

INTRODUCTION

The organization and structure of health care systems in Europe are closely related to the idea of providing universal access to health care services for the overall population as the main goal of social policy.

Germany was the first country in which the state provided social insurance for its citizens. The formal starting point dates back to 1883 when public health insurance was introduced by Chancellor Otto von Bismarck. In the succeeding years, other European countries adopted welfare policies and regulations to insure their citizens in cases of accidents, illness, old age, and unemployment.

The establishment of social insurance systems not only allowed for increased participation of workers in the production process but also provided financial means to develop the health care system itself. Today, most developed countries have a sophisticated health care system with numerous players who seek to protect their interests while serving the public and its health care needs.

The objectives of any health care system usually are based on some general principles which include the following:

- Equal access to health care for everyone
- Cost-efficient production of health services
- Effective medical care and patient management
- Cost-control of public expenditures for medical services[1]

As with many other objectives, these demands are not easy to meet. Due to the fast growing health care market that depends heavily on the progress of medical science and technology, new conflicts and obstacles appear that require new regulatory decisions. During the past two centuries many attempts have been made to regulate the provision of health care and especially the drug market to control the growing discrepancy between health care needs and availability of financial resources.

Throughout Europe the health care sector faces challenges which include the following:

- The aging population with its increased health care needs and life expectancy
- Medical and pharmaceutical progress leading to more expensive technology and drugs
- An increase in supplier-induced demand
- Insufficient quality and integration of treatment processes
- Inappropriate drug use by physicians and consumers

In a competitive environment, each of the players focuses on their own interest. This also applies for the health care and drug market:

- Patients: have nearly unlimited claims on scarce resources
- Physicians: defend their freedom to choose therapy for a patient
- Pharmacists: direct patients' decision with regard to self medication
- Wholesalers: using differences in price across the European Union via parallel import of drugs
- Pharmaceutical industry: seeks profits to support R & D
- Sickness funds: try to control costs spent for health care and medicines
- Media: reflect opinions of all advocacy groups

Although these challenges are seen worldwide, the solutions to them are very often based on national experience and tradition. Furthermore, it has to be emphasized that Europe is not a unique but is a rather diverse region that is currently undergoing a substantial political transition.

Therefore, health care systems in the European Union differ in terms of financing, the scope of benefits and purchasing structures in health services, the quality of care, the degree of freedom to choose and personal responsibility for preserving one's health, the skill mix of health professionals' education and training, and the set of incentives to regulate the provision of health services.[2]

Due to continuous reform efforts and different historical roots in all member states of the European Union, it remains difficult to classify European health care systems. Nevertheless, historically two models of financing and organizing the health care system can be differentiated. One model is oriented on a system of social health insurance (SHI) named after the former German chancellor as "Bismarck model" versus the so called National Health Service (NHS) model, also called the Beveridge model after the British civil servant who outlined the principles on which this model is based. The National Health Service model can be characterized by mainly tax financing, whereas the SHI model is financed through the employees by payroll taxes. The Beveridge model is also called the Anglo-Saxon model, the liberal model, or the residual welfare model.

Besides these two general models, several European countries use mixed approaches with elements of tax financing and employer's payroll taxes at a time. Furthermore, statutory and private insurance may also coexist in some countries, as for instance in Germany where the private insurance covers about 10 percent of the population, but the other 90 percent are covered by a statutory social health insurance. More recently, the statutory health insurances in Germany are allowed to offer a private complementary insurance in addition to the social health insurance to cover special services, as, for instance, the guarantee for a single hospital room. Table 30.1 gives some characteristics by which health care systems in the European Union can be distinguished.

The differences between the Bismarck and the Beveridge models have become less clear over time as countries show an increasing mix of different elements from the two models.[3] To understand this process the general principles of both models will be described.

The Beveridge model aims at a more or less complete equality of supply (basic principle of social solidarity) for all citizens. As funds available for health care are limited at any given time the allocation of financial means prefers those who are in greatest need. Therefore, the majority of national health care systems following this model operate with waiting lists, restriction in "the freedom to choose" of a specialist doctor, and additional insurances that must be financed privately.[4] Freedom of choice also means that a patient has access to any accredited doctor without paying an extra fee. In countries relying on a National Health Service system the patient has limited choices, because everybody is assigned to a general practitioner and hospital where they live. Especially the latter fact contradicts the demand for an equality of supply. National Health Care Systems, another term used for the Beveridge model, are based on public structures in terms of providing and administrating health care services.

TABLE 30.1. Overview of the European health care systems

Characteristic	Social health insurance (SHI)/ Bismarck model	National health service (NHS) Beveridge model
Financing and coverage	Employers and employees payroll taxes/contributions, solidarity principle, nearly universal	General tax revenues, universal access for all
Benefits	Benefits in kind and cash	Benefits in kind
Delivery	Public and private	Public and private
Steering	Collective barging and state regulation	Public administration of budgets, parliament
Administration	Self-governmental bodies	Public administration
Role of the patient	Freedom to choose providers, treatment and insurances (some countries restrict the freedome to choose insurances)	Public planning and setting priorities

Source: Adapted from Knieps (1998), p. 42; Schaub (2001), p. 23; Neugebauer (2003), p. 79.

The Bismarck model focuses on those who are active in the labor market and their family members. (Other terms used for this model are Central European or the conservative model.) Countries with an orientation toward this model show a heterogeneous picture, because some of them follow a more competitive model whereas others focus more on a corporatist model. The corporatist model relies on self-government of health insurance funds in administration. This self-governmental structure implies that in addition to the health insurance funds, the insured and the employers are integrated, whereas the public governmental bodies only exercise the task of overall control. The competitive models then allow for a competition between different statutory social health insurances. In general, the financing of these systems is based on the insurance principle with individual contributions proportional to payroll taxes.

Complementing these two basic models—both of which show an increasing trend to require or rely on out-of-pocket copayments by patients—is an approach in which social responsibilities are to be solved within the family, or as close to the family as possible. This model is also called the subsidiary model, the Southern European, or the Catholic model.

In practice it is often found that tax-financed systems such as the Beveridge model are comparatively successful in controlling health expenditure because of the centralized administration of the health care system by health authorities. On the other hand, competition in a state-financed system with public provision of services is obviously quite small. Therefore, the efficiency of the system in terms of quality of care is relatively low, and efforts to assess the needs of consumers are less rewarded. On the contrary, providers who attempt to make procedures more effective risk being punished by having their budgets cut by the amount saved for the next period. Such systems always run the risk of underfunding, as the health sector is subject to political debate on its budget each year.[5]

Statutory social health insurance such as the Bismarck model is typically financed by income-related contributions from employer and employee. Thus, the contributions are not based on risk (as the premiums of private insurance companies are), but on the ability to pay. Regulation includes description of the beneficiaries, the benefit scheme, the internal organization of the fund (including responsibilities and decision-making authority), terms of financing by the contributors, and payment to the providers. The benefits are usually set on a national level, and the contributions are calculated to finance the overall cost of these benefits.[6]

Seen more geographically, the Scandinavian as well as the Anglo-Saxonian countries are to a large degree based on general tax revenues, whereas the countries of Southern European show a mixture between general tax revenues and contributions in financing their system. The countries of the Western part of Europe rely on contributions; however, even in most of these countries the health care system receives public subsidies from the overall national budget.

The new Middle and Eastern European member states of the European Union were formerly influenced by the so-called Siemiaszko model based on a centralized socialist model with a focus on equality, central planning, and national ownership of all health care facilities.[7] After the political and economic breakdown of the former socialist countries the Middle and Eastern European countries have followed different pathways and can no longer be described as one model. Some of those countries tried to establish a Bismarckian type of model or a Beveridge model or even elements of both depending on which country they used as their model.

To sum up, the European member states share a common set of fundamental principles and values that include providing necessary health care services to their population and following the principle of solidarity although to a different extents. Differences are also reflected in their understanding of social justice and the necessity to view health care expenditures as an investment in human capital. Nonetheless, even systems with elements of competition claim to pursue a well regulated and socially bounded competition. One key difference from the United States in this respect is the claim of the European systems to allow all citizens more or less equal access and to offer at least a European wide health care system based on minimum quality standards. [8,9,10,11,12]

HEALTH CARE DATA FROM DIFFERENT EUROPEAN COUNTRIES

Stimulated by World Health Organization (WHO) and its general aim of providing quality health care to all member states, a continuous survey of health care expenditures in different countries is undertaken. The crucial question in this respect is whether high health care expenditures result in better health outcomes or health status for the citizens.

The health status is determined by a set of complex multicausal factors, which are partially individual, structural, demographic, socioeconomic, and medical. To illustrate the interrelation between objectives and goals, one has to disaggregate by groups of persons or diseases. However, to a significant degree, individual health status is mainly influenced by behavior. For instance, promoting preventive medicine in this context means to interfere in a person's autonomy and introducing incentives to change lifestyle, even when the quality of life is affected. In a broader context, a successfully implemented antismoking campaign reduces the number of cancer deaths and means a decline in costs. However, smokers would probably claim a loss in their quality of life.

This also leads to a more methodological question: Due to the complexity of health care and the individual variation in the responses to or outcomes of treatment it is difficult to establish a clear relationship between health care services and health care expenditures, respectively, and their effect on the health status of a certain country.

To begin with we want to consider data about health care expenditure and its variation in different European countries. The standardized Organization for Economic Co-operation and Development (OECD) data show health care expenditures as a percentage of gross domestic product (GDP). Large differences exist in ratios for the European Union member states reaching from 11 percent (Germany) to approx. 7 percent (Ireland). Analyzing the ratio of health care expenditure of the Middle and Eastern European countries, 4.9 percent to almost 8 percent can be seen. However, many Middle and Eastern European countries still have some degree of informal payments, which is difficult to assess (see Tables 30.2 and 30.3). Informal payments mean that in addition to the health insurance, the patient has to pay the physician out of pocket for any additional treatment.[13] Slightly different results can be seen when expenditures on health care across countries are expressed as payments per capita in U.S. dollars.

TABLE 30.2. Health care expenditures as a percent of GDP for European Union member states.

Countries	1999	2000	2001	2002
Austria	7.8	7.7	7.6	7.7
Belgium	8.7	8.8	9	9.1
Czech Republic	6.6	6.6	6.9	7.1
Cyprus	5.9	6.0	6.2	6.4
Denmark	8.5	8.4	8.6	8.8
Estonia	6.1	5.5	5.1	5.1
Finland	6.9	6.7	7	7.3
France	9.3	9.3	9.4	9.7
Germany	10.6	10.6	10.8	10.9
Greece	9.6	9.7	9.4	9.5
Hungary	7.4	7.1	7.4	7.8
Ireland	6.3	6.4	6.9	7.3
Italy	7.8	8.1	8.3	8.5
Latvia	5.2	4.8	5	4.9
Lithuania	6	6	5.7	5.7
Luxembourg	6.2	5.5	5.9	6.2
Malta	8.31	8.81	8.92	9.69
Netherlands	8.2	8.2	8.5	9.1
Poland	5.9	5.7	6	6.1
Portugal	8.7	9.2	9.3	9.3
Slovakia	5.8	5.5	5.6	5.7
Slovenia	7.7	8	8.2	...
Spain	7.5	7.5	7.5	7.6
Sweden	8.4	8.4	8.8	9.2
United Kingdom	7.2	7.3	7.5	7.7
European Region	6.24	6.37	6.41	6.53
EU members since May 2004	6.24	6.06	6.3	6.44

Source: Adapted from World Health Organization (2005). Health for all database. Available at http://www.euro.who.int/hfadb.

Despite an increasing number of studies trying to evaluate the outcomes of single health care interventions, no clear evidence yet exists that increasing health care expenditures necessarily improve the health status on a broader base. Generally accepted indicators such as life expectancy, death rates (especially infant death rates), disease rates, and self-assessment of health vary in different countries over time. To use them as a rational base for resource allocation remains difficult due to the various impact factors on

TABLE 30.3. Total health expenditure, PPP$ per capita

Countries	1999	2000	2001	2002
Austria	2,069	2,147	2,174	2,220
Belgium	2,139	2,288	2,441	2,515
Cyprus	. . .	. . .	1,313	1,161
Czech Republic	932	977	1,083	1,118
Denmark	2,297	2,351	2,523	2,580
Estonia	509	553	518	625
Finland	1,641	1,698	1,841	1,943
France	2,306	2,416	2,588	2,736
Germany	2,563	2,640	2,735	2,817
Greece	1,517	1,617	1,670	1,814
Hungary	820	847	961	1,079
Ireland	1,623	1,774	2,059	2,367
Italy	1,853	2,001	2,107	2,166
Latvia	325	338	386	451
Lithuania	399	426	482	588
Luxembourg	2,734	2,682	2,900	3,065
Malta	1,262	1,521	1,173	1,709
Netherlands	2,098	2,196	2,455	2,643
Poland	571	578	629	654
Portugal	1,424	1,570	1,662	1,702
Slovakia	578	591	633	698
Slovenia	1,230	1,389	1,404	. . .
Spain	1,467	1,493	1,567	1,646
Sweden	2,119	2,243	2,370	2,517
United Kingdom	1,725	1,839	2,012	2,160
EU	1,821	1,910	2,030	2,130
EU members before May 2004	2,028	2,127	2,256	2,364
EU members since May 2004	665	688.46	750	799

Source: Adapted from World Health Organization (2005). Health for all database. Available at http://www.euro.who.int/hfadb.

the health status. Furthermore, disparities exist among different ethnic groups as well as by gender, which cannot be explained easily.

The OECD, a not-for-profit, nongovernmental international organization, initiated a Health Care Quality Indicators Project in 2004 in order to collect internationally comparable data reflecting the health outcomes and health improvements that can be attributed to health care in their member countries. As a result, health care policymakers might be able to base their decision making on a more rational base of evidence and allow qualified benchmarking. Expert panels have described indicators in five priority areas, which are primary care and prevention, patient safety, cardiac care, diabetes care, and mental health. Initial results are expected in 2006.

Meanwhile, many OECD countries have already started to collect technical quality indicators in their own countries, which, however, are not necessarily internally comparable. Therefore, the international discussion will go on until an international agreement on the most suitable indicators is achieved.

At the same time the process of health care system comparison is channeled by the European Commission of the European Union using the so called "open method of coordination." The future goal is to find a set of common indicators across the European Union for a benchmark system of health care systems that will allow a bottom-up convergence of the various health care systems in the European Union. Some general indicators everyone can likely comply with are equal access for everyone, and sustainable and fair financing of the health care system. However, until now this process of finding suitable indicators is still under way, and experts from all European Union member states are working together with the European Commission on these issues. The following section focuses on general principles of the relation between insured patients, payers, and health care providers in order to describe the situation of health care in Europe.

RELATIONSHIP BETWEEN INSURED PATIENT, PAYER, AND HEALTH CARE PROVIDER

From an economic point of view, four major stakeholder groups in the health care system can be identified: the health care providers, the citizen/patient, the health insurance funds/third party payer, and the government as regulator. Each of these stakeholders pursues certain objectives: insured patients expect high quality health care services, the insurance funds have to control costs based on their financial resources. Health care providers are willing to meet their patient demands but at the same time are under control of the sickness funds with regard to the budget available for health care. The function of the state is to regulate all processes in order to avoid failure of the health care system due to inadequate resources and to secure social equity in the use of health care services (see Figure 30.1). To use market mechanisms for regulation, most European governments promote competition between different kinds of sickness (insurance) funds. Sickness funds, public and private, offer different services at different fees, thus bringing about changes from one sickness fund to the other, at least for pa-

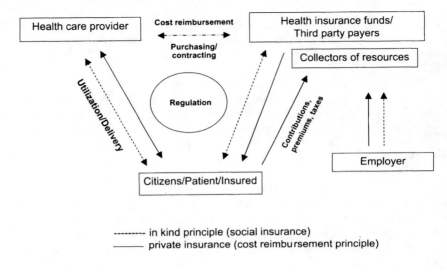

FIGURE 30.1. Key stakeholders in health care systems.

tients who are looking for good services at reasonable fees. However, it is often difficult for individuals to evaluate whether the relation between services offered and fee to be paid is worthwhile and advantageous.

In a market-oriented system, different submarkets exist that follow their own rules. Furthermore, between the stakeholders in Figure 30.1 we find so-called asymmetric information as one side is always better informed than the other. For example, the insurance can only assess the risk profile of the insured to a certain degree because the possibility of the insurance to gain sufficient information is limited since the individual knows best about his or her lifestyle and family background. The patient will more often visit the physician since the burden of the cost will be shared by all insured without an individual extra fee. Malpractice and misconduct can be the consequence of the asymmetric distribution of information.

In the context of private insurance plans, in most circumstances no direct link between the provider and insurances exists. The patient is covered by a private insurance contract and depending on the agreed package of benefits and mode of reimbursement while submitting the bills (cost reimbursement principle).

On the other end of the supply chain are a growing number of patient organizations that act on regional as well as on national and European levels. They focus on communication and support for those who have fallen ill by helping to get and evaluate qualified information, especially via the Internet in order to help patients cope with the disease and its treatment. The political impact of these patient organizations, however, is still limited with regard to their influence on health policy decisions.

Targeting pharmaceutical expenditures is at the center of actions by most governments in the EU member states. All European Union member states face the challenge to reform their health care systems in the context of an aging society and a rather low level of economic growth and scarce resources.

STATUS AND CURRENT DEVELOPMENT OF THE EUROPEAN HEALTH CARE SECTOR

With regard to medicines, all European Union member states try to regulate their own health care markets. As a matter of fact pharmaceutical markets are regulated more than any other, market mainly due to the nature of the product and services. Governments and regulatory bodies have to balance several but partly conflicting objectives: protecting public health, guaranteeing patient access to safe and effective medicines, improving quality of care, and at the same time keeping costs under control.[14] Due to the reasons previously indicated, not only health care in general but also medicines are becoming more expensive while the financial means to meet health care demands are limited at any time. Therefore, European countries, too, put their focus on cost containment rather than increasing the available health care budget.

Instruments used to regulate the pharmaceutical market differ with respect to the position of the regulatory body—usually the government—and the stage of the supply chain where interventions are effective. Among those instruments used or at least discussed in several European countries are shown in Exhibit 30.1.

An important driver of change in the European health care systems is the increasing influence resulting from the application of the European Competition Law and rulings by the European Court of Justice. All European member states have to comply with these ruling. The following aspects reflect an approximation of health care services within Europe.

In outpatient care the patients/consumers of health care service enjoy the access to a European wide supply of health care service providers, which is increasingly accepted especially when it results in cost savings either for sickness funds or for patients. With regard to inpatient care, the authorization of the national health insurance prior to the treatment is mandatory for reimbursement. Especially patients living in European member states operating with waiting lists and open ratings such as in systems with National

EXHIBIT 30.1. Selected instruments to regulate the pharmaceutical market along the supply chain

General approaches

- Establishment of Institutes for Quality assurance, evidence based medicine or health technology assessment (e.g., in the UK and Germany)
- Public discussion about the ethics of health care with regard to legitimate demands and allocation of resources

Focus on the producers

- Regulations prior to the approval (e.g., patent monopolies, orphan drug regulation, cost effectiveness)
- Reference price regulations (when the patent of a drug has expired and generic drugs are already on the market)
- Negative lists (listing drugs which are not reimbursed by the sickness funds)
- Positive lists (listing only those drugs which can be prescribed and will be reimbursed)
- Pricing principles (any regulation with an influence on market prices)
- Regulations for advertising medicines

Focus on the distributors

- Allowance or even promotion of parallel an re-importation

Focus on the health care professionals

- Promoting rational prescribing of drugs
- Setting a budget for prescribing physicians
- Benchmarking prescribing physicians with regard to cost-containment
- Introducing elements of managed care and integrated care
- Allowance of mail order pharmacies and call centres

Focus on the consumers

- Promoting rational use of drugs, including compliance
- out of pocket payment (prescription fees)
- Rx to OTC switch
- Self empowerment

Health Care services rely increasingly on services offered by other European Union member states. Examples in which this kind of transnational service is already used (sometimes referred to as "health care tourism") include dental care, eye surgery, hip replacement, rehabilitation, and wellness. However, patients who come from a well developed health care environment expect the same quality of treatment service as in their home country. For this reason some countries and their sickness funds, respectively, have started to sign bilateral contracts to regulate transnational health care services with regard to medical and quality standards as well as liability. With regard to pharmaceuticals, the individuals of the European Union member states are allowed to buy drugs all across the Union according to the reimbursement measures of their home country.

This trend is supported by recent developments in the IT (information technology) sector, which allows long-distance communication of health care data and information. Plans to introduce individual smart cards containing all relevant information about a patient's health will also promote a Europe-wide use of health care services as long as the cost savings balance out other inconveniences such as separation from the patient's usual social environment. Nowadays most European countries use these smart cards already on a national level.

Regulation of Pharmaceutical Market Prices

The approaches in regulation of pharmaceutical market prices show similarities as well as differences in different European countries. Some countries rely on direct negotiation of prices, whereas others regulate profits of the pharmaceutical industry or maximum price for reimbursements as well as volume agreements. The majority of countries have introduced lists (positive or negative) to determine under which circumstances drugs are reimbursable by the health insurances. In addition, deductibles and copayments (percentage of packages, fixed fee per item/prescription) transfer the financial burdens to the patients.

Most of the European countries have some sort of direct price control (except Denmark and Germany). Some countries regulate the patented (single source) market directly but exclude the off-patent (multiple source) market (France and Italy). Free pricing exists in Germany and the United Kingdom for patented pharmaceuticals only. A system of reference pricing (a system that relates prices of competitive drugs to the price of the innovator patent holder) is used for off-patent pharmaceuticals in Belgium, Denmark, France, Germany, Italy, Portugal, Spain, and the Netherlands, where patented products are also included. Nearly all countries except Germany and the UK use international price comparisons. In addition, the UK controls the profit of the pharmaceutical industry according to the Pharmaceutical Price Regulation Scheme, which has been in effect in various forms since 1957.[15] The approaches to defining reference prices is described in Table 30.4. In addition, agreements of different types exist between government and pharmaceutical industry in some countries to keep the growth of health care expenditures under control. Examples can be found in Table. 30.5.[16]

TABLE 30.4. Comparative definitions of reference price in selected EU schemes.

Country	Since	Definition of reference price
Germany	1989	Statistically derived median price for drugs containing the same active substance and having comparable efficacy
Netherlands	1991	Average price of drugs with similar pharmacotherapeutic effects
Denmark	1996	Lowest priced generic equivalent available on the market
Spain	2000	Arithmetic mean of the three lowest cost-per-treatment-day grouped by formulation and calculated by defined daily dose (DDD)
Belgium	2001	Equal to a price that is 26 percent lower than the price of the original brand for generic equivalent products
Italy	2001	Lowest priced generic equivalent available on the market
Portugal	2003	Lowest priced generic equivalent available on the market

Source: Adapted from Mrazek and Mossialos (2004).

TABLE 30.5. Examples of government-industry agreements in selected EU member states.

Country	Agreement
Austria	Agreement on drug expenditure targets for the Social Insurance Institution; growth to be slowed through price reductions
Denmark	Agreement on reduction in overall price level such that overall expenditure on subsidized pharmaceuticals is kept constant
France	sector-based agreements on issues including exchange of information, Promotion of compliance with national objectives, rational drug use and others
Ireland	Agreement on supply terms, conditions and prices of medicines for the health service
Portugal	Agreement to cap NHS drug expenditures and repay excess
Spain	Multiple agreements covering price cuts, expenditure targets and company Repayment if spending targets are exceeded
UK	Pharmaceutical Price Regulation Scheme

During recent years, and due to additional measures such as an allowance for parallel importation between EU member states, an approximation of prices for pharmaceuticals could be observed within Europe. However, compared with the U.S. price level for pharmaceuticals European prices for medicines are still moderate. This is one important reason for multinational pharmaceutical companies to increase their export orientation especially toward the U.S. market with a certain repercussion upon the research expenditure in the respective countries.

Another issue of discussion with regard to the national and international price level of medicines is the value-added tax (VAT) (a tax based on a percentage of the cost of the goods sold), which is differently applied in the European Union countries (see Table 30.6).

TABLE 30.6. Value-added taxes (VATs) in the European Union.

Country	VAT for goods (percent)	VAT for medicines (percent)
UK	17.5	(only 17.5 on medicines purchased by hospitals)
Sweden	25	–
Finland	22	8
Slovak Republic	19	19
Slovenian Republic	20	8.5
Portugal	19	5
Poland	22	7
Austria	20	20.0
The Netherlands	19	6
Malta	18	–
Hungary	25	5
Luxembourg	15	3
Lithuania	18	5
Latvia	18	5
Cyprus	15	5
Italy	20	10
Ireland	21	21
France	19.6	2.1 reimbursable and rest 5.5
Spain	16	4
Greece	18	8
Estonia	18	5
Germany	16	16
Denmark	25	25
Czech Republic	19	25
Belgium	21	6

Reimbursement of Pharmaceuticals

In practice, decisions about reimbursement of pharmaceuticals determine physicians' prescribing behavior as well as patients' access to medicines as much as the price of the medicine itself. In the first line, reimbursement decisions are a regulative measure that can be based on rational data such as cost-effectiveness studies or refer to simple administrative definitions, as in case of off-label use, which are usually not reimbursed in EU countries. Thus, reimbursement levels reflect the outcome of negotiations between players in health care. On the other hand, they have to consider that resources for out-of pocket copayments by patients are limited, too.

Medicines eligible for reimbursement are usually listed in so-called positive lists, those not eligible for reimbursement are found on so-called negative lists. Most of these lists further differentiate medicines into different categories of drugs, usually with reference to efficacy information and/or prices of the product. Evidence about a therapeutic benefit is usually addressed when a new drug is introduced, e.g., an application for its marketing authorization is put forward. A tendency seems to exist to add only those innovative medicines to positive lists when they have proven not only their therapeutic benefit but an advantage as compared with other drugs already on the market.

All listing schemes have advantages and disadvantages: They guarantee a certain level of quality, efficacy, and therapeutic benefit for included products. On the other hand they lack flexibility for the integration of innovative drugs and build another hurdle for achieving reimbursement by a health insurance, thus hampering as well research from the pharmaceutical industry into new biologically active substances.

Against this background, regulatory bodies require and the pharmaceutical industry increasingly provides pharmacoeconomic evaluation prior to approval. Thus, pharmacoeconomic assessment is diffusing quickly across OECD countries putting an increasing emphasis on value-for-money, especially for new drugs in line with their price negotiations. So far, only the UK and the Netherlands have released national guidelines on pharmacoeconomics. Most other countries have agreed on some sort of consensus about methodological issues of pharmacoeconomic studies. Although not yet legally required, many pharmaceutical companies use pharmacoeconomic studies to strengthen the base of evidence for their products and to justify their pricing decisions. In addition, an increasing awareness and utilization of economic evaluation within the regulatory context exists as well. This move tries to link price, cost, and outcome data but goes along with preferably methodological concerns, especially about the suitability of outcome parameters such as quality adjusted life years (QALYs).[17]

In all EU countries is a strong focus on pharmacoeconomic research issues and increasing attempts to consider patient reported outcomes and the patient perspective. Although this reflects an increased awareness of cost-effectiveness for pharmaceutical products, the health care market still requires additional methods of cost containment. Among these other approaches to deal with rising health care costs adopted by most of the European countries, the most promising are the introduction of structured care programs and measures to assure quality of health care. In addition, an increasing trend exists to make the best possible use of European resources and to harmonize regulatory procedures.

With regard to the regulation of pharmaceuticals, the role of the European Agency for the Evaluation of Medicinal Products (EMEA), which was established in 1995, is eminent since the agency is regulating the market access of pharmaceutical products (harmonized market authorization). This allows companies in principle to introduce their new drugs no longer into the market of single states only but throughout all EU member states more or less at the same time. However, the European Commission does not hold the power to interfere in national price control measurements or with industry profits, but the central approval by EMEA is binding for all European member states. Especially biotechnical products or orphan drugs are mandatory to be approved by the EMEA. Through the European competition law, parallel importing is encouraged by the European Commission in accordance with the basic principle of free movement of citizens and products within the European internal market.

ASSURING THE QUALITY OF HEALTH CARE

As most countries pursue the policy of keeping contributions or taxes stable, they have to look for other methods and instruments to keep the cost development in health care under control in order to guarantee equal access and high quality care and avoid unacceptable rationing.[18] Therefore, the introduction of quality standards is a key concern for many EU countries. Some countries, such as the UK and Germany, have already established institutes for quality assurance and evidence-based medicine or health technology assessment.

General strategies to improve quality in health care have also become more relevant as a reaction to the expanding cost-containment programs. They aim at using available resources more efficiently in order to avoid a decrease in quality due to financial undercoverage. Some of these approaches originated in the United States but have been adapted to the social and economic environment in Europe. Again, their degree of implementation differs from country to country, although the general aim to bridge the gap between rising health care costs and limited financial resources is the same for all European countries. Some strategies and approaches most commonly used to control costs in health care while maintaining high quality are described in the following sections.

Influencing the Prescription Behavior of Physicians, Especially General Practitioners

Both organizations of physicians as well as sickness funds have introduced tools to analyze and compare prescription behavior in order to improve the quality of prescribing with regard to rational decision making. For example, to support this process, so-called quality circles have been established in Germany that meet on a regular base to discuss under the auspices of a moderator the cases of single patients and the best way to treat them. Although advice and peer-based discussion builds support for this movement, a threat also exists from the sickness funds to hold single physicians financially responsible if they exceed their budget. Most of these quality circles allow only physicians to be members. In some, however, physicians and pharmacists cooperate, which is common practice only in the Netherlands.

Introduction of Disease Management Programs and Promotion of Integrated Care

Although seen as a strategy for cost containment, disease management programs (originally designed to better coordinate and manage patient's treatment with chronically diseases) have stimulated other important developments and raised questions with regard to outcomes, methods, and logistics. For example, disease management has stimulated research in and the acceptance of evidence-based medicine as the rational base of therapeutic guidelines. Indirectly, disease management programs initiate changes in the health care structure, improving opportunities for cooperation and networking as well as a stronger regulation of health care processes itself. One important issue in this respect is the coordination between in- and outpatient care in order to reduce costs due to unnecessary hospital stays. Still, the time a patient stays in hospital is in European countries in general longer than in the United States.

Many disease management programs or therapeutic guidelines recommend a preferred list of medicines to be used for the rational treatment of a disease. A repercussion of this on the pharmaceutical industry is that whether a specific drug is recommended by a guideline has a significant impact on sales and revenues. Therefore, new drugs that are pushed into the market are increasingly under pressure to provide evidence not only for their efficacy against a disease but also for their effectiveness compared with those drugs already on the market. This has also raised other questions about therapeutic benefit and how to measure it.

Implementing Pharmaceutical Care into Hospital and Community Pharmacies

As in other countries, the year 1993 when WHO released its *Guide to Good Pharmacy Practice* marked the beginning of the introduction of pharmaceutical care into pharmacy in most of the European countries. One year later in 1994 the Pharmaceutical Care Network Europe (PCNE) was founded to support and coordinate scientific studies throughout Europe. The development of more patient-orientated care is found in most European countries, although it is following different time frames.[19] The crucial point, however, is the acceptance by the payers and the sickness funds, respectively, and reimbursement of the additional and in many cases time-consuming service that pharmacies offer. For the time being, an insufficient recognition of pharmaceutical care services is the main reason for the lacking enthusiasm of the pharmaceutical profession to provide care on a broad and regular base. However, signs exist that this situation may change for the better, as in Germany where first contracts about the provision of pharmaceutical care services have been agreed on between pharmacist organizations and several sickness funds.

Patient Empowerment and Prevention

Strengthening the patients' responsibility for their own health is an important issue in all European Union countries. It is closely related to implementing preventive matters and educational programs. In this context a special interest exists on discovering methods to raise the compliance of these matters, because the benefits of preventive action such as nonsmoking or health food can only be observed in the long run.

Strategies such as promoting prevention may be associated with higher costs for education and communication in the beginning. They surely contribute to a prolongation of a healthy life with a later onset of chronic diseases and a decrease or postponement of life threatening events such as myocardial infarction or stroke. Thus prevention in the end is contributing to an aging society with increased demands for general health care. This also raises an important question that all European societies have to deal with: Does society have to pay for an individual benefit such as a prolonged healthy life span, and where are the borders or limits between the individual demand and available resources? This applies as well to medical treatment or drugs that are used preferably for this purpose, especially in an environment in which individuals are used to a high standard of health care, such as in Europe, and therefore are prone to behavior that is described as moral hazard (meaning that insured patients may try to get as much as possible out of the health care systems for their insurance fee. This can also apply to a high risk health behavior for example with regard to alcohol, tobacco, or other drugs that lead to drug dependence) because individuals can be sure that the society or the health care system will care for them in case of emergency. This is one more example of the relationship between individuals, payers, and health care providers beings characterized by different conflicts of interest.

Educational programs that try to raise the public level of knowledge about the general subject of health and disease now try to make use of the Internet as do other providers of health and health care information. Patient empowerment therefore includes that patients must learn to evaluate information they receive and consume or at least be able to decide when they have to seek for additional professional advice. The lead in this respect was taken by the UK and the University of Oxford, respectively, by developing an instrument for the evaluation of health related information by laymen (www.discern.org.uk). The instrument provides sixteen questions that are to allow the evaluation of the reliability of a publication with a focus on treatment choices, and it has also been translated into German.

Increasing Patient Safety by Improved Risk Management

Patient safety has as well become an important aim of health care in Europe, although the issue of medication errors has been more openly addressed only recently, again with the exception of the UK, which is more in the U.S. tradition in this respect. This development is supported by the harmonization of the pharmacovigilance systems in Europe under the leadership of the EMEA. Improved risk management also benefits from technological progress, such as the increasing availability of electronic medical records and electronic prescribing amended by structured health care programs such as disease-management programs and pharmaceutical care. Moreover, data on metabolic pathways and genetic variations in the response to drugs that can cause measurable differences in clinical endpoints such as rates of cure, morbidity, side effects, and death are available in the scientific literature. They demonstrate that genetic variability can affect significantly changes in medical outcomes. If considered prior to decisions about the prescription of drugs, they can improve the desired outcome and reduce possible harm, especially for so-called slow metabolizers. However, the transmission of this kind of information into daily routine is not yet satisfactory.

Benefits from Progress in Biotechnology, Genomics, and Information Technology

Recent developments in biotechnology, especially in the field of genomics, open the horizon to new opportunities for an individualized treatment of diseases, some of which were not treatable before. Progress in this respect will find its own limit regarding the costs associated with this strategy, thus increasing the gap between what is possible from a scientific point of view and what can be realized and paid for. Although it certainly will take time to develop and produce more individualized medicines, it may be worthwhile to pay more attention to relevant genetic variations influencing the metabolism of drugs in patients as described above.

Progress in information technology (IT) refers to two different issues: First, this allows and at the same time requires a qualified documentation of individual data relevant for health care, for instance on smart cards. When aggregated or pooled these data are available for specific analysis, evaluation, and decision making. Based on these data the outcome and effectiveness of health care services is expected to improve. However, concerns about data protection slow down the development when the public is afraid that this kind of data can be misused in sensible personals areas. The main concern in this respect is that information about a person's health status can be referred to with regard to decisions about employment or dismissal.

Another IT issue relates to the performance of health care services itself. The Internet-based communication and transformation of health care data allows new forms of treatment such as surgery advice and technical support from experts over long distances. Small devices that patients at risk can carry with them will be used for monitoring changes in their health status such as arrhythmia in post-myocardial patients in order to react more quickly in cases of emergency. In general, a strong movement exist in Europe to drive this technological development, which also requires reliable technical and logistical solutions.

SUMMARY AND OUTLOOK

All European member states strive to realize more patient orientation, equal access to medicines, and a high level of quality assurance in health care. To achieve this different strategies are followed. In general, it is assumed that high quality health care reduces the risk for costly health problems, e.g., myocardial infarction or apoplectic insults. The better the health status, the less must be spent on the consumption of health care services, which strengthens the argument for a continuous prevention. On the other hand, diseases and health conditions are unequally distributed among the population and predetermined by genes as well as behavior, which is often influenced by social class. Therefore, it also lies in the state's responsibilities to care for an environment that promotes health and healthy living.

The main objective of health policy aims at an optimal allocation of scarce resources. Interventions to meet health care demands are very complex. As instruments target pricing, volume regulation and financial and nonfinancial incentives are applied. In most countries measurements taken combine all of these actions while their governments must balance contrasting objectives: On the one hand they must guarantee access to cost-effective medicine, protection of public health, safe and effective medicine, and quality assurance. On the other hand, they are expected to promote drug research and development, the pharmaceutical industry as employer, and their export performance.

In most developed EU countries the health and social service sector accounts for almost 10 percent of the overall employment. Furthermore, aging populations who suffer from chronic diseases have strong needs for treatment. Therefore, the health care sector can be seen as a growth market with a high potential for further development.

The challenges for health care in the future are not too different from those Europe faces today. The need to finance the medical-technical process is pushed forward by the science and the health care industry and also by political bodies and the public. Coping with the consequences of developments such as an ageing society with increasing chronic diseases will require a restructuring of the whole health care sector. This process will take time since some of the current structures of care such as individual doctors' offices and independent pharmacies have their roots in the Middle Ages. Therefore, integrated health care delivery systems, networking, managed care, and case management as well as telemedicine are keywords for the future logistics of health care. To improve quality of care, the role of evidence-based medicine and pharmacy will increase. This requires standardized and qualified documentation and the development and concomitant use of suitable methods for the analysis and evaluation of relevant health care data that respect the patients' rights for data protection.

Various new attempts will be made by traditional and new players in the health care market to introduce logistic solutions for the situation previously described. In accommodating conflicting interests of different health care players, only those who contribute to optimize the whole health care process and—most import of all—serve legitimate patients' need will be successful in the long run.

NOTES

1. Schulenburg, J.-M. Graf v.d. (2004 *Versicherungsökonomik.* Karlsruhe, Germany: Verlag Versicherungswirtschaft GmbH.

2. Henke KD (1992). Financing a national health insurance. *Health Policy* 20(3): 253-268.

3. Maydell BB v., Borchardt K., and Henke K.-D. (2005) *Social Europe.* Bad Neuenahr-Ahrweiler: Europäische Akademie.

4. Mossialos E and McKee M (2002). *The Influence of EU Law on the Social Character of Health Care Systems.* Brussels, Belgium: Peter Lang.

5. Schulenburg, J.-M. Graf v.d. (2004).

6. Schulenburg, J.-M. Graf v.d. (2004).

7. Figueras J, McKee M, Cain J, and Lessof S (2004). *Health Systems in Transition: Learning from Experience.* Copenhagen, Denmark: European Observatory on Health Care Systems and Policies.

8. Henke KD (1999). Socially bounded competition in the German health care system. *Health Affairs* 18: 203-205.

9. Brown L and Amelung V (1999). "Manacled competition" in Germany. *Health Affairs* 18(3): 76-92.

10. Shalala DE and Reinhardt UE (1999). Viewing the U.S. health care system from within: Candid talk from HHS (Health and Human Science). Health Affairs 18(3): 47-55.

11. Mossialos E and McKee M (2002).

12. Leidl R (1999). Was leisten ökonomische Methoden in der Gesundheitssystemforschung? In König HH and Stillfried D (Hrsg.), *Gesundheitssystemforschung in Wissenschaft und Praxis* (pp. 24-32). Stuttgart, Germany: Schattauer Verlag.

13. Organization for Economic Co-operation and Development OECD (2004). OECD-Gesundheitdaten 2004, Vergleichendaten Analyse von 30 Ländern, CD-Version, 2004.

14. Mossialos E, Mrazek M, Walley T (2004). *Regulating Pharmaceuticals in Europe: Striving for Efficiency, Equity and Quality.* European Observatory on Health Systems and Policies Series. Berkshire, UK: Open University Press.

15. Mossialos E, Mrazek M, Walley T (2004).

16. Mossialos E, Mrazek M, Walley T (2004).

17. McGuire AJ, Drummond M, and Rutten F (2004). Reimbursement of pharmaceuticals in the European Union. In E Mossialos, M Mrazek, and T Walley (eds.), *Regulating Pharmaceuticals in Europe: Striving for Efficiency, Equity, and Quality.* Berkshire, UK: Open University Press.
18. Henke KD and Borchardt K (2003). Reform proposals for health-care systems: Capital funded versus pay-as-you-go in health-care financing reconsidered. *CESifo DICE Report* 3: 3-8.
19. Schaefer M and Verheyen F (2003). The diffusion of pharmaceutical care: A European perspective. In CH Knowlton and RP Penna (Eds.), *Pharmaceutical care,* Second edition (pp. 313-326). Bethesda, MD: American Society of Health System Pharmacists.

FURTHER READING

European Commission (2003) The social situation in the European Union, Brussels.
European Federation of Pharmaceutical Industries and Associations (EFPIA) (2005) The Pharmaceutical Industry in Figures, Key Data, update.
Health for all database 2005.
Knieps F (1998) EU-Gesundheitssysteme-Von Bismarck bis Beveridge, Gesundheit und Geselllschaft, Heft 10, pp. 40-46.
Knowlton CH, Penna R (2003) Pharmaceutical Care (2nd edition), American Society of Health-System Pharmacists.
Neugebauer G (2003) Wettbewerb der europäischen Gesundheitssysteme aus ökonomischer Sicht, in: Klausen, N (Hrsg.) Europäischer Binnenmarkt und Wettbewerb—Zukunftsszenarien für die GKV, Beiträge zum Gesundheitsmanagement, Band 3, Baden-Baden.
Schaub VE (2001) Grenzüberschreitende Gesundheitsversorgung in der Europäischen Union, Band 7, Europäische Schriften zu Staat und Wirtschaft, Baden-Baden.

SELECTED INTERNET LINKS

http://www.discern.org.uk
http://www.observator.dk
http://www.oecd.org

Index

Page numbers followed by the letter "f" indicate figures; those followed by the letter "t" indicate tables.